Field Wilderness Medicine

FIFTH EDITION

Paul S. Auerbach,
MD, MS, FACEP, MFAWM, FAAEM
Redlich Family Professor
Department of Emergency Medicine
Stanford University School of Medicine
Stanford, California

Benjamin B. Constance,
MD, MBA, FACEP, FAWM, DiMM
President and CFO
Tacoma Emergency Care Physicians
Tacoma, Washington;
Instructor
University of Washington School of Medicine
Seattle, Washington

Luanne Freer,
MD, FACEP, FAWM
Medical Director, Yellowstone National Park and
Midway Atoll NWR
Medcor, Inc.
Founder and Director
Everest Base Camp Medical Clinic
Himalayan Rescue Association
Big Sky, Montana

ELSEVIER

ELSEVIER

1600 John F. Kennedy Blvd.
Ste. 1600
Philadelphia, PA 19103-2899

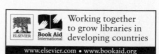

Working together
to grow libraries in
developing countries

www.elsevier.com • www.bookaid.org

Field Guide to
Wilderness
Medicine

This book is dedicated to every person who takes the time to assist others in need of care, whether in the wilderness, on the battlefield, or in relief after a catastrophic event. At a time of worldwide concern about the intentions of men and women toward their fellow humans, we applaud those who are brave, skilled, and compassionate.

Preface

Accompanying the seventh edition of the textbook *Auerbach's Wilderness Medicine*, this fifth edition of *Field Guide to Wilderness Medicine* continues the tradition of providing a concise guide for medical practitioners committed to caring for persons in austere wilderness settings. Guided by advances in knowledge, comments from readers, and the astute authorship of Drs. Benjamin Constance and Luanne Freer, this book supports trained healthcare providers to practice medicine in the field.

As always, this guide relies on the collected wisdom of contributors to the textbook. They remain generous and remarkable experts. Although directed toward trained healthcare providers, the *Field Guide to Wilderness Medicine* offers useful information for any level of wilderness responder.

Seek every opportunity to help others. We hope this field guide makes you more confident and effective as you do your best to practice the science and art of wilderness medicine. Accidents and illnesses afflict all of us, and the best-prepared rescuers offer the most useful assistance. As you minister to your patients, also pay attention to planet Earth. To preserve the wilderness, we each must fulfill our responsibilities to understand global environmental science and be proactive in preserving the landscape.

—Paul S. Auerbach

Acknowledgments

The wilderness medicine community includes many extraordinary individuals. For the creation of this edition, I thank all of the contributors over the years to the textbook *Wilderness Medicine*, with heartfelt remembrance of Warren Bowman and Bruno Durrer.

—*Paul S. Auerbach*

Thank you to the men and women of Tacoma Mountain Rescue — what you do matters. To Agatha, my partner and amazing wife, your support and encouragement make everything possible. Thank you to Jackson and Landon for making life new again through the eyes of a child. Explore, enjoy, live and love this amazing planet!

—*Benjamin B. Constance*

I thank my family of friends in Yellowstone National Park for showing me the relevance of wilderness medicine, the Wilderness Medical Society for the opportunity to learn from the best, and the growing community of wilderness medicine enthusiasts for reminding me that there is always more to learn.

—*Luanne Freer*

Contents

Color plates follow page xii

High-Altitude Medicine

DEFINITIONS
- High altitude: 1500 to 3500 m (4921 to 11,483 ft). This altitude is marked by decreased exercise performance and increased ventilation at rest. Altitude illness is common with rapid ascent above 2500 m (8202 ft).
- Very high altitude: 3500 to 5500 m (11,483 to 18,045 ft). Arterial partial pressure of oxygen (PaO_2) falls below 60 mm Hg and maximal arterial oxygen saturation (SaO_2) drops below 90%. Extreme hypoxia may occur during exercise or sleep and with altitude sickness. Severe high-altitude illness (e.g., high-altitude pulmonary edema [HAPE] and high-altitude cerebral edema [HACE]) occurs most commonly at very high altitude.
- Extreme altitude: above 5500 m (18,045 ft). Marked hypoxemia and hypocapnia occur, and successful acclimatization is impossible. Abrupt ascent to extreme altitude without supplemental oxygen is quite dangerous.

HIGH-ALTITUDE ILLNESS
High-Altitude Headache
Signs and Symptoms
- Often the first symptom of altitude exposure
- May be the only symptom following altitude exposure
- May or may not portend the development of acute mountain sickness (AMS; see later)

Treatment
1. Oxygen beginning at low flow rates (0.5 to 2 L/min by nasal cannula to raise arterial SaO_2 to greater than 90%) is usually very effective, if available.
2. Nonsteroidal antiinflammatory drugs (NSAIDs), such as ibuprofen 400 mg q8h, acetaminophen 500 mg q4h, or both, are generally effective for both treatment and prevention. Avoid narcotics because they may suppress ventilation and predispose to AMS. AMS treatment agents, such as acetazolamide and dexamethasone (see later), may be used to prevent or treat high-altitude headache.

Acute Mountain Sickness
AMS can be quantified by using the Lake Louise score (LLS)—see Appendix D.

Primary Signs and Symptoms

Headache, usually throbbing, bitemporal or occipital; worse at night, with Valsalva maneuver, or when stooping over; with one or more of the following:

- Anorexia
- Nausea or vomiting
- Dizziness or lightheadedness
- Fatigue, lassitude

Absence of Altitude Diuresis

There may be absence of altitude diuresis expected with normal acclimatization. During acclimatization, diuresis is expected; for example, a well-hydrated person who is acclimatizing appropriately should awaken at least once during the night to urinate. A person who does not awaken to urinate or infrequently urinates during the daytime is possibly dehydrated and also should be watched closely for signs of AMS.

Natural Course

- Natural course is highly variable.
- Symptoms may start within 2 hours after arrival at altitude.
- Symptoms rarely start after 48 hours at a given altitude.
- Most AMS resolves within 3 days.
- Some patients worsen despite remaining at a fixed altitude (e.g., nausea and headache do not resolve with rest or the symptoms worsen in intensity without progressing to HACE).

Treatment (Box 1.1)

1. Do not proceed to a higher sleeping altitude unless/until all symptoms completely resolve.
2. Monitor the patient for progression of illness (to pulmonary or cerebral edema).
3. If symptoms worsen despite an additional 24 hours of acclimatization at the same altitude, descend. Descent of 500 to 1000 m (1640 to 3281 ft) is often sufficient to achieve clinical improvement and resolution of symptoms.
4. Immediately descend if the patient suffers ataxia, altered consciousness, or pulmonary edema.
5. For mild AMS, halt the ascent and wait (12 hours to 3 days) for acclimatization to occur. Administer acetazolamide, 250 mg PO bid (pediatric dose: 2.5 mg/kg/dose bid to a maximum dose of 250 mg) for 2 days while at altitude or until symptoms have diminished.
6. Oxygen beginning at low flow rates (0.5 to 2 L/min by nasal cannula to raise arterial SaO_2 to greater than 90%) is usually very effective, if available.
7. *Ginkgo biloba* 100 mg PO bid started 5 days before ascent has been shown in some studies to prevent and reduce symptoms

> **BOX 1.1** Field Treatment of High-Altitude Illness
>
> **High-Altitude Headache and Mild Acute Mountain Sickness**
> Stop ascent, rest, and acclimatize at same altitude
> Acetazolamide, 125 to 250 mg bid, to speed acclimatization
> Symptomatic treatment as needed with non-narcotic analgesics
>   and antiemetics
> OR descend 500 m (1640 ft) or more
>
> **Moderate to Severe Acute Mountain Sickness**
> Low-flow oxygen (0.5 to 2 L/min by nasal cannula to raise arterial
> SaO_2 to greater than 90%)
> Acetazolamide, 250 mg bid (pediatric dose: 2.5 mg/kg/dose bid to
>   a maximum dose of 250 mg)
> Hyperbaric therapy
> OR immediate descent of at least 1000 m (3281 ft) (or more if
>   feasible)
>
> **High-Altitude Cerebral Edema**
> Immediate descent or evacuation
> Oxygen by nasal cannula to raise arterial SaO_2 to greater than 90%
> Dexamethasone, 8 mg PO, IM, or IV, then 4 mg q6h (pediatric
>   dose 0.15 mg/kg/dose q6h to a maximum dose of 4 mg)
> Hyperbaric therapy
>
> **High-Altitude Pulmonary Edema**
> Minimize exertion and keep warm
> Oxygen (by nasal cannula or mask) to achieve SaO_2 greater
>   than 90%
> If oxygen is not available:
>   Nifedipine sustained release, 20 mg PO q8h or 30 mg PO q12h
>   Consider sildenafil, 50 mg PO q8h or tadalafil, 10 mg PO q12h
>   Hyperbaric therapy
>   OR immediate descent
>
> **Periodic Breathing**
> Acetazolamide, 62.5 to 125 mg PO in the evening

of AMS, but most reports indicate that gingko is a less reliable prophylactic drug than acetazolamide.

8. Administer aspirin, 650 mg; acetaminophen, 650 mg; or ibuprofen, 400 to 600 mg PO for headache.
9. Administer an antiemetic (e.g., ondansetron, prochlorperazine, promethazine, metoclopramide) for nausea and vomiting.
10. Avoid sedative-hypnotic drugs and alcohol.
11. Minimize exertion.
12. Consider promptly descending 500 to 1000 m (1640 to 3281 ft) if medications are ineffective or unavailable or if illness is severe.
13. If readily available and in unlimited supply, consider administering oxygen 0.5 to 1.5 L/min by nasal cannula or simple (open

type) face mask during sleep. This is particularly effective for headache.

14. Consider administering dexamethasone 8 mg PO/IM/IV, then 4 mg q6h (pediatric dose: 0.15 mg/kg/dose q6h to a maximum dose of 4 mg) *in conjunction with descent*, for progressive neurologic symptoms or ataxia, or if the patient cannot tolerate acetazolamide. Even if symptoms resolve with use of dexamethasone, it is unwise to remain at high altitude or to ascend while taking dexamethasone, because signs of progression to HACE could be masked.

15. Consider undertaking a 2- to 6-hour treatment in a portable hyperbaric bag (e.g., Gamow bag) inflated to 2 psi. Maintaining 2 psi inside the bag is equivalent to a descent of 1000 to 3000 m (3281 to 9843 ft), depending on the starting altitude. The hyperbaric bag can be used with or without supplemental oxygen. Most portable bags require constant pumping, so recruit additional persons for assistance (see Box 1.1).

High-Altitude Cerebral Edema
Signs and Symptoms
- Ataxic gait is the hallmark of diagnosis. Ataxia in the face of recent ascent to high altitude is HACE until proven otherwise.
- Altered consciousness (confusion, drowsiness, stupor, coma)
- Severe lassitude
- Headache
- Nausea and vomiting
- Hallucinations (rare)
- Hypoxemia associated with concomitant pulmonary edema
- Seizures (rare)

Focal neurologic deficits are only rarely found in HACE and in the setting of normal consciousness suggest an alternate diagnosis.

Treatment
1. Immediately descend at least 500 to 1000 m (1640 to 3281 ft) or more. There is no upper limit to descent rate or distance. For example, if a person is able to descend rapidly to sea level, this is preferred.

2. Administer dexamethasone 8 mg IV, IM, or PO, followed by 4 mg q6h (pediatric dose: 0.15 mg/kg/dose q6h to a maximum dose of 4 mg).

3. Administer oxygen 2 to 4 L/min by nasal cannula or simple (open type) face mask, to maintain SaO_2 greater than 90%. Higher O_2 concentrations and a nonrebreather mask may be required.

4. If the patient is comatose, manage the airway and drain the bladder.

5. Only after descent or if descent is not feasible, consider undertaking a 2- to 6-hour treatment in a portable hyperbaric bag (e.g., Gamow bag) inflated to 2 psi. Maintaining 2 psi inside the bag is equivalent to a descent of 1000 to 3000 m (3281 to 9843 ft),

depending on the starting altitude. The hyperbaric bag can be used with or without supplemental oxygen. Most portable bags require constant pumping, so recruit additional persons for assistance (see Box 1.1).
6. If neurologic symptoms persist despite treatment with oxygen, steroids, and descent, a cerebrovascular accident may be present. Evacuate for definitive evaluation and care.

High-Altitude Pulmonary Edema
Signs and Symptoms
- Decreased exercise performance and increased recovery time
- Dyspnea on exertion that progresses to dyspnea at rest
- Cough (mild and dry initially, becoming productive late in the disease)
- Tachycardia and tachypnea at rest
- Fatigue, weakness, and lassitude
- Low-grade fever
- Symptoms of AMS occur in approximately 50% of cases
- Cyanotic nail beds and lips
- Audible chest rales, classically beginning in the right middle lobe (auscultate right lateral chest between fourth and sixth intercostal spaces) and becoming bilateral and diffuse
- Pink or blood-tinged sputum (late finding)
- Mental status changes, ataxia, decreased level of consciousness, and coma may signify extreme hypoxemia or signal coexisting HACE
- Hypoxemia determined by pulse oximetry. It is difficult to precisely define a "normal" pulse oximetry reading at high altitude. Because variables are constant for traveling companions on the same itinerary, one strategy is to average the readings among well companions and consider substantially lower readings (10% or more) in persons who are unwell as tantamount to hypoxemia.

Treatment
1. Immediately descend at least 500 to 1000 m (1640 to 3281 ft). Because of augmented pulmonary hypertension and greater hypoxemia with exercise, exertion must be minimized.
2. Administer oxygen 2 to 4 L/min by nasal cannula or simple (open type) face mask to maintain SaO_2 greater than or equal to 90%. Higher O_2 concentrations and a nonrebreather mask may be required.
3. If supplemental oxygen is not available, consider giving nifedipine 20 mg sustained-release capsule q8h or 30-mg sustained-release capsule q12h to reduce pulmonary arterial pressure.
4. Keep the patient warm because cold stress elevates pulmonary arterial pressure.
5. Consider using pursed-lip breathing or continuous positive airway pressure (CPAP) delivered by face mask.
6. Consider undertaking a 2- to 6-hour treatment in a portable hyperbaric bag (e.g., Gamow bag) inflated to 2 psi. Maintaining

2 psi inside the bag is equivalent to a descent of 1000 to 3000 m (3281 to 9843 ft), depending on the starting altitude. The hyperbaric bag can be used with or without supplemental oxygen. Most portable bags require constant pumping, so recruit additional persons for assistance (see Box 1.1).

7. Consider a phosphodiesterase-5 (PDE-5) inhibitor, such as sildenafil 50 mg q8h or tadalafil 10 mg q12h. This recommendation is not yet well studied for treatment but is effective for prevention, discussed next.

8. Consider dexamethasone 8 mg q12h, which is not yet studied for treatment, but has been shown to be effective for prevention and may treat coexisting HACE.

Prevention

Anecdotal evidence suggests that acetazolamide 125 to 250 mg PO bid or 500-mg sustained-release capsule q24h prevents HAPE in persons with a history of recurrent episodes. Agents that limit hypoxic pulmonary hypertension might block the onset of HAPE. One example is nifedipine 20-mg sustained-release capsule q8h or 30-mg sustained-release capsule q12h. Studies suggest that the inhaled β-adrenergic agonist salmeterol metered-dose inhaler (MDI) two puffs q8-12 h may prevent HAPE. The PDE-5 inhibitors sildenafil 50 mg q8h, or tadalafil 10 mg q12h may effectively prevent HAPE. Dexamethasone has been shown to prevent HAPE in susceptible subjects. The dose used was 8 mg q12h starting 2 days before exposure.

OTHER ALTITUDE DISORDERS
Sleep Disturbances

Sleep disturbances are common at high altitude, where there is a shift from deeper sleep to lighter sleep, and more time is spent awake, with significantly increased arousals. Disturbed sleep may be only minimally related to the common phenomenon of periodic breathing at altitude.

Signs and Symptoms
- Increased wakefulness
- Periodic breathing
- Frequent arousal
- Decreased rapid eye movement (REM) sleep

Periodic Breathing
Signs and Symptoms
Nocturnal hyperpnea followed by apnea

Treatment of Sleep Disturbances and Periodic Breathing
1. Administer acetazolamide 62.5 mg to 125 mg PO in the evening.
2. Use sedative-hypnotic sleep aids cautiously (especially in patients with altitude sickness) because of the potential for respiratory depression.

3. If acetazolamide is not effective or unable to be used, consider the PO use of temazepam 10 mg, or zolpidem 5 to 10 mg.

Peripheral Edema
Signs and Symptoms
Edema of the hands, face, and ankles, which may occur in the absence of any altitude illness

Treatment
1. Examine the patient for signs of AMS, HAPE, or HACE.
2. Acetazolamide 125 to 250 mg may be used if the symptoms are bothersome to the patient. Expect spontaneous resolution with acclimatization.

High-Altitude Pharyngitis and Bronchitis
Signs and Symptoms
- Reddened and painful throat
- Chronic cough (dry or productive)
- Dry or cracking nasal passages

Treatment
1. Maintain adequate hydration.
2. Suck on lozenges or hard candies.
3. Use an antitussive agent (codeine 30 mg PO q8-12 h).
4. Administer steam inhalation, taking care to avoid facial burns.
5. Use nasal saline spray prn.

High-Altitude Retinal Hemorrhages
Common in trekkers and climbers above 5000 m (16,404 ft)

Signs and Symptoms
- Usually asymptomatic
- If bleeding is perimacular, field deficits may occur
- Requires an ophthalmoscope for definitive diagnosis

Treatment
1. No specific treatment is known.
2. If visual field deficit(s) occurs (with or without objective ophthalmoscopic evidence or abnormality), descent is recommended to prevent progression.

Focal Neurologic Conditions Without Cerebral Edema
Various localizing neurologic signs occur that are usually transient and do not necessarily occur in the setting of AMS. Syndromes include the following:
- Migraine headache
- Transient ischemic attack (TIA)
- Stroke with permanent focal neurologic dysfunction

Factors contributing to stroke at altitude may include polycythemia, dehydration, increased intracranial pressure, cerebrovascular spasm, and coagulation abnormalities.

Signs and Symptoms
- Transient hemiplegia
- Hemiparesis
- Transient global amnesia
- Unilateral paresthesias
- Aphasia
- Scotoma
- Cortical blindness

Treatment
1. Supportive measures
2. Supplemental oxygen to maintain pulse oximetry saturation at approximately 90% to 94%
3. Descent to definitive care
4. Steroids may be effective for treatment of possible underlying HACE
5. Patients with signs and symptoms of TIA (fluctuating or resolving neurologic symptoms that are not consistent with the presence of a hemorrhagic stroke) at high altitude may benefit from administration of aspirin, but a risk assessment (considering time to advanced imaging, which would exclude hemorrhage that could be worsened by aspirin administration) should be taken into consideration. For instance, a patient with a presentation classic for TIA or embolic stroke who is hours from imaging might tip the risk/benefit ratio in favor of administration of 325 mg aspirin PO, but a patient with a presentation that could be consistent with hemorrhage might be considered higher risk; therefore waiting to administer aspirin until imaging makes the diagnosis clear would be the wiser course of action.

High-Altitude Flatus Expulsion
Signs and Symptoms
Excessive flatulence

Treatment
1. Administer oral simethicone, 80 mg PO prn.
2. Encourage a carbohydrate diet.
3. Apologize to tentmates.

High-Altitude Deterioration
Signs and Symptoms
- Acclimatization is impossible, with patient's condition marked by weight loss, lethargy, weakness, headache, and poor-quality sleep
- Very common at extreme high altitude of 7500 m (24,606 ft) and above

- More common in persons with chronic diseases, particularly those associated with hypoxemia

Treatment
The only definitive treatment is descent to a lower altitude.

Ultraviolet Keratitis ("Snowblindness")
Signs and Symptoms
- Eye pain
- Sensation of grittiness in the eyes
- Photophobia
- Tearing
- Conjunctival erythema
- Chemosis
- Eyelid swelling

Treatment
1. Remove contact lenses and do not reinsert these until all symptoms have resolved.
2. Use a topical anesthetic (e.g., tetracaine ophthalmic 0.5%, one to two drops) for evaluation but do not use repetitively (inhibits corneal reepithelialization).
3. Administer aspirin 500 mg q4h, or ibuprofen 400 mg q4h PO.
4. Use external cool compresses.
5. If the patient is able to maintain eye rest and sun protection, instill a short-acting mydriatic-cycloplegic agent (e.g., cyclopentolate ophthalmic 0.5% or 1%, one or two drops administered once) to reduce ciliary spasm and dilate the pupil, the latter to prevent synechiae.
6. Consider a topical NSAID (e.g., ketorolac 0.5% ophthalmic solution, one drop four times daily).
7. Avoid topical corticosteroids.
8. Patch the affected eye(s) for 24 hours; then reexamine. Do not patch the eye if there is a purulent discharge, facial rash consistent with herpes zoster, or any suggestion of corneal ulcer.
9. If the patient has both eyes affected and must use one eye, patch the more severely affected eye.
10. Encourage the patient to rest.

Acclimatization
Acclimatization is the key to successful habitation at high altitude. Beginning at an altitude of 1500 m (4921 ft), the following physiologic changes are noted:
1. Increased ventilation, which decreases alveolar carbon dioxide and increases alveolar oxygen. This is mediated in part by the hypoxic ventilatory response (carotid body), which can be affected positively by respiratory stimulants (progesterone, almitrine) and negatively by alcohol, sedative-hypnotics, and fragmented sleep. Acetazolamide is a respiratory stimulant that acts on the central respiratory center.

2. Renal bicarbonate excretion in response to increased ventilation, hypocapnia, and the resulting respiratory alkalosis. Without this correction in pH, the alkalosis would inhibit the central respiratory center and limit ventilation. Ventilation reaches a maximum after 4 to 7 days at the same altitude. Acetazolamide facilitates this process.

3. Hypoxic pulmonary vasoconstriction leads to increased pulmonary artery pressure. This is not completely ameliorated by administration of supplemental oxygen at altitude.

4. Red blood cell mass increases over a period of weeks to months. This may lead to polycythemia. Long-term acclimatization also leads to increased plasma volume.

How to Acclimatize to Altitude

1. Avoid abrupt ascent to sleeping altitudes above 3000 m (9843 ft).

2. Spend two or three nights at 2500 to 3000 m (8202 to 9843 ft) before further ascent.

3. Add an extra night of acclimatization for every 600 to 900 m (1969 to 2953 ft) of ascent.

4. Make day trips to a higher altitude, with a return to lower altitude for sleep.

5. Avoid alcohol and sedative-hypnotics for the first two nights at a new higher altitude.

6. Be aware that mild exercise may be beneficial and extreme exercise deleterious.

7. Administer acetazolamide 125 mg PO bid (pediatric dose: 2.5 mg/kg/dose bid to a maximum dose of 125 mg), beginning 24 hours before ascent. An alternative dose is one 500-mg sustained-release capsule q24h.

   a. Continue taking acetazolamide during the ascent and until acclimatization has occurred (generally for 48 hours at maximum altitude).

   b. Do not use acetazolamide in patients with history of anaphylaxis or severe reaction to sulfa or penicillin derivatives. Although acetazolamide is usually tolerated well by persons with a history of sulfa antibiotic allergy, approximately 10% of persons with a history of sulfa allergy may have an allergic reaction, so it is wise to be cautious in persons with a history of allergy, especially anaphylaxis, to either sulfa or penicillin. Many experts recommend a trial dose of the medication in a controlled setting well before the altitude sojourn, to determine if the drug is tolerated well. Although the usual allergic reaction is a rash starting a few days after ingestion, anaphylaxis to acetazolamide does rarely happen.

   c. Side effects include peripheral paresthesias, polyuria, nausea, drowsiness, impotence, myopia, and altered (bitter) taste of carbonated beverages. Another side effect is transient bone marrow suppression.

   d. Dexamethasone 4 mg PO q12h can be used if acetazolamide is contraindicated. Because of a higher incidence of side effects than with acetazolamide and possible rebound phenomenon, dexamethasone is best reserved for treatment rather than for prevention of AMS, or used for prophylaxis when necessary in persons intolerant of or allergic to acetazolamide, or when a sudden ascent is required and acclimatization is impossible (e.g., during rapid deployment to high-altitude to accomplish a rescue).

e. Studies with *G. biloba* have shown inconsistent results. Some studies show that ginkgo (nonprescription) 100 mg PO bid taken 5 days before ascent and continued for 2 days at the highest altitude attained may be effective for preventing symptoms. Potency and quality of preparations vary. ConsumerLab.com at http://www.consumerlab.com compares available preparations. Acetazolamide is a superior agent to ginkgo for acclimatization.

f. Ibuprofen in an adult dose of 600 mg PO q8h has been shown to be effective for prophylaxis against AMS at altitudes of up to 3500 m (11,700 ft). It has not been studied at higher or more extreme altitudes. If it is used for this purpose, it should be administered until the highest altitude is attained for 48 hours.

COMMON MEDICAL CONDITIONS AND HIGH ALTITUDE

Persons with certain preexisting illnesses might be at risk for adverse effects on ascent to high altitude, either because of exacerbation of their illnesses or because their illnesses might affect acclimatization and susceptibility to altitude illness. Certain populations, such as pregnant women and older adults, require special consideration (Box 1.2).

BOX 1.2 Advisability of Exposure to High and Very High Altitude for Common Conditions (Without Supplemental Oxygen)

Probably No Extra Risk
Young and old (no age limitations)
Fit and unfit
Diabetes
After coronary artery bypass grafting (without angina)
Mild COPD
Well-controlled asthma
Low-risk pregnancy (should not travel above 2500 m [8202 ft])
Mild obstructive sleep apnea
Controlled hypertension
Controlled seizures
Stable psychiatric disorders
Neoplastic diseases
Inflammatory conditions

Continued

> **BOX 1.2**   Advisability of Exposure to High and Very High Altitude for Common Conditions (Without Supplemental Oxygen)—cont'd
>
> **Caution**
> Moderate COPD
> Compensated CHF
> Severe sleep apnea syndrome
> Cystic fibrosis (FEV 30%–50% predicted)
> Mild pulmonary hypertension
> Troublesome arrhythmias
> Stable angina/CAD (consider functional evaluation before travel)
> Sickle cell trait
> Cerebrovascular diseases
> Any cause for restricted pulmonary circulation
> Poorly controlled seizures
> Radial keratotomy surgery
> Morbid obesity
>
> **Contraindicated**
> High-risk pregnancy
> Recent unstable cardiac condition (e.g., CAD, uncompensated
>   CHF, arrhythmias)
> Pulmonary hypertension (systolic PAP >60 mm Hg)
> Untreated cerebrovascular aneurysms or arteriovenous
>   malformations
> Cerebral space-occupying lesions
> Recent stroke <90 days
> Sickle cell anemia (with history of crises)
> Severe COPD
> Pulmonary hypertension

CAD, Coronary artery disease; *CHF,* congestive heart failure; *COPD,* chronic obstructive pulmonary disease.

Based on available research, it seems prudent to recommend that only women with normal, low-risk pregnancies undertake sojourns to high altitude. For these women, exposure to an altitude (up to 2500 m [8202 ft]) at which SaO_2 will remain above 85% most of the time appears to pose no risk for harm, but further study is necessary to place these recommendations on more solid scientific footing.

The Wilderness Medical Society published updated consensus guidelines for the treatment of altitude illness in 2014 (available for free download at http://www.wemjournal.org/article/S1080-6032(14)00257-9/pdf).

Avalanche Safety and Rescue

The factors that contribute to avalanche release are terrain, weather, and snowpack. Terrain factors are fixed; however, the state of the weather and snowpack change daily, even hourly. Precipitation, wind, temperature, snow depth, snow surface, weak layers, and settlement are factors that contribute to avalanche potential. Comprehensive review of snowpack evaluation and route finding is beyond the scope of this chapter. Anyone venturing into avalanche terrain must be familiar with avalanche hazard evaluation and appropriate route selection.

AVALANCHE SAFETY AND RESCUE EQUIPMENT

Traveling safely in avalanche terrain requires special preparations, including education and carrying safety and rescue equipment. Safety equipment should include the following:

Snow Shovel

The snow shovel is an essential piece of equipment for anyone traveling in avalanche country. All persons should carry one.
- It can be used to dig snow pits for stability evaluation and snow caves for overnight shelter.
- A shovel is necessary for digging in avalanche debris because such snow is far too firm for digging with hands or skis.
- The shovel should be sturdy and strong enough, yet light and small enough to fit into a pack. Shovels are made of aluminum or high-strength polycarbonate and can be collapsible.
- Extricating someone buried beneath 1 m (3.3 ft) of snow requires removing about 1 to 1.5 tons of snow.
- Seven to 10 minutes is needed to uncover someone buried 1 m (3.3 ft) deep. A 2-m (6.6-ft) burial requires 15 to 30 minutes.

Probe

- This may be used to assist in pinpointing a victim following a transceiver (rescue beacon) search and is essential if the victim is without a transceiver.
- Organized rescue teams keep rigid poles in 3- to 4-m (10- to 12-ft) lengths as part of their rescue equipment caches.
- The recreationist can buy collapsible probe poles of tubular aluminum or carbon fiber that come in 45-cm (18-inch) sections that attach quickly by pulling a stiffening cable to construct a full-length probe.
- Ski poles with removable grips and baskets can be screwed together to make an avalanche probe. These are largely inferior to dedicated commercial probes.

- Although markedly suboptimal, a tent pole, the tail of a ski, or a ski pole with the basket removed can substitute for this piece of equipment in an absolute emergency.

Avalanche Rescue Transceivers (Beacons)

- The term *transceiver* differentiates avalanche transceivers from satellite emergency notification devices, such as personal locator beacons and SPOT devices (satellite personal tracker that transmits a person's location via satellite to friends or emergency services).
- Avalanche rescue transceivers are the best devices to quickly find a buried companion.
- Transceivers emit an electromagnetic signal on a worldwide standard frequency of 457 kHz.
- A buried person's transceiver emits the signal, and the rescuer's unit can be set to receive the signal.
- The signal carries a distance of 30 to 50 m (100 to 150 ft) and, when used properly, can guide searchers to the buried transceiver in less than 5 minutes.
- Modern transceivers generally use a computer chip to process the signal, displaying a digital readout of the distance and general direction to the buried unit.
- Newer triple-antenna transceivers provide data about distance, direction, and signal strength and can more easily identify multiple burials and their approximate location in relation to each other.
- It is essential to confirm that all members of the party have their transceivers set to "transmit" before travel.
- Merely possessing a transceiver does not ensure its lifesaving capability. Frequent practice is required to master a transceiver-guided search.
- Beacons should be strapped close to the body under a layer of clothing or in a secure, beacon pocket (commonly on the pant thigh).
- Always check batteries before trips and carry extra batteries. Use high-quality batteries.
- Never use rechargeable batteries in an avalanche rescue transceiver. The transceiver could lose power without warning or prior indication of low power.
- Transceivers should be turned "on" at the start of the day and turned "off" at the end of the day.
- Check every party member's transceiver periodically throughout the trip.
- Keep the device dry and free from battery corrosion.
- Avalanche rescue transceiver searches have become highly specialized, and search technique depends largely on the specific model and type. It is essential to practice and learn the specifics of any model used before using it in an actual rescue.
- Box 2.1 provides a generic overview of a search, but these instructions should not take the place of the unit's type-specific instructions.

BOX 2.1   Avalanche Transceiver Search

Initial Search
1. Safely access the slide path and debris area, and have everyone switch their transceivers to "receive" and turn the volume to "high."
2. If enough people are available, post a lookout to warn others about possible additional slides.
3. Should a second slide occur, have rescuers immediately switch their transceivers to "transmit."
4. Have rescuers space themselves no more than 30 m (100 ft) apart and walk abreast along the slope.
5. If a single rescuer is searching within a wide path, he or she should zigzag across the rescue zone and limit the distance between crossings to 30 m (100 ft).
6. For multiple victims, when a signal is picked up, have one or two rescuers continue to focus on that victim while the remainder of the group continues to search for additional victims.
7. For a single victim, when a signal is picked up, have one or two rescuers continue to locate the victim while the remainder of the group prepares shovels, probes, and medical supplies for the rescue.

Avalanche Airbag System (Fig. 2.1)

- Although airbags were originally designed for guides and ski patrollers, airbags can be used by anyone venturing into avalanche terrain.
- The airbag is based on the principle of "inverse segregation," which causes larger particles to rise to the surface. A person is already a large particle. The airbag makes the user an even larger particle.
- During partial burial, the brightly colored balloons hopefully become easily visible on the surface, making a transceiver search unnecessary.
- The airbag is integrated into a special backpack or vest, and the user deploys it by pulling a ripcordlike handle.
- Airbags are of two types: dual bags, one on each side of the pack; or a behind-the-head, pillow-like single bag.
- Empiric data suggest that an inflated avalanche airbag system (ABS) reduces by approximately 50% the likelihood of dying because of avalanche burial.
- Deployment failure or noninflation is typically due to user error, mainly inability to reach or pull the inflation cord.
- Avalanche risk increases when users view airbags as a "magic shield." The reality is that ABS protection is certainly not foolproof. This device should never be used to justify taking additional risks.

AvaLung (Fig. 2.2)

- The AvaLung is an emergency breathing device that prevents rebreathing expired air, which is a major cause of asphyxiation

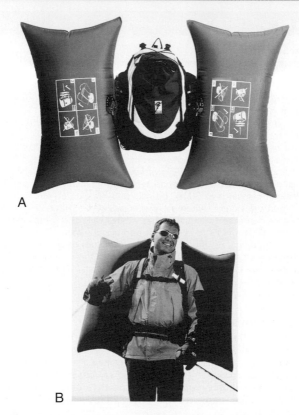

FIGURE 2.1   A, A small avalanche airbag system (ABS) backpack with deployed airbags. The airbags are stowed in outside pockets of the backpack. **B,** Integrated into a backpack, the avalanche ABS is deployed by pulling the white T handle. (Courtesy Peter Aschauer, GmbH.)

during avalanche burial, by diverting expired air away from inspired air that is drawn from the snowpack.
- It is worn as an independent device over the outer layer of clothing or incorporated into various-sized backpacks with a stowable mouthpiece kept in the shoulder strap.
- If buried, the person can breathe through a mouthpiece and flexible tube connected to the device.
- The person inhales oxygenated air coming from the surrounding snow, which passes through a membrane in the device.
- The exhaled air passes through a one-way valve and into another area of the snow posterior to the person to greatly reduce the effects of carbon dioxide contaminating the airspace.

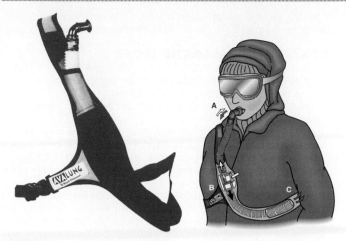

FIGURE 2.2   Left, The AvaLung 2 is a breathing device intended to prolong survival during avalanche burial by diverting expired air away from inspired air drawn from the snowpack. **Right,** *A,* The person can breathe through a mouthpiece and flexible tube connected to the vest. *B,* The person inhales oxygenated air coming from the surrounding snow, which passes through a membrane in the vest. *C,* The exhaled air passes through a one-way valve and into another area of the snow posterior to the person to greatly reduce the effects of carbon dioxide contaminating the airspace.

- The AvaLung has worked well in simulated burials, allowing the person to breathe for 1 hour in tightly packed snow. It has been effective in actual avalanche burials.
- This device should never be used to justify taking additional risks.

Recco Rescue System

This two-part system consists of the Recco reflector, which is a small, Band-Aid–sized tab integrated into outerwear, boots, and helmets; and the Recco detector, which is a special handheld detector used by organized rescue teams (either on the ground or from helicopters).

- The detector sends out a radio signal that is doubled in strength and reflected by the specially tuned reflector.
- The reflected signal provides directional pinpointing of the person's location.
- The search strategies with the detector are like those using avalanche rescue transceivers. However, the Recco system does not replace transceivers.
- For people equipped with transceivers, the reflector becomes a backup system. For novices who might not even know they should carry a transceiver, the reflector provides a basic rescue system.

- Through air, the signal range is up to 200 m (656 ft); in snow, the range is up to 20 m (66 ft); liquid water attenuates the signal.

CROSSING AN AVALANCHE SLOPE

Travel through avalanche terrain always involves risk. Before crossing a potential avalanche slope, take the following precautions.

1. Never ski alone in dangerous conditions.
2. Tighten up clothing, fasten zippers, and wear hat, gloves, and goggles.
3. If wearing a heavy mountaineering pack, loosen it before crossing so that it can be jettisoned if necessary. A heavy pack may increase potential for traumatic injury. Conversely, a lighter pack or "day pack" may protect the spine and may continue to be worn.
4. Remove ski pole straps and ski runaway straps because attached poles and skis will add to potential for trauma and may act like anchors, trapping a person beneath the surface. In avalanche terrain, always use releasable bindings on snowboards and mountaineering (including telemark skis).
5. Check transceiver batteries, and be sure that all rescue transceivers are set to "transmit."
6. Anticipate an avalanche. Plan your escape route ahead of time.
7. Cross slopes at a high point, and stay on ridges. The person highest on a slope runs the least risk for being buried should the slope slide.
8. If crossing below the slope, cross far out from runout zones. Avalanches can be triggered from the flats below steep slopes. The warning signs to this danger typically include collapsing snow and "whumpfing" sounds. In exceptionally unstable snow conditions, avalanches have been triggered in valleys up to 0.8 km (0.5 mile) from the slope.
9. Cross one person at a time. This exposes only a single individual to danger and puts less weight on the snow. Watch this person carefully as he or she crosses.
10. Cross potential avalanche slopes as quickly as possible. Never stop moving in the middle of an avalanche slope.
11. When climbing or descending an avalanche path, stay close to the sides. This makes it easier to escape to the side should the slope begin to slide. Try to move toward natural islands of safety free from avalanche dangers, such as large rock outcroppings or dense trees. Although avalanches may not start in dense trees, avalanches can run into or through dense timber.

SURVIVING AN AVALANCHE

1. Escape to the side. The moment the snow begins to move, try to escape by skiing or moving quickly to the side of the avalanche, like the method a swimmer uses to ferry to the side of a river. Turning skis or a snow machine downhill to outrun the avalanche invariably fails because the avalanche will overtake you.

2. Shout "avalanche!" to alert companions, then close your mouth to prevent snow inhalation.
3. If wearing an AvaLung, the mouthpiece should be quickly placed in the mouth, which also helps to prevent oropharyngeal snow impaction. If wearing an ABS, the ripcord should be pulled and airbag activated.
4. If knocked off your feet, kick off your skis and toss away ski poles.
5. Although skiers should try to discard their gear, snowmobile riders should try to stay on their snow machines. Once they are off their machines, riders are twice as likely to be buried as are their machines.
6. Try to grab on to a fixed object (hanging on allows more snow to go past, reducing odds of burial).
7. Once knocked off your feet, get your hands up to your face. Reach across the face and grab a jacket collar or the pack strap where it crosses the shoulder. This may not position your hands directly in front of your face, but you can use the crook of your elbow to create an air pocket.
8. Attempting to place your hands immediately in front of your face increases the probability of maintaining airspace in a tumbling ride. It also allows your hands to create a breathing space around your mouth and nose after the avalanche stops.
9. Once the avalanche stops, it is nearly impossible to move the hands to the face to create an air pocket. Without an air pocket, the consequences of a burial are usually fatal, unless the person is uncovered in minutes.
10. Creating an air pocket is the key to survival, but some persons, sensing themselves to be near the surface, have thrust a hand or foot toward the surface. Any clue on the surface that gives the rescuers something to see greatly improves an individual's odds of survival.

Initiate Search and Scan for Clues

The International Commission for Alpine Rescue deems avalanche burial to be a medical emergency. Early notification of rescue teams may be key to assisting companions. Call for help, but do not leave the site. A buried person's best chances of survival are in the hands of his or her companions. When a person is observed caught in an avalanche:

1. Stop and assess the danger. Do not make the situation worse by triggering a second avalanche.
2. Assign a leader. Someone must take charge and confirm how many persons are missing and what will be the rescue plan.
3. Call for help. Use a cell phone, satellite phone, or emergency locator to alert rescuers. See Calling for Help for additional information.
4. If enough rescuers are available, one may stay on the phone to coordinate with rescue teams. This person can also keep an eye out to alert searchers if other people—potential triggers—move into the adjacent avalanche starting zones or trigger a second avalanche.

5. Safely access the avalanche debris, and go to the victim's last seen area. Mark this location.
6. Spread searchers out to effectively scan the debris. Look and listen for clues, such as any equipment or body parts that may be sticking out of the snow.

Rescue Transceivers and Probing After Transceiver Search

1. With transceivers: Have all survivors immediately switch their units to "receive." Confirm that this step has been done. With skilled rescuers, when a signal is received, the search can be quickly narrowed and the person pinpointed within a few minutes. For specific transceiver search technique, refer to the manual that came with your unit and practice often (at least several times during the ski season) (Fig. 2.3; see Box 2.1).
2. Without a transceiver: Search the fall line below the person's last-seen location for clues. Make shallow probes at likely burial areas with an avalanche probe, ski pole, or tree limb. Likely burial spots are the uphill sides of trees, rocks, benches, or bends in the slope where snow avalanche debris is concentrated. The "toe" of the debris is also a place where many victims come to rest.
3. Alert others when a clue is found or transceiver signal is heard. Pull the clue out of the snow, and leave it visible on the surface.
4. When the victim's location has been pinpointed, probing should begin. The probe should be placed perpendicular to the slope at the location of the highest transceiver signal and pushed deeply, usually 2 to 3 m (6.6 to 10 ft; most probe lengths).
5. When the victim is located by a probe strike, the probe should be left in place and shoveling begin.
6. Shovel fast and efficiently. See Shoveling to use effective techniques to move snow quickly.

Probe Line Search (Only Applicable in the Initial Search if the Victim Is Without a Transceiver)

When a surface search reveals enough clues so the likely burial area can be identified, companions should systematically probe the area. Optimal probing is performed with three holes per step.
1. Probers stand with arms out, wrist to wrist.
2. Probers first probe between their feet, and then probe 50 cm (20 inches) to the right and 50 cm (20 inches) to the left (Fig. 2.4).
3. At a command from the leader, the line advances 50 cm (20 inches) (one step).
4. This method gives an 88% chance of finding the person on the first pass.
5. It is most helpful to use a guidon cord (marked with 50-cm intervals) suspended between two rescuers.

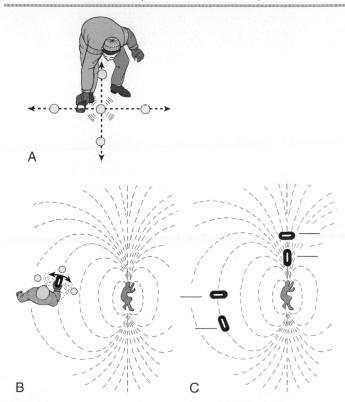

FIGURE 2.3 Induction ("tangent") line search method. **A,** The arrangement of the electromagnetic flux lines (induction lines) emitted from a buried victim. The signal received by the searching transceiver along the transmitted flux line is strongest when it is oriented in parallel and weakest when it is oriented perpendicularly. **B,** The searcher moves in short (3 to 5 m [9.8 to 16.4 ft]) "tangents" and then orients the transceiver to the strongest signal. In this way, the receiving transceiver follows a flux line toward the victim. The sensitivity (loudness) of the beacon should be adjusted downward as the victim is approached so that the searcher can discern the strongest signal before proceeding in a new direction. **C,** The "pinpoint" search is performed when the buried victim is within 3 m (9.8 ft); this typically occurs when the transceiver is at its loudest with the sensitivity turned all the way down. It is a "grid" search on a much smaller scale that is carried out close to the snow surface. The loudest signal is found along one axis (E to W) and followed by the perpendicular axis (N to S) to the likely burial position. A probe is then used to confirm the victim's location and depth.

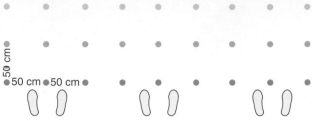

FIGURE 2.4   Fine avalanche probing (three-hole-per-step method).

6. The goal is to rescue someone alive, but all too often, probe lines are too slow and function as a body recovery method.

Shoveling

In companion rescue, the shoveling component will take much longer than a well-performed transceiver search. Depending on the number of rescuers and the technique used, this shoveling could be the difference between life and death. Unburying an avalanche victim is the most time-consuming component of the rescue. Teaching efficient shoveling techniques should be included in all avalanche rescue courses and practiced as often as transceiver searches to reduce the total time to extrication. Before detailing two specific techniques, here are some helpful guidelines:

- The person's depth and precise position should be rapidly pinpointed by final probe placement (remember, it is faster to probe than to dig).
- Although speed is essential when digging, try to do the following:
  - Leave the probe in place as a marker.
  - Avoid standing on top of the person, which may collapse the person's airspace.
  - Move snow only once.
  - Sweep or paddle snow to the sides or downhill rather than lifting and tossing.
  - Upon reaching the person, free the head and chest of snow.
  - Ensure an open and adequate airway immediately upon uncovering the patient's head.

Strategic Shoveling

1. During companion rescue, where typically only one to three shovelers might be available and the debris is often softer, the strategic shoveling technique increases digging efficiency (Fig. 2.5).
2. Avoid standing over the buried person. Begin digging downslope from the probe, lift snow as little as possible by throwing it to the side, and move snow only once.
3. With the probe left in place, shovelers begin digging downslope about 1 to 1.5 times the burial depth (as determined by the probe).

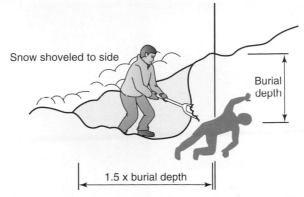

FIGURE 2.5   Strategic shoveling technique for one or two rescuers. (Courtesy Dale Atkins and the National Ski Patrol, Lakewood, CO.)

4. Quickly dig a waist-deep starter hole about one arm span wide (i.e., the distance between the fingertips when one's arms are held out to the sides).
5. If two shovelers are digging, they should work in tandem and side by side rather than one digging behind the other.
6. Throw snow to the sides.
7. Move to the starter hole, and continue digging downward and forward. As depth increases, snow can be cleared to the back rather than lifted and tossed to the sides.
8. When close to the person, use a scraping action to clear snow. Use the first body part to estimate the location of the head, and then use one's hands to clear away snow from the person's face and airway, while continuing to clear snow off his or her chest.
9. The most important feature of efficient shoveling is to create a ramp or platform in the snow that leads to the probe (and the person) instead of digging a hole down around the probe. In this way, extrication and resuscitation of the person are made easier by having a flat surface available, the air pocket is not compromised, there is space to work on the person, and raising up the person is not necessary.

Snow Conveyor Belt

If a delay occurs that necessitates an organized rescue effort, the debris is often much harder because of age hardening than what is experienced by companion rescuers. Typically, more shovelers are available. In this situation, the conveyor belt method works effectively to clear snow quickly (Fig. 2.6). The snow conveyor belt can be used by just a few companions, just as strategic shoveling can be used by rescue teams.

1. The lead shoveler chops out blocks of snow and scoops the snow downslope.

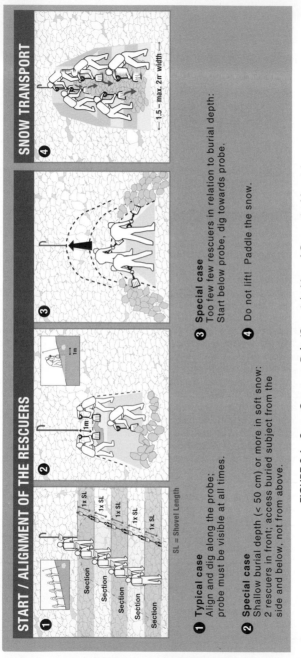

FIGURE 2.6 Snow Conveyor Belt. (Copyright Manuel Genswein. Mountain-Safety.info 2018.)

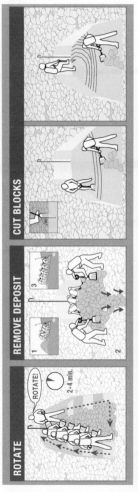

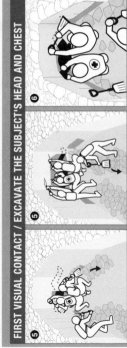

⑤ First visual contact
- No more rotation
- Two rescuers at the subject, kneeling with shortened shovel shafts, enlarging the cavity

⑥ Stop using the shovel in close proximity to the head. Airway status? Vital signs?

FIGURE 2.6, cont'd

2. The other shovelers use paddling-like motions to clear out snow.
3. When getting close to the buried person, an additional shoveler may join the lead shoveler to increase the working space.
4. Shovelers may rotate clockwise every 5 minutes to decrease fatigue.
5. After the victim is reached, locate his or her head and chest, and use one's hands to clear the airway.

CALLING FOR HELP

- Mobile phones and other emergency notification devices should be tried immediately when a burial is known or suspected. If contact cannot be made, then companions must decide whether and when to go for help. If the accident occurs in or near a ski area and there are several companions, one person can be sent to notify the ski patrol immediately. If only one or two companions are present, the correct choice is more difficult. The best advice is to search the surface quickly but thoroughly for clues before anyone leaves to notify the ski patrol.
- Cell phones are the most effective and efficient method of calling for help because contact can be made without losing manpower for continued companion rescue and the phones allow for two-way communications. In the United States, the Next Generation 9-1-1 system is being implemented in some areas to support text messages, images, and video. However, cell phones do not work in all mountain areas.
- If a voice connection cannot be made, try sending a text message. Ask the recipient to confirm your message.
- If the avalanche occurs in the backcountry far from any organized rescue team, all companions should remain at the site and search until they can do no more or until they put themselves in danger by remaining at the scene. The guiding principle in backcountry rescues is that companions search until they cannot or should not continue.
- When deciding when to stop searching, the safety of companions must be weighed against the decreasing survival chances of the buried person.

ORGANIZED RESCUE

Organized rescue is no longer always a separate action that occurs after companion rescue has failed to locate the buried person. Companion rescue and organized rescue often work hand in hand. Immediate notification of rescue teams when a burial is known or suspected means faster searches, faster rescues, better medical care, and faster evacuations. Rescue teams prefer to be called too often than too late.

AVALANCHE VICTIM (Table 2.1)

Avalanches kill in two ways:
- Asphyxiation secondary to airway occlusion by snow, increased inhaled air carbon dioxide levels, pressure of snow on the thorax, and formation of an ice mask around the nose and mouth after burial.

Table 2.1 Injuries in Survivors of Avalanche Burial (Partial and Total)		
	UTAH	**EUROPE**
Total Injuries	**9 (Total, 91 Avalanche Accidents)**	**351 (Total, 1447 Avalanche Accidents)**
Major orthopedic	3 (33%)	95 (27%)
Hypothermia requiring treatment at hospital arrival	2 (22%)	74 (21%)
Skin/soft tissue	1 (11%)	84 (24%)
Craniofacial	—	83 (24%)
Chest	3 (33%)	7 (2%)
Abdominal	—	4 (1%)

From Grossman MD, Saffle JR, Thomas F, Tremper B: Avalanche trauma. *J Trauma* 29:1705, 1989.

- Trauma secondary to the wrenching action of snow in motion and impact with trees, rocks, loose equipment, and cliffs. Prognostic features for low survival potential include the following:
- Complete burial of the person. Survival probabilities greatly diminish with increasing burial depth, probably because of increased digging time. Very few avalanche victims in the United States have survived burials deeper than 2 m (6.6 ft).
- Time is the enemy of the buried person. In the first 15 minutes after the avalanche, more persons are found alive than dead. Within 15 to 30 minutes, an equal number of people are found dead and alive. After 30 minutes, more people are found dead than alive, and the survival rate rapidly diminishes as time increases thereafter. However, a very few, lucky persons have survived burials of many hours.
- A factor that affects survival is the position of the person's head (i.e., whether the person was buried face up or face down). The most favorable position is face up. If buried face up, an airspace forms around the face as the back of the head melts into the snow; if buried face down, an airspace cannot form as the face melts into the snow.
- Avalanche victims seldom die from hypothermia, but nearly all buried persons suffer hypothermia. Be ready to insulate and protect an injured person from the environment.

CARE OF THE PATIENT (Fig. 2.7)
Medical Treatment and Resuscitation of Avalanche Burial Victims
1. An initial impression of the level of consciousness is made as the head and chest are exposed and cleared of snow.

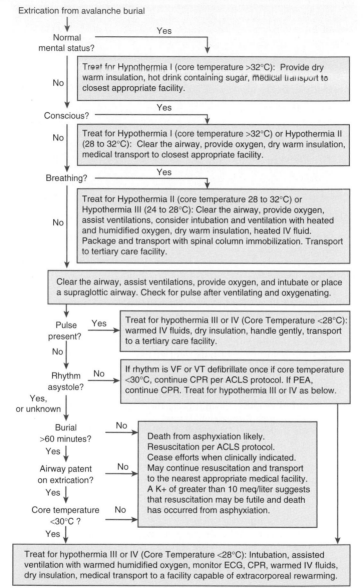

Extrication from avalanche burial

Normal mental status? — Yes →

No ↓

Treat for Hypothermia I (core temperature >32°C): Provide dry warm insulation, hot drink containing sugar, medical transport to closest appropriate facility.

Conscious? — Yes →

No ↓

Treat for Hypothermia I (core temperature >32°C) or Hypothermia II (28 to 32°C): Clear the airway, provide oxygen, dry warm insulation, medical transport to closest appropriate facility.

Breathing? — Yes →

No ↓

Treat for Hypothermia II (core temperature 28 to 32°C) or Hypothermia III (24 to 28°C): Clear the airway, provide oxygen, assist ventilations, consider intubation and ventilation with heated and humidified oxygen, dry warm insulation, heated IV fluid. Package and transport with spinal column immobilization. Transport to tertiary care facility.

Clear the airway, assist ventilations, provide oxygen, and intubate or place a supraglottic airway. Check for pulse after ventilating and oxygenating.

Pulse present? — Yes →

Treat for hypothermia III or IV (Core Temperature <28°C): warmed IV fluids, dry insulation, handle gently, transport to a tertiary care facility.

No ↓

Rhythm asystole? — No →

If rhythm is VF or VT defibrillate once if core temperature <30°C, continue CPR per ACLS protocol. If PEA, continue CPR. Treat for hypothermia III or IV as below.

Yes, or unknown ↓

Burial >60 minutes? — No →

Death from asphyxiation likely.
Resuscitation per ACLS protocol.
Cease efforts when clinically indicated.
May continue resuscitation and transport to the nearest appropriate medical facility.
A K+ of greater than 10 meq/liter suggests that resuscitation may be futile and death has occurred from asphyxiation.

Yes ↓

Airway patent on extrication? — No →

Yes ↓

Core temperature <30°C ? — No →

Yes ↓

Treat for hypothermia III or IV (Core Temperature <28°C): Intubation, assisted ventilation with warmed humidified oxygen, monitor ECG, CPR, warmed IV fluids, dry insulation, medical transport to a facility capable of extracorporeal rewarming.

Notes:
Burial for 60 minutes: The provider should use the 60-minute threshold as a general, but not absolute, guide. Circumstances such as a presumed large air pocket could allow for a longer survival time without development of severe hypothermia. Core temperature: Providers may not have access to core temperature thermometers in the field. In this circumstance, the severity of hypothermia may be estimated with the use of Swiss hypothermia stages I through IV as determined by the clinical presentation (see Box 4.2).

FIGURE 2.7 Assessment and medical care of extricated avalanche burial victim. *ACLS,* Advanced cardiac life support; *CPR,* cardiopulmonary resuscitation; *ECG,* electrocardiogram; *IV,* intravenous; *PEA,* pulseless electrical activity; *VF,* ventricular fibrillation.

2. Opening the airway and ensuring adequate breathing are the primary medical interventions. Every effort should be made to clear the airway of snow as soon as possible and to provide assistance if breathing is absent or ineffective. These measures should be instituted as soon as possible and not await extrication of the entire body.

3. If injury to the spinal column is suspected or if there is evidence of head or facial trauma, then the spinal column is immobilized as the airway is opened, adequate breathing ensured, and oxygen provided.

4. If endotracheal intubation is required for the unconscious apneic patient who is not yet fully extricated from snow burial, then the inverse intubation technique may be required. With this technique, the laryngoscope is held in the right hand while straddling the patient's body and facing the head and face. While facing the patient, insert the laryngoscope blade into the oropharynx with the right hand so that the larynx and cords can be visualized by leaning over and looking into the patient's mouth; the endotracheal tube is then passed through the vocal cords with the left hand.

5. After an adequate airway and breathing are established and supplemental oxygen provided, circulation is assessed. The conscious patient is assumed to have a perfusing rhythm, and further treatment is directed at treating injuries and mild hypothermia.

6. A person who is found unconscious but with a pulse may have moderate or severe hypothermia and should be handled gently to avoid precipitating ventricular fibrillation. The medical treatment of this patient is focused on ensuring adequate oxygenation and ventilation, either noninvasively with a bag-valve-mask, supraglottic airway device, or endotracheal tube while simultaneously immobilizing the spinal column for transport and treating manifestations of trauma.

7. Intravenous access may be obtained and warmed isotonic fluids infused. Provide for thermal stabilization. Handle the patient gently in anticipation of hypothermia. Hypothermia treatment is described in Chapter 3.

8. If a pulse is not present after opening the airway and ventilating the patient or is absent after checking for up to 1 minute, cardiopulmonary resuscitation (CPR) is begun. Avalanche burial victims may be hypothermic, which causes peripheral vaso-constriction and makes pulses difficult to palpate. In addition,

moderate to severe hypothermia causes bradycardia and respiratory depression. To reiterate, before initiating the chest compressions of CPR, palpation for a pulse should be done for a period that is sufficiently long (up to 60 seconds) to ensure that spontaneous circulation is not present.

9. In a pulseless avalanche burial victim, electrocardiographic monitoring should be used to assess cardiac rhythm, or, alternatively, an automated external defibrillator (AED) may be applied. In the moderately or severely hypothermic patient in ventricular fibrillation with a core body temperature below 30°C (86°F), defibrillation should be performed according to standard guidelines, with the caveat that after unsuccessful defibrillation attempt(s), further defibrillation may be deferred until rewarming is underway as chest compressions continue. Drugs may be administered as part of advanced cardiac life support in accordance with standard guidelines, noting that they may be less or not effective in the hypothermic patient.

10. An air pocket for breathing and patent airway must be present for an avalanche burial victim to survive long enough to develop severe hypothermia. If an air pocket for breathing is not present or if the airway is obstructed, the avalanche victim who is extricated from snow burial in cardiac arrest has most likely died from trauma or asphyxiation. This is not meant to discourage initial attempts at resuscitation but rather to suggest that prolonged CPR may be a futile exercise. It is always warranted to initially start CPR to see if return of spontaneous circulation can be achieved in a reasonable time. This is because the rescuer can never know precisely when the avalanche burial victim suffered cardiac arrest.

11. When laboratory testing equipment is available, serum potassium level can be used as a prognostic indicator for the avalanche burial victim in cardiac arrest. In a hypothermic adult avalanche victim in cardiac arrest, a serum potassium level of greater than 10 mmol/L indicates that resuscitation efforts should be terminated.

12. Provide for evacuation.

DEFINITION

Accidental hypothermia is the unintentional decline of at least 2°C (3.6°F) from normal human core temperature of 37.2°C to 37.7°C (99°F to 99.9°F) that occurs in the absence of any primary central nervous system causation. It is both a symptom and clinical disease entity and can occur in all seasons. Hypothermia is classified as mild, moderate, severe, or profound (Table 3.1) and presents as either a primary disorder resulting from environmental exposure or secondary to other causes, such as trauma, infection, or metabolic disease. When sufficient heat cannot be generated to maintain homeostasis and core temperature drops below 30°C (86°F), the patient becomes poikilothermic and cools to ambient temperature.

GENERAL TREATMENT

- Consider rescuer scene safety factors, including unstable snow, ice, and rock fall.
- Handle all patients suspected of having moderate or severe hypothermia carefully to avoid unnecessary jostling or sudden impact. Rough handling can cause ventricular fibrillation. Consider aeromedical evacuation.
- The rescuer should stabilize injuries, protect the spine, splint fractures, and cover open wounds (Box 3.1).
- Prevent further heat loss; insulate the patient from above and below (Fig. 3.1 and Box 3.2).
- Anticipate an irritable myocardium, hypovolemia, and large temperature gradient between the periphery and core.
- Anticipate problematic intravenous (IV) access, and carry intraosseous (IO) infusion systems, which are compatible with crystalloids, colloids, and medications.
- Treat hypothermia before treating frostbite.
- Reconsider the decision to perform cardiopulmonary resuscitation (CPR) in the field if there is evidence of asphyxia, lethal injury, or a rigid thorax precluding chest compressions.

DISORDERS

Mild Hypothermia

Mild hypothermia is diagnosed when the core body temperature is between 37°C (98.6°F) and 33°C (91.4°F).

Signs and Symptoms

- Shivering
- Dysarthria
- Poor judgment, perseveration, or neurosis

- Amnesia
- Apathy or moodiness
- Ataxia
- Initial hyperreflexia, tachypnea, tachycardia, elevated systemic blood pressure
- Hunger, nausea, fatigue, dizziness

Table 3.1	Characteristics of the Four Zones of Hypothermia		
Stage	**CORE TEMPERATURE**		
	°C	**°F**	**Characteristics**
Mild	37.6	99.7 ± 1	Normal rectal temperature
	37.0	98.6 ± 1	Normal oral temperature
	36.0	96.8	Increases in metabolic rate, blood pressure, and preshivering muscle tone
	35.0	95.0	Urine temperature 34.8°C (94.6°F); maximal shivering thermogenesis
	34.0	93.2	Development of amnesia, dysarthria, and poor judgment; maladaptive behavior; normal blood pressure; maximal respiratory stimulation; tachycardia, then progressive bradycardia
	33.30	91.4	Development of ataxia and apathy; linear depression of cerebral metabolism; tachypnea, then progressive decrease in respiratory minute volume; cold diuresis
Moderate	32.0	89.6	Stupor; 25% decrease in oxygen consumption
	31.0	87.8	Extinguished shivering thermogenesis
	30.0	86.0	Development of atrial fibrillation and other arrhythmias; poikilothermia; cardiac output two-thirds normal; insulin ineffective
	29.0	84.2	Progressive decrease in level of consciousness, pulse, and respiration; pupils dilated; paradoxical undressing

Table 3.1   Characteristics of the Four Zones of Hypothermia—cont'd

Stage	CORE TEMPERATURE °C	°F	Characteristics
Severe	28.0	82.4	Decreased ventricular fibrillation threshold; 50% decrease in oxygen consumption and pulse; hypoventilation
	27.0	80.6	Loss of reflexes and voluntary motion
	26.0	78.8	Major acid-base disturbances; no reflexes or response to pain
	25.0	77.0	Cerebral blood flow one-third normal; loss of cerebrovascular autoregulation; cardiac output 45% of normal; pulmonary edema may develop
	24.0	75.2	Significant hypotension and bradycardia
	23.0	73.4	No corneal or oculocephalic reflexes; areflexia
	22.0	71.6	Maximal risk of ventricular fibrillation; 75% decrease in oxygen consumption
Profound	20.0	68.0	Lowest temperature for mechanical resumption of cardiac electromechanical activity; pulse 20% of normal
	19.0	66.2	Electroencephalographic silencing
	18.0	64.4	Asystole
	13.7	56.7	Lowest adult accidental hypothermia survival
	15.0	59.0	Lowest infant accidental hypothermia survival
	10.0	50.0	92% decrease in oxygen consumption
	9.0	48.2	Lowest therapeutic hypothermia survival

> **BOX 3.1**   Preparing Hypothermic Patients for Transport
>
> 1. The patient must be dry. Gently remove or cut off wet clothing, and replace it with dry clothing or a dry insulation system. Keep the patient horizontal, and do not allow exertion or massage of extremities.
> 2. Stabilize injuries (e.g., place spine fractures in correct anatomic position). Open wounds should be covered before packaging.
> 3. Initiate heated fluid infusions (intravenous or intraosseous) if feasible; bags can be placed under the patient's buttocks or in a compressor system. Administer a fluid challenge.
> 4. Active rewarming should be limited to heated inhalation and truncal heat. Insulate hot water bottles in stockings or mittens before placing them in the patient's axillae and groin.
> 5. The patient should be wrapped (see Fig. 3.1). Begin building the wrap by placing a large plastic sheet on the available surface (floor, ground), and upon this sheet place an insulated sleeping pad. A layer of blankets, sleeping bag, or bubble wrap insulating material is laid over the sleeping pad. The patient is then placed on the insulation. Heating bottles are put in place along with fluid-filled bags intended for infusion, and the entire package is wrapped layer over layer, with the plastic as the final closure. The patient's face should be partially covered, taking care to create a tunnel to allow access for breathing and monitoring.

Treatment

If the patient is awake:

1. Gently remove all wet clothing, and replace it with dry clothing.
2. Insulate the patient with sleeping bags, cloth pads, bubble wrap, blankets, or other suitable material.
3. Always insulate the patient from the ground up. Use adequate insulation underneath the patient (see Fig. 3.1).
4. If the patient is capable of purposeful swallowing (will not aspirate), encourage drinking of warm and sweet drinks such as warm gelatin (Jell-O), reconstituted fruit beverages, juice, or decaffeinated tea or cocoa, because carbohydrates fuel shivering. Avoid heavily caffeinated drinks to prevent further diuresis.
5. If a mildly hypothermic patient is well hydrated and insulated from further cooling, he or she can often walk out to safety.

Moderate Hypothermia

Moderate hypothermia is diagnosed when core body temperature is between 32°C (89.6°F) and 29°C (84.2°F).

Signs and Symptoms

- Stupor progressing to unconsciousness
- Loss of shivering reflex
- Atrial fibrillation and other arrhythmias, including bradycardia

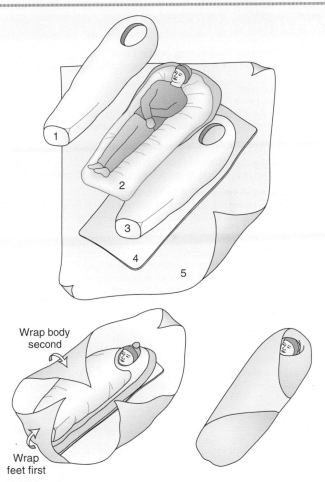

Wrap body
second

Wrap
feet first

FIGURE 3.1   An insulation wrap consists of multiple layers of insulation *(1–3)* on top of a foam pad or inflatable insulation pad *(4)*, covered in a windproof and waterproof layer *(5)*. Heating bottles, IVs, and monitoring equipment (e.g., blood pressure cuff, pulse oximeter) can be placed in the wrap to access through the layers. A tunnel should be created through the insulation to the face to access the airway for monitoring during transport.

- Poikilothermy
- Mild to moderate hypotension
- Diminished respiratory rate and effort, bronchorrhea
- Dilated pupils
- Diminished neurologic reflexes and voluntary motion
- Decreased ventricular fibrillation threshold

BOX 3.2   Rewarming Options

Passive External Rewarming in the Field

1. Cover the patient with dry insulating materials in a warm environment.
2. Block the wind.
3. Keep the patient dry.
4. Insulate the patient from the ground (e.g., use a foam pad).
5. Use a windproof tarp, tent fly, or aluminized (reflective) body cover, such as a "space blanket."
6. Rescue groups typically carry specialized casualty evacuation bags. These are often windproof, waterproof, and well insulated. Many offer specialized zippers and openings for patient access.

Active External Rewarming in the Field

1. Apply hot water bottles, chemical heat packs, or warmed rocks to areas of high circulation, such as around the neck, in the axillae, and in the groin. Take care to avoid thermal burns by insulating the heated objects.
2. Use skin-to-skin contact by putting a normothermic rescuer in contact with the patient inside a sleeping bag. This method may suppress shivering and reduce rewarming rates in mildly hypothermic persons. However, it may be one of few options in remote locations or with severely hypothermic, nonshivering patients, especially when evacuation will be delayed.
3. Use a forced-air warming system within a sleeping bag.
4. Immerse the patient in a warm (40°C [104°F]) water bath. Be cautious with immersion warming in the field because this may increase core temperature afterdrop.
5. Place just the hands and feet in warm (40°C [104°F]) water if whole-body warming is not possible.
6. Do not rub or massage cold extremities to rewarm them.

Core Rewarming in the Field

NOTE: The impact of these modalities on the rate of rewarming in the field may not be significant.

1. Use heated (40°C to 45°C [104°F to 113°F]), humidified oxygen inhalation.
2. Administer heated (40°C to 42°C [104°F to 107.6°F]) intravenous solutions.

- Prolonged PR, QR, and QTc intervals; J (Osborn) wave
- Paradoxical undressing

Treatment

A patent airway and presence of respirations must be established (Fig. 3.2). If the patient is confused, stuporous, or unconscious but shows obvious signs of life:

1. Handle gently and immobilize the patient (reduces the potential for ventricular fibrillation).
2. Consider aeromedical evacuation to prevent jostling.

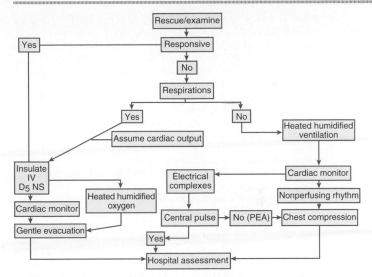

FIGURE 3.2 Prehospital life support. *IV D$_5$ NS*, Intravenous 5% dextrose in normal saline; *PEA*, pulseless electrical activity.

3. Maintain the patient in a horizontal position to avoid orthostatic hypotension.
4. Do not encourage ingestion of oral fluids. The small contribution to hydration and rewarming is outweighed by the risk for aspiration.
5. Do not massage or vigorously manipulate the patient's extremities.
6. Provide oxygenation commensurate with the patient's clinical condition.
   a. Options include simple administration of oxygen by nasal cannula or face mask, bag-valve-mask ventilation, or endotracheal intubation.
   b. If endotracheal intubation is performed, avoid overinflation of the tube cuff with frigid air, which may later expand upon warming and obstruct the tube or cause laryngeal injury.
7. If IV or IO capability exists, initiate access and administer 250 to 500 mL of heated (37°C to 41°C [98.6°F to 105.8°F]) 5% dextrose in normal saline (NS) solution. If NS solution is unavailable, use any crystalloid, preferably containing dextrose. However, avoid lactated Ringer solution because a cold liver poorly metabolizes lactate. The IV fluid can be warmed by any of the following techniques:
   a. Use commercially available products, such as Thermal Angel, Wilderness IV Warmer, and Ultimate Hot Pack.

b. Place the IV bag underneath the patient's back, shoulder, or buttocks.

c. Tape heat-producing packets (e.g., hand warmers, meals ready to eat [MRE] heating packs) to the fluid bag.

d. If heated fluids are unavailable, administer fluid heated to the rescuer's skin temperature (i.e., >86°F [30°C]). This can be accomplished by carrying plastic fluid-filled bags next to the skin during rescue.

8. Use a fluid bag–compressor inflatable cuff.

9. Consider treatment of hypoglycemia with 50% dextrose, 25 g IV or IO.

10. Stabilize the patient's body temperature.

a. Remove wet clothing, and replace it with dry clothing; insulate the patient from above and below.

b. Be cautious with immersion warming in the field because this may cause core temperature afterdrop.

c. Place hot water bottles or padded heat packs in the axillae and groin areas and around the neck. Wrap hot water bottles with insulation (e.g., fleece) to prevent thermal burns.

d. Initiate external warming using blankets, sleeping bags, or shelter. Patients in the field should be wrapped. The wrap starts with a large plastic sheet upon which is placed an insulated sleeping pad. A layer of blankets, sleeping bag, or bubble wrap insulating material is laid over the sleeping bag. The patient is placed on the insulation, the heating bottles are put in place along with fluid-filled bags intended for infusion, and the entire package is wrapped layer over layer. The plastic is the final closure. The face should be partially covered in a manner that allows a tunnel to be created to allow access for breathing and monitoring of the patient (see Fig. 3.1).

e. A warmed-air–circulating heater pack may be used as an adjunct.

f. Consider heated, humidified oxygen if personnel are well trained in its use.

Severe Hypothermia
Severe hypothermia is diagnosed when core body temperature falls below 28°C (82.4°F).

Signs and Symptoms
- Absent neurologic reflexes (deep tendon, corneal, oculocephalic)
- Absent response to pain
- Pulmonary edema
- Acid-base abnormalities
- Coagulopathy, thrombocytopenia
- Significant hypotension
- Significant risk for ventricular fibrillation
- Flat electroencephalogram
- Asystole

Treatment

When the patient is confused, stuporous, or unconscious but shows signs of life, follow the treatment guidelines for moderate hypothermia. When no immediate signs of life are present, do the following:

1. Determine if the patient is breathing.
   a. Because chest rise may be difficult to discern, listen and feel carefully around the nose and mouth. A "vapor trail" is usually absent. If a stethoscope is available, auscultate for breath sounds.
   b. If the patient is not breathing, assist with oxygenation and ventilation by endotracheal intubation or supraglottic airway device (e.g., laryngeal mask airway, King airway).
   c. Avoid overzealous assisted ventilations, which can induce hypocapnic ventricular irritability.
2. Feel for a pulse (best done at the carotid or femoral arteries). Do this for at least 1 minute. If there is no palpable pulse and a stethoscope is available, auscultate for heart sounds. If a portable ultrasound device is available, assess for heart wall motion.
3. Avoid unnecessary chest compressions of CPR because these may initiate ventricular fibrillation.
4. Apply a cardiac monitor-defibrillator.
   a. If ventricular fibrillation or asystole is determined, defibrillate one time with 2 joules/kg up to 200 joules. Use benzoin to affix nonadherent electrodes. Do not defibrillate if electrical complexes indicating an organized rhythm are seen on a cardiac monitor. Defibrillation rarely succeeds below a core temperature of 30°C (86°F). If the patient remains in asystole or ventricular fibrillation, begin CPR.
   b. If electrical complexes indicating an organized rhythm are seen on a cardiac monitor, assess for a central pulse to determine if the patient has pulseless electrical activity (PEA). This is a difficult judgment call. The patient may have a low blood pressure that cannot be appreciated by the rescuer, in which case the chest compressions of CPR might initiate ventricular fibrillation.
4. If resuscitation is not successful in the field, continue warming and CPR until the patient arrives at a hospital or you cannot continue because of fatigue or danger to yourself.
5. If the resuscitation is successful, follow the preceding protocol for moderate or severe hypothermia.

CARDIOPULMONARY RESUSCITATION

Basic and advanced life support recommendations in hypothermia continue to evolve (Fig. 3.3). Cardiac output generated with closed-chest compressions maintains viability in certain patients with hypothermia.

1. Carefully determine the patient's cardiopulmonary status.
   a. Feel for a carotid or femoral pulse for at least 1 minute.
   b. Watch the chest for motion (breathing) for at least 30 seconds.

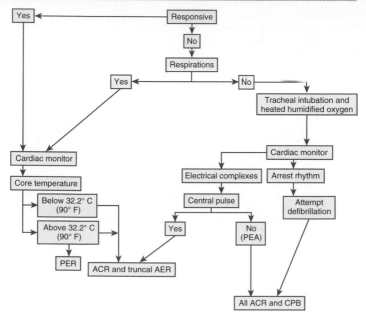

FIGURE 3.3 Emergency department algorithm. *ACR,* Active core rewarming; *AER,* active external rewarming; *CPB,* cardiopulmonary bypass; *PEA,* pulseless electrical activity; *PER,* passive external rewarming.

    c. Listen with the ear close to the patient's nose for breathing for at least 30 seconds.
2. If a hypothermic patient has any sign of life, do not begin the chest compressions of CPR, even if a peripheral pulse cannot be appreciated.
3. Manage the airway.
    a. If the patient is breathing at a suboptimal rate, assist with mouth-to-mouth or mouth-to-mask technique.
    b. Perform endotracheal intubation or place a supraglottic airway for standard indications (oxygenation, ventilation, and protection of the airway).
    c. Heated, humidified oxygen can prevent further heat loss and improve oxygenation.
4. If the patient is without any sign of life, begin standard CPR.
    a. Differentiating between bradycardia with difficult-to-feel pulses, asystole, and shockable rhythms in the field may be impossible without a portable cardiac monitor or defibrillator.
    b. A single rescuer who is fatigued may continue at slower rates of compression and artificial breathing with some expectation that these may be adequate because of the protective effects of hypothermia.

    c. Continue CPR until the patient is brought to a hospital, the rescuer is fatigued, or the rescuer is endangered.

5. Do not begin CPR if the patient has suffered obviously fatal injuries.

    a. A serum potassium (K^+) level greater than 10 mEq/L in the presence of hypothermia is a strong prognostic marker for death.

    b. Remember that a patient who appears dead may recover from hypothermia. Fixed and dilated pupils, dependent lividity, rigid muscles, and absence of detectable vital signs may be seen in patients with profound hypothermia. If in doubt, begin the resuscitation.

6. Begin rewarming concurrently with assisted ventilations or CPR.

    a. All patients will benefit from passive external rewarming (PER) and active external rewarming (AER).

    b. Patients with electrical complexes but no central pulses are assumed to suffer from PEA and may benefit from active core rewarming (ACR) or cardiopulmonary bypass (CPB) and should be transported to facilities with this capability whenever possible (see Fig. 3.3).

4

Frostbite and Other Cold-Induced Tissue Injuries

FROSTBITE
DEFINITIONS

With superficial frostbite, there is little or no expected tissue loss, whereas with deep frostbite, substantial tissue loss is expected. This definition of frostbite is based on the appearance of the frozen part after rewarming and is therefore useful in a field setting. In a more detailed classification, based on retrospective observation or advanced imaging, frostbite severity is divided into first, second, third, and fourth degrees. Superficial frostbite likely correlates with first- and second-degree signs and symptoms and deep frostbite with third and fourth degree signs and symptoms. Frostnip is a superficial temporary condition that results in tissue blanching and paresthesias that resolve with rewarming and does not cause permanent tissue damage. The following sections describe the appearance of frostbite after rewarming.

First-Degree Frostbite (see Plate 1)
Signs and Symptoms
- Numbness
- Erythema
- White or yellowish plaque
- Edema

Second-Degree Frostbite (see Plate 2)
Signs and Symptoms
- Blisters filled with clear or milky fluid develop after rewarming.
- Erythema and edema surround blisters.

Third-Degree Frostbite (see Plate 3)
- Deeper injury involves the dermis.
- Blisters filled with bloody fluid and edema develop after rewarming.

Fourth-Degree Frostbite (see Plate 4)
Signs and Symptoms
- Injury extends through the dermis into muscle and deeper; there may be no blistering and minimal edema, with characteristic cyanotic appearance without capillary refill after rewarming.
- The tissue dies and typically mummifies, with eschar development over a period of weeks.

FIELD PROGNOSIS

Favorable (Suggesting Superficial Injury) Prognostic Signs (After Rewarming)

- Sensation to pinprick
- Normal color
- Warmth
- Clear or milky fluid-filled blisters

Unfavorable (Suggesting Deep Injury) Prognostic Signs (After Rewarming)

- Dark fluid- or blood-filled blisters
- Minimal or no edema
- Cyanosis that does not blanch with pressure

FIELD TREATMENT

A decision must be made whether to actively rewarm the frostbitten tissue, because refreezing rewarmed tissue is more damaging than delaying rewarming. If, during evacuation, frostbitten tissue thaws spontaneously, all efforts should be made to keep the tissue thawed and not allow refreezing.

Strategies for field treatment are dictated largely by the presence of one of two scenarios:

Scenario 1: The frostbitten tissue has the potential to refreeze and will not be actively rewarmed.

Scenario 2: The frostbitten part can be rewarmed and kept thawed with minimal risk for refreezing until arrival at definitive care.

For Both Scenarios

1. Protect the patient from the environment, and provide appropriate shelter.
2. Treat systemic hypothermia (see Chapter 3).
3. Transfer or evacuation arrangements must protect the patient from cold exposure.
4. Frostbitten tissue should be protected from further freezing or additional trauma but allowed to spontaneously thaw if conditions make thawing unavoidable (i.e., do not intentionally keep frozen but do not actively rewarm.) Do not rub or apply ice or snow to the affected area. Remove jewelry or constrictive clothing. Replace constrictive and wet clothing with dry, loose wraps or garments, anticipating substantial edema formation.
5. Treat dehydration and maintain hydration. Vascular stasis that accompanies frostbite is worsened by dehydration.
6. Oral ibuprofen blocks or decreases production of inflammatory mediators that lead to vasoconstriction and dermal ischemia. Administer 12 mg/kg/day (up to 2400 mg/day if also used as an analgesic).

7. To minimize local trauma, apply bulky, clean, and dry gauze or sterile cotton dressings to frostbitten tissue, taking care to pad between affected toes and fingers.
8. If it is necessary to walk on a frostbitten foot to evacuate, this may cause more trauma. If it is possible for the patient to be carried or evacuated without having him or her walk on frostbitten feet, this is optimal. If the patient is carried, keep injured extremities elevated to minimize swelling.
9. Prohibit the use of tobacco products.
10. Antibiotics, anticoagulants, and vasodilators are not indicated for field treatment of frostbite.

Additional Treatment in Scenario 2

1. Field rewarming in a warm (37°C to 39°C [98.6°F to 102.2°F]) water bath should be performed if definitive care is more than 2 hours away and the tissue can be kept thawed in transit. If water temperature cannot be measured by thermometer, use an uninjured hand to judge warmth by keeping it immersed in the warmed water for at least 30 seconds to confirm that the water will not scald. Circulate water around the frozen tissue, and add warm water as needed to maintain the proper temperature. Rewarming is usually accomplished within 30 minutes. Air dry or gently blot dry the injured tissue.
2. Give analgesic medications (ibuprofen at the dosing indicated earlier and/or opiates) to control pain associated with rewarming.
3. If active rewarming is not indicated or possible, spontaneous thawing should be allowed.
4. Tense, clear fluid-filled blisters at risk for rupture during an evacuation may be aspirated and dry gauze dressing applied to minimize infection. Hemorrhagic bullae should not be aspirated or débrided electively in the field.
5. Aloe vera lotion or gel improves frostbite outcome by (weakly) reducing inflammatory mediators and if available should be applied to thawed tissue before applying dressings.
6. Supplemental oxygen (if available) should be administered if the patient is hypoxic (oxygen saturation <90%) or at high altitude above 4000 m (13,123 ft). It is otherwise not indicated solely for the treatment of frostbite.

Evacuation Timing and Destination Concerns

• Angiography performed within 24 hours of deep frostbite injury that reveals no perfusion may guide thrombolytic treatment in selected cases.
• Thrombolysis and iloprost infusions have shown promise in studies of deep frostbite injury, but they should be used only in advanced care facilities and guided by imaging.
• Be aware that thrombolytic and iloprost therapies should be initiated within 24 hours of deep injury, so prompt evacuation of persons with deep injuries is optimal.

- Radioisotope scanning or other diagnostic modalities may be used to aid prognosis at 2 to 3 weeks following injury. Magnetic resonance angiography or triple-phase bone scan performed at day 2 has been used to provide insight into prognosis and guide early surgery.

PREVENTION

- Maintain adequate systemic hydration.
- Wear properly fitted, nonconstrictive dry clothing, particularly footgear.
  - Avoid wrinkles in socks.
  - Keep mittens, gloves, and footgear dry.
  - Wear mittens in preference to gloves.
  - Keep fingernails and toenails properly trimmed.
  - Carry extra garments.
- Do not handle cold liquids or metals. (NOTE: Fuel and metal cameras are common culprits.)
- Maintain good nutrition.
- Avoid fatigue and sleep loss.
- Maintain oxygenation, using supplemental oxygen at extreme altitude.
- Do not excessively wash skin; allow natural oils to accumulate.
- Wind and high altitude greatly increase risk.
- Avoid ingested alcohol and inhaled tobacco.
- Persons with preexisting Raynaud phenomenon or prior cold injury should exercise special caution.
- Physical activity (providing severe fatigue can be prevented) will raise core and peripheral temperatures and can prevent frostbite.
- Chemical or electric warmers may be used to maintain peripheral warmth. (NOTE: Warmers should be close to body temperature before being activated.)
- Perform buddy "cold checks." If extremity numbness develops, apply warmth to the axillae and groins, and attempt to transfer adjacent body heat from a companion.
- Minimize cold exposure, particularly at environmental temperatures less than −15°C (5°F) (even with low wind speeds).

Many of the recommendations for prevention and treatment of frostbite were taken from updated consensus guidelines published by the Wilderness Medical Society (http://www.wemjournal.org/article/S1080-6032(14)00280-4/pdf).

TRENCH FOOT OR IMMERSION FOOT

Trench foot follows exposure to nonfreezing cold and wet conditions over a number of hours to days, leading to neurovascular damage without ice crystal formation.

OVERVIEW

- Injury occurs when tissue is exposed to cold and wet conditions at temperatures ranging from 0°C to 15°C (32°F to 59°F).

- Injury may extend proximally and involve the knees, thighs, and buttocks, depending on the depth of immersion.
- Symptoms are usually insidious in onset.

Signs and Symptoms

- Prehyperemic phase: Blanched pale skin that becomes extremely edematous; loss of sensation and proprioception are common. Capillary refill is slow, peripheral pulses may be absent, and muscle cramping is common.
- Hyperemic phase: Skin becomes reddened, very painful, and edematous. Pulses may return but capillary refill remains sluggish.
- After 2 to 7 days: hyperemia is predominant, with regional skin temperature variation, edema, blisters, and ulceration.
- Posthyperemic phase: After 7 days: nature of the pain changes to "shooting or stabbing." Sensory deficits may diminish, but paresthesias continue; anesthesia may remain extensive and hyperhidrosis is often present.

Treatment

1. Keep the affected area dry and warm.
2. Initial treatment is similar to that for frostbite, with the exception that rapid rewarming (thawing) is not necessary.
3. As with frostbite, elevate the affected extremity.
4. Recovery during the "posthyperemic" phase may be hastened by physiotherapy.

Prevention

- Maintain body core temperature.
- Remain active; encourage blood flow to the feet.
- Make certain footgear fits properly and does not constrict.
- Keep feet dry, continually changing socks (up to 2 or 3 times per day in some situations).
- Limit sweat accumulation.
- Take special care if wearing "vapor barrier boots."
- Prophylactic treatment with silicone preparations has proven effective in clinical studies.

5

Heat Illness

DEFINITIONS

The term *heat illness* encompasses a spectrum of syndromes ranging from muscle cramps to heatstroke, which is a life-threatening emergency. Predisposing factors include the following:

- Environmental temperature exceeding 35°C (95°F) with humidity level greater than 80% and lack of air movement
- Dehydration (one indicator in the field is dark-colored urine)
- Obesity
- Poor physical fitness
- Cardiovascular disease
- Fever
- Hyperactivity
  - Seizures
  - Psychosis
  - Cocaine or amphetamine intoxication
- Muscular exertion
- Burns (including sunburn)
- Drugs
  - Anticholinergic agents (antihistamines, phenothiazines, antispasmodics)
  - β-Adrenergic blockers, angiotensin-converting enzyme (ACE) inhibitors, diuretics
  - Stimulants
  - α-Adrenergic agonists
- Extremes of age
- Fatigue or lack of sleep
- Excessive clothing
- Electrolyte abnormalities (e.g., hyponatremia, hypokalemia)
- Sweat gland disorders

DISORDERS

Heat Edema

Signs and Symptoms

Peripheral edema develops during the first few days in a hot environment in unacclimatized travelers.

Treatment

The edema is usually self-limited and does not require medical therapy. Diuretics should be avoided because the dehydration that may ensue predisposes a person to more serious heat illness syndromes.

"Prickly Heat" (Miliaria Rubra)
Signs and Symptoms
- Erythematous, papular, and pruritic rash caused by sweat gland obstruction
- In dry climates, the rash is confined to skin sufficiently occluded by clothing to produce local sweating

Treatment
1. Cool and dry affected skin.
2. Administer antihistamine (diphenhydramine, adult dose 25 to 50 mg q4-6h) to relieve itching.
3. Topical mild corticosteroid may be helpful to reduce irritation.
4. Desquamation of the affected epidermis and recovery of sweat gland function occurs in 7 to 10 days.

Heat Syncope
Signs and Symptoms
Syncope occurs after prolonged standing in a hot environment or after rapidly standing up from a lying or sitting position.

Treatment
1. Perform a full secondary assessment after the primary survey to assess for any trauma that may have occurred because of a fall.
2. Place the patient in the Trendelenburg position.
3. Cool the patient, and administer oral fluids when he or she is awake and alert. The body can absorb a carbohydrate-containing beverage, such as Gatorade, faster than plain water. The concentration of carbohydrates in such a beverage should not exceed 6%; otherwise, gastric emptying and fluid absorption by the intestines may be delayed. Responders should target an intake for the patient of 1 to 2 L (1.1 to 2.1 qt) over the first hour.
4. Patients with heat syncope usually recover rapidly with treatment. If the patient does not improve or worsens, he or she should be evaluated for heatstroke or other potential cause of syncope and transported to a hospital immediately.

Heat Cramps
Heat cramps result from fluid and electrolyte deficits and occur most often in persons who have not been fully acclimated to a combination of intense muscular activity and environmental heat. Individuals who are susceptible to heat cramps are often believed to be profuse sweaters who sustain large sweat sodium losses.

Signs and Symptoms
- Painful, spasmodic muscle cramps that usually occur in heavily exercised muscles

- Recurrent cramps that may be precipitated by manipulation of the muscle
- Onset during or after exercise

Treatment
1. Administer an oral fluid containing sodium chloride (see later). Avoid salt tablets.
2. The affected muscles often respond to passive stretching to "work out" the cramp.
3. Allow the patient to rest in a cool environment.
4. Ingesting pickle juice, magnesium supplements, wasabi, or HOTSHOT is recommended by some to be beneficial.

Heat Exhaustion
Signs and Symptoms
- Nonspecific symptoms (malaise, fatigue, dizziness, headache, weakness, nausea, anorexia)
- Vomiting
- Orthostatic hypotension
- Tachycardia
- Core body temperature is usually less than 38°C to 40°C (100.4°F to 104°F) and may be normal
- Sweating is present
- Normal mental status and normal findings on neurologic examination

Treatment
1. Stop all exertion, and move the patient to a cool and shaded environment.
2. Remove restrictive clothing.
3. Administer oral fluids (see Heat Cramps, earlier). In severely dehydrated individuals, administer intravenous rehydration.
4. Cool the patient by placing ice or cold packs on the neck, chest wall, axillae, and groin. Do not place ice directly against skin, to avoid frostbite injury. Fanning the patient, while spraying with tepid water, is also an effective cooling method.
5. In general, patients recover rapidly, and hospitalization is not necessary.

Heatstroke
Although classic and exertional heatstrokes differ in certain characteristics, the field treatment approach is the same. Environmental heatstroke can be regarded as the end stage of heat exhaustion when compensatory mechanisms for dissipating heat have failed. There is usually a history of exposure to hot and humid weather or vigorous physical activity. The transition from heat exhaustion to heatstroke is often recognized when a patient begins to show abnormal mental status and neurologic function. Mental status changes in an individual who is performing exertion in the heat should be the defining characteristic of heatstroke. Sweating is still

likely to be present in the early stages of heatstroke. Heatstroke is a true medical emergency; if not promptly and effectively treated, morbidity and mortality are high. This necessitates immediate cooling measures.

Signs and Symptoms
- Elevated core body temperature, usually above 40°C (104°F)
- Altered neurologic state (confusion, combativeness, disorientation, bizarre behavior, ataxia, seizures, coma). Loss of coordination is one of the earliest manifestations.
- Tachycardia
- Hypotension
- Tachypnea
- Sweating may be present or absent.

Treatment
1. Cool the patient rapidly. Prognosis is a function of the magnitude and duration of hyperthermia. The faster cooling is accomplished, the lower the morbidity and mortality.
   a. Place the patient in the shade and remove restrictive clothing.
   b. Place ice or cold packs on the neck, axillae, chest wall, and groin. Take care to avoid creating a frostbite injury.
   c. Wet the patient with tepid (not cold) water, then fan rapidly to facilitate evaporative cooling.
   d. Wrap the patient in cold wet sheets. Be sure to cover the head and soak the sheets every few minutes to recool them.
   e. Immerse the patient in cold (ice) water if available. Provide constant hands-on supervision.
2. Protect the airway, and do not give anything by mouth because of the risk for vomiting and aspiration.
3. Administer fluid intravenously (1 to 2 L of normal saline solution as an initial bolus in adults and 20 to 40 mL/kg in children).
4. Treat seizures and combative behavior with a benzodiazepine (diazepam 0.1 to 0.3 mg/kg IV or IM adult dose; midazolam 0.2 mg/kg IV or IM adult dose).
5. Suppress shivering by administering a benzodiazepine (diazepam 5 to 10 mg IV adult dose) or chlorpromazine (25 to 50 mg IM or IV adult dose).
6. Evacuate the patient immediately to the nearest medical facility. Continue to cool the patient during transport until his or her core body temperature has fallen to 38°C to 39°C (100.4°F to 102.2°F).
7. Recheck the temperature at least every 30 minutes.
8. Do not give aspirin or any nonsteroidal antiinflammatory drug.
9. Do not use alcohol sponge baths.

Hyponatremia
Symptomatic hyponatremia is diagnosed when serum sodium level is less than 130 mEq/L and is generally caused by drinking

large volumes of water or markedly hypo-osmotic fluids. It may be difficult to differentiate in the field between heat illness and hyponatremia from water intoxication because of considerable overlap of symptoms. One hint is that, in heat illness, core body temperature is greater than 39°C (102.2°F), whereas in hyponatremia, core temperature is usually normal or close to normal. During an athletic event in which there will be marked sweating, it is useful to weigh the participants prior to the event. If they later present with altered mental status and have gained weight during the event, it is likely due to excessive water drinking without adequate electrolytes, and a clue that dilutional hyponatremia is present.

Signs and Symptoms
- Weakness
- Anorexia
- Vomiting
- Muscle cramps
- Altered neurologic state (lethargy, apathy, confusion, disorientation, agitation, psychosis, seizures, coma)

Treatment
1. If the patient is mentating normally and capable of safely consuming oral liquids, have him or her drink a full-strength sports beverage, such as Gatorade.
2. Administer 2 L of IV normal saline, initially at 500 to 1000 mL/h.
3. If severe dilutional hyponatremia is confirmed or strongly suspected, as an alternative to normal saline, administer hypertonic (3%) saline in 100 mL aliquots up to 3 times.

PREVENTION OF HEAT ILLNESS
The best indicator of environmental heat stress is the wet bulb globe temperature (WBGT). Although a regular thermometer measures the dry-air temperature, a wet bulb thermometer (WBT) measures the effect of humidity as well as temperature. The standard dry bulb thermometer temperature by itself is a poor predictor of heat stress because humidity is such an important factor in heat dissipation accomplished by sweating. Because the WBGT is complex and 70% of the value is derived from the WBT, a simple alternative in the field is to use a sling psychrometer. This instrument has a thermometer with a wick surrounding the bulb attached to an aluminum frame with a hinged handle. After the wick is moistened, the psychrometer is slung over the head for approximately 2 minutes. Air passing over the wetted thermometer bulb cools the bulb in inverse proportion to the humidity. The WBGT can be used as a guide for recommended activity levels (Table 5.1). These guidelines incorporate work intensity, environment, work-to-rest cycles, and fluid intake. These guidelines use WBGT to mark levels of environmental heat stress and emphasize both the need for sufficient fluid replacement during heat stress and concern for the dangers

Table 5.1 Wet Bulb Globe Temperature and Recommended Sports Activity Levels		
°C	°F	RECOMMENDATIONS
<10	<50	Low risk for hyperthermia but a possible risk for hyperthermia.
<18.3	<65	Low risk for heat illness.
18.3–22.8	65–73	Moderate risk toward the end of the workout. Maintain adequate hydration.
22.8–27.8	73–82	Those at high risk for heat injury should not continue to train. Everyone exercise in shorts and T-shirts. If unacclimatized, curtail exercise and avoid hiking, sports, and sun exposure.
27.8–28.9	82–84	Acclimatized exercise with caution; rest periods and water breaks every 20–30 min for everyone.
28.9–31.1	84–88	Unacclimatized: stop training; cancel outdoor exercise in heavy clothing. Acclimatized: exercise with extreme caution and constant observation.
31.1–32.2	88–90	Limited brief activity for acclimatized, fit persons only. Light clothing only.
>32.2	>90	Stop all training.

of overhydration. These recommendations specify an upper limit for hourly and daily water intake, which safeguards against over-drinking and water intoxication. The guidelines do not account for individual physiologic variability.

The National Academy of Medicine provides general guidance for composition of "sports beverages" for persons performing prolonged physical activity in hot weather. It recommends that fluid replacement beverages contain approximately 20 to 30 mEq/L sodium (chloride as the anion), approximately 2 to 5 mEq/L potassium, and approximately 6% carbohydrate. The sodium and potassium are used to help replace sweat electrolyte losses, while sodium also helps to stimulate thirst, and carbohydrate provides energy and facilitates intestinal absorption. These components can also be consumed using nonfluid sources such as gels, energy bars, and other foods. Drinks containing sodium, such as sports beverages, may be helpful, but many foods can supply the needed electrolytes. A little extra salt may be added to meals and recovery fluids when sweat sodium losses are high. Table 5.2 presents the electrolyte and carbohydrate contents of common sport drinks, tablets, and powdered additives that can be used to help replace electrolytes lost during activity or exercise.

PRODUCT	SERVING SIZE	CHO (G)	NA⁺ (MG)	K⁺ (MG)	CA²⁺ (MG)	MG²⁺ (MG)
CeraSport	8 fl oz (0.2 L)	5	200	100	0	0
Ensure	8 fl oz (0.2 L)	42	200	460	375	62.5
Elete Electrolyte Add-In	0.5 tsp (2.5 mL)	0	125	130	0	45
Elete Tablytes	1 tab	0	150	95	40	30
Gatorade (G2 Series)	8 fl oz (0.2 L)	14	110	30	0	0
Gatorade (Pro Series)	8 fl oz (0.2 L)	14	200	90	0	0
Lucozade Lite	8 fl oz (0.2 L)	5	0	0	92.5	0
Nutrilite	8 fl oz (0.2 L)	14	110	30	0	0
Pedialyte	8 fl oz (0.2 L)	6	253	192	25	2.5
Powerade	8 fl oz (0.2 L)	14	100	25	0	0
Powerade Zero	8 fl oz (0.2 L)	0	55	35	0	0
Vitaminwater Essential	8 fl oz (0.2 L)	13	0	70	50	0
Vitalyte	8 fl oz (0.2 L)	10	68	92	2.1	1.6

Table 5.2 Electrolyte and Carbohydrate Contents of Common Sport Drinks, Tablets, and Powdered Additives

CHO, Carbohydrate; NA^+, sodium; K^+, potassium; CA^{2+}, calcium; MG^{2+}, magnesium.

ACCLIMATIZATION

Physiologic acclimatization to a hot environment is an important adaptive response. It usually requires 8 to 14 days to reach maximum benefit and is facilitated by a minimum amount of daily exercise (90 min/day). During initial exposure to a hot environment, workouts should be moderate in intensity and duration. A gradual increase in the time and intensity of physical exertion over 8 to 14 days should allow for optimal acclimatization. As with physical conditioning, there are limits to the degree of protection that acclimatization provides from heat stress. Given a sufficiently hot and humid environment, no one is immune to heat injury. It is important to note that heat acclimatization is specific to the climate and activity level. If individuals will be working in a hot, humid climate, heat acclimatization should be conducted under similar conditions.

Once heat acclimatization is achieved, skin vasodilation and sweating are initiated at a lower core temperature threshold, and higher sweat rates can be sustained without the sweat glands becoming "fatigued." Although an unacclimatized individual secretes sweat with a sodium concentration of approximately 60 mEq/L (or higher), the concentration of secreted sodium from the sweat glands of an acclimatized individual is significantly lower, at approximately 5 mEq/L. Provided that fluids are not restricted during physical activities, heat-acclimated individuals will be better able to maintain hydration during exercise. Thirst is a poor indicator of adequate hydration because it is not stimulated until plasma osmolarity rises 1% to 2% above normal.

6

Wildland Fires

SENSIBLE LAND DEVELOPMENT PRACTICES TO PROTECT AGAINST WILDFIRE

- Create access to adequate water sources.
- Do not stack firewood next to houses.
- Do not pile slash (e.g., branches, stumps, logs, and other vegetative residues) on home sites or along access roads.
- Do not build structures on slopes with unenclosed stilt foundations.
- Remove trees and shrubs growing next to structures, under eaves, and among stilt foundations.
- Do not create roads that are steep, narrow, winding, unmapped, unsigned, unnamed, and bordered by slash or dense vegetation because these are prone to be difficult, if not impossible, for fire suppression vehicles to negotiate.
- Do not place a dwelling or group of dwellings in an area without at least two or more access roads for simultaneous ingress and egress.
- Do not create roads and bridges without the grade, design, and width to permit simultaneous evacuation by residents and access by firefighters and emergency medical personnel and their equipment.
- Do not place dwellings and other structures on excessive slopes, within continuous or heavy fuel situations, or in box canyons.
- Place constructed firebreaks and fuel breaks around home sites and within clusters of dwellings.
- Be certain to prune and thin landscape, or otherwise reduce living fuels, vegetation, and litter that readily contribute to spot fire development and fire intensity. Keep the grass cut and yard cleaned up.
- Do not construct homes with flammable building materials such as wooden shake shingles.
- Do not expose propane tanks to the external environment.
- Create a system that will allow delivery of water effectively before and during passage of a fire front in and around the structure.

URBAN VERSUS WILDLAND FIRES

1. Heat rises to upper stories. Toxic gases and smoke rise to the ceiling and work their way down to the victim. Smoke obscures exit routes and causes oxygen deprivation.
2. As the fire consumes oxygen, the ambient oxygen content drops. When the oxygen content drops to less than 8%, death by asphyxiation occurs.

3. Ambient air temperatures rise rapidly from even small fires.
4. Smoke, heat, and gases are more concentrated.
5. Smoke contains toxic compounds.

EARLY WARNING SIGNALS OR INDICATORS ASSOCIATED WITH EXTREME FIRE BEHAVIOR

Fuel
- Continuous fine fuels, especially fully cured (dead) grasses
- Large quantities of medium and heavy fuels (e.g., deep duff layers, dead-down logs)
- Abundance of bridge or ladder fuels in forest stands (e.g., branches, lichens, suspending needles, flaky or shaggy bark, small conifer trees, tall shrubs extending from the ground surface upward)
- Tight tree crown spacing in conifer forests
- Presence of numerous snags
- Significant amounts of dead material in elevated, shrubland fuel complexes
- Seasonal changes in vegetation (e.g., frost kill)
- Fire, meteorologic, or insect and disease impacts (e.g., preheated canopy or crown scorch; snow-, wind-, or ice-damaged stands; drought-stressed vegetation; or mountain pine beetle–killed stands)

Weather
- Extended dry spell
- Drought conditions
- High air temperatures
- Low relative humidity
- Moderately strong, sustained winds
- Unstable atmosphere (visual indicators include gusty winds, dust devils, good visibility, and smoke rising straight up)
- Towering cumulus clouds
- High, fast-moving clouds
- Battling or shifting winds
- Sudden calm
- Virga (a veil of rain beneath a cloud that does not reach the ground)

Topography
- Steep slopes
- South- and southwest-facing slopes in northern hemisphere
- North- and northeast-facing slopes in southern hemisphere
- Gaps or saddles
- Chutes, chimneys, and narrow or box canyons

Fire Behavior
- Many fires that start simultaneously
- Fire that smolders over a large area

- Rolling and burning pine cones, agaves, logs, hot rocks, and other debris igniting fuel downslope
- Frequent spot fires developing and coalescing
- Spot fires occurring ahead of the main fire early on
- Individual trees readily candling or torching out
- Fire whirls that cause spot fires and contribute to erratic burning
- Vigorous surface burning with flame lengths starting to exceed 1 to 2 m (3.3 to 6.6 ft)
- Sizable areas of trees or shrubs that begin to readily burn as a "wall of flame"
- Black or dark, massive smoke columns with rolling, boiling vertical development
- Lateral movement of fire near the base of a steep slope

CONDITIONS THAT PRODUCE A CROWN FIRE
- Dry fuel
- Low humidity and high temperatures
- Heavy accumulations of dead and downed fuels
- Small trees in the understory, or "ladder fuels"
- Steep slope
- Strong winds
- Unstable atmosphere
- Continuous crown layer

TEN STANDARD FIREFIGHTING ORDERS
1. Keep informed of fire weather conditions, changes, and forecasts and how they may affect the area where you are located.
2. Know what the fire is doing at all times through personal observations, communication systems, or scouts.
3. Base all actions on current and expected behavior of the fire.
4. Determine escape routes and plans for everyone at risk, and make certain that everyone understands routes and plans.
5. Post lookouts to watch the fire if you think there is any danger of being trapped, of increased fire activity, or of erratic fire behavior.
6. Be alert, keep calm, think clearly, and act decisively to avoid panic reactions.
7. Maintain prompt and clear communication with your group, firefighting forces, and command and communication centers.
8. Give clear, concise instructions, and be sure that they are understood.
9. Maintain control of the people in your group at all times.
10. Fight the fire aggressively, but provide for safety first.

"WATCH OUT!" SITUATIONS IN THE WILDLAND FIRE ENVIRONMENT
- You are moving downhill toward a fire but must be aware that fire can move swiftly and suddenly uphill. Constantly observe

fire behavior, fuels, and escape routes, assessing the fire's potential to run uphill.

- You are on a hillside where rolling, burning material can ignite fuel from below. When below a fire, watch for burning materials, especially cones and logs, that can roll downhill and ignite a fire beneath you, trapping you between two coalescing fires.
- Wind begins to blow, increase, or change direction. Wind strongly influences fire behavior, so be prepared to respond to sudden changes.
- The weather becomes hotter and drier. Fire activity increases, and its behavior changes more rapidly as ambient temperature rises and relative humidity decreases.
- Dense vegetation with unburned fuel between you and the fire. The danger in this situation is that unburned fuels can ignite. If the fire is moving away from you, be alert for wind changes or spot fires that may ignite fuels near you. Do not be over-confident if the area has burned once, because it can reignite if sufficient fuel remains.
- You are in an unburned area near the fire where terrain and cover make travel difficult. The combination of fuel and difficult escape makes this dangerous.
- You are traveling or working in an area you have not seen in daylight. Darkness and unfamiliarity create a dangerous combination.
- You are unfamiliar with local factors influencing fire behavior. When possible, seek information on what to expect from knowledgeable people, especially those from the area.
- By necessity, you must make a frontal assault on a fire with tankers. Any encounter with an active line of fire is dangerous because of proximity to intense heat, smoke, and flames, along with limited escape opportunities.
- Spot fires occur frequently across the fire line. In general, increased spotting indicates increased fire activity and intensity. The danger is that of entrapment between coalescing fires.
- The main fire cannot be seen, and you are not in communication with anyone who can see it. If you do not know the location, size, and behavior of the main fire, planning becomes difficult.
- An unclear assignment or confusing instructions have been received. Make sure that all assignments and instructions are fully understood.
- You are drowsy and feel like resting or sleeping near the fire line in unburned fuel. This may lead to fire entrapment. No one should sleep near a wildland fire. If resting is necessary, choose a burned area that is safe from rolling material, smoke, reburn, and other dangers or seek a wide area of bare ground or rock.
- Fire has not been scouted and sized up.
- Safety zones and escape routes have not been identified.
- You are uninformed on strategy, tactics, and hazards.

- No communication link with crew members or supervisor has been established.
- A line has been constructed without a safe anchor point.

WILDLAND-URBAN "WATCH OUT!" SITUATIONS

- Access is poor (e.g., narrow roads, twisting and single-lane routes).
- Local bridges are narrow and/or have light or unknown load limits.
- Winds are strong, and erratic fire behavior is occurring.
- The area contains garages with closed, locked doors.
- The water supply is inadequate to attack the fire.
- Structure windows are black or smoked over.
- There are septic tanks and leach lines.
- A structure is burning with puffing rather than steady smoke.
- Construction of structures includes wood, with shake shingle roofs.
- Natural fuels occur within 9 m (29.5 ft) of the structures.
- Known or suspected panicked individuals are in the vicinity.
- Structure windows are bulging, and the roof has not been vented.
- Additional fuels can be found in open crawl spaces beneath the structures.
- Firefighting is taking place in or near chimney or canyon situations.
- Elevated fuel or propane tanks are present.

VEHICLE BEHAVIOR IN A FIRE SITUATION

- The engine may stall and not restart.
- The vehicle may be rocked by convection currents.
- Smoke and sparks may enter the cab.
- The interior, engine, or tires may ignite.
- Temperatures increase inside the cab because heat is radiated through the windows.
- Metal gas tanks and containers rarely explode.
- If it is necessary to leave the cab after the fire has passed, keep the vehicle between you and the fire.
- If smoke obstructs visibility, turn on the headlights and drive to the side of the road away from the leading edge of the fire. Try to select an area of sparse vegetation offering the least combustible material.
- Attempt to shield your body from radiant heat energy by rolling up the windows and covering up with floor mats or hiding beneath the dashboard. Cover as much skin as possible.
- Stay in the vehicle if possible. Unruptured gas tanks rarely explode, and vehicles usually take several minutes to ignite.
- Grass fires create about 30 seconds (maximum) of flame exposure, and chances for survival in a vehicle are good. Forest fires create higher-intensity flames lasting 3 to 4 minutes (maximum) and lowering changes for survival. Staying in a vehicle improves chances for surviving a forest fire. Remain calm.

- A strong, acrid smell usually results from burning paint and plastic materials, caused by small quantities of hydrogen chloride released from breakdown of polyvinyl chloride. Hydrogen chloride is water soluble, and discomfort can be relieved by breathing through a damp cloth. Urine is mostly water and can be used in emergencies.

GUIDANCE FOR PEOPLE IN A VEHICLE DURING A WILDLAND FIRE
Advance Preparation
1. Always carry woolen blankets, leather gloves, and a supply of water in the vehicle.
2. Dress in nonsynthetic clothing and shoes, including a hat.

Encountering Smoke or Flames
1. If you see a wildland fire in the distance, carefully pull over to the side of the road to assess the situation. If it is safe to do so, turn around and drive to safety.
2. If you have been trapped by a wildland fire, find a suitable place to park the car and take shelter from the fire.

Positioning Your Car
1. Find a clearing away from dense brush and high ground-fuel loads.
2. Minimize exposure to radiant heat by parking behind a natural barrier, such as a rocky outcrop.
3. Position the car facing toward the oncoming fire front.
4. Park the car off the roadway to avoid collisions in poor visibility.
5. Do not park close to other vehicles.

Inside Your Car
1. Stay inside your car because it offers the best level of protection from radiant heat as the fire front passes.
2. Turn headlights and hazard warning lights on to make the car as visible as possible.
3. Tightly close all windows and doors.
4. Shut all the air vents, and turn off the air conditioning.
5. Turn off the engine.
6. Get down below the window level into the foot wells, and shelter under woolen blankets.
7. Drink water to minimize the risk for dehydration.

As the Fire Front Passes
1. Stay in the care until the fire front passes and the temperature outside the car has dropped.
2. Fuel tanks are unlikely to explode.
3. As the fire front approaches, the intensity of the heat will increase, along with the amount of smoke and embers.

4. Smoke will gradually enter the car, and fumes will be released from the interior of the car. Stay as close to the floor as possible to minimize inhalation, and cover the mouth with a moist cloth.
5. Tires and external plastic parts may catch on fire. The car interior may catch on fire.
6. Once the fire front has passed and the temperature has dropped, cautiously exit the car.
7. Move to a safe area, such as a strip of land that has already burned.
8. Stay covered in woolen blankets, continue to drink water, and await assistance.

GUIDANCE FOR PEOPLE IN A BUILDING DURING A WILDLAND FIRE

The decision to evacuate a building or remain and defend is not an easy one. Several principles should guide the evacuation decision:

- A fire within sight or smell is a fire that endangers you.
- More unattended houses burn down.
- Evacuation when fire is close is too late; evacuation must be done well before danger is apparent.
- More people are injured and killed in the open than in houses.
- Learn beforehand about community refuges.
- Evacuate only to a known safe refuge.

Before fire approaches a dwelling, take the following precautions:

1. If you plan to stay, evacuate your pets and livestock and all family members not essential to protecting the home well in advance of the fire's arrival.
2. Be properly dressed to survive the fire. Wear long pants and boots, and carry for protection a long-sleeved shirt or jacket made of cotton fabrics or wool. Synthetics should not be worn because they can ignite and melt. Wear a hat that can offer protection against radiation to the face, ears, and neck areas. Wear leather or natural-fiber gloves, and have a handkerchief handy to shield the face, water to wet it, and safety goggles.
3. Remove combustible items from around the house, including lawn and poolside furniture, umbrellas, and tarp coverings. If they catch fire, the added heat could ignite the house.
4. Ensure that anything that might be tossed around by strong fire-induced winds is secured.
5. Ensure that the areas around any external propane tanks are fuel free for a considerable distance. Direct the pressure relief valve away from buildings and access ways.
6. Close outside attic, eave, and basement vents to eliminate the possibility of sparks blowing into hidden areas within the house. Close window shutters.
7. Place large plastic trash cans or buckets around the outside of the house, and fill them with water. Soak burlap sacks,

small rugs, and large rags to use in beating out burning embers or small fires. Inside the house, fill bathtubs, sinks, and other containers with water. Toilet tanks and water heaters are important water reservoirs.

8. Place garden hoses so that they will reach any place on the house. Use the spray gun type of nozzle, adjusted to spray. Avoid laying the hose over combustible objects.

9. If you have portable gasoline-powered pumps to take water from a swimming pool or tank, make sure they are operating and in place.

10. Place a ladder against the roof of the house opposite the side of the approaching fire. If you have a combustible roof, wet it down or turn on any roof sprinklers. Turn on any special fire sprinklers installed to add protection. Do not waste water. Waste can drain the entire water system quickly. Divert water from gutters back into the firefighting supply.

11. Back your car into the garage and roll up the car windows. Disconnect the automatic garage door opener (otherwise, in case of power failure, you cannot remove the car). Close all garage doors and seal them with wet rags.

12. Place valuable papers and mementos inside the car in the garage for quick departure, if necessary. In addition, place all pets in the car.

13. Close windows and doors to the house to prevent sparks from blowing inside. Close all doors inside the house to prevent drafts. Open the damper on any fireplace to help stabilize outside-inside pressure, but close the fireplace screen so that sparks will not ignite the room. Turn on a light in each room to make the house more visible in heavy smoke. Have flashlights handy.

14. Turn off the main gas supply to stoves and furnaces.

15. If you have time, take down drapes and curtains. Close all Venetian blinds or noncombustible window coverings to reduce the amount of heat radiating into the house. This provides added safety in case the windows give way because of heat or wind.

16. As the fire approaches, go inside the house. Stay calm; you are in control of your immediate environment. Wear goggles to protect your eyes from smoke. Move around continually to check the house. Avoid areas with a single way to exit.

17. After the fire passes, check the roof immediately. Extinguish any sparks or embers. Then check the attic for hidden burning sparks. If you have a fire, enlist your neighbors to help fight it. For several hours after the fire, recheck for smoke and sparks throughout the house.

IF YOU CANNOT ESCAPE AN APPROACHING WILDFIRE

1. Select an area that will not burn—the bigger the better or, failing that, an area with the least amount of combustible material, and

one that offers the best microclimate (e.g., depression in the ground).

2. Use every means possible (e.g., boulders, rock outcrops, large downed logs, trees, snags) to protect yourself from radiant and convective heat emitted by the flames.
3. Protect your airway from heat at all costs, and try to minimize smoke exposure.
4. Try to remain as calm as possible.
5. If you are caught out in the open and are likely to be entrapped or burned over by a wildfire and not able to take refuge in a vehicle, building, or fire shelter:
   a. Retreat from the fire, and reach a safe haven.
   b. Burn out a safety area.
   c. Hunker in place.
   d. Pass through the fire edge into the burned-out area.

SURVIVING A WILDLAND FIRE ENTRAPMENT OR BURNOVER

When entrapment or burnover by a wildland fire appears imminent, injuries or death may be avoided by following these basic emergency survival principles and procedures:

1. *Acknowledge the stress you are feeling.* Most people are afraid when trapped by fire. Accept this fear as natural so that clear thinking and intelligent decisions are possible. If fear overwhelms you, judgment is seriously impaired and survival becomes more a matter of chance than of good decision making.
2. *Protect yourself against radiation at all costs.* Many victims of forest fires die before the flames reach them. Radiant heat quickly causes heatstroke. Find shielding to reduce heat rays quickly in an area that will not burn, such as a shallow trench, crevice, large rock, running stream, large pond, vehicle, building, or the shore water of a lake. Do not seek refuge in an elevated water tank. Avoid wells and caves because oxygen may be used up quickly in these restricted places; consider them a last resort. To protect against radiation, cover the head and other exposed skin with clothing or dirt.
3. *Regulate your breathing.* Avoid inhaling dense smoke (which can impair both your judgment and eyesight). Keep your face near the ground, where there is usually less smoke. Hold a dampened handkerchief over the nose. Match your breathing with the availability of relatively fresh air. If there is a possibility of breathing superheated air, place a dry, not moist, cloth over the mouth. The lungs can withstand dry heat better than moist heat.
4. *Do not run blindly or needlessly.* Unless a clear path of escape is indicated, do not run. Move downhill and away from the flank of the fire at a 45-degree angle, where possible. Conserve your strength. If you become exhausted, you are much more prone to heatstroke and may easily overlook a place of safe refuge.

5. *Burn out fuels to create a safety zone if possible.* If you are in dead grass or low shrub fuels and the approaching flames are too high to run through, burn out as large an area as possible between you and the fire edge. Step into the burned area and cover as much of your exposed skin as possible. This requires time for fuels to be consumed and may not be effective as a last-ditch effort, nor does this work well in an intense forest fire.

6. *Lie prone on the ground.* In a critical situation, lie face down in an area that will not burn. Your chance of survival if the fire overtakes you is greater in this position than standing upright or kneeling.

7. *Enter the burned area whenever and wherever possible.* Particularly in grass, low shrubs, or other low fuels, do not delay if escape means passing through the flame front into the burned area. Move aggressively and parallel to the advancing fire front. Choose a place on the fire's edge where the flames are less than 1 m (3.3 ft) deep and can be seen through clearly, and where the fuel supply behind the fire has been mostly consumed. Cover exposed skin and take several breaths, then move through the flame front as quickly as possible. If necessary, drop to the ground under the smoke for improved visibility and to obtain fresh air.

PERSONAL GEAR FOR A RESCUE MISSION ON A WILDLAND FIRE INCIDENT

- Boots (leather, high top, lace up, nonslip soles, extra leather laces)
- Socks (cotton or wool, at least two pairs)
- Pants (natural fiber, flameproof, loose fitting, hems lower than boot tops)
- Belt or suspenders
- Shirt (natural fiber, flameproof, loose fitting, long sleeves)
- Gloves (natural fiber or leather, extra pair)
- Hat (hard hat and possibly a bandana, stocking cap, or felt hat)
- Jacket
- Handkerchiefs or scarves
- Goggles
- Sleeping bag and ground cover
- Map
- Protective fire shelter
- Food
- Canteen
- Radio (AM radio will receive better in rough terrain; FM is more line of sight; emergency personnel should have a two-way radio)
- Bolt cutters (carried in vehicles to get through locked gates during escape from flare-ups or in the rescue of trapped people)
- Miscellaneous items (mess kit, compass, flashlight, extra batteries, toilet paper, pencil, notepaper, flagging tape, flares, matches

[windproof], can opener, washcloth, toiletries, insect repellent, plastic bags, knife, first-aid kit, and lip balm)

HOW TO REPORT A WILDLAND FIRE TO LOCAL AUTHORITIES

A caller should be prepared to provide the following information when reporting a fire:

- Name of person giving the report
- Where the person can be reached immediately
- Where the person was at the time the fire was discovered
- Location of the fire; orient the fire to prominent landmarks such as roads, creeks, and mileposts on the highways
- Description of the fire: color and volume of the smoke, estimated size, and flame characteristics if visible
- Whether anyone is fighting the fire at the time of the call

PORTABLE FIRE EXTINGUISHERS

Extinguishers are chosen based on the three major classes of fires:

Class A fires: fueled by ordinary combustible materials such as wood, paper, cloth, upholstery, and many plastics—use water, dry chemical, or liquefied gas extinguishers

Class B fires: fueled by flammable liquids and gases such as kitchen greases, paints, oil, and gasoline—use carbon dioxide or dry chemical extinguishers

Class C fires: fueled by live electrical wires or equipment such as motors, power tools, and appliances—use dry chemical or liquefied gas extinguishers

7 | Burns and Smoke Inhalation

Thermal burns are classified into minor, moderate, and major, largely based upon burn depth and size in proportion to the patient's total body surface area (TBSA). Burn size can be calculated by the "rule of nines." Each upper extremity accounts for 9% TBSA, each lower extremity accounts for 18%, the anterior and posterior trunk each account for 18%, the head and neck account for 9%, and the perineum accounts for 1% (Fig. 7.1). Children less than 4 years old have larger heads and smaller thighs in proportion to body size than do adults. In an infant, the head accounts for approximately 18% of the TBSA; body proportions do not fully reach adult percentages until adolescence. For smaller burns, an accurate assessment of burn size can be made by using the patient's hand. The entire palmar surface of the hand, fingers included, represents 1% TBSA. Reassessment of burn size and depth is important, particularly early in the management of burn patients, because the extent of injury may not be initially apparent.

TYPES OF BURNS
Scald Burns
Scalds, usually resulting from hot water, are the most common cause of burns. Water at 60°C (140°F) creates a deep partial-thickness or full-thickness burn in 3 seconds. At 68.9°C (156°F), the same burn occurs in 1 second. Boiling water usually causes deep burns, and soups and sauces, which are thicker in consistency, remain in contact longer with the skin and often cause very deep burns. In general, exposed areas tend to be burned less deeply than areas covered with thin clothing. Clothing retains the heat and keeps the liquid in contact with the skin longer. Scald burns from grease or hot oil are generally deep partial thickness or full thickness. Cooking oil and grease, when hot enough to use for cooking, may be as hot as 204.4°C (400°F).

Flame Burns
Flame burns in an outdoor setting may occur from wildland fires, using cooking stoves fueled by white gasoline, taking lanterns into tents, smoking in sleeping bags, and starting or improving campfires with gasoline or kerosene. Most accelerants, whether gasoline, kerosene, propane, or diesel, behave similarly with ignition temperatures of 210°C to 280°C (410°F to 536°F) and therefore burn at a high temperature with rapid tissue injury and full-thickness burns.

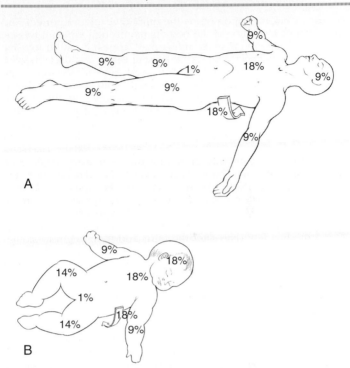

FIGURE 7.1 Rule of nines used for estimating burned body surface. **A,** Adult. **B,** Infant.

Flash Burns

Explosions from natural gas, propane, gasoline, and other flammable liquids cause intense heat for a very brief time. Flash burns generally have a distribution over all exposed skin, while unignited clothing tends to protect the skin. Flash burns are usually partial thickness but may be associated with significant thermal damage to the upper airway.

Contact Burns

In the wilderness setting, the most common contact burn is from hot coals, which are often as hot as 538°C (1000°F). Even though the injured areas may be small, they can be deep and devastating when the hiker must walk a considerable distance on burned feet.

Electrical Burns

Electrical burns are thermal burns from very high intensity heat. As electricity meets the resistance of body tissues, it is converted to heat in direct proportion to the amperage of the current and the electrical resistance of the body parts through which it passes. Although cutaneous manifestations may appear limited, massive underlying tissue necrosis may be present because muscle, nerves, blood vessels, and bones can be burned beyond recovery. The intense muscle contractions associated with electrical burns may cause traumatic injuries, such as fractures of the lumbar vertebrae, humerus, or femur or dislocation of the shoulders or hips.

Chemical Burns

Chemical burns are usually caused by strong acids or alkalis and, in contrast to thermal burns, cause progressive damage until the chemicals are inactivated by reaction with the tissue or by dilution using copious irrigation with water. A full-thickness chemical burn may appear deceptively superficial, appearing as only a mild brownish surface discoloration. The skin may appear intact during the first few days after the burn and then begin to slough spontaneously. Chemical burns, especially alkali burns, should be considered deep partial thickness or full thickness until proved otherwise.

GENERAL TREATMENT

1. Remove the patient from the source of the burn.
   a. If clothing is on fire, roll the patient on the ground or wrap him or her in a blanket to extinguish the flames.
   b. Any hot or burned clothing, jewelry, and obvious debris should immediately be removed to prevent further injury and enable accurate assessment of the extent of burns.
   c. If the burn is chemical, use large amounts of water (minimum 10 minutes of active rinsing) to wash off the agent(s). Do not apply a specific neutralizing agent (e.g., alkali to neutralize acid), which may generate heat and worsen the injury.
   d. If the burn is from hydrofluoric acid, first copiously irrigate the burn with water, then apply topical calcium gluconate gel as 3.5 g of 2.5% calcium gluconate mixed with 5 oz of water-soluble lubricant, 4 to 6 times a day for 3 to 4 days.
   e. If the eyes are involved, copiously irrigate them with the cleanest available water.
   f. Because phosphorus ignites on contact with air, keep any phosphorus still in contact with the patient's skin covered with water. Embedded particles of phosphorus can be located by using ultraviolet light, which causes phosphorescence.
2. Perform a primary and secondary survey. Evaluate the airway for smoke inhalation. If present, administer oxygen by face mask, 5 to 10 L/min, and transport the patient to a medical facility (see Smoke Inhalation and Thermal Airway Injury, later). Be alert for vomiting into the face mask.
3. Treat burns by rapidly applying cool water (1°C to 5°C [33.8°F to 41°F]) for about 30 minutes. Local cooling of less than 10%

of TBSA can be continued longer than 30 minutes to relieve pain; however, prolonged cooling of a larger TBSA burn may cause hypothermia and macerate skin. Cooling has no therapeutic benefit, other than pain control, if delayed more than 30 minutes after the burn injury.

4. Remove any jewelry from burned areas, fingers, and toes to avoid difficult removal later and tourniquet effect.
5. Update tetanus immunization as soon as possible.
6. Immediate evacuation to a burn center should be arranged when injuries meet the criteria for major burns (see later).

BURN CLASSIFICATION

Burns are classified by increasing depth as first degree, superficial partial thickness, deep partial thickness, full thickness, and fourth degree. Many burns, however, have a mixture of characteristics that give the rescuer an imprecise diagnostic ability. Treatment recommendations are based on the estimation of burn depth and size.

Superficial Burn (First-Degree Burn)
Signs and Symptoms
- Only involves the epidermis
- Erythema and pain without blisters
- Prototype: mild sunburn
- When over a large surface area: fever, weakness, chills, vomiting

Treatment
1. Immediately cool the burn with cold water or wet compresses. Do not use ice directly on skin.
2. Apply aloe vera gel or lotion in concentrations of at least 60% topically to the burn. Aloe vera has antimicrobial properties and is an effective analgesic.
3. Administer ibuprofen, aspirin, or another nonsteroidal antiinflammatory drug. An adult dose is ibuprofen 800 mg q8h for 48 hours.
4. Erythema and pain should subside over 2 to 3 days. By day 4, injured epithelium desquamates ("peels").

Superficial Partial-Thickness Burn (Second-Degree Burn)
Signs and Symptoms
- It involves the upper layer of dermis and creates clear fluid-filled blisters.
- Blisters may not appear until several hours after injury.
- When blisters are removed, the skin is moist and erythematous, blanches with pressure, and is hypersensitive to touch.
- If infection is prevented, the burn heals spontaneously within 3 weeks without functional impairment.

Deep Partial-Thickness Burn (Second-Degree Burn)
Signs and Symptoms
- Damage to hair follicles and sweat glands.
- Blisters form, but the wound surface is usually mottled pink and white immediately after injury or may be dry with a cherry-red appearance. By the second day, the wound may be white and is dry.
- Wound is possibly less sensitive to touch than surrounding normal skin. The patient complains of discomfort rather than pain.
- When pressure is applied to the burn, capillary refill returns slowly or is absent.
- If infection is prevented, the burn heals in 3 to 9 weeks with scar formation. Physical therapy should be continued throughout the healing period to avoid motion impairment and hypertrophic scarring.

Treatment
1. Irrigate gently with cool water or saline solution to remove all loose dirt and loose, devitalized skin. Wash the burn gently with plain soap and water, and gently dry with a clean towel. Wash water should be suitable for drinking (e.g., disinfected) but does not need to be sterile or bottled.
2. Peel off or trim any necrotic skin with sharp debridement.
3. Drain large (>2.5 cm [1 inch]), thin, fluid-filled blisters, and trim the dead skin if a sterile dressing can be applied.
4. Leave small, thick blisters intact.
5. Apply a topical chemotherapeutic agent to the wound. Commonly used topical agents include bacitracin, Neosporin, Polysporin, and double- or triple-antibiotic ointment. Silver sulfadiazine is a widely used agent because it is soothing to the wound, has a good antimicrobial spectrum, and has almost no systemic absorption or toxicity. The patient should be questioned about allergy to sulfa drugs before their use, because allergic reactions are encountered in about 3% of patients. If a commercial agent is not available, honey can also be used. Topical butter for burns is not recommended.
6. Cover the burn with a nonadherent dressing such as Telfa or Adaptic, and change the dressing at least once per day. Other dressings (hydrogels, silver-coated dressings, silicone gel sheets, calcium alginate) designed to minimize the frequency of dressing changes and promote healing are available but are not necessary and are more expensive. No dressing has been shown conclusively to accelerate the healing of burn wounds. The dressing should cover the entire burned area, leaving no burned skin exposed to air, and should not limit the patient's ability to actively flex and extend all burned extremities and digits. In the absence of a burn dressing, use fine gauze impregnated with antiseptic ointment, or a covering of clean, white cotton.

Cover all burned skin. Avoid dependent positioning of the burned body part.

7. Change dressings daily. Remove all exudates and crusts. Keep the wound moist, but do not allow unburned skin to become macerated. Once the healing burn shows epithelialization, it may benefit from the application of moisturizing lotion. Other topical substances that may be used include aloe (at least 60%), vitamin E, oat beta glucan, Aquaphor, Vaseline, A+D ointment, or melaleuca. Superficial partial-thickness burns may benefit from dressings that contain elemental silver.

8. Promote early motion, particularly of joints, during healing to prevent contractures and lessen hypertrophic scar formation.

9. Patients with burns that involve less than 10% TBSA generally do not require fluid resuscitation. They should stay well hydrated but should not be encouraged to force fluids. Patients with burns that involve 10% to 20% TBSA usually do not require intravenous (IV) fluid resuscitation. They should be encouraged to drink fluids that contain electrolytes. Hydration status in these patients should be monitored by ensuring that the oral mucous membranes are moist and that urine output is normal (at least 1 mL/kg/h) with light-colored urine.

10. Patients with burns that involve more than 20% TBSA should receive IV fluid resuscitation with crystalloid solution (normal saline or lactated Ringer's solution) until they reach a medical facility. Because of the high incidence of septic thrombophlebitis, lower extremities should be avoided as IV portals. Upper extremities are preferable, even if the IV line must pass through burned skin.

    a. Administer 4 mL/kg per % TBSA per 24 hours. Half the calculated 24-hour fluid total is given over the first 8 hours from the time the burn occurred (not the time the IV line was established). The second half is infused over the remaining 16 hours. The rate should be adjusted to support the patient's vital signs and maintain a urine output of at least 1 mL/kg per hour.

    b. Intraosseous infusion of fluids is useful when there is difficulty achieving a percutaneous IV line.

11. Avoid hypothermia in the patient by placing a clean sheet under the person and then covering with another clean sheet, followed by clean blankets.

12. Antibiotics should be administered only if the burn becomes infected.

    a. Infection is manifested by pus, foul odor, cloudy blisters, increased redness and swelling in the normal skin around the burn, and fever greater than 38.3°C (101°F).

    b. If an antibiotic is necessary, give dicloxacillin (adult dose 500 mg PO q6h) or cephalexin (adult dose 500 mg PO q6h).

13. Partial thickness burns can be excruciatingly painful. Administer pain medication such as hydrocodone/acetaminophen 5/325

(adult dose is 1 to 2 tablets PO q4–6 h prn) or oxycodone/acetaminophen 7.5/325 (adult dose is 1 to 2 tablets PO q6h prn).

Full-Thickness Burn (Third-Degree Burn)
Signs and Symptoms
- Involves all layers of the dermis and can heal only by wound contracture, epithelialization from the wound margin, or skin grafting.
- Leathery, firm, depressed when compared with adjoining normal skin, and insensitive to light touch or pinprick.
- Rarely blanches with pressure; may have a dry, white ("waxy") appearance with or without small clotted blood vessels that appear as purple or maroon lines under the surface. An immersion scald may have a red appearance, but it does not blanch with pressure.
- Can be difficult to differentiate from a deep partial-thickness burn.
- Develops classic burn eschar that separates from underlying viable tissue.

Treatment
See Treatment section under Fourth-Degree Burn.

Fourth-Degree Burn
Signs and Symptoms
- Deep injuries that extend through the skin into underlying tissues such as fascia, muscle, and/or bone.
- Almost always has a charred appearance.

Treatment
1. Follow the same instructions as for second-degree burn.
2. Immediate evacuation to a burn center is recommended.
3. Field considerations for fourth-degree burns are the same as for full-thickness burns.
4. Escharotomy of the neck or chest may be required if mechanical constriction from eschar prevents adequate respiration. Decompressive escharotomy of an extremity may be required for circumferential full-thickness burns if edema causes constriction and distal ischemia. Even in the wilderness, escharotomy should be performed if respiration is impaired or there is compromised distal perfusion. Escharotomy does not require an anesthetic. The burned area should be rinsed well and cleansed with soap and water. A scalpel is used to perform an incision through the eschar into the subcutaneous tissue. Ideally only the eschar is incised because subcutaneous fat is often viable and can cause bleeding. A "give" is felt as the scalpel passes through the eschar and into the fat. After the long initial incision is made, a short, push-type maneuver is performed by laying the belly of the scalpel blade along the entire length of the incision to ensure

that all constricting tissue has been freed. A popping open of the incision occurs as the scalpel moves from one end of the incision to the other. For extremity escharotomy, the first incision is made along the lateral aspect of the extremity. The extremity should soften, and any signs or symptoms of ischemia should resolve within a few minutes. If this does not occur, a second incision should be made along the medial aspect of the extremity. On completion of the procedure, a moist dressing such as antibiotic/antiseptic cream or ointment should be applied. A compression wrap and elevation of the extremity after the procedure will assist in maintaining hemostasis.

DISPOSITION

1. A burn less than 10% TBSA in adults and less than 5% in young or old (<10 or >50 years old) can be treated in a wilderness setting if adequate first-aid supplies are available and wound care is performed diligently. Exclusions are deep burns of the face, hands, feet, perineum, or circumferential burn of an extremity.
2. Patients with moderate burns should be admitted to a hospital. Moderate burns are defined as any of the following:
   a. In adults, 10% to 20% TBSA
   b. In young or old, 5% to 10% TBSA burn
   c. Full-thickness burn of 2% to 5% TBSA
   d. High-voltage injury
   e. Suspected inhalation injury
   f. Circumferential burn
   g. Patient with medical problems predisposing to infection (e.g., diabetes, sickle cell disease, immunosuppression)
3. A major burn patient should be evacuated immediately to a burn center. A major burn is defined as any of the following:
   a. Greater than 20% TBSA burn in adults
   b. Greater than 10% TBSA in young or old
   c. Greater than 5% TBSA full-thickness burn
   d. High voltage burn
   e. Known inhalation injury
   f. Any significant burn to face, eyes, ears, genitalia, or joints
   g. Significant associated injuries (fracture or other major trauma)

CARBON MONOXIDE POISONING

Carbon monoxide is a colorless, odorless, and tasteless gas that has an affinity for hemoglobin 200 times greater than that of oxygen. Carbon monoxide poisoning is a serious complication of burns and inhalation injuries because it displaces oxygen and limits the oxygen-carrying capacity of blood.

Signs and Symptoms

- If resulting from a fire: dyspnea, burns of the mouth and nose, singed nasal hairs, sooty (from smoke) sputum, harsh cough
- Headache, nausea, vomiting, tachypnea, dizziness, loss of manual dexterity

- Sometimes subtle perception and memory abnormalities or frank confusion and lethargy
- Unconsciousness leading to coma
- Possible cardiac arrest
- Late complications (after first 48 hours): personality disorders, chronic headaches, seizures, Parkinson's disease (generally after 2 to 40 days)

Treatment
1. Administer 100% oxygen by a nonrebreather mask.
2. Evacuate the patient immediately to the nearest medical center.
3. Hyperbaric oxygen therapy may reduce neurologic sequelae if initiated less than 24 hours after the patient is removed from the CO source.

SMOKE INHALATION AND THERMAL AIRWAY INJURY
Signs and Symptoms
- Facial burns
- Intraoral or pharyngeal burns
- Singed nasal hairs
- Soot in the mouth or nose, carbonaceous sputum
- Hoarseness, inspiratory stridor with a barking sound that seems to originate in the neck, or expiratory wheezing
- Shortness of breath and coughing that produces carbonaceous black sputum
- Muffled voice, drooling, difficulty swallowing
- Swollen tongue

Treatment
1. Once the injury has occurred, no measures can be taken to limit its progress, so evacuate the patient immediately.
2. Administer humidified 100% oxygen by a nonrebreather mask.
3. Consider initiating intubation and ventilation if stridor or dyspnea is present. Note that progressive edema can produce complete airway obstruction.
4. If the patient loses his or her airway, and intubation is not possible, perform immediate surgical cricothyroidotomy (see Chapter 10).
5. Administer a bronchodilator (albuterol, 200 to 400 mcg [2 to 8 full inhalations, depending on preparation] by metered-dose inhaler with a spacer q15–20 min prn).

8

Solar Radiation and Photoprotection

Erythemogenic doses of ultraviolet (UV) energy are defined as multiples of the minimal erythema dose (MED), which is the lowest dose to elicit perceptible erythema. In a day's time, a person can receive 15 MEDs of ultraviolet B (UVB) but only 2 to 4 MEDs of ultraviolet A (UVA). So, although humans are exposed to 10-fold to 100-fold more UVA than UVB, more than 90% of sunlight-induced erythema is attributable to UVB. However, UVA exposure contributes significantly to development of skin cancer. Almost all ultraviolet C (UVC) is absorbed by the earth's ozone layer.

Wind augments sunburn. In mice, exposure to wind plus UV radiation (UVR) results in more erythema than does exposure to UVR alone. In humans, wind reduces heat perception and encourages longer exposure. Altitude profoundly influences UVB exposure; there is an 8% to 10% increase in UVB for each 305-m (1000-ft) rise above sea level.

ACUTE SUNBURN
Sunburn is a local cutaneous inflammatory and vascular-mediated reaction. UVB erythema has its onset 2 to 6 hours after exposure, peaks at 12 to 36 hours, and fades over 72 to 120 hours. UVA erythema has its onset within 4 to 6 hours, peaks in 8 to 12 hours, and fades in 24 to 48 hours.

Signs and Symptoms
- Painful erythema of skin
- Skin blistering, low-grade fever, chills, nausea, vomiting, and diarrhea in severe cases

Treatment (Box 8.1)
Sunburn is self-limited, and its treatment is largely symptomatic.
1. Cool-water soaks or compresses may provide immediate relief. Moisturizers are sometimes helpful.
2. Topical anesthetics are sometimes useful. It is generally preferable to use nonsensitizing preparations containing menthol, camphor, and pramoxine rather than potentially sensitizing preparations containing benzocaine and diphenhydramine. Refrigerating topical anesthetics before application provides added relief.
3. Anecdotal remedies (controlled studies are lacking) include topical aloe, baking soda, or oatmeal (Aveeno).
4. Topical steroids (e.g., triamcinolone 0.1% cream applied bid when erythema first appears) may blanch reddened skin but should not be used on blistered skin. The combined use of

---

BOX 8.1   Sunburn Treatments

Pain Control
Nonsteroidal antiinflammatory drugs (e.g., aspirin 500 mg PO q4h, ibuprofen 400 mg PO q4h)
Nonsteroidal antiinflammatory drug topical (e.g., diclofenac 1.0% gel applied 6 h and 10 h after exposure)

Skin Care
Cool soaks, compresses
Nonmedicated moisturizers
Topical anesthetics
• Prax lotion (pramoxine)
• Sarna antiitch lotion (menthol plus camphor)
• Aveeno antiitch concentrated lotion (pramoxine plus camphor plus calamine)
• Neutrogena Norwegian formula soothing relief moisturizer (lidocaine plus camphor)

Steroids
Topical
Systemic

---

topical steroids and oral nonsteroidal antiinflammatory drugs (NSAIDs) slightly decreases erythema during the first 24 hours if these drugs are administered before exposure or shortly after exposure, before sunburn becomes clinically apparent.
5. Systemic steroids (e.g., 3 to 5 days of prednisone) have anecdotal support but are not proven by any clinical trial.
6. Diclofenac 1.0% gel, a NSAID, alleviates pain, erythema, and edema for up to 48 hours when applied at 6 and 10 hours after exposure.
7. Oral NSAIDs, including aspirin, provide analgesia and may reduce sunburn erythema.

PHOTOPROTECTION
The essential element in avoiding UVR-induced injury is a comprehensive approach to protection.

Sunscreens
Sun Protection Factor (Table 8.1)
• The ability of a sunscreen to protect the skin from UVR-induced erythema is indicated by the sun protection factor (SPF).
• The SPF is defined as a ratio. The numerator is the UVR required to produce minimal erythema (1 MED) in sunscreen-protected skin, and the denominator is the UVR required to produce minimal erythema in unprotected skin.
• SPF 15 sunscreen or clothing blocks 93% of UVB. Histologically, an SPF 30 sunscreen provides better protection against sunburn cell formation than does an SPF 15 sunscreen.

SPF	UVB ABSORPTION (%)
2	50.0
4	75.0
8	87.5
15	93.3
30	96.7
50	98.0

Table 8.1 Skin Protection Factor and Ultraviolet B Absorption

SPF, Skin protection factor; *UVB*, ultraviolet B.

- Although UVB is primarily responsible for the burning effects from the sun, both UVB and UVA radiation can cause skin cancer. In addition, UVA rays penetrate more deeply into the skin and are largely responsible for premature wrinkles, aged skin, and photosensitivity. Broad-spectrum sunscreens that include UVA and UVB protection with SPF 15 or greater are recommended.

Sunscreen Vehicles
- Sunscreen vehicles affect efficacy.
- The ideal vehicle spreads easily; maximizes skin adherence; minimizes interaction with the active sunscreening agent; and is noncomedogenic, nonstinging, nonstaining, and inexpensive.
- Sunscreens are a leading cause of photoallergic contact dermatitis. Oxybenzone is the most commonly implicated agent.
- Para-aminobenzoic acid (PABA) sensitizes approximately 4% of exposed subjects.
- Creams and lotions (emulsions) spread easily and penetrate well.
- Oils spread easily, but thinly; certain oils are comedogenic.
- Ointments and waxes may be preferable for extreme conditions; they resist chapping.
- Gels are nongreasy but wash or sweat off easily; alcohol-containing gels may cause stinging.
- Stick waxes are impractical for large surface areas.
- Aerosols are wasteful and may form an uneven layer.
- Sunscreens are incorporated into many cosmetics.
- There are environmental consequences of sunscreen choice: as little as one drop of sunscreen containing oxybenzone is enough to damage fragile coral reef systems by leaching nutrients and bleaching coral.

Sunscreen Application
- The protection provided by a sunscreen is related to the amount of product applied. Sunscreens are typically applied at much

lower concentrations than the 2 mg/cm^2 at which they are tested; when used ad lib, sunscreens are typically applied in concentrations of 0.5 to 1 mg/cm^2, and the resultant SPF is typically about 50% of the labeled SPF for chemical sunscreens. Newly available sunscreens that contain disappearing colorants are popular because they provide visible assurance of complete coverage.

- Adequate coverage of just the face, ears, and dorsal hands requires 2 to 3 g, which requires an 8-oz (0.2-L) bottle of sunscreen every 80 to 120 days.
- Apply liberally and frequently. Apply 15 to 30 minutes before water exposure. Reapply after every exit from the water.
- Cover all exposed areas.
- Take care to avoid having sunscreen run into the eyes.
- The concomitant use of sunscreen and insect repellent containing DEET can lower effective SPF by 34%.
- Safe Sea jellyfish-safe sunblock, available in SPF 15 or 30, contains chemical agents that inhibit stings by jellyfish and other nematocyst-bearing stinging creatures.

Ultraviolet A Protection
Recently, more efficient UVA blocking agents have become available.
- Common UVA blocking agents include avobenzone, ecamsule, and micronized TiO$_2$ and ZnO.
- No accepted standard exists for UVA protectiveness.
- Sunscreens with a labeling claim of UVA protection may allow transmission of 6% to 52% of UVA.

Ultraviolet A/Ultraviolet B Combined Protection
The U.S. Food and Drug Administration's directives require that products labeled "broad spectrum" and "SPF 15" (or higher) demonstrate protection against both UVB and UVA radiation.

Substantivity
- The ability of a sunscreen to resist water wash-off is referred to as *substantivity*. "Water-resistant (40 minutes)" sunscreens retain their SPF after 20 minutes of immersion plus 15 minutes drying repeated once, and "water-resistant (80 minutes)" sunscreens retain activity after the process is repeated twice more.
- By applying sunscreen 15 to 30 minutes before water exposure, substantivity can be increased.
- Reapplication after swimming or sweating helps ensure protection.
- Cold churning water, sand abrasion, and toweling may add to sunscreen loss.

Stability
- Keep sunscreens out of glove compartments and similar locations where they are exposed to extreme temperatures for prolonged periods.

- Shelf life is presumed to be at least 1 year for most commercially available sunscreens; however, data are lacking.

Clothing Protection

- Clothing varies considerably in its ability to block UV.
- Standardized testing of clothing has produced the ultraviolet protection factor (UPF), analogous to SPF in sunscreens.
- The single most important factor in determining SPF is the tightness of the weave, followed by the actual fabric. For instance, Lycra blocks nearly 100% of UVR when lax and only 2% when maximally stretched. Other determinants include wetness and color. Dry, dark fabrics have a higher SPF than do otherwise identical wet, white fabrics. A typical dry, white cotton T-shirt has a SPF of 5 to 9. Women's hosiery generally has a SPF of less than 3.
- In the United States, sun-protective clothing is regulated as a medical device. For example, one approved product, Solumbra, is made of tightly woven nylon with advertised SPF of 100+.
- A hat with a brim wide enough to protect the nose, cheeks, and chin is highly protective.

Table 8.2 Sunglasses Selection Criteria for Mountaineering	
SUBJECT	**CHARACTERISTICS**
UV absorption	99%–100%
Visible light transmittance	5%–10%*
Lens material	Polycarbonate or CR-39[†]
Optical quality	Clear image without distortion[‡]
Frame design features	Large lenses; side shields or "wraparound" design; fit close to face; good stability on face during movement; lightweight; durable
Color	Gray[§]

*Glasses with less than 8% transmittance of visible light should not be worn while driving. Sunglasses or any tinted lenses with visible light transmittance of less than 80% should not be worn while driving at night.

[†]Glass lenses typically have very good optical clarity and scratch resistance but are heavier and more expensive.

[‡]Hold the sunglasses at arm's length and move them back and forth. If the objects are distorted or move erratically, the optical quality is less than desirable. Also, compare the image quality between several different pairs of sunglasses to get a basis for comparison.

[§]Colored lens tints can alter color perception and possibly compromise visibility of traffic signals. Neutral gray absorbs light relatively constantly across the visible spectrum and avoids these problems.

UV, Ultraviolet.

Sunglasses

- Glasses, contact lenses, and sunglasses protect the corneas from most UVB and variable amounts of UVA.
- Acute exposure to high levels of UVR may result in acute UV photokeratitis.
- UVR is implicated in myriad ocular disorders, including cataracts, macular degeneration, and retinitis pigmentosa.
- Standard sunglasses transmit 15% to 25% of visible light; mountaineering sunglasses transmit 5% to 10%, which is necessary to reduce luminance to a comfortable range.
- Side shields or deeply wrapped lens designs should be used in mountaineering environments. Table 8.2 provides desirable characteristics in selecting sunglasses for environments with high levels of luminance and UVR.

Sun Avoidance

- Avoid excessive midday sun, from 10 a.m. to 3 p.m.
- Seek shade whenever possible. Overhead shade cloths provide more protection than clothing made of the same fabrics.
- Automobile windshields typically block UVB and some UVA, whereas side windows block only UVB. Transparent plastic films can be applied to block more than 99% of UVR.
- Apply sunscreens liberally, and begin their use early in life.

9

Lightning Injuries

Although the chances of being struck by lightning are minimal, 200 to 400 persons are victims of lightning strikes in the United States each year, resulting in a recent average of 30 deaths per year. Worldwide estimates are up to 240,000 annual injuries with up to 24,000 deaths. Lightning is the electrical discharge associated with thunderstorms. An initial electrical stroke can show a potential difference between the tip and the earth that ranges from 10 to 200 (average 30) million volts. Up to 30 strokes that constitute a single lightning flash give lightning its flickering quality. The main stroke usually measures 2 to 3 cm in diameter, and its temperature at the hottest has been estimated to range from 8000°C to 50,000°C (14,432°F to 90,032°F), or up to four times as hot as the surface of the sun. Thunder results from the shock waves generated by the nearly explosive expansion of the heated and ionized air. Thunder is seldom heard over distances greater than 10 miles (16 km).

Lightning can cause injury by:

- Direct hit
- Splash (lightning bolt first hits object, then jumps to victim)
- Contact with a conductive material that is hit or splashed by lightning
- Step voltage
- Ground current
- Surface arcing
- Upward streamer current
- Blunt trauma from the explosive force of the positive and negative pressure waves (thunder) it produces

The "flashover phenomenon" describes the situation wherein the electrical current of lightning travels appreciably over the body's surface, rather than through it. This likely accounts for vaporized moisture on the skin and unique skin burn patterns.

DISORDERS

Box 9.1 lists the types of immediate injuries that can occur with any of the effects of lightning, which is best described as a unidirectional massive current impulse.

Signs and Symptoms

- Generally, a history of a lightning strike or near strike
- Disarray of clothing and belongings
- Lichtenberg figure (pathognomonic sign of lightning injury that self-resolves and needs no treatment) (see Plate 5)

BOX 9.1   Types of Immediate Injuries Attributable to Lightning

- Cardiopulmonary arrest
  - Immediate cardiac arrest that may be brief because of inherent automaticity
  - Respiratory arrest, caused by paralysis of the medullary respiratory center, which leads to secondary cardiac arrest from hypoxia
- Neurologic injury
  - Seizures
  - Deafness
  - Confusion or amnesia
  - Blindness
  - Dizziness
  - Extremity paralysis
  - Headache, nausea, and postconcussion syndrome
- Contusions and fractures
- Chest pain and muscle aches
- Tympanic membrane rupture
- Superficial punctate and feathering burns (Plates 5 and 6)
- Partial-thickness burns

- Linear or punctate (see Plate 6) burns with tympanic membrane rupture and confusion in an outdoor setting
- Confusion, amnesia, or unconsciousness in a person found indoors after or during a thunderstorm
- Muscle aches and body tingling
- Keraunoparalysis (a temporary self-resolving state characterized by skin mottling, extremity paralysis, and diminished or absent extremity pulses)

Treatment

Note that lightning victims are not "charged" and thus pose no hazard to rescuers.

1. Assess and treat first those victims who appear dead, because they may ultimately recover if properly resuscitated.
   a. As with any cardiac arrest, the first steps are addressing chest compressions (circulation), airway, and breathing.
   b. Perform cardiopulmonary resuscitation (CPR) if indicated. If no pulse is obtained within 20 to 30 minutes of initiating resuscitation, it is reasonable to stop CPR. Be aware that dilated pupils should not be taken as the sole sign of brain death in the lightning victim.
   c. If you successfully obtain a pulse with CPR, continue ventilation until spontaneous adequate respirations resume, the person is pronounced dead, continued resuscitation is deemed not feasible, or you are in danger.
2. Stabilize and splint any fractures.

3. Be aware that the patient may have been thrown a considerable distance by the strike. Initiate and maintain spinal fracture precautions as indicated.
4. Administer oxygen and intravenous fluids. Apply a cardiac monitor.
5. Prepare for transport to a medical facility.

Prevention

Many experts recommend using the 30-30 rule: if you see lightning, then hear thunder before you can count to 30 seconds, you should be seeking shelter. Activities should not be resumed for at least 30 minutes after the last lightning is seen and the last thunder heard. Because this rule may be difficult to remember, the latest advice from the United States National Weather Service is "when thunder roars, go indoors." A link to current recommendations may be found at http://www.lightningsafety.noaa.gov.

- Lightning may travel nearly horizontally as far as 10 miles (16 km) or more in front of a thunderstorm. When a thunderstorm threatens, seek shelter in a substantial building or inside a metal-topped vehicle (not a tent or a convertible automobile). If you are in a car, roll up all windows and stay in it. If it is a convertible and there is no other shelter, huddle on the ground at least 45 m (49 yards) away from the vehicle.
- If you are in a tent, stay as far away from the poles and wet tent material (e.g., fabric) as possible.
- Do not count on rubber-soled shoes or raincoats to provide protection. Similarly, the rubber tires on a car do not provide any protection. Electrical energy travels along the outside of the car body and dissipates into the ground.
- Do not stand under a tall tree in an open area or on a ridge or hilltop.
- Move away from open water, and do not stand near a metal boat. If you are swimming, get out of the water.
- Move away from tractors and other metal farm equipment. Avoid tall objects, such as ski lifts, boat masts, flagpoles, and power lines.
- Get off motorcycles, bicycles, and golf carts. Put down golf clubs, umbrellas, and fishing poles.
- Stay away from wire fences, clotheslines, metal pipes, and other metallic paths that could carry lightning to you from a distance.
- Avoid standing in small, isolated sheds or other small structures in open areas.
- Once you are indoors, avoid being near windows, open doors, fireplaces, or large metal fixtures. Be aware that a cellular telephone can transmit loud static that can cause acoustic damage.
- In a forest, seek shelter in a low area under a thick growth of saplings or small trees. Avoid the tallest trees, staying a distance from the tree at least equal to the tree's height. Avoid the entrances to caves.

- In an open area, go to a low place such as a ravine or valley.
- If you are totally in the open:
  - Stay far away from single trees to avoid lightning splashes.
  - Drop to your knees and bend forward, putting your hands on your knees.
  - If it is available, place insulating material (e.g,, sleeping pad, life jacket, rope) between you and the ground. Do not lie flat on the ground.
- If your hair stands on end, you hear high-pitched or crackling noises, or you see a blue halo around objects, there is electrical activity around you that typically precedes a lightning strike. If you can, leave the area immediately. If you are unable to do this, crouch down on the balls of your feet and tuck your head down. Do not touch the ground with your hands.
- When a thunderstorm is about to pass, maintain a cautious approach because this continues to be a dangerous time.

10 | Emergency Airway Management

Emergency airway management encompasses assessment, establishment, and protection of the airway in combination with effective oxygenation and ventilation. Airway management in the wilderness must often be provided in austere or unusual environments under less-than-ideal circumstances, so improvisation may prove invaluable.

The conscious or semiconscious person with an airway emergency instinctively seeks an optimal position for breathing. The unconscious person, unless deeply anesthetized, paralyzed, or profoundly hypoxic, continues effort to breathe until death is very near. If a patient can speak, the airway is likely intact. Even if a patient's chest wall is moving, there may still be an upper airway obstruction. It is important to assess chest excursions and breath sounds to assure a patent airway. If a patient is making no respiratory effort at all, consider initiating cardiopulmonary resuscitation (CPR).

RECOGNITION OF AIRWAY OBSTRUCTION

Cyanosis can be present without airway compromise, and significant airway compromise can be present without cyanosis.

Signs and Symptoms

The two most important aspects of respiratory assessment are the following:

- The presence or absence of respiratory effort (assesses the integrity of the central nervous system).
- If attempts to breathe are being made, assess the work of breathing and make positional changes to optimize air exchange.

Additional Signs and Symptoms

- Labored respirations are typified by a rate that is forcefully rapid, irregular, or gasping.
- Unusual sounds or noisy respirations (stridor) may be present.
- Accessory muscles of the chest wall, shoulders, neck, and abdomen strain with the effort.
- In the obstructed airway, expiration tends to be prolonged.
- Partial obstruction can be recognized by the following:
  - Decreased volume exchange (decreased air entry by auscultation or decreased chest rise by inspection).
  - Increased transit time during inhalation or exhalation.
- No pause between breaths is an ominous sign. This suggests that there is a significant airway obstruction.

Head and Tongue Positioning

The most common causes of upper airway obstruction are the following:

- A floppy tongue and lax pharyngeal muscles from decreased muscle tone of the genioglossus muscle, which contracts to move the tongue forward during inspiration and dilate the pharynx.
- Soft tissue enlargement from infection, edema, or hypertrophy.
- Teeth play an important role in preserving the size and patency of the oropharynx. Edentulous persons (the young, older adults, persons with poor dentition, and recently traumatized persons) are vulnerable to upper airway obstruction.

Treatment of Airway Obstruction

Upper airway obstruction is almost always improved by optimal head positioning, mouth opening, clearing of nasal passages, and/or tongue manipulation.

1. Open the mouth of an unconscious person.
2. Note the position of the tongue and the presence of vomitus, foreign debris, or pooled secretions. Suction the airway if required and available (see section "Suctioning," later).
3. Listen to the quality and consistency of lung and airway sounds.
4. In the obtunded infant or small child, the site of upper airway obstruction is usually between the tip of the tongue and the hard palate in the front of the mouth.
5. In an obtunded adult, the site of upper airway obstruction is usually between the base of the tongue and the posterior oropharynx (Fig. 10.1).

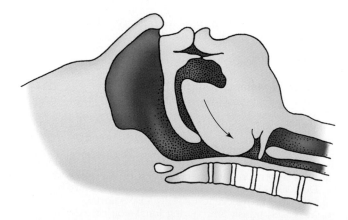

FIGURE 10.1 Tongue position in the unconscious adult. Note airway obstruction by the base of the tongue against the posterior pharyngeal wall with closure of the epiglottis over the trachea.

6. When the tongue is retrodisplaced, it causes the epiglottis to fold over and close off the tracheal opening, which results in a secondary site of upper airway obstruction.

7. Relief of both sources of obstruction can be obtained by lifting the jaw forward (Fig. 10.2) to simultaneously open the mouth and move the tongue from obstructing the oropharynx.

8. The optimal head position for airway alignment and patency varies with age. However, no matter the person's age, the most desirable posture is maintaining a "neutral" (neither flexion nor hyperextension) head position with the chin jutted forward: nose in the "sniffing" position, mouth open, tongue resting on the floor of the mouth, and angle of the mandible perpendicular to the ground.

9. The least desirable head position in any age group is with the neck flexed and chin pointed toward the chest. Flexion also increases unfavorable stresses on a potentially unstable cervical spine.

10. Extreme hyperextension of the head in any age group stresses ligaments and angulates the airway and is to be avoided.

11. Because of prominence of the cranial occiput in an infant, an infant's airway is best supported with a shoulder roll or built-up surface for the back.

12. The child does best without a pillow or with a built-up cushion for the back and only a small pad for the occiput.

13. The adult's airway is best supported in the "sniffing" position with a small pillow under the head, the chin pointed in the air, and preserved natural lordosis of the cervical spine.

14. If the mechanism of injury or physical examination suggests a possible cervical spine injury, efforts to stabilize the neck and head should be undertaken. The patient should be spared

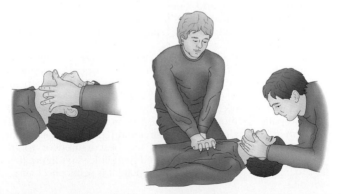

FIGURE 10.2 Triple-maneuver airway support: Maintain axial alignment of the cervical spine, lift on the angle of the mandible, and hold open the mouth. Located midway between the chin and the angle of the mandible, the facial artery pulse may be monitored at the same time.

neck flexion, hyperextension, or lateral rotation. Fortunately, the best head position for the airway is also good for the cervical spine. If a cervical spine immobilization method is employed, the airway should be evaluated for obstruction both before and after application.

Body Positioning

The supine position may be neither desirable nor achievable. Because of gravity, some airways are better maintained in a side-lying or prone position. Nontraditional positioning for stabilization and transport may be necessary because of burns, vomiting, management of secretions, or location of impaled objects. Principles of transport for patients in nonsupine positions relate to preservation of good perfusion and mechanical alignment in all body parts under pressure, maintaining neck straightness, and ensuring the ability of the rescuer to monitor airway patency. In a nonsupine position, the same airway posture is desirable: minimal torsion of the cervical spine, neck in a sniffing position, mouth open, and tongue on the floor of the mouth (Fig. 10.3).

MANUAL AIRWAY TECHNIQUES

If the upper airway is obstructed, there are four basic noninvasive airway-opening maneuvers. All noninvasive airway maneuvers except tongue traction and the internal jaw lift can be conjoined with rescue breathing or bag-valve-mask (BVM) assisted ventilation.

1. Head tilt, chin lift. The heel of one of the rescuer's hands is pressed down on the patient's forehead, and the fingers of the other hand are placed under the chin to lift it up. The intended result is the sniffing position. Problems arise if the mouth is closed or soft tissues are folded inward because of the chin lift. In addition, downward pressure on the forehead tends to lift the eyebrows and open the eyelids, so measures may need to be taken to protect the eyes. This technique should not be employed in patients suspected of having a cervical spine injury.
2. Jaw thrust (Fig. 10.4A). Pressure is applied to the angle of the mandible to move it upward while forcefully opening the mouth. This is painful, and the conscious or semiconscious patient will object by clamping down or writhing.
3. Internal jaw lift (see Fig. 10.4B). The rescuer's thumb is inserted into the patient's mouth under the tongue, and the mandibular mentum (chin) is lifted, thus stretching out the soft tissues and opening the airway. This is the best maneuver for the unconscious patient with a shattered mandible. The internal jaw lift is dangerous to the rescuer if the patient is semiconscious and can bite.
4. A fourth noninvasive airway maneuver takes some practice but serves several purposes and is the best maneuver if done correctly. In this two-handed maneuver, the head is held between two hands to prevent lateral rotation and maintain neck control. The

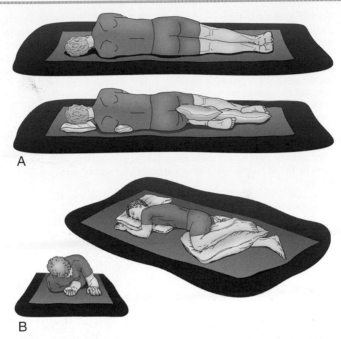

FIGURE 10.3 **A,** Patient lying on side with airway/neck in good position and pressure points protected. Flexing the down-side leg stabilizes the torso. The pillow and axillary roll help maintain the spine in good alignment. **B,** Patient positioned semiprone to facilitate gravity drainage of secretions. A pillow under the head keeps the spine in relative alignment. With no pillow under the head, the width of the shoulder inclines the pharynx downward at a steeper angle.

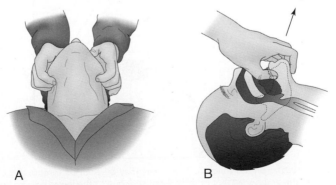

FIGURE 10.4 **A,** External jaw thrust. **B,** Internal jaw lift.

fourth and fifth fingers are hooked behind the angle of the mandible to dislocate the jaw upward, and the thumbs ensure that the mouth is maintained open (see Fig. 10.2). The third finger may be positioned over the facial artery as it comes around the mandible so that the pulse can be monitored at the same time. For greatest stability, the rescuer's elbows should rest on the same surface on which the patient is lying.

Improvised Tongue Traction Technique

If the patient is unconscious, the airway may be opened temporarily by attaching the anterior aspect of the patient's tongue to the lower lip with one or two safety pins (Fig. 10.5). An alternative to piercing the lower lip is to pass a string through the safety pins and exert

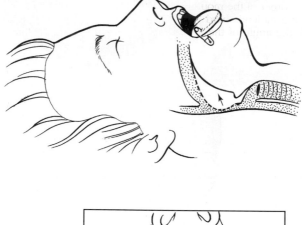

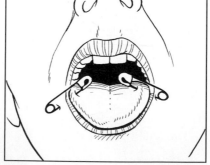

FIGURE 10.5   Tongue traction. The airway may be opened temporarily by attaching the anterior aspect of the patient's tongue to the lower lip with two safety pins.

traction on the tongue by securing the end of the string to the patient's shirt button or jacket zipper (Fig. 10.6).

MECHANICAL AIRWAY ADJUNCTS

Several airway adjuncts are available to maintain airway patency while freeing up the rescuer to perform other tasks or improve assisted ventilation. Basic and advanced airway equipment are important considerations in a wilderness medical kit (Box 10.1).

Oropharyngeal Airway

The oropharyngeal airway (OPA) holds the tongue off the posterior pharyngeal wall (Fig. 10.7). These devices are most effective in unconscious and semiconscious patients who lack a gag reflex or cough. The use of an OPA in a patient with a gag reflex or cough is contraindicated because it may stimulate retching, vomiting, or laryngospasm.

The proper OPA size is estimated by placing the OPA's flange at the corner of the mouth so that the bite-block segment is parallel with the patient's hard palate; the distal tip of the airway should reach the angle of the jaw.

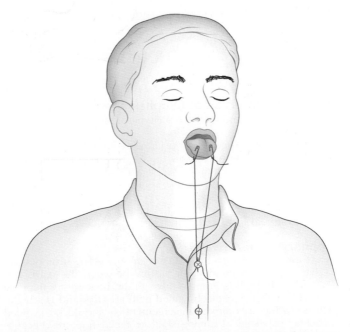

FIGURE 10.6 Tongue traction. An alternative to piercing the lower lip is to pass a string through the safety pins and exert traction on the tongue by securing the end of the string to the patient's shirt button or jacket zipper.

> **BOX 10.1**   Sample Contents of a Wilderness Airway Management Kit
>
> **Basic Airway Equipment**
> Laordal pocket mask
> Cardiopulmonary resuscitation microshield barrier
> Nasal airway kit
> Oral airway kit
> Stethoscope
> Bulb suction device
>
> **Advanced Airway Equipment**
> Bag-mask ventilation device with pediatric and adult masks
> Manual suction device
> Endotracheal tubes with stylet
> Compact and battery-operated video laryngoscope system
> Laryngoscope handles and blades
> Magill forceps
> Esophageal detector device
> Colorimetric end-tidal carbon dioxide detector
> Laryngeal mask airway or King LT airway
> Needle cricothyrotomy catheter or device
> Commercial cricothyrotomy kit
> Oxygen cylinder with toggle handle
> Nasal cannula, oxygen mask with strap, and nonrebreather bag
> Oxygen tubing
> Pulse oximeter

Technique for Insertion of Oropharyngeal Airway

1. Open the mouth, and clear the pharynx of any secretions, blood, or vomitus.
2. Insert the OPA upside down or at a 90-degree angle to avoid pushing the tongue posteriorly during insertion. Slide it gently along the roof of the mouth. As the oral airway is inserted past the uvula or crest of the tongue, rotate it so that the tip points down the patient's throat.
3. The flange should rest against the patient's lips, and the distal portions should rest on the posterior pharyngeal wall.

Nasopharyngeal Airway

The nasopharyngeal airway (NPA) is an uncuffed, trumpet-like tube that provides a conduit for airflow between the nares and pharynx (Fig. 10.8). It is inserted through the nose rather than the mouth. This device is better tolerated than an OPA and is a better choice for wilderness airway management. It should be avoided in patients suspected of having skull or facial fractures because intracranial placement may occur.

Proper NPA length is determined by measuring the distance from the tip of the patient's nose to the tragus of the patient's ear.

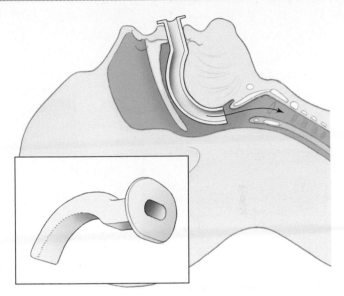

FIGURE 10.7 Oropharyngeal airway. (Redrawn from Mahadevan SV, Garmel GM, editors: *An introduction to clinical emergency medicine*, Cambridge, UK, 2012, Cambridge University Press. Copyright Chris Gralapp, http://www. biolumina.com.)

Technique for Insertion of Nasopharyngeal Airway

1. Lubricate the NPA with a water-soluble lubricant.
2. Place the NPA in the nostril with the bevel directed toward the nasal septum.
3. Gently push the NPA straight back along the floor of the nasal passage. As the NPA passes through the turbinates, there will be mild resistance, but once the tip has entered the nasopharynx, there will be sensation of a "give."
4. If you meet persistent resistance, rotate the tube slightly, reattempt insertion through the other nostril, or try a smaller-diameter tube. Do not force the tube.
5. Following insertion, the flange should rest on the patient's nostril and the tube should be visible in the oropharynx as it passes behind the tonsils. The tip should come to rest behind the base of the tongue but above the vocal cords.
6. Complications of NPAs include failure to pass through the nose (usually resulting from a deviated septum), epistaxis, accidental avulsion of adenoidal tissue, mucosal tears or avulsion of a turbinate, submucosal tunneling (the tube tunnels out of sight behind the posterior pharyngeal wall), and creation of pressure sores.

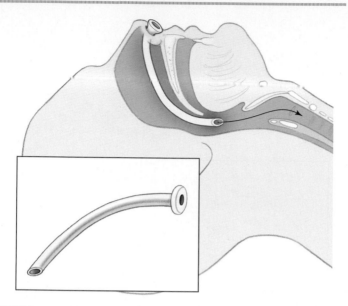

FIGURE 10.8   Nasopharyngeal airway. (Redrawn from Mahadevan SV, Garmel GM, editors: *An introduction to clinical emergency medicine*, Cambridge, UK, 2012, Cambridge University Press. Copyright Chris Gralapp, http://www. biolumina.com.)

7. If the NPA or any nasal tube is left in place for more than several days, impedance to normal drainage may predispose the patient to sinusitis or otitis media.

Improvised Mechanical Airways

Any flexible tube of appropriate diameter and length can be used as an improvisational substitute for a NPA. Examples include a Foley catheter, radiator hose, solar shower hose, siphon tubing, or inflation hose from a kayak flotation bag or sport pouch. An endotracheal tube (ETT) can be shortened and softened in warm water to allow passage through the nose and function as an NPA. The flange can be improvised using a safety pin through the nostril end of the tube (Fig. 10.9).

FOREIGN BODY ASPIRATION

Foreign bodies may cause partial or complete airway obstructions. A patient with a partial airway obstruction can usually phonate or produce a forceful cough to expel the foreign body. A person with a complete airway obstruction cannot speak, exchange air, or cough. Failure to relieve the obstruction can lead to respiratory collapse and cardiac arrest. For techniques in relieving an airway obstruction, see Chapter 25.

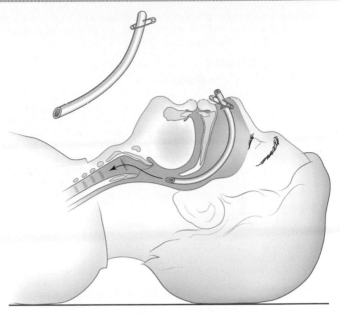

FIGURE 10.9   Improvised nasopharyngeal tube.

SUCTIONING

In the wilderness, one must remove secretions typically without the benefit of electric suction deceives used in most hospitals and ambulances. Several innovative, lightweight, and hand-operated products such as the Suction-Easy Device or V-Vac Suction are on the market for this purpose.

- Sweep debris from the mouth with a finger wrapped in a T-shirt or other available cloth.
- Position patient so that gravity facilitates drainage of blood, vomit, saliva, and mucus. Something absorbent or basin-like can be placed at the side of the mouth to catch drained effluvia.
- Turkey basters can be included in an expedition first-aid kit for extraction of secretions and for gentle wound irrigation and moisturizing burn dressings or wet compresses. The rubber self-inflating bulbs marketed for infant nasal suctioning can also be used to suction out debris from the mouths and noses of adults.
- A "mucus trap" suction device can be improvised from a jar with two holes poked in its lid and two tubes or straws duct-taped into the holes. One straw goes to the rescuer, who provides suction, and the other is directed toward whatever has accumulated in the airway. The jar serves to trap the removed secretions so that the rescuer is protected from bodily fluids or foreign substances.

- Secretion removal by gravity or suctioning is key to the management of epistaxis and for maintaining the airway of a patient with mandibular fractures (see Chapter 17).

RESCUE BREATHING
Mouth-to-Mouth Ventilation

Mouth-to-mouth ventilation is an efficient approach to assisting ventilation. Failure to use a barrier device during mouth-to-mouth ventilation places the rescuer at risk for exposure to infectious bodily fluids. The rescuer should use a non-rebreathing flap-valve to permit air to be pushed into the patient through one aperture while exhaled air and secretions are exhausted through a separate route, thus helping minimize exposure to infectious substances. These one-way valves are small, lightweight, and inexpensive and are easy to tuck into a small container, along with gloves and a face barrier.

Technique

1. Open the airway using the head tilt with chin lift approach if cervical spine trauma is not suspected.
2. If needed, clear the airway of vomitus, secretions, and foreign bodies.
3. Pinch the patient's nostrils closed with the finger and thumb of one hand; the heel of that same hand may be placed on the forehead to maintain the head tilt.
4. Support the patient's chin with the other hand, and hold the patient's mouth slightly open.
5. Take a deep breath.
6. Place your mouth over the properly placed barrier device (or around the patient's mouth if a barrier device is unavailable), and make a tight seal with your lips against the patient's face.
7. Exhale slowly into the valve or patient's mouth until you see the patient's chest rise and feel resistance to the flow of your breath.
8. Break contact with the patient to allow passive exhalation.

Mouth-to-Mask Ventilation

Mouth-to-mask ventilation is the safest and most effective technique for rescue breathing. The mask has a one-way valve in the stem to prevent exhaled gases and bodily fluids from reaching the rescuer. In addition, a disposable high-efficiency particulate air filter may be inserted into the pocket mask to trap infectious air droplets and secretions. The pocket face mask is made of a soft plastic material and can be folded and carried in a pocket. Some masks are available with an oxygen inlet to allow for supplemental oxygen administration.

Despite optimal cushion inflation, however, some facial shapes provide special challenges. Poor face-mask fit on heavily bearded individuals may be improved by first applying petroleum jelly or other thick ointment to allow the mask to fit on the film and prevent air leaks. Adult-sized masks can be inverted with the nosepiece at the chin to allow coverage over the entire face of an infant or small child.

To select the most widely adaptable "first-aid kit" mask-and-valve product, look for the following features:

- Transparent and easily bendable mask body materials that retain little "memory" of residing in their carrying positions and that do not become stiff, brittle, or nondeformable in cold temperatures
- An inflatable cushion seal that can be adjusted for changes in temperature and altitude
- A flexible, high-volume, low-pressure cushion seal able to conform to many different face sizes and shapes
- A mask span that can be used on both small and large patients, tough materials resistant to cracks and punctures, and a compact mask or carrying case that does not take up disproportionate space in the first-aid kit

Technique

1. Open the airway using the head tilt with chin lift approach if cervical spine trauma is not suspected.
2. Connect the one-way valve to the mask.
3. If available, connect oxygen tubing to the inlet port, and set the flow rate at 15 L/min.
4. Position yourself at the head of the patient.
5. Clear the patient's airway of vomitus, secretions, and foreign bodies, if necessary.
6. Insert an oral or NPA.
7. Place the mask on the patient's face.
8. Apply pressure to both sides of the mask with the thumb side of the palms to create an airtight seal. Apply upward pressure to the mandible (i.e., jaw thrust) using the index, middle, and ring fingers of both hands while maintaining a head tilt.
9. Take a deep breath, exhale into the port of the one-way valve, and observe for chest rise.
10. Allow the patient to passively exhale between breaths.

Bag-Valve-Mask Ventilation

The self-inflating ventilation bag with face mask (i.e., BVM ventilation device) provides a means for emergency ventilation with high concentrations of oxygen. When it is attached to a high-flow (15 L/min) oxygen source, the BVM device can supply an oxygen concentration of nearly 100% (see Chapter 11). The adapter of the face mask is interchangeable with an ETT, so the same bag can be used after intubation. The BVM device can be used by a single rescuer but is easier and more successful when used by two persons. Successful ventilation depends on an adequate mask seal and patent airway. Placement of an oral airway should always be considered before BVM. Slow and gentle ventilation minimizes the risk for gastric inflation and subsequent regurgitation. Smaller BVM devices are employed for infants and children to prevent overinflating the lungs and subsequent barotrauma.

SUPRAGLOTTIC/ALTERNATIVE AIRWAY DEVICES

In certain wilderness conditions and settings, tracheal intubation may be difficult or impossible. Under such circumstances, alternative airway adjuncts or techniques may be employed to provide an airway. Alternative airways that require blind passage of the device into the airway may be simpler to master than passing an ETT under direct visualization. To achieve good outcomes with these devices and techniques, health care providers must maintain a high level of knowledge and skills through frequent practice and field use. Although there are many alternative airway devices on the market, only the laryngeal mask airway (LMA) and King LT airway will be discussed because they are the most widely employed.

Laryngeal Mask Airway

The LMA is a modified ETT with an inflatable, oval cuff ("laryngeal mask") at its base (Fig. 10.10). It is ideal for wilderness use. The LMA is inserted blindly into the pharynx and advanced until resistance is felt as the distal portion of the tube locates in the laryngopharynx. Inflation of the collar provides a seal around the laryngeal inlet, facilitating tracheal ventilation. The LMA provides ventilation equivalent to that with a tracheal tube. The LMA may have advantages over traditional endotracheal intubation when access to the patient is limited, when the possibility of unstable neck injury exists, or when appropriate patient positioning for tracheal intubation is impossible.

King LT Airway

The King LT airway is a single-lumen, dual-cuffed airway with ventilation outlets between the pharyngeal and esophageal cuffs. The King LT airway is inserted blindly. A single port with a pilot balloon inflates both cuffs simultaneously. Ventilation capability seems to be like that of the LMA. The device's airway seal may be lost after insertion and require deflation of the balloons and repositioning. The King LT airway is available in newborn through adult sizes.

DEFINITIVE AIRWAY MANAGEMENT

The presence of a definitive airway implies patency and protection. Provision of a definitive airway requires a tube in the trachea with the cuff inflated, secured in place, and attached to an oxygen-rich ventilation device. Whether in the wilderness or at the hospital, inability or failure to secure a timely and definitive airway can lead to disastrous or fatal consequences for the patient.

Approaches to definitive airway management include immediate oral endotracheal intubation, awake oral intubation, rapid-sequence oral intubation, nasotracheal intubation, and surgical airways (e.g., cricothyrotomy). Only experienced providers with appropriate

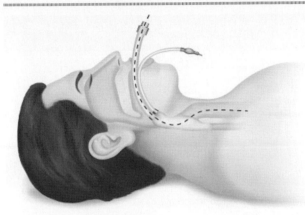

FIGURE 10.10   Correct placement of laryngeal mask airway. (From Strauss RA, Noordhoek R: Management of the difficult airway. *Atlas Oral Maxillofacial Surg Clin North Am* 18(1):11-28, 2010, Elsevier.)

equipment should attempt placement of a definitive airway, because basic airway maneuvers are often effective and provide immediate and reliable ventilation and oxygenation. Although the ultimate decision to endotracheally intubate a patient can be complicated and may depend on a variety of factors, the following are indications for definitive airway management:

- Failure of ventilation or oxygenation
- The patient's inability to maintain or protect the airway
- The potential for deterioration based on the patient's clinical presentation
- Patient safety and protection

Assessing the Airway

To assess for the safety of rapid sequence intubation (RSI), evaluate for potential (1) difficult laryngoscopy, (2) difficult rescue mask ventilation, (3) difficult placement or use of an extraglottic device (EGD), and (4) difficult cricothyrotomy. Although specialist backup, difficult airway devices, and rescue techniques may be limited in wilderness settings, knowledge of the four aspects of assessment is crucial to successful planning. Preintubation discovery of difficult airway characteristics is highly predictive of a challenging intubation. Providers should *always* be ready for a difficult-to-manage airway. Aspects of a difficult airway are recalled by the mnemonics LEMON (Box 10.2), MOANS (Box 10.3), RODS (Box 10.4), and SMART (Box 10.5).

Immediate Oral Intubation ("Crash" Intubation)

Patients in cardiorespiratory arrest or with agonal vital signs require immediate oral intubation. These patients often have little or no

> **BOX 10.2**   LEMON Mnemonic for Evaluation of Difficult Direct Laryngoscopy
>
> Look externally for signs of obvious difficulty
> Evaluate the 3 3 2 rule
> Mallampati classification
> Obstruction or Obesity
> Neck mobility (reduced)

> **BOX 10.3**   MOANS Mnemonic for Challenging Rescue Bag-and-Mask Ventilation
>
> Mask seal (beard or altered anatomy)
> Obstruction or Obesity
> Aged (>55 years old)
> No teeth
> Stiffness (resistance to ventilation or intrinsic lung pathology)

> **BOX 10.4**   RODS Mnemonic for Potentially Difficult Extraglottic Device Placement and Use
>
> Restricted mouth opening
> Obstruction or Obesity
> Distorted anatomy
> Stiffness (resistance to ventilation)

muscular tone and can be intubated without the need for RSI drugs.

1. Attempt immediate intubation without medications.
2. If intubation is unsuccessful (e.g., due to residual muscular contraction and limited mouth opening), use a neuromuscular blocking agent (NMBA) followed by another intubation attempt.
3. If an ETT has not been placed after three attempts, place an EGD.
4. If at any point the oxygen saturation drops and cannot be maintained with an EGD or rescue ventilation technique, move quickly to create a surgical airway.

Rapid Sequence Intubation

If a patient does not require an immediate (crash) airway intervention and assessment does not predict a sufficiently difficult airway such that neuromuscular blockade might be contraindicated, pursue RSI. RSI follows a coordinated series of steps to allow safe and effective airway management without interposed BVM. It is the method of choice for most acutely ill or injured patients.

> **BOX 10.5**   SMART Mnemonic for Evaluation of Difficult Cricothyrotomy
>
> Surgery
> Mass (head and neck cancer, hematoma)
> Access/anatomy problems (obesity, edema)
> Radiation
> Tumor

Technique Using the *Seven Ps of RSI*

1. Prepare all your equipment and medications for use during airway management.
2. Preoxygenate the patient with high flow nasal cannula or nonrebreather face mask oxygen at 100% for 3 minutes of normal breathing.
3. Pretreatment with fentanyl for cardiovascular emergencies or head injured patients may be considered but is controversial and without clear consensus guidelines.
4. Paralysis and induction of deep sedation with medications given as an intravenous bolus to facilitate unconsciousness and neuromuscular blockade.
   a. Induction agents cause deep sedation and should be given prior to neuromuscular blockade (Table 10.1).
   b. Neuromuscular blockage agents induce rapid, transient paralysis to facilitate laryngoscopy and ETT placement. These agents do not provide analgesia, sedation, or amnesia (Table 10.2).
5. Position the patient by placing rolls, daypack, or even shoes under the shoulders and posterior occiput to achieve the "sniffing position" and align the external auditory meatus of the ears to the sternal notch. This aligns the oral, pharyngeal, and laryngeal axis and maximizes visualization of the glottis.
6. Place the ETT through the vocal cords once the patient is fully paralyzed under direct or video laryngoscopy.
7. Prove (verify) the ETT is in the trachea using at least 2 of the following methods:
   a. Listen over the stomach for absence of gurgling and confirm breath sounds in all lung fields
   b. Monitor pulse oximetry
   c. Monitor end-tidal CO_2 or calorimetry device
   d. Use an ETT aspiration confirmation device

Postintubation Management

Successful airway management does not end with intubation. Be sure to complete the following:

1. Verify correct ETT placement within the trachea after every patient movement.

Table 10.1 Clinical Characteristics of Induction Agents

INDUCTION AGENT	INDUCTION DOSE (INTRAVENOUS)*	ONSET OF ACTION	DURATION OF ACTION	BENEFITS	PRECAUTIONS
Midazolam	0.2–0.3 mg/kg	30–60 s	15–30 min	Readily available Amnestic Anticonvulsant	Slow onset, apnea and hypotension No analgesia Often underdosed for rapid sequence intubation
Etomidate	0.3 mg/kg	15–45 s	3–12 min	Decreased intracranial pressure Rarely, decreased blood pressure	Myoclonic jerks Vomiting No analgesia
Ketamine	1–2 mg/kg	45–60 s	10–20 min	Increased blood pressure and bronchodilation Dissociative amnesia and pain control	Increased secretions Emergence phenomenon
Propofol	1.5 mg/kg	30–60 s	2–5 min	Reversible, rapid offset; anticonvulsant	Apnea and hypotension; variable dosing

*All doses should be halved in the setting of profound refractory shock to prevent circulatory collapse.

Table 10.2	Neuromuscular Blocking Agents*		
AGENT	**INTUBATING DOSE (INTRAVENOUS)**	**ONSET**	**DURATION**
Depolarizing Agent			
Succinylcholine	1.5 mg/kg (adult) 2 mg/kg (child) 3 mg/kg (infant)	45–60 s	6–12 min
Nondepolarizing Agents			
Rocuronium	1 mg/kg	50–70 s	30–60 min
Vecuronium	0.15 mg/kg	90–120 s	60–75 min

*May require refrigeration. See manufacturer's recommendations.
Adapted from Mahadevan SV, Garmel GM, editors: *An introduction to clinical emergency medicine: guide for practitioners in the emergency department*, Cambridge, UK, 2005, Cambridge University Press.

2. Secure the ETT (i.e., tape or tie it) to prevent movement or migration.
3. Closely monitor the patient's vital signs.
   a. Bradycardia after intubation is worrisome for hypoxia.
   b. Gastric distention should prompt detection of a possible esophageal intubation.
   c. Hypertension after intubation suggests inadequate sedation.
   d. Hypotension after intubation may result from a tension pneumothorax, decreased venous return, large induction agent dose, or cardiac cause.
4. If a longer-acting neuromuscular blocker (e.g., rocuronium or vecuronium) is used, sedation is mandatory.
   a. An IV benzodiazepine (e.g., midazolam [0.05 to 0.1 mg/kg], diazepam [0.2 mg/kg], or lorazepam [0.05 to 0.1 mg/kg]) may be administered initially for sedation and repeated for any sign of awakening with awareness.
   b. Propofol (0.3 mg/kg) and ketamine (1 to 2 mg/kg) are increasingly popular as both induction agents and postintubation sedatives.
   c. An opioid agent, such as fentanyl (3 to 5 μg/kg) or morphine sulfate (0.1 mg/kg), may also be administered for additional patient comfort.
5. Nondepolarizing NMBAs (e.g., pancuronium [0.1 mg/kg] or vecuronium [0.1 mg/kg]) may be used for long-term paralysis.
   a. If any motor activity is detected after 45 to 60 minutes, give a repeat dose that is one-third the initial dose.
   b. Ensure adequate sedation when long-acting paralysis is employed.

CRICOTHYROTOMY

If the upper airway is completely obstructed and obstruction cannot be relieved or bypassed, the only way to avoid death is to create an air passage directly into the trachea. The most accessible and least complicated access site is through the cricothyroid membrane. Even in experienced hands, the relatively high complication rates (10% to 40%) for emergent cricothyrotomy are still less than those for tracheotomy. Complications include bleeding, puncture of the posterior trachea and esophagus, creation of a false passage, inability to ventilate, aspiration, subcutaneous and mediastinal emphysema, vocal cord injury, and subsequent tracheal stenosis.

Technique

1. The cricothyrotomy hole may be made percutaneously with a trocar or needle, or surgically with a knife blade.
2. If a syringe containing 1 mL of water or lidocaine is attached to the needle used for puncture, bubbles may be seen during gentle aspiration as the needle tip enters the trachea.
3. When the trachea is successfully entered, a gush of air will exit, often with a cough.
4. Once the cricothyroid membrane is punctured, it is essential to maintain patency of the tract and identify the hole with a tube, bougie, stylet, obturator, tweezers, wire, or another temporary place marker. It is very easy to lose the tract and create a false passage while trying to instrument or cannulate the route.
5. Making a small (1- to 1.5-cm [0.4 to 0.6 inches]) vertical incision in the skin over the cricothyroid membrane facilitates the ease of the next step: puncture through the lower third of the dime-sized membrane. Vertical skin incisions have advantages over horizontal incisions because vertical incisions tend to be more controlled and better positioned in reference to landmarks.
6. The needle/catheter is advanced in the midline of the neck at a 45-degree angle aiming toward the lower back.
7. Once the needle or introducer aspirates air, the catheter is slid off the stylet and the stylet is withdrawn.
8. Taking care not to kink a flexible catheter at the insertion site, the hub may be secured in place with tape or sutures or may be attached to a Luer-Lok syringe-adapter mechanism.
9. With anything other than a commercial cricothyrotomy set or ETT, provision of positive pressure ventilation requires creative assembly of an adapter connecting the apparatus in the trachea to the female connector on an Ambu bag. Fig. 10.11 shows an example of the step-up series of connections needed for this type of extension.
10. If the catheter in the trachea is to be replaced by a stiffer or bigger cannula, a guidewire is inserted through the catheter several centimeters down the trachea, the catheter is withdrawn

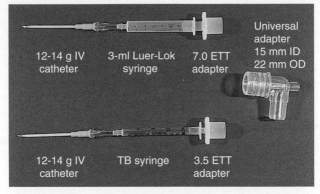

FIGURE 10.11 Combination of catheter assemblies to allow connection of a needle cricothyrotomy to a 15/22-mm (0.6/0.9-inch) standard adapter for Ambu ventilation. *ETT*, endotracheal tube. (Courtesy Anne E. Dickison, MD.)

with the guidewire remaining, and a dilator is advanced over the guidewire and then withdrawn.

11. Next, the intended cannula is threaded over the guidewire until it is seated with its flanges flush to the skin. The Seldinger technique is the process of identifying a lumen with an introducer, marking the lumen with a guidewire, dilating the entry site, and placing the final apparatus over the guidewire. The procedure of replacing a smaller tube with a larger one is termed a *dilational cricothyrotomy.*

12. A temporary cricothyrotomy trocar and tube can be fashioned from a tuberculin or 3-mL syringe that has been cut on the diagonal and then forcefully inserted through the cricothyroid membrane (Fig. 10.12). Because the improvised trocar point of the syringe is sharp and irregular, insertion is likely to be traumatic. Care must be taken to not lacerate the posterior tracheal wall or create a tracheoesophageal fistula.

13. Even with a universal adapter (15/22-mm [0.6/0.9-inch]) connection, without a jet ventilation device or cricothyrotomy tube of the proper diameter, curvature, and length, it is extremely difficult to ventilate a patient with positive pressure through a needle catheter or improvisational substitute. The patient has the best chances for survival if spontaneous respiratory effort can be preserved; it is easier for the patient to draw air in through a critically small opening than it is for a rescuer to generate the pressure needed to force air in through the same aperture. Pressures sufficient to make the chest rise can be generated by a rescuer blowing through the needle catheter, but such efforts rapidly lead to rescuer fatigue.

14. Temporary transtracheal oxygenation and ventilation through a 12- or 14-gauge needle can be provided using a flow rate of 15 L/min or by jet ventilation (40 psi) at a slow intermittent rate of 6 breaths/min and an inspiratory-to-expiratory ratio of 1 · 14 The very long expiratory time is necessary to allow passive expiration through a restrictive channel.

15. Packaged dilator cricothyrotomy sets such as those manufactured by Melker and Arndt contain a scalpel blade, syringe with an 18-gauge over-the-needle catheter and/or a thin introducer

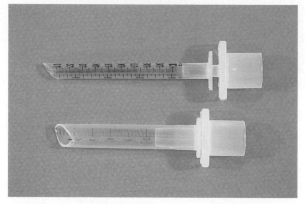

FIGURE 10.12   A tuberculin or 3-mL syringe can be cut on the diagonal to improvise a combination trocar-cricothyrotomy tube. Caution must be taken with insertion to avoid traumatizing the posterior pharyngeal wall. (Courtesy Anne E. Dickison, MD.)

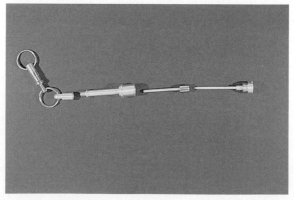

FIGURE 10.13   LifeStat key-chain emergency airway set. (Courtesy Anne E. Dickison, MD.)

needle, guidewire, appropriately sized dilator, and a polyvinyl airway cannula. The Patil set, Portex Mini-Trach II, and military version of the Melker set are sold without the guidewire and appeal to prehospital providers unfamiliar with the Seldinger technique. The Pertrach is similar in concept, except the guidewire and dilator are forged as a single unit so that a

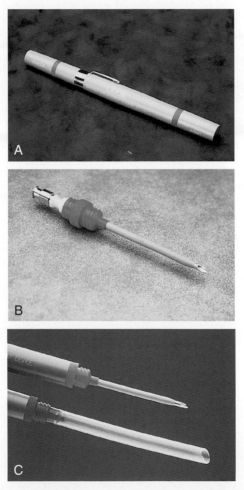

FIGURE 10.14   A, Wadhwa Emergency Airway Device. **B,** Wadhwa transtracheal catheter with removable stylet and Luer-Lok connection for jet ventilation. **C,** Internal components of the Wadhwa Emergency Airway Device. Both the transtracheal catheter and the nasopharyngeal airway screw into the case for an extension with a 15-mm (0.6-inch) adapter. (Courtesy Cook, Inc.)

finder catheter cannot be used and the introducer must be peeled away. The Nu-Trake device is complicated to use, has a rigid airway that risks trauma to the posterior trachea, and is difficult to secure.

16 In terms of expedition kit portability, three transtracheal puncture emergency airway devices deserve special mention.

   a. LifeStat manufactures a key-chain emergency airway set that consists of a sharp-pointed metal trocar introducer that fits through a straight metal cannula that screws into a metal extension with a universal 15-mm (0.6-inch) male adapter. Lightweight and less than 76 mm (3 inches) long, the three-component apparatus is attached to a separate and detachable key chain (Fig. 10.13).

   b. Cook Critical Care offers a 6-French reinforced-catheter emergency transtracheal airway catheter with a molded Luer-Lok connection for jet ventilation or added assembly of a 15-mm (0.6-inch) adapter for standard modes of positive pressure ventilation.

   c. Cook Critical Care also offers the Wadhwa Emergency Airway Device. This lightweight, impact-resistant assembly is 184 mm (7.25 inches) long and the diameter of a highlighter pen (Fig. 10.14). It disassembles to yield a 12-French Teflon-coated cricothyrotomy catheter with removable metal stylet (with a molded plastic Luer-Lok connection for oxygen or jet ventilation), plus a flexible NPA adhered to a molded plastic flange. Both the cricothyrotomy catheter and the NPA screw into the Wadhwa case to provide a low-resistance extension and a 15-mm (0.6-inch) (male) connection for standard positive pressure ventilation equipment.

11 Emergency Oxygen Administration

Emergency medical oxygen (O_2) administration is a critical part of wilderness emergency care, when available. Every provider of wilderness medicine must be familiar with the therapeutic value, indications, hazards, equipment, and technique of oxygen administration (Box 11.1).

INDICATIONS

Indications for the use of supplemental O_2 include (but are not limited to) the following:

- Shock
- Tissue hypoxia
- Hypoxemia
- Pulmonary gas exchange impairment caused by trauma, edema, asthma, infection, or embolism
- Decompression illness (DCI), including both decompression sickness (DCS) and arterial gas embolism (AGE)
- Acute mountain sickness
- High-altitude pulmonary edema (HAPE)
- High-altitude cerebral edema (HACE)
- Carbon monoxide (CO) poisoning
- Respiratory or cardiopulmonary arrest

CONTRAINDICATIONS

In an acutely hypoxic patient, there is no absolute contraindication to administration of supplemental O_2. In patients with severe chronic obstructive disease (COPD), prolonged administration of O_2 may cause hypercapnia, so close monitoring of ventilation is important.

Pulmonary Oxygen Toxicity

- If a high concentration of supplemental O_2 is administered for many hours, pulmonary O_2 toxicity is possible, particularly if a diver with DCI subsequently requires hyperbaric oxygen therapy (HBOT).
- First symptoms of pulmonary O_2 toxicity are caused by tracheobronchitis, which is characterized by substernal burning, chest tightness, and cough.
- Continued exposure may result in dyspnea and adult respiratory distress syndrome (ARDS).
- Pulmonary O_2 toxicity is usually reversible with cessation of O_2 therapy or reduction in inspired concentration.
- In some individuals, continuously breathing 100% O_2 at normal atmospheric pressure (1 atmosphere [atm]) may cause symptoms to appear as soon 6 hours.

BOX 11.1   How to Administer Oxygen in General

1. Place the cylinder upright. Open and close the tank valve slowly ("crack the tank") with a wrench to remove debris from the outlet.
2. Close the tank valve and attach a regulator to the tank. Tighten the regulator to the tank securely by hand. Never use a regulator without the proper oxygen washer. *Never use tape to hold a loose regulator in place.*
   a. Ideally, the depressurized regulator should remain attached to the tank always. This ensures that the equipment is ready to use and free of debris.
3. Open tank valve slowly, one full turn.
4. Attach an O_2 delivery device to the regulator, either to the DISS (diameter index safety system) threaded port or to the constant flow nipple on the end of the regulator. Attach a breathing mask or nasal cannula to the other end of hose or tubing, if it is not already attached.
5. Adjust the constant flow controller to the desired flow rate in liters per minute when using a constant flow mask.
   a. When using a demand-style mask connected to the DISS threaded port, it is not necessary to adjust the flow rate.
   b. A regulator marking of "low" indicates 2 to 4 L/min, "medium" is 4 to 8 L/min, and "high" is 10 to 15 L/min. Flow rate for a nonrebreather mask should be no less than 6 L/min; flow rate for a nasal cannula should be no more than 6 L/min.
   c. To ensure proper oxygenation, the recipient should receive high-flow O_2 (10 to 15 L/min) whenever feasible.
6. Position the mask or cannula on the patient's face. Adjust for comfort. Observe the patient to be certain that the device is tolerated, and that the reservoir bag fills properly.

- Most people can safely breathe O_2 at a fractional inspired concentration (F_{IO_2}) of 1.0 for 12 hours.
- Rate of onset of symptoms can be reduced by using periodic "air breaks," during which the patient breathes air for 5 to 10 minutes.

Central Nervous System Oxygen Toxicity

Central nervous system (CNS) O_2 toxicity can only occur when a person is exposed to O_2 at ambient pressures greater than 1 atm (e.g., while diving underwater or during HBOT in a hyperbaric chamber).

Signs and symptoms of CNS O_2 toxicity are most likely to appear at P_{IO_2} greater than 1.6 and may include:
- Sweating
- Bradycardia
- Mood changes
- Nausea
- Visual field constriction

- Twitching
- Syncope
- Seizures

During HBOT, implementation of periodic 5-minute air breaks reduces the likelihood of CNS O_2 toxicity. Oxygen seizures occur at 1.3 per 10,000 treatments for HBOT at 2.4 atmospheres of air pressure absolute (ATA) (0.7 per 10,000 when hypoglycemic seizures are excluded). With air breaks and a resting patient, treatment with 100% O_2 at almost 3 ATA is possible. If the individual were performing physically exerting exercise (e.g., swimming), such high concentrations would not be safe because it would raise the incidence of oxygen seizures to an unacceptable level.

EQUIPMENT
Cylinders

Medical O_2 cylinders or tanks are made of aluminum or steel and come in a variety of sizes (Table 11.1). In the United States, any pressure vessel that is transported on public roads is subject to US Department of Transportation (DOT) regulations. The DOT requires that cylinders be visually and hydrostatically tested every 5 years and either be destroyed if they fail or be stamped and labeled appropriately if they pass. Gas suppliers will not fill cylinders that have not been appropriately tested and stamped. The working pressure of steel medical O_2 cylinders is 2015 psi (13,893 kPa). The working pressure of aluminum O_2 cylinders is either 2015 psi or 2216 psi (13,893 kPa or 15,279 kPa), depending on the type. High-pressure, lightweight cylinders used for high-altitude climbing are not discussed here.

Cylinders come in two practical field sizes: D (50 cm [20 inches] in length; carries 360 L of oxygen) and E (75 cm [30 inches] in length; carries 625 L of oxygen). Time during which oxygen can be delivered is calculated by dividing tank capacity by flow rate.

Valves

Valves for medical O_2 cylinders sold in the United States are designed to accept only medical O_2 regulators to avoid the possibility of using a medical O_2 regulator with an incompatible gas (e.g., acetylene). Two types of valves are available in the United States: CGA-870 and CGA-540. CGA-870 is also known as the "pin-index" valve and used on smaller, portable cylinders (e.g., D, E). CGA-540 is used primarily on larger, nonportable cylinders (e.g., H, M), such as those mounted in ambulances.

Outside the United States, several other medical O_2 valve types are manufactured and used. Adapters are available to make a US pin-index regulator fit on an Australian bull-nose valve. Using adapters is discouraged by the US Compressed Gas Association (CGA).

Some O_2 cylinders come with built-in O_2 regulators. These cylinders offer simplicity but may limit flow options.

Table 11.1	Common Portable Medical Oxygen Cylinder Specifications					
CYLINDER SIZE	ALLOY	WORKING PRESSURE (PSI)	VOLUME (L, FT³)	LENGTH (CM, INCHES)	DIAMETER (CM, INCHES)	WEIGHT (KG, LB)
M9	Aluminum	2015	8.7, 246.3	27.7, 10.9	11.1, 4.4	1.8, 3.9
D	Aluminum	2015	15, 424.7	41.9, 16.5	11.1, 4.4	2.5, 5.5
D*	Steel	2015	14.5, 410.4	42.5, 16.75	11.1, 4.4	3.4, 7.5
Jumbo D	Aluminum	2216	22.9, 648.3	43.2, 17	13.3, 5.3	4.1, 9.0
E	Aluminum	2015	24, 679.4	65.0, 25.6	11.1, 4.4	3.6, 8.0
E*	Steel	2015	24.1, 682.0	65.4, 25.75	11.1, 4.4	4.8, 10.5

*Steel cylinder specifications provided by Pressed Steel Tank Co.
Note: Aluminum cylinder specifications provided by Luxfer Inc.

Regulators

A regulator functions to reduce peak pressures within the tank to a usable O_2 flow rate. It is typically mounted directly to the cylinder with a compatible valve. A regulator consists of a pressure gauge, pressure-reducing valve, and flowmeter. It reduces the high pressure of the oxygen inside the tank (>2000 psi) to approximately 50 psi and allows delivery at flow rates between 1 and 15 L/min. Regulators are primarily of three types: constant flow only, demand/flow-restricted oxygen-powered ventilator (FROPV) only, or multifunction, which has both constant flow and demand/FROPV capability.

A pressure gauge allows the user to monitor the amount of O_2 in the cylinder. In a tank with a maximum operating pressure of 2000 psi, a reading of 500 psi indicates that there remains one-quarter of the tank's O_2.

Devices for Assisted Ventilation

If a patient is not adequately oxygenating or ventilating, assisted ventilation devices can be used (Box 11.2). When used on a nonintubated patient, these devices all depend on adequate mask seal to ensure optimal O_2 delivery and ventilatory support. Use of a device minimizes direct patient contact and reduces risk for disease transmission. Personal protective equipment (e.g., gloves, goggles) and standard precaution practices should always be employed.

Bag-Valve-Mask Device

A bag-valve-mask (BVM) device consists of a mask, bag, and valves that direct flow of air and O_2. As with the FROPV, different mask sizes can be used to accommodate different faces or be attached directly to an endotracheal tube (ETT). The volume of the bag is 1600 mL in most commercially available models.

- The BVM works best with supplemental O_2 but will function on room air if O_2 supply is depleted.
- The BVM requires training and practice to use effectively. Even with proper training, it is difficult to maintain adequate mask seal, maintain airway patency, and ventilate sufficient volumes (600 to 1000 mL) when only one rescuer is available.

BOX 11.2   Preferences for Ventilating a Person in Respiratory Arrest

1. Bag-valve-mask unit with two rescuers and supplemental O_2
2. Resuscitation mask with supplemental O_2
3. Flow-restricted oxygen-powered ventilator
4. Bag-valve-mask unit with one rescuer and supplemental O_2
5. Mouth-to-mouth ventilation is the last choice and not an option for professional rescuers because of the risk for disease transmission

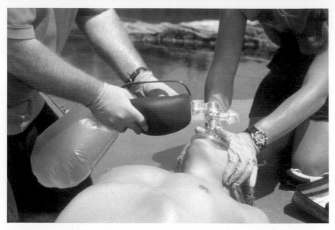

FIGURE 11.1 Bag-valve-mask devices deliver 100% oxygen and are best used with two rescuers. This device is ideal in wilderness settings because it provides adequate ventilation even without an oxygen source.

- The BVM should be used first with two rescuers (one maintaining mask seal and patency of the airway, the other squeezing the bag Fig. 11.1).
  To use a BVM:
1. Attach the O_2 tubing from the BVM to the constant flow barbed outlet on the O_2 regulator. Expand the bag (which is often stored collapsed).
2. Set the constant flow controller to 10 to 15 L/min.
3. Establish airway patency by direct visualization. Suction or manually clear as able.
4. Position one rescuer at the patient's head to maintain the airway and ensure mask seal.
   a. The second rescuer should ventilate the patient by squeezing the bag with both hands. Gentle, steady force on the bag should result in chest rise.
   b. If excessive force on the bag is required, or chest does not rise, have the first rescuer reassess airway patency. Reposition mask and airway. Attempt to ventilate again.
   c. If ventilation remains inadequate, check for airway obstruction; consider using an airway adjunct (e.g., nasopharyngeal airway, oral airway) and initiating an airway obstruction protocol.
5. Ventilations should last 1 second as part of cardiopulmonary resuscitation (CPR).
6. Alternate 30 chest compressions with two ventilations, or ventilate with uninterrupted compressions at a rate of 10 breaths/min.
7. Ventilate with sufficient speed and force to make the patient's lower chest and upper abdomen rise.
8. It is not necessary to empty the bag with each ventilation.

Resuscitation Mask

A pocket-type resuscitation mask is a clear, flexible plastic mask designed to fit over the patient's mouth and nose while the health care provider ventilates by exhaling forcefully through the "chimney." Typically, a one-way valve directs the rescuer's breath into the patient while directing the patient's exhaled breath away from the rescuer. This simple device requires minimal training and is lightweight, easily packed, and available both with and without an outlet for supplemental O_2.

When using the pocket-style resuscitation mask to deliver O_2:

1. Remove the O_2 tubing from a nonrebreather mask.
2. Stretch out the hose to be certain there are no kinks.
3. Attach the O_2 tubing to the constant flow barbed outlet on the O_2 regulator.
4. Connect the other end of the tubing to the O_2 inlet on the resuscitation mask.
5. Set the constant flow controller to 10 to 15 L/min.
6. The rescuer should ensure a proper mask seal by positioning the mask over the patient's mouth and nose, lifting the jaw up into the mask.
7. The rescuer should inhale away from the mask and then breathe into the one-way valve on the mask to make the patient's lower chest and upper abdomen rise.
8. Ventilations should last 1 second as part of CPR.
9. Alternate 30 chest compressions with two ventilations.
    a. If the ventilations do not go in, reposition the patient's airway.
    b. If the ventilations still do not go in, check for airway obstruction, and initiate an airway obstruction protocol.

Flow-Restricted Oxygen-Powered Ventilator/Positive-Pressure Demand Valve

Older-style positive-pressure demand valves (PPDVs), such as the LSP 063-05 or Elder CPR Demand valve, function both in positive-pressure mode (pushing the button to ventilate a nonbreathing patient) and demand mode.

It is a misconception that a PPDV will easily cause pulmonary overpressurization injury; this valve has fallen out of favor with some health care providers. In positive-pressure mode, all PPDVs manufactured in the United States have an overpressure relief valve that stops the flow of gas at 55 to 65 cm H_2O (a pressure at which lung overpressurization is unlikely). MTV-100 FROPV (LSP/Allied) has two overpressure-relief valves, the first set at 60 cm H_2O and the second at 65 to 80 cm H_2O.

A mask adapter is a standard 15-mm fitting that fits a variety of masks and can also be used directly with an ETT. A FROPV requires a supply of pressurized O_2.

When using an FROPV:

1. Connect the FROPV to the DISS threaded port on the O_2 regulator.

2. It is not necessary to adjust the O_2 flow rate on the regulator.
3. Position one rescuer at the patient's head to maintain the airway and ensure a mask seal.
4. The second rescuer should ventilate the patient by depressing the button on the FROPV.
5. The second rescuer should also place a second hand on the patient's upper abdomen and lower chest to monitor chest rise.
6. Ventilations should last 1 second as part of CPR.
7. Alternate 30 chest compressions with two ventilations.
   a. If the ventilations do not go in, have the first rescuer reposition the patient's airway.
   b. If the ventilations still do not go in, check for airway obstruction, and initiate an airway obstruction protocol.

Demand-Only, or Flow-Restricted Oxygen-Powered Ventilators in Demand Mode

Use of demand mode requires spontaneous respirations. To use in demand mode, hold the mask to the patient's face. Negative pressure of inhalation opens the valve and then gas flows. Flow stops when the person stops inhaling, like other demand systems, such as scuba and aviation regulators. This is the first choice for O_2 delivery when there is critical need for a high concentration of inspired O_2 or gas supplies are limited.

When using a demand-only valve:
1. Connect the demand valve to the DISS threaded port on the O_2 regulator.
2. It is not necessary to adjust the O_2 flow rate on the regulator.
3. Ask the patient to breathe normally from the mask.
4. Monitor the patient to ensure breathing.
5. Watch the clear mask to make sure it fogs with each exhalation.
6. If the patient is not conscious or is breathing adequately to activate the demand-only valve, it is necessary to switch to a constant flow delivery device, such as the nonrebreather mask.

Constant Flow Devices for Adequately Breathing Patients
Nonrebreather Mask

A nonrebreather mask consists of a mask, reservoir bag, and series of one-way valves, one separating reservoir from the mask and others on the sides of the mask.

When using a nonrebreather mask:
1. Open the nonrebreather mask packaging; stretch out the tubing to make sure there are no kinks.
2. Connect the tubing on the nonrebreather mask to the constant flow, barbed outlet on the O_2 regulator.
3. Set the constant flow controller to 10 to 15 L/min.
4. Place a thumb over the one-way valve between the mask and the reservoir bag.

5. Allow the bag to fill completely before placing the mask on the patient.
6. Position the mask over the patient's mouth and nose.
7. Pinch the nose clip over the patient's nose.
8. Pull on the elastic straps to tighten the mask to the patient's face, and pull the skin into the mask.
9. Ask the patient to breathe normally from the mask.
10. Monitor the patient to ensure breathing.
11. Watch the clear mask to make sure it fogs with each exhalation.

Nasal Cannula

A nasal cannula may be used when a patient will not tolerate a mask or when high inspired O_2 concentrations are not required. A nasal cannula delivers Fio_2 of only 0.24 to 0.29.

Flow rates for a nasal cannula are limited to 1 to 6 L/min for extended durations. Flow rates exceeding 6 L/min for long periods of time are uncomfortable and may result in drying of the nasal mucosa. Limited use of flow rates exceeding 6 L/min up to greater than 15 L/min may be effective for passive, or apneic oxygenation during the peri-intubation period.

When using a nasal cannula:
1. Open the cannula packaging; stretch out the tubing to make sure there are no kinks.
2. Connect the tubing to the constant flow, barbed outlet on the O_2 regulator.
3. Set the constant flow controller to 4 to 6 L/min.
4. Position the prongs in the patient's nostrils.
5. Position the hose behind the patient's head and tighten the straps.
6. Ask the patient to breathe normally through the nose.
7. Monitor the patient.
8. If oxygen supplies are limited, titrate O_2 flow to improved symptoms. At high altitude, maintain O_2 saturation above 90% to 92%.

Oxygen Rebreathers

Rebreather devices are designed to reuse exhaled O_2-rich air, and remove CO_2 and exchange it for additional oxygen. Rebreather devices all have the same basic components: mask, breathing circuit (like anesthesia equipment), and canister with an absorbent chemical, usually soda lime. Soda lime chemically removes CO_2 from the exhaled gas, allowing O_2 to be rebreathed. Supplemental O_2 is added at approximately 1 L/min to replace metabolized O_2. Using this system, an O_2 tank that would supply a nonrebreather mask for 45 minutes, or an on-demand device for approximately 1 hour, can provide a patient an Fio_2 of 0.85 to 0.99 for more than 8 hours.

Rebreather devices require significant training and contain parts (typically the breathing circuit and absorbent canister) that are often single-patient use. Adequate mask seal is required to function effectively; otherwise, dilution of inhaled gas with air results in a lower FIO_2. Compared with a constant flow mask, increased breathing resistance may be experienced.

Emergency Oxygen Administration at High Altitude

Atmospheric pressure and partial pressure of oxygen (PO_2) decrease with altitude. Oxygen can be used to treat high-altitude pulmonary or cerebral edema. Definitive treatment is descent to a lower altitude. Supplemental O_2 is indicated if it will not delay descent, or if immediate descent is not possible. Increased partial pressure of available O_2 is achieved by increasing the O_2 concentration or increasing the barometric pressure.

Many climbers use O_2 when climbing above 8000 m (26,247 ft). O_2 sets for climbing, typically continuous flow open circuits with rebreather reservoirs, are suitable for emergency O_2 delivery. Portable hyperbaric chambers that increase barometric pressure and therefore available O_2 are used to treat various high-altitude syndromes.

Oxygen Generator Systems

Oxygen generators produce O_2 using a chemical process. O_2 concentrators typically use electrical power and are not readily portable for field use. These devices often produce 3 to 4 L/min over a 15-minute cycle, with a peak flow of up to 6 L. Although insufficient for some emergency needs, these rates can be employed to fill an O_2 cylinder to operational pressure. In established remote clinics with electrical supply, O_2 generators provide abundant O_2 stores without need for distant and costly resupply.

HAZARDS

Oxygen does not burn, but it greatly accelerates combustion. Concentrated O_2 facilitates conversion of sparks or embers (e.g., lit cigarettes) into vigorous fires. O_2 should only be used in open, well-ventilated areas and never in the presence of burning materials. Use care when handling O_2 equipment to avoid allowing contaminants (e.g., petroleum products) to come in or around the orifices on the cylinder or regulator through which O_2 flows. Cylinders should not be exposed to temperatures above 52°C (125°F).

Trauma Emergencies: Assessment and Stabilization

ESTABLISHING PRIORITIES

There are three immediate priorities in managing wilderness trauma:

1. *Control oneself.* It is normal to feel anxious when confronted with an injured patient. However, anxiety must not be transmitted to the patient or other members of the expedition team.

2. *Control the situation.* Ensure the safety of uninjured members of the party. Expeditious evacuation of a patient requires that all expedition members function at maximal efficiency; even minor injuries to other members in the group can jeopardize physical strength, functional manpower, and success of the evacuation. Although the physician member of the team may not be the expedition leader, their position is automatically elevated during a medical crisis. However, this does not mean that the medical provider should dominate the evacuation process. Although the expedition leader must rely on the medical assessment provided by the medical provider, the leader is best prepared to plan the evacuation.

3. *Obtain an overview of the situation.* The patient's general condition should be evaluated. Is the patient in immediate distress from a condition that requires relatively straightforward management, such as airway control? Is the patient in such a precarious environmental situation that he or she needs to be moved prior to any attempt at resuscitation? Scene security may be integral to safety of the injured person and caregiver. Is the patient properly protected from the elements, including sun, wind, cold, and water?

BASIC PRINCIPLES OF WILDERNESS TRAUMA MANAGEMENT

1. *Primary survey:* Rapidly identify immediate life threats to the patient by assessing "ABCDE"—airway; breathing; circulation; disability and neurologic status, including possible cervical spine injury; and environmental exposure.

2. *Resuscitation:* Stabilize any conditions discovered during the primary survey.

3. *Secondary survey:* Complete a basic medical history and head-to-toe examination of the patient to discover all injuries.

4. *Definitive plan:* Create a treatment and evacuation plan for the patient.

5. *Packaging and transfer preparation:* Protect the patient from environmental exposure, and evacuate the patient or prepare for rescue assistance.

UNIVERSAL PRECAUTIONS IN THE WILDERNESS

Every victim in the wilderness must be assumed to carry a communicable disease, and every effort should therefore be made to approximate universal precautions, particularly protection of the hands and eyes. The Centers for Disease Control and Prevention have established a set of standard precautions to be applied in all cases of contact with human body fluids, which may need to be improvised in a wilderness setting.

- Goggles (alternatively ski goggles, sunglasses)
- Gloves (alternatively insulating gloves or plastic bags)
- Fluid-impervious gowns (alternatively rain jacket and pants)
- Shoe covers and fluid-impervious leggings
- Mask (alternatively bandana or buff)
- Head covering (alternatively hat)

PRIMARY SURVEY

The focus of the primary survey is to identify immediately life-threatening injuries based on the mechanisms of injury, vital signs, and treatment priorities. Even if monitoring equipment, such as blood pressure and oxygen saturation monitors, is unavailable, use observation to regularly assess the patient's mental status, heart rate, respiratory rate, and skin temperature and color.

Assess the Scene

1. Ensure the safety of noninjured members of the party.
2. Assess the scene for further hazards such as falling rocks, avalanche, and dangerous animals before rendering first-aid care.
3. Avoid approaching the patient from directly above if falling rock or a snowslide is possible.
4. Do not allow your sense of urgency to transform an accident into a risky and foolish rescue attempt.

Airway

1. If the patient is unresponsive, immediately determine if they are breathing.
   a. If the patient's position prevents adequate assessment of the airway, roll the patient onto the back as a single unit, supporting the head and neck (Fig. 12.1).
   b. Place your ear and cheek close to the patient's mouth and nose to detect air movement while looking for movement of the chest and abdomen (Fig. 12.2). In cold weather, look for a vapor cloud and feel for warm air movement.
2. If no movement of air is detected, clean out the mouth with your fingers and use the chin lift (Fig. 12.3) or jaw thrust technique to open the airway.
   a. Perform the jaw thrust by kneeling with your knees on either side of the patient's head, placing your hands on either side of the patient's mandible, and pushing the base of the jaw up and forward (Fig. 12.4).

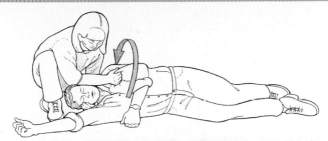

FIGURE 12.1   One-Person Roll.

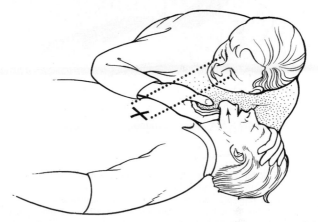

FIGURE 12.2   Listening for breathing and watching for movement of chest and abdomen.

b. Note that the jaw thrust and chin lift techniques are labor intensive and occupy your hands. If you are alone and the situation is critical, you can establish a temporary airway by pinning the anterior aspect of the patient's tongue to the lower lip with a safety pin (see Fig. 10.5), noting that this can result in significant bleeding and is perceived by some observers as a maneuver of last resort. An alternative to puncturing the lower lip is to pass a string or shoelace through the safety pin and hold traction on the tongue by securing the other end to the patient's shirt button or jacket zipper (see Fig. 10.6).

3. Adjunctive devices, such as oropharyngeal and nasopharyngeal airways, can be useful to maintain a patient's airway (see Chapter 10). These, however, do not constitute a definitive airway and do not protect against aspiration of saliva or emesis.

4. Patients who have an unprotected airway due to altered level of consciousness, or require positive pressure ventilation, may

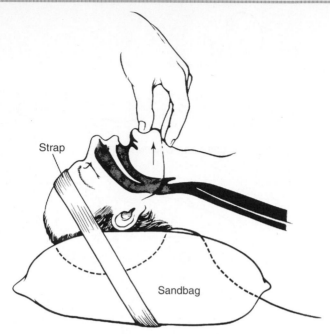

FIGURE 12.3 Chin Lift. This procedure optimally uses two rescuers. One person stabilizes the patient's neck. The other person opens the patient's airway using the thumb to grasp the patient's chin just below the lower lip, while fingers of the same hand are placed underneath the patient's anterior mandible and the chin is gently lifted.

require assisted ventilation. This may be accomplished with a pocket mask, supraglottic device (such as a laryngeal mask airway or King airway device), or endotracheal intubation (see Chapter 10).

5. If an unstable patient is unable to be oxygenated or ventilated through the nose or mouth due to an obstructed upper airway or severe facial trauma, a cricothyroidotomy may need to be performed (also see Chapter 10).

   a. Locate the cricothyroid membrane by palpating the patient's neck, starting at the top. The first and largest prominence felt will be the thyroid cartilage ("Adam's apple"); the second felt is the cricoid cartilage (below the thyroid cartilage). The small space between these two, noted by a small depression, is the cricothyroid membrane (Fig. 12.5A).

   b. With the patient lying on his or her back, cleanse the neck around the cricothyroid membrane with an antiseptic.

   c. Put on protective gloves. Make a vertical 2.5-cm (1-inch) incision through the skin with a knife over the membrane

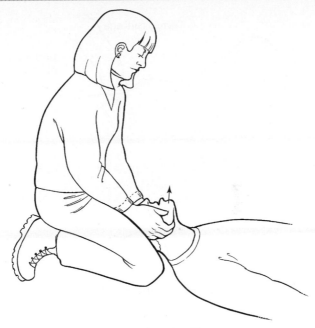

FIGURE 12.4   Jaw Thrust.

(go a little bit above and below the membrane) while using the fingers of your other hand to pry the skin edges apart. Anticipate bleeding from the wound (see Fig. 12.5B and C).

d. After the skin is incised, puncture the membrane by stabbing it with your knife or other pointed object.

e. Stabilize the larynx between the fingers of one hand, and insert an improvised cricothyrotomy tube (Box 12.1) through the membrane with your other hand while aiming caudally (toward the buttocks). Secure the object in place with tape. You can also insert the improvised tube through the tape before placing it through the cricothyroid membrane.

Complications associated with this procedure include hemorrhage at the insertion site, subcutaneous or mediastinal emphysema caused by faulty placement of the tube into the subcutaneous tissues rather than into the trachea, and perforation through the posterior wall of the trachea with placement of the tube in the esophagus.

Breathing and Ventilation

Expose the patient's chest, and assess for chest wall movement, breath sounds, and signs of breathing, such as condensation of water vapor emanating from the nose and mouth. If the patient is

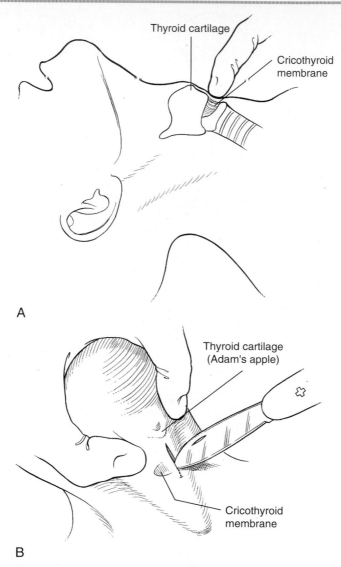

FIGURE 12.5   Cricothyroidotomy (Cricothyrotomy). A, Locate the cricothyroid membrane in the depression between the thyroid cartilage (Adam's apple) and the cricoid cartilage. **B,** Make a vertical 1-cm (0.4-inch) incision through the skin.

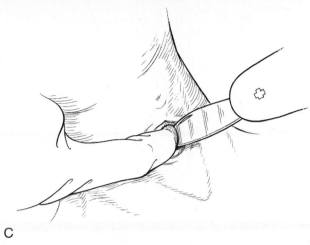

C

FIGURE 12.5, cont'd   C, Locate the cricothyroid membrane with a gloved finger, and puncture it with the tip of a knife or other pointed object.

BOX 12.1 Improvised Cricothyrotomy Tubes

1. *Syringe barrel:* Cut the barrel of a 1- or 3-mL syringe with the plunger removed at a 45-degree angle at its midpoint. The proximal flange of the syringe barrel helps secure the device to the neck and prevents it from being aspirated (Fig. 12.6).
2. *IV administration set drip chamber:* Cut the plastic drip chamber of a macrodrip (15 drops/mL) IV administration set at its halfway point with a knife or scissors. Remove the end protector from the piercing spike and insert the spike into the cricothyroid membrane. The plastic drip chamber is nearly the same size as a 15-mm (0.6-inch) endotracheal tube adapter and fits snugly in the valve fitting of a bag-valve device (Fig. 12.7).
3. *Any small hollow object:* Examples include a small flashlight or penlight casing, pen casing, small pill bottle, and large-bore needle or IV catheter. Several commercial devices are available that are small and sufficiently lightweight to be included in the first-aid kit.

---

not adequately breathing, you may need to provide rescue breaths (see Chapters 10 and 11). If the patient demonstrates tachypnea, dyspnea, resonant hemithorax, absence of breath sounds, asymmetric chest movement, hypotension, or hypoxia, the patient may have a tension pneumothorax. Treatment of a hemodynamically unstable patient with a tension pneumothorax is needle decompression (Box 12.2).

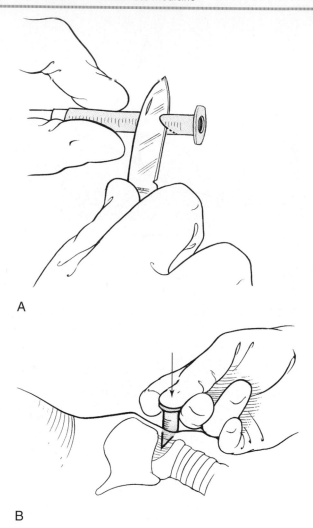

A

B

FIGURE 12.6 A and **B,** Cut the barrel of a syringe at a 45-degree angle, and insert the pointed end through the membrane.

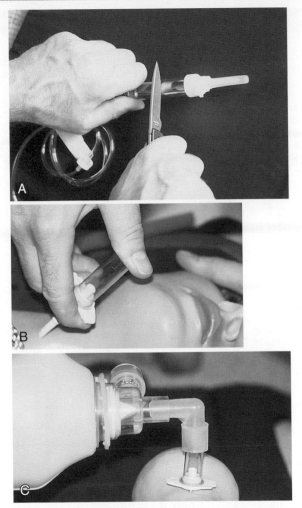

FIGURE 12.7   A, Cut the plastic drip chamber at its halfway point. **B,** Insert the spike from the drip chamber into the cricothyroid membrane. **C,** The bag-valve device will fit over the chamber for ventilation.

BOX 12.2   Needle Decompression of a Tension Pneumothorax

1. Expose the chest.
2. Insert a large (16–14 gauge) IV catheter or long needle (>5 cm [2 inches]) directly above the third rib into the second intercostal space until the pneumothorax is decompressed. This is often accompanied by a release ("rush") of air.
3. Alternatively, you can place the IV catheter or needle directly above the sixth rib in the fifth intercostal space in the axillary line at the traditional site for a thoracostomy tube (Fig. 12.8).
4. If an IV catheter is used, advance the catheter over the needle and leave it in place as you withdraw the needle.

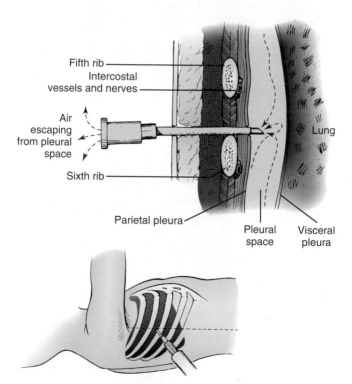

FIGURE 12.8   Needle decompression of a tension pneumothorax.

Circulation

In the event of active bleeding or hemodynamic instability (heart rate >100 beats/min, no palpable arterial pulse, altered mental status), bleeding should be immediately controlled, and if possible, vascular or osseous access obtained. Initial boluses of crystalloid fluid should be given in an amount of 1 to 2 L in adults, or 20 mL/kg initially, and up to 60 mL/kg in children. Recommendations for fluid administration resuscitation protocols are in evolution, so they should be reviewed by clinicians regularly.

External Bleeding

1. Carefully check the patient for signs of profuse bleeding. Be sure to feel inside any bulky clothing and check underneath the patient for signs of bleeding.
2. Control bleeding with direct pressure.
3. Hemostatic dressings, such as HemCon and QuickClot, can be applied directly to the site of bleeding and are lightweight and useful for stopping difficult to control bleeding.
4. Apply a tourniquet only as a last resort when bleeding cannot be stopped by direct pressure.
   a. A tourniquet is a band applied directly on the skin around an extremity so tightly that all blood flow distal to the site is stopped.
   b. Rescue teams should carry and apply commercially available tourniquets, such as the Combat Application Tourniquet (CAT) and Special Operations Forces Tourniquet (SOFT).
   c. Tourniquets can be improvised from clothing, towels, or tent material (Box 12.3).
   d. If the tourniquet is left on for more than 3 to 6 hours, tissue distal to the tourniquet may die and the extremity may require amputation.
   e. The tourniquet may be loosened every 60 minutes to see if pressure alone will staunch the bleeding. However, this should be done with extreme caution, because there is always the risk that when a tourniquet is released, there will be significant blood loss.
5. In a healthcare setting, consider tranexamic acid (TXA).
   a. Loading dose is 1000 mg in 100 mL of 0.9% NaCl infused IV over 10 minutes.
   b. Maintenance is 1000 mg in 500 mL of 0.9% NaCl infused IV over 8 hours.

Internal Bleeding

Life-threatening internal bleeding can occur in the chest, abdomen, pelvis, retroperitoneum, and thighs.
1. Avoid unnecessary movement of the patient.
2. Splint all fractured extremities.
3. Apply traction to a femur fracture (see Chapter 18).

BOX 12.3 How to Apply a Tourniquet

1. Tourniquet material should be wide and flat to prevent crushing tissue. Use a firm bandage, belt, or strap 7.5–10 cm (3–4 inches) wide that will not stretch. Never use wire, rope, or any material that will cut the skin.
2. Wrap the bandage snugly around the extremity several times as close above the wound as possible, and tie an overhand knot.
3. Place a stick or similar object on the knot, and tie another overhand knot over the stick (Fig. 12.9A).
4. Twist the stick until the bandage becomes tight enough to stop the bleeding. Tie or tape the stick in place to prevent it from unraveling (see Fig. 12.9B).
5. Mark the patient with a "TK" where it cannot be missed, and note the time the tourniquet was applied.
6. If you are more than an hour from medical care, loosen the tourniquet very slowly at the end of 60 min, while maintaining direct pressure on the wound. If bleeding is again heavy, retighten the tourniquet. If bleeding is now manageable with direct pressure alone, leave the tourniquet in place but do not tighten it again unless severe bleeding starts.

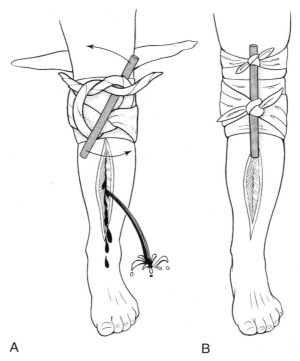

A   B

FIGURE 12.9 Applying a tourniquet. A, Place a stick or similar object on the knot and tie another overhand knot over the stick. **B,** Twist the stick until the bandage becomes tight enough to stop the bleeding. Tie or tape the stick in place to prevent it from unraveling.

BOX 12.4 Applying an Improvised Pelvic Sling

1. Ensure that objects have been removed from the patient's pockets and that any belt has been removed so that pressure of the sheet or object does not cause discomfort by pressing items against the pelvis.
2. Gently slide the improvised material under the patient's buttocks, and center it under the bony prominences of the hips (greater trochanters) (Fig. 12.10A).
3. Cross the object over the front of the pelvis, and tighten the sling by pulling both ends and securing with a knot, clamp, or duct tape (see Fig. 12.10B and C).
4. Another tightening technique is to wrap the sling snugly around the pelvis and tie an overhand knot. Place tent posts, a stick, or similar object on the knot, and tie another overhand knot. Twist the poles or stick until the sling becomes tight.
5. If a Therm-a-Rest pad or other inflatable sleeping pad is available, fold it in half so that it approximates the size of the pelvis. Gently slide the pad under the patient's buttocks, and center it under the greater trochanters and symphysis pubis. Secure the pad with duct tape, then inflate the pad as you would normally until it produces a snug fit.

---

4. Apply a circumferential compression pelvic sling to a pelvic fracture (Box 12.4). There are manufactured devices available, such as the SAM Pelvic Sling (see Fig. 18.23), or a sling can be improvised from available materials (see Fig. 18.24).
   a. Unstable pelvic fractures are associated with significant blood loss.
   b. Pelvic reduction and stabilization in the early posttraumatic phase will mitigate venous hemorrhage.
   c. Clothes, sheets, a sleeping bag, pads, air mattress, tent, or tent fly can be used to improvise an effective pelvic sling in the backcountry. The object should be wide enough so that it does not cut into the patient when tightened.

VASCULAR ACCESS

Obtaining vascular access is a basic tenet of trauma care. Many rescue reams carry vascular access supplies. If available, initial access should be attempted with two large-bore IVs in the antecubital fossae. The external jugular (EJ) vein or lower extremity veins can be used as an alternative. Often in trauma, however, IV access is difficult due to hypovolemia, hypothermia, or shock physiology.

Intraosseous (IO) fluid and medication administration is an acceptable alternative to IV. There are numerous IO devices, ranging from simple needle kits to battery operated IO drills (i.e., EZ-IO device). If peripheral IV access is not obtained after two attempts, consider IO placement if available.

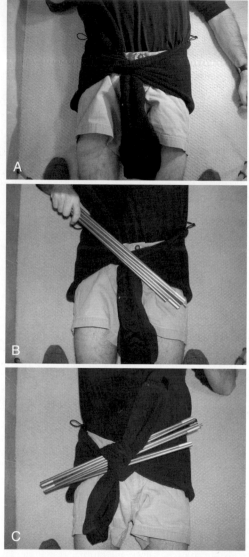

FIGURE 12.10   Improvised pelvic sling. A, Gently slide the improvised material under the patient's buttocks and center it under the bony prominences of the hips (greater trochanters). **B** and **C,** Cross the object over the front of the pelvis and tighten the sling by pulling both ends and securing with a knot, clamp, or duct tape.

Cardiopulmonary Resuscitation and Circulation (See Also Chapter 25)

If a trauma patient is pulseless and apneic, cardiopulmonary resuscitation (CPR) is not likely to be successful unless the patient has a tension pneumothorax that can be relieved. Efforts should be focused on identifying and treating reversible causes of cardiopulmonary arrest. A short period of CPR (10 to 15 minutes, unless the patient is hypothermic) is recommended.

Disability and Neurologic Assessment

1. Neurologic assessment during the primary survey should be rapid and efficient.
2. Establish the level of consciousness (alert, responds to verbal stimuli, responds to painful stimuli only, or unresponsive).
3. Assess bilateral pupil size and reactivity.
4. Assess the Glasgow Coma Scale (GCS; see Appendix B) or other repeatable scale for neurologic function.
5. Deterioration in mental status is a poor prognostic sign. Patients with a suspected head injury or abnormal GCS should be reevaluated every hour for status changes.

Cervical Spine

1. Initiate and maintain spine immobilization if a spinal injury is suspected after trauma with a concerning mechanism for severe multisystem trauma (Table 12.1).
2. Any patient with neurologic signs or symptoms suspected of having a spinal injury should receive full immobilization.
3. Many patients with minor trauma, no midline neck pain, and a normal neurologic examination may be transported in a position of comfort.
4. Patients with mild to moderate trauma and a normal neurologic examination but with midline neck pain should be transported supine on a gurney or vacuum mattress with or without support.
5. If a cervical spine injury is suspected, immobilize the patient's head and neck and prevent any movement of the torso (Box 12.5).
6. Avoid moving the patient with a suspected spinal injury if they are in a safe location. The patient will likely benefit from organized rescue and evacuation.

Exposure and Environmental Control

1. The victim should be fully undressed and exposed, if possible in a protected environment.
2. Garments and gear should be removed if necessary by cutting them away, unless the garments can be dried and are essential for future protection from the environment.
3. Wet clothing must be removed early to prevent hypothermia.
4. Cover the patient immediately after removal of clothing. Hypothermia and its effects on mental status, cardiovascular function,

Table 12.1 Recommendations for Field Spinal Immobilization

Spinal Immobilization Chart—Trauma

	NO MIDLINE NECK PAIN/TENDERNESS	MIDLINE NECK PAIN/TENDERNESS	NEUROLOGIC SIGNS/SYMPTOMS	ALTERED MENTAL STATUS
Ambulatory	Position of comfort	Gurney—position of comfort with/without support	Full	Position of Comfort
Non-ambulatory	Position of comfort	Gurney—position of comfort with/without support	Full	Full
Severe multisystem trauma	Full	Full	Full	Full

BOX 12.5   Immobilization Aids

Cervical Collar
The cervical collar is always viewed as an adjunct to full spinal immobilization and is preferentially not used alone.

Properly applied and fitted, the cervical collar is primarily a defense against axial spine loading, particularly in an evacuation that involves tilting the patient's body uphill or downhill.

After the collar is placed around the neck, secure plastic bags, stuffed sacks, socks filled with sand or dirt, or rolled-up towels and clothing on either side of the head and neck to prevent any lateral movement.

SAM Splint Cervical Collar (Fig. 12.11)
Create a bend in the SAM Splint approximately 15 cm (6 inches) from the end of the splint. This bend will form the anterior post. Next, create flares for the mandible. Apply the anterior post underneath the chin, and bring the remainder of the splint around the neck. Take up circumferential slack by creating lateral posts. Finally, squeeze the back to create a posterior post and secure with tape.

Closed-Cell Foam System
Fold the pad longitudinally into thirds, and center it over the back of the patient's neck. Wrap the pad around the neck and under

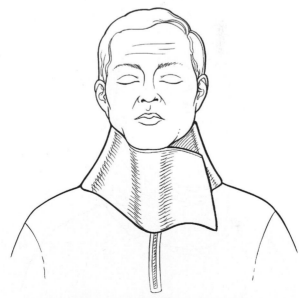

FIGURE 12.11   SAM Splint cervical collar.

BOX 12.5 Immobilization Aids—cont'd

the chin. If the pad is not long enough, tape or tie on extensions (Fig. 12.12).

Blankets, beach towels, or a rolled plastic tarp can be used in a similar manner. Avoid small, flexible cervical collars that do not optimally extend the chin-to-chest distance.

Padded Hip Belt
Remove the padded hip belt from a large internal- or external-frame backpack, and modify it to function as a cervical collar. Diminish the width by overlapping the belt and securing the excess material with duct tape.

Clothing
Use bulky clothing as a collar.

Prewrap a wide, elastic ("Ace-type") bandage around a jacket to help compress the material and make it more rigid and supportive.

Spine Boards
Internal-Frame Pack/Snow Shovel System
Modify an internal-frame backpack by inserting a snow shovel through the center-line attachment points (the shovel's handgrip may need to be removed first).

Tape the patient's head to the lightly padded shovel, which serves as a head bed.

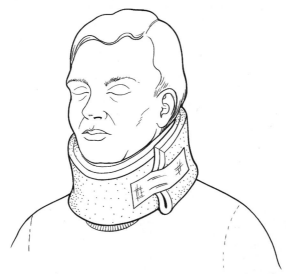

FIGURE 12.12 Ensolite pad used as a cervical collar.

BOX 12.5   Immobilization Aids—cont'd

Use the remainder of the pack suspension system to secure the shoulders and torso as if the patient were wearing the pack.

Inverted Pack System
Make an efficient short board using an inverted internal- or external-frame backpack.

Use the padded hip belt as a head bed and the frame as a short board in conjunction with a cervical collar (Fig. 12.13).

Snowshoe System
Make a snowshoe into an improvised short board.
Be sure to pad the snowshoe first.

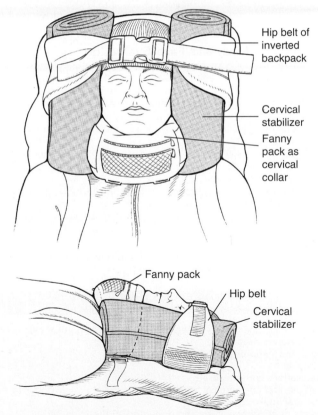

Hip belt of inverted backpack

Cervical stabilizer

Fanny pack as cervical collar

Fanny pack

Hip belt

Cervical stabilizer

FIGURE 12.13   Inverted pack used as a spine board.

and coagulation are among the most underappreciated entities in care of the trauma victim.

5. Assessment of an area of injury should be performed, but clothing should be left to cover the patient to ensure that the body temperature is maintained.

SECONDARY SURVEY

After the primary survey is complete, perform a comprehensive head-to-toe examination of the patient. Begin with examination of the head, and move in a systematic fashion through a more detailed examination of the face, neck, chest, abdomen, pelvis, extremities, and skin.

History

The patient's brief medical history should be assessed during the secondary survey. Consider the SAMPLE history mnemonic (Box 12.6) for this purpose. Knowledge of the mechanism of injury and any comorbidities or allergies may enhance understanding of the patient's physiologic state.

Neurologic, Head, and Face Evaluation

1. Estimate the GCS or another neurologic status scoring system (if not done in the primary survey), and repeat at a minimum hourly if initially abnormal and circumstances permit.
2. Perform a more detailed examination, searching for focal neurologic deficits.
   a. Sensory defects follow the general dermatome patterns shown in Fig. 12.14.
   b. Changes in reflexes not accompanied by altered mental status do not mandate evacuation unless the patient also has a spinal cord injury.
3. Palpate the scalp thoroughly, seeking tenderness, depressions, and lacerations.
   a. Immediately evacuate any patient with suspected depressed skull fracture or basilar skull fracture accompanied by penetrating scalp trauma.
   b. Administer a broad-spectrum antibiotic for suspected skull fractures or penetrating head injuries.

BOX 12.6   SAMPLE History Mnemonic

The SAMPLE mnemonic is a useful way to remember pertinent elements of the trauma history:
Signs and symptoms
Allergies
Medications currently used
Past medical and surgical history
Last oral intake
Events or environment leading or related to the injury

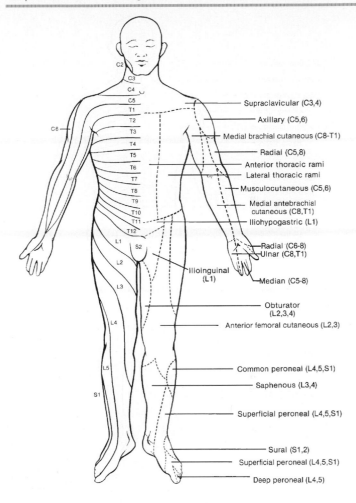

Dermatomes—anterior

FIGURE 12.14 Dermatome pattern of skin area stimulated by spinal cord elements. Sensory deficits follow general dermatome patterns.

Continued

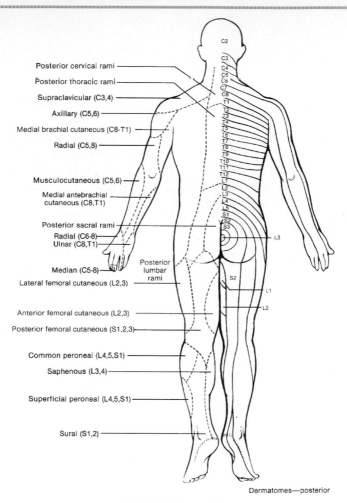

Dermatomes—posterior

FIGURE 12.14, cont'd

c. Do not remove any impaling foreign bodies piercing the head or neck. Pad and secure these to prevent motion that would cause further injury.

Evaluation of the Body

1. Undress the patient sufficiently to perform a proper head-to-toe examination. Keep in mind the weather conditions and appropriate concern for patient modesty. Check for a medical information bracelet or tag and in the patient's wallet or pack for a medical identification card.

2. Have the patient attempt to move any body part suspected of injury before you move it. If the patient resists because of pain or weakness, you should suspect a fracture or spinal cord injury. Never force the patient to move.
3. Examine the patient's skin for sweating and color, while locating injuries such as bruises, rashes, burns, bites, or lacerations. Check inside the patient's lower eyelids for pale color, which can indicate anemia or internal hemorrhage. Note abnormal skin temperature.
4. Examine the chest, watching the patient breathe to see if the chest expands completely and equally on both sides. Examine the chest wall for tenderness and deformities or foreign objects. Auscultate for breath sounds.
5. Gently press all areas of the back and abdomen to find areas of tenderness. Examine the buttocks and genitals.
6. Examine the patient's bony structure. Gently press on the chest, pelvis, arms, and legs to reveal areas of tenderness. Run your fingers down the length of the clavicles and press where they join the sternum. Evaluate the integrity of each rib, and observe for areas of deformation or discoloration.
7. Measure the patient's temperature.
8. Record all findings of your examination.

13 | Shock

DEFINITION
Shock is a life-threatening condition in which blood flow and oxygen delivery to body tissue are inadequate. This can be caused by inadequate blood volume, inadequate arterial pressure, or inadequate heart function to circulate blood.

The priorities are to stabilize the patient, control bleeding, and arrange for immediate transport to definitive medical care.

DISORDERS
Box 13.1 outlines the types of shock.

Signs and Symptoms
- Pale, cool, and diaphoretic skin
- Erythematous and warm skin may be present in septic shock
- Decreased pulse pressure
- Capillary refill greater than 4 seconds
- Tachycardia
- Tachypnea
- Decreased urine output
- Hypotension
- Altered mental status (anxiety, confusion, combativeness, restlessness)
- Unresponsiveness

Treatment
As there may be little the rescuer can do little in the field, recognition of shock is important so that transportation to a medical facility is not delayed.

1. Keep the patient lying supine. If the patient experiences dyspnea because of heart failure and pulmonary edema, raise the shoulders or, if tolerated, support in a sitting position.
2. Elevate the legs only if bleeding is controlled and there is no concern for spinal cord injury. This may transiently improve cardiac output in noncardiogenic shock.
   a. You can elevate the legs by allowing the patient to recline with the feet uphill.
   b. If the patient has internal bleeding, avoid any unnecessary movement.
   c. With pulmonary edema, the patient may be more comfortable with the head and shoulders raised slightly.
3. Do not elevate the patient's legs if there is a severe head injury, difficulty breathing, a broken leg, neck or back injury, uncontrolled bleeding, or if doing so causes pain.

BOX 13.1   Types of Shock

Hypovolemic Shock
- Not enough circulating blood, causing inadequate blood return to the heart
- External bleeding
- Internal bleeding
  - Bleeding from a ruptured or lacerated organ (painful and tender abdomen may be present)
  - Bleeding from a fractured pelvis or femur
- Profound dehydration (often from diarrhea)

Cardiogenic Shock
- Heart function inadequate to maintain circulation
- Patient may have chest pain or dyspnea
- Patient may have distended neck veins or swollen ankles

Vasogenic Shock
- Vasodilation causing transient, relative hypovolemia
- Patient may have bradycardia or "normal" pulse
- Sometimes called *psychogenic shock*

Neurogenic Shock
- Loss of vascular tone secondary to decreased autonomic nervous system innervation
- Caused by a spinal cord injury above the level of the sixth thoracic vertebra (T6)
- Patient will manifest bradycardia, rather than tachycardia, despite concomitant hypotension
- Patient is paralyzed
- Skin may be warm and flushed instead of pale and cool
- Male patient may have priapism

Septic Shock
- Distributive process causing relative hypovolemia and hypotension
- Fever may be present
- The skin may be warm and flushed
- Evidence of an infected wound, abdominal pain, pain and frequency of urination, or signs and symptoms of a respiratory infection may exist

Anaphylactic Shock
See Chapter 26

4. Keep the patient covered and warm. Particularly try to keep the patient's head, neck, and hands covered. Take the patient out of harsh weather conditions, and insulate from the ground. If you cannot locate sufficient covering for warmth, lie next to the patient and share body heat.
5. Attempt to control external bleeding with direct pressure. If that is not successful, a tourniquet(s) may become necessary.

6. Loosen restrictive clothing.
7. Splint all fractures. If the femur is fractured, apply and maintain traction (see Chapter 18). Apply a pelvic binder for suspected pelvic fractures (see Chapter 12).
8. Administer intravenous (IV) fluid resuscitation.
   a. This is not recommended in suspected cardiogenic shock because fluid administration may cause worsening heart failure and pulmonary edema.
   b. Insert a large-gauge IV catheter (preferably 18 to 14 gauge), and administer initially 1 to 2 L normal saline or lactated Ringer's solution for adults. For children administer 20 mL/kg IV over 10 to 20 minutes and repeat as necessary every 30 to 60 minutes, up to 60 mL/kg.
   c. If transport to a medical center will take longer than 6 hours and the patient is likely suffering from noncardiogenic shock, you may attempt oral fluid resuscitation as tolerated. The patient should not be given oral fluids if he or she has altered mental status or is vomiting.
9. Do not administer oral fluids to a patient with suspected intra-abdominal or thoracic hemorrhage.
10. Administer high-flow oxygen (10 to 15 L/min by face mask) if available.
11. For septic shock, start early empiric antibiotic coverage for suspected organisms. Combination therapy directed at gram-positive, gram-negative, and anaerobic organisms may be indicated for unknown or multiple sites of infection. All initial antibiotics in septic shock should be administered intravenously if possible. The following are examples of combination therapy in adults:
    • Ceftriaxone 1 g IV over 3 to 5 minutes **PLUS** clindamycin 600 to 900 mg IV
    • Metronidazole 500 mg IV over 1 hour **OR** ciprofloxacin 400 mg IV; **PLUS** clindamycin 600 to 900 mg IV
12. For massive soft tissue damage or open fracture, administer a cephalosporin (e.g., cefazolin 1 g IV) over 3 to 5 minutes. Oral antibiotics can be given if IV antibiotics are unavailable.
13. In a diabetic patient, consider hypoglycemia (see Chapter 29). If the patient is conscious and can swallow adequately, administer glucose paste or a sugar-sweetened liquid in small sips. Otherwise, do not give the patient anything to eat or drink unless he or she is alert and hungry or thirsty.
14. If the patient appears to be suffering from an allergic reaction to a bite or sting (see Chapters 26 and 38), address the cause of that reaction.
15. Because patients suffering from shock cannot be effectively diagnosed and treated in the field, transport them to a medical facility as quickly as possible.

14 Head Injury

Head injury assessment begins with the primary survey, in which life-threatening conditions, such as airway compromise and severe bleeding, are recognized and simultaneous management is begun. For the purposes of wilderness assessment and management, head injuries can be subdivided into three risk groups that help guide decisions about the need for and urgency of evacuation.

GENERAL TREATMENT

1. Because potential problems include airway compromise from obstruction caused by the tongue, broken teeth, vomit, or blood, make a quick inspection of the patient's mouth as part of the primary survey.
2. Logroll the patient to clear the mouth without jeopardizing the spine (Fig. 14.1). Be aware that head trauma may be accompanied by spine injury.
3. Primary survey of the head-injured patient involves rapid assessment of level of consciousness using the mnemonic AVPU (alert, verbal stimuli response, painful stimuli response, or unresponsive).
4. Secondary survey includes a more detailed neurologic examination, including pupillary examination (Table 14.1), Glasgow Coma Scale (GCS) or Simplified Motor Score (SMS), and a more detailed neurologic examination.

EVALUATION OF THE HEAD-INJURED PATIENT

Scores that quantify the effects of traumatic brain injury (TBI) are used to triage patients to the correct level of care and to follow the clinical progress of injured patients. Although the GCS is most commonly used, TBI is not the indication for which it was designed, and there may be more applicable scoring methodologies.

GLASGOW COMA SCALE

The GCS (see Appendix B) is the most widely used method of defining a patient's level of consciousness and obviates use of ambiguous terminology such as lethargic, stuporous, and obtunded. The GCS is a neurologic scale that aims to give a reliable, objective way of recording the state of consciousness of a person for initial and continuing assessment. A patient is assessed against the criteria of the scale, and the resulting points give the GCS score (see later). The patient's best motor, verbal, and eye-opening responses determine the GCS score. A patient who is able to follow commands, is fully oriented, and has spontaneous eye-opening is assigned a

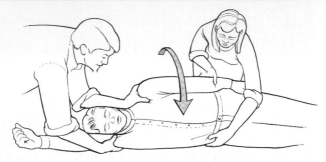

FIGURE 14.1   Logrolling patient to clear the mouth without jeopardizing the spine.

Table 14.1 Interpretation of Pupillary Findings in Head-Injured Patients		
PUPIL SIZE	**LIGHT RESPONSE**	**INTERPRETATION**
Unilaterally dilated	Sluggish or fixed	Third nerve compression secondary to tentorial herniation
Bilaterally dilated	Sluggish or fixed	Inadequate brain perfusion; bilateral third nerve palsy
Unilaterally dilated or equal	Cross-reactive (Marcus Gunn)	Optic nerve injury
Bilaterally constricted	Difficult to determine; pontine lesion	Opiates
Bilaterally constricted	Preserved	Injured sympathetic pathway

GCS score of 15; a patient with no motor response, eye opening, or verbal response to pain is assigned a GCS score of 3. Patients with a GCS score of 8 or less are considered being in "coma." Head-injury severity is generally categorized into three levels on the basis of the GCS score after initial resuscitation. A "mild" GCS score is 13 to 15; "moderate" GCS score is 9 to 12; and "severe" GCS score is 3 to 8. Any patient with a GCS score less than 15 who has sustained a head injury should be evacuated as soon as possible. A declining GCS score suggests increasing intracranial pressure or other cause of worsening traumatic brain injury.

Elements of the Glasgow Coma Scale Explained
Eye Response
Four grades exist:

4—Eye(s) opening spontaneously
3—Eye(s) opening to speech (not to be confused with arousing a sleeping person; such a patients receives a score of 4, not 3)
2—Eye(s) opening in response to pain (patient responds to pressure on his or her fingernail bed; if this does not elicit a response, supraorbital and sternal pressure or rub may be used)
1—No eye opening

Verbal Response
Five grades exist:

5—Oriented (patient responds coherently and appropriately to questions such as the patient's name and age, where he or she is located and the reason; the year, month, etc.)
4—Confused (patient responds to questions coherently, but there is some disorientation and confusion)
3—Inappropriate words (random or exclamatory articulated speech, but no conversational exchange)
2—Incomprehensible sounds (moaning but no words)
1—None

Motor Response
Six grades exist:

6—Obeys commands (patient does simple things as asked)
5—Localizes to pain (purposeful movements toward changing painful stimuli [e.g., hand crosses midline and gets above clavicle when supraorbital pressure applied])
4—Withdraws from pain (pulls part of body away when pinched; normal flexion)
3—Flexion in response to pain (decorticate response)
2—Extension to pain (decerebrate response: adduction, internal rotation of shoulder, pronation of forearm)
1—No motor response

The GCS has limited applicability to children, especially younger than the age of 36 months (because the verbal performance of even a healthy child would be expected to be poor).

SIMPLIFIED MOTOR SCORE
The GCS can be complex and is prone to poor interrater reliability; the newer SMS has proven more user friendly and as reliable as GCS for predicting outcome from TBI. The three-point score is

as follows: 2 points—obeys commands; 1 point—localizes pain; 0 points—withdraws to pain or worse.

HIGH RISK FOR TRAUMATIC BRAIN INJURY: IMMEDIATE EVACUATION

Any head-injured patient with any of the following is at high risk for TBI and requires immediate evacuation to a medical facility: *GCS score of 13 or less, SMS less than 2, focal neurologic signs, or decreasing level of consciousness.* Patients with suspected skull fracture, epidural hematoma, or prolonged unconsciousness also fall into the high-risk category.

Skull Fracture

Fracture of the skull is not in itself life threatening, but skull fracture may be associated with underlying brain injury or severe bleeding.

Signs and Symptoms

- Severe headache
- Deformity, step-off, or crepitus on palpation of the scalp; "boggy" swelling in the soft tissue overlying the fracture
- Blood or clear fluid draining from the ears or nose without direct trauma to those areas
- Ecchymosis around the eyes (raccoon eyes) or behind the ears (Battle's sign)
- In a patient with a skull fracture, observe for seizures, unequal or nonreactive pupils, weakness, or altered level of consciousness from an underlying brain injury (quantify with GCS or SMS).

Treatment

1. Evacuate the patient to a medical facility as soon as possible.
2. Keep the patient with the head slightly uphill or elevated to reduce cerebral edema.
3. In any person with a serious head injury, immobilize the cervical spine in anticipation of an injury to this area.

Epidural Hematoma

Signs and Symptoms

- Patient who wakes up from unconsciousness and appears completely normal, then becomes drowsy or disoriented or lapses back into unconsciousness (usually within 30 to 60 minutes)
- Unconscious patient with one pupil significantly larger than the other

Treatment

Because these are indications of bleeding from an artery inside the skull, which causes an expanding blood clot (epidural hematoma) that compresses the brain, this injury requires immediate evacuation to a medical facility.

Prolonged Unconsciousness
Signs and Symptoms
Loss of consciousness for more than 5 to 10 minutes may indicate significant brain injury.

Treatment
1. Immediate evacuation to a medical center is mandatory.
2. During transport, maintain cervical spine precautions and keep the patient's head uphill on sloping terrain. On a flat surface, elevate the head of the litter 30 degrees. Do not compromise overall patient safety to attain these positions.
3. Be prepared to logroll the patient if the patient vomits.
4. Continually monitor the airway for signs of obstruction and decreasing respiratory rate.
5. Administer oxygen, if available.

MODERATE RISK FOR TRAUMATIC BRAIN INJURY: BRIEF LOSS OF CONSCIOUSNESS OR CHANGE IN CONSCIOUSNESS AT TIME OF INJURY
Patients with a predisposition to bleeding (e.g., anticoagulated or with clotting disorders) need a much more aggressive approach requiring evacuation and evaluation at a higher level of care. Despite a normal examination, these bleeding-predisposed persons should be considered at moderate risk for TBI.

Signs and Symptoms
- Short-term unconsciousness, in which the patient wakes up after 1 or 2 minutes and gradually regains normal mental status and physical abilities, indicating concussion (which may be initially assessed using the Sport Concussion Assessment Tool 5 [SCAT5] for an adult or Child SCAT5; see Appendix C)
- Confusion or amnesia for the event and repetitive questioning by the patient even in the absence of history of loss of consciousness
- Progressive headache or vomiting

Treatment
1. Be aware that the safest strategy is to evacuate the patient to a medical center for evaluation and observation.
2. Interrupt the patient's normal sleep every 2 hours briefly to see that the condition has not deteriorated and he or she can be easily aroused.
3. If a patient is increasingly lethargic, confused, or combative or does not behave normally, and if these signs are present in isolation and the evacuation can be completed in less than 12 hours, evacuation should proceed. If evacuation is impossible or will require longer than 12 hours, the patient should be closely observed for 4 to 6 hours. If the examination improves

to normality during the observation period, it is reasonable to continue observation.

LOW RISK FOR TRAUMATIC BRAIN INJURY: MAY BE OBSERVED AND DOES NOT REQUIRE IMMEDIATE EVACUATION

The low-risk group includes persons who have suffered a blow to the head but are asymptomatic or minimally symptomatic.

Signs and Symptoms

Head injury without any loss of consciousness or altered mental status is rarely indicative of a serious injury to the brain. Mild stable headache or dizziness may be present. GCS score should be 15, and SMS should be 2. A concussion may have occurred. This is indicated by headache, blurry vision, photophobia, nausea and vomiting, difficulty concentrating, and malaise.

Treatment

1. Inspect the scalp for evidence of lacerations, which generally bleed copiously, and apply pressure as needed.
2. If the patient appears normal (can answer questions appropriately, including name, location, and date; walks normally; appears to have coordinated movements; and has normal muscle strength), no immediate evacuation is required.
3. If the patient develops any signs or symptoms of brain injury (Box 14.1), evacuate the patient immediately.
4. If a child has suffered a head injury, then begins to vomit, refuses to eat, becomes drowsy, appears apathetic, or in any other way seems abnormal, evacuate him or her to a medical facility as soon as possible.
5. Close observation of these patients includes awakening the patient from sleep every 2 hours and avoidance of strenuous activity for at least 24 hours. The following signs indicate that more advanced medical care is necessary: (1) inability to awaken

---

BOX 14.1 Brain Injury Checklist

- Increasing headache
- Changing level of consciousness (increasing somnolence or confusion)
- Difficulty with vision
- Urinary or bowel incontinence
- Persistent or projectile vomiting
- Bleeding from ears or nose (without direct injury to those areas), cerebrospinal fluid rhinorrhea
- Raccoon eyes or Battle's sign
- Seizure
- Weakness or numbness involving any part of the body

the patient; (2) severe or worsening headaches; (3) somnolence or confusion; (4) restlessness, unsteadiness, or seizures; (5) difficulties with vision; (6) vomiting, fever, or stiff neck; (7) urinary or bowel incontinence; and (8) weakness or numbness involving any part of the body.

6. Generally one should not return to an environment in which concussion is a risk (e.g., contact sports) until symptoms have been absent for 4 weeks.
7. The SCAT5 is a standardized method of evaluating injured persons 13 years of age and older for concussion. Use the Child SCAT5 for children ages 5 to 12 years. Compared to a baseline SCAT5, the test can be used to indicate the possible presence of a concussion (see Appendix C).

SCALP LACERATIONS

Scalp lacerations are common after head injuries and tend to bleed vigorously because of the scalp's rich blood supply.

Treatment

1. Apply direct pressure to the wound with your gloved hand. It might be necessary to hold pressure for up to 30 minutes.
2. If you are faced with a bleeding scalp laceration and the patient has a healthy head of hair, tie the wound closed using the patient's own hair (see Chapter 20). This should not be expected to control the bleeding but will approximate the edges of the wound.

SCALP BANDAGING

Scalp wounds often require a dressing placed over hair, making adhesion difficult. The dressing can be secured with a triangular bandage in a method that allows for considerable tension should pressure be necessary to stop bleeding (see Fig. 20.7).

HEAD INJURY AND SCUBA DIVING

Any significant head injury that increases the risk for late seizures is a contraindication for scuba (self-contained underwater breathing apparatus) diving. Such injuries include a significant brain contusion, subdural hematoma, skull fracture, loss of consciousness, or amnesia for greater than 24 hours. In case of minor head injury that does not have any associated symptoms and that does not require anticonvulsant medication, scuba diving can be considered after 6 weeks.

15 Chest Trauma

In the wilderness environment, blunt thoracic injuries usually result from falls or direct blows to the chest. Penetrating injuries result from gun, knife, or arrow wounds; impalement after a fall; or a rib fracture. Immediate, life-threatening thoracic injuries include flail chest, pneumothorax/hemothorax, tension pneumothorax, open ("sucking") chest wound, and pericardial tamponade.

DISORDERS
Rib Fracture
Signs and Symptoms
- Pain in the chest after blunt chest trauma
- Pain that worsens with inspiration
- Point tenderness over the fractured rib(s)
- Crepitus and deformity, occasionally detected on palpation
- Fractured ribs usually occur along the side of the chest. Pushing on the sternum while the patient lies supine will produce pain at the fracture site, instead of at the point of contact.

Treatment
1. Care for any open chest wounds.
    a. Cover the wound quickly, especially if there is air bubbling, to avoid "sucking" chest wound (see Open ["Sucking"] Chest Wound, later).
    b. Use a petrolatum-impregnated gauze, heavy cloth, or adhesive tape for the dressing.
2. Treat an isolated rib fracture.
    a. Administer an oral analgesic, and instruct the patient to rest.
    b. Note that thoracic taping and splinting are contraindicated so that the patient can take full unimpeded inspirations.
    c. Encourage the patient to cough or deep-breathe at least 10 times per hour to prevent atelectasis.
3. Treat multiple rib fractures.
    a. Be aware that multiple fractures are associated with higher risk for serious underlying injuries.
    b. Cushion the patient in a position of comfort, and frequently reevaluate the patient's ability to breathe.
    c. Do not tape or tightly wrap the ribs because this might prevent complete reexpansion of the lung with inspiration, leading the patient to take only shallow, inadequate breaths and possibly leading to atelectasis and pneumonia. Provide analgesics so that the patient may take at least 10 deep breaths or give one good cough every hour.

d. Evacuate the patient as soon as possible. If the chest injury is on one side, transport the patient with the injured side down to facilitate lung expansion and oxygenation of the blood on the uninjured side.

Flail Chest
Signs and Symptoms
- A portion of the chest wall that is mechanically unstable, indicating that a series of three or more ribs is fractured in both the anterior and posterior planes
- Unstable segment that paradoxically moves inward during inspiration, thereby inhibiting ventilation

Treatment
1. Immediately arrange for evacuation of the patient. A small or moderate flail segment can be tolerated for 24 to 48 hours, after which it may need to be managed with mechanical ventilation.
2. Administer intercostal nerve block(s) (Fig. 15.1) to assist in short-term management of pain and pulmonary toilet.
3. Place a bulky pad of dressings, rolled-up extra clothing, or small pillow gently over the site, or have the patient splint the arm against the injury to stabilize the flail segment and relieve some of the pain.
   a. Use soft and lightweight materials.
   b. Use large strips of tape to hold the pad in place.
   c. Do not tape entirely around the chest because this will restrict breathing efforts.
   d. Do not allow the object to restrict breathing in any manner.
4. If the patient is unable to walk, transport him or her lying on the back or injured side.
5. If the patient is severely short of breath, assist with mouth-to-mouth rescue breathing. Time your breaths with those of the patient, and breathe gently to provide added air during the patient's inspirations.

Pneumothorax/Hemothorax
Signs and Symptoms
- Pain that worsens with inspiration
- Tachypnea
- Unilateral decreased or absent breath sounds
- Resonance on percussion with a pneumothorax; flat or dull on percussion with a hemothorax
- Subcutaneous emphysema (in the case of pneumothorax)
- Pneumothorax can be identified by loss of the "comet tails" or loss of pleural sliding on ultrasound examination.

Treatment
1. Evacuate the patient immediately.
2. Monitor closely for the development of a tension pneumothorax.
3. Administer analgesics as needed.

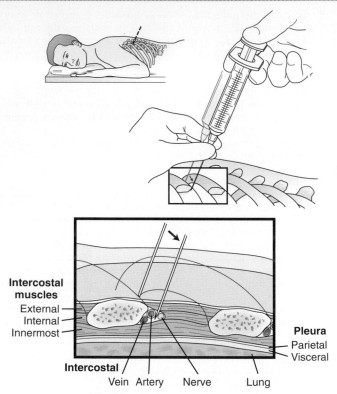

Intercostal muscles
External
Internal
Innermost

Intercostal
Vein   Artery   Nerve   Lung

Pleura
Parietal
Visceral

FIGURE 15.1   Technique for Intercostal Nerve Block. With the patient seated or lying prone, skin prepped ideally using sterile technique, identify the posterior angle of the rib (6 to 8 cm [2.4 to 3.1 inches] from the spinous processes). The 25-gauge needle is advanced with 20 degrees of cephalad angulation and to the inferior margin of the rib. The needle is then walked off the inferior rib margin while maintaining cephalad angulation and advanced 2 to 3 mm to lie adjacent to the intercostal nerve. The intercostal nerve lies inferior to the intercostal vein and artery. Inject 3 to 5 mL bupivacaine 0.25% to 0.5%, lidocaine 1% to 2% with epinephrine 1:200,000 to 1:400,000, or ropivacaine 0.5% to 0.75%.

Tension Pneumothorax
Signs and Symptoms

- Distended neck veins (may not be present if patient is hypovolemic)
- Tracheal deviation away from the side of the pneumothorax
- Unilateral, absent, or grossly diminished breath sounds

- Hyperresonant hemithorax to percussion
- Subcutaneous emphysema
- Respiratory distress, cyanosis, cardiovascular collapse

Treatment

1. Use rapid pleural decompression if the patient appears to be decompensating (Box 15.1; Fig. 15.2). A premade kit such as a Heimlich Chest Drain Valve kit (Chinook Medical Gear, Durango, CO) can be used for decompression. Possible complications include infection and profound bleeding from puncture of the heart, lung, or major blood vessel.
2. Arrange for immediate evacuation.
3. Administer analgesics as needed.

Open ("Sucking") Chest Wound

Signs and Symptoms

- Traumatic defect of the chest wall usually caused by penetrating injury, at least two-thirds the diameter of the trachea.
- This injury causes decreased ventilation owing to preferential movement of air through the chest wall defect instead of the major airway.

BOX 15.1   How to Perform Pleural Decompression

1. Swab the entire chest with povidone–iodine or other antiseptic, such as chlorhexidine.
2. If sterile surgical gloves are available, put them on after washing hands.
3. If local anesthesia is available, infiltrate the puncture site down to the rib and over its upper border.
4. Insert a large-bore (14-gauge) intravenous catheter, needle, or improvised pointed, sharp object into the chest just above the third rib in the midclavicular line (midway between the top of the shoulder and the nipple in a line with the nipple approximates this location; see Fig. 15.2A). If you hit the rib, move the needle or knife upward slightly until it passes over the top of the rib, thus avoiding the intercostal blood vessels that course along the lower edge of every rib (see Fig. 15.2B). The chest wall is 3.8 to 6.4 cm (1.5 to 2.5 inches) thick, depending on the individual's muscularity and the amount of fat present. A gush of air signals that you have entered the pleural space; do not push the penetrating object in any further. Releasing the tension converts the tension pneumothorax into an open pneumothorax.
5. Leave the needle or catheter in place (see Fig. 15.2C), and place the cut-out finger portion of a surgical glove with a slit cut into the end over the external opening to create a unidirectional flutter valve that allows continuous egress of air from the pleural space (see Fig. 15.2D and E).

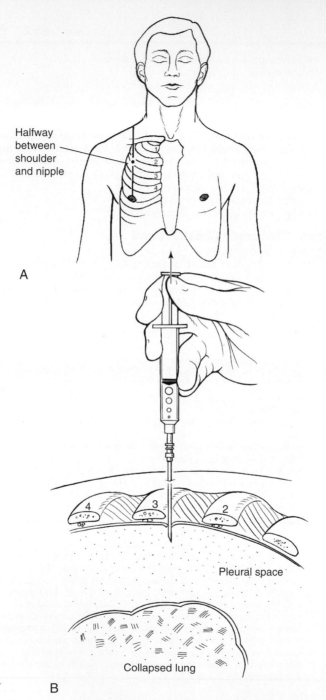

Halfway between shoulder and nipple

A

Pleural space

Collapsed lung

B

FIGURE 15.2 For legend see opposite page

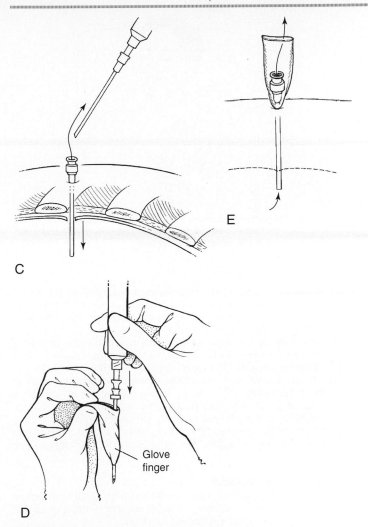

FIGURE 15.2, cont'd   Pleural Decompression. A, Insertion point for pleural decompression. **B,** "Walk" needle over the top of the rib to avoid intercostal vessels. **C,** Catheter in place. **D,** Finger of a glove is attached to the needle or catheter to create a flutter valve. **E,** Flutter valve allows air to escape but collapses to prevent air entry.

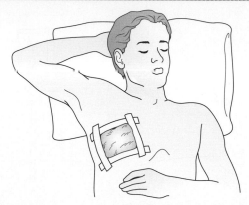

FIGURE 15.3   Treatment of Sucking Chest Wound. Sealing the wound with a gel defibrillator pad works best because this pad adheres to wet or dry skin. Petrolatum gauze or plastic wrap also works well.

Treatment
1. Place a petrolatum-impregnated gauze pad on top of the wound, cover it with a 4 × 4 inch gauze pad, and tape it on all four sides (Fig. 15.3).
2. Observe closely for signs of tension pneumothorax, and treat as described earlier, with pleural decompression.
3. If a penetrating object remains impaled in the chest, do not remove it. If necessary, carefully shorten the external portion of the penetrating object (e.g., break off the arrow). Place a petrolatum gauze dressing next to the skin around the object, and stabilize it with layers of bulky dressings or pads.
4. A patient with an open chest wound below the nipple line may also have an injury to an intraabdominal organ (see Chapter 16).

Pericardial Tamponade
Blunt or penetrating cardiac injury leading to pericardial tamponade is uncommon but life threatening. A small amount of intrapericardial blood can severely restrict diastolic function.

Signs and Symptoms
• The triad of distended neck veins, hypotension, and muffled heart sounds is present in only one-third of patients.
• Pulsus paradoxus, an increase in the normal physiologic decrease in blood pressure with inspiration, may be present.

Treatment
1. The only temporizing measure pending evacuation is pericardiocentesis. This procedure should be done in the wilderness

only if there is a high index of suspicion, coupled with shock (and impending death) unresponsive to other resuscitative efforts.

2. Advance a long (≈15 cm [5.9 inches]), 16- to 18-gauge needle with an overlying catheter through the skin 1 to 2 cm (0.4 to 0.8 inches) below and to the left of the xiphoid. The needle is advanced at a 45-degree angle with the tip directed at the tip of the left scapula.

3. After the pericardial sac is entered, aspirate blood with a syringe until the patient's condition improves. Once the blood is aspirated, the needle is removed and ideally the catheter left in place and secured. Repeat aspiration may be required according to the hemodynamic status as the patient is being evacuated for definitive care. Repeat aspiration as the patient's condition warrants.

4. Immediately evacuate the patient.

16 | Intraabdominal Injuries

Intraabdominal injuries may have been caused by penetrating or blunt mechanisms

PENETRATING INJURIES
Gunshot Wound
- Low caliber: small entrance and often no exit wound
- High caliber, high velocity: relatively innocuous entrance wound, small and nondisfiguring to large and disfiguring exit wound, extensive internal injuries

Signs and Symptoms
- Wound as above
- Abdominal pain
- Signs of shock may be present (see Chapter 13)

Treatment
1. Immediately make plans to evacuate the patient.
2. Anticipate and treat for shock (see Chapter 13).
3. If violation of the peritoneum is suspected, administer a broad-spectrum antibiotic (e.g., ciprofloxacin 500 to 750 mg PO bid) until emergent delivery to definitive care.
4. Do not push extruded bowel back into the abdomen. Keep the exteriorized bowel moist and covered at all times (apply sterile dressing and moisten every 2 hours ideally with sterile saline, alternatively with potable water, and then cover with thin, clingy plastic wrap).
5. Keep patient NPO except for sips of water with antibiotic.

Stab Wound
Signs and Symptoms
Deep wound laceration caused by knife, or impalement by piton, ski pole, tree limb, or other sharp object

Treatment
1. If the wound extends into subcutaneous tissue and deeper penetration is in question, the evacuation decision may rest on results of local wound exploration. This procedure is simple to perform, even in the wilderness environment, but can be done safely only for wounds that lie between the costal margin and the inguinal ligament. Infiltrate skin and subcutaneous tissue with lidocaine 1% with epinephrine, and extend the laceration several centimeters to clearly visualize the underlying anterior

fascia. The wound should never be probed with any instruments, particularly if overlying the ribs.
2. If thorough exploration of the wound shows no evidence of anterior fascial penetration, and if the patient demonstrates no evidence of peritoneal irritation, the wound can be closed with tape (e.g., Steri-Strips) or adhesive bandages, dressed, and the evacuation process delayed. Physical examination should be performed every few hours for the next 24 hours. If no peritoneal signs develop and the patient feels constitutionally strong, a remote expedition may resume with caution and an eye to evacuation should the patient become ill.
3. If a patient is impaled by a retained object, do not remove the object, but instead shorten (e.g., break off the arrow) if possible to effect evacuation.
4. Control external bleeding.
5. Anticipate and treat for shock (see Chapter 13).
6. Administer a broad-spectrum antibiotic (e.g., ciprofloxacin 500 to 750 mg PO bid) if the wound extends deeper than the subcutaneous tissue.
7. Do not push extruded bowel back into the abdomen. Keep the exteriorized bowel moist and covered at all times (apply sterile dressing, and moisten every 2 hours ideally with sterile saline, alternatively with potable water, and then cover with thin, clingy plastic wrap).
8. If anticipating evacuation, keep the patient NPO except for sips of water with antibiotics.

Blunt Injuries
Signs and Symptoms
- Signs of shock (tachypnea, tachycardia, delayed capillary refill, weak or thready pulse, cool or clammy skin)
- Abdominal distention
- Pain or muscle guarding elicited on palpation
- Percussion tenderness
- Pain referred to the left shoulder (ruptured spleen)
- Gross hematuria
- Abdominal pain with movement
- Fever

Treatment
1. Immediately evacuate the patient.
2. Anticipate and treat for shock (see Chapter 13).

17 | Maxillofacial Trauma

Maxillofacial trauma ranges from simple lacerations to massive injuries with extensive bleeding, fractures, and airway obstruction. In general, the ability to treat these injuries in the wilderness is limited. Among the disorders that may be stabilized are lacerations, mandibular fracture, midface (Le Fort) fracture, orbital floor fracture, nasal fracture, and epistaxis.

GENERAL TREATMENT

1. Perform a primary survey, paying attention to airway compromise from aspiration of blood, avulsed teeth or dental appliance, direct trauma and swelling, or a regressive tongue secondary to a mobile mandibular fracture. The most important part of care for maxillofacial trauma is maintenance of a clear airway. If the airway is threatened by edema or inability of the patient to keep the airway clear, early intubation is recommended. Cricothyrotomy (see Chapter 10) may be necessary.
   a. Remove any loose material (teeth, clots, soft tissue, foreign material) from the oropharynx to clear the airway.
   b. Note any deformity or asymmetry of the facial structures, which may indicate underlying bone fracture.
   c. Enophthalmos may be one sign that an orbital blowout fracture is present.
   d. Look for malocclusion or a step-off in the teeth as an indication of mandibular or maxillary fracture.
   e. Observe the position and integrity of the nasal septum. If the septum is bulging on one side into the nasal cavity, it could indicate a septal hematoma. A septal hematoma can be drained in the field by making a small incision into the septum with a safety pin or point of a knife, allowing the blood to drain out.
   f. Examine soft tissue injuries, looking for foreign bodies, including avulsed teeth.
   g. Test motor and sensory function by checking for sensation on each side of the face and by having the patient wrinkle the forehead, smile, bare the teeth, and close the eyes tightly.
   h. Gently palpate the facial structures, noting areas of tenderness, bony defects, crepitus, and false motion.
   i. Test dental integrity by grasping the front and bottom anterior teeth and checking for motion.
   j. If the patient is unconscious but breathing well and shows no sign of hemorrhaging into the airway, you can use an oropharyngeal or nasopharyngeal airway to ensure airway patency.

2. Anticipate cervical spine trauma, and immobilize the spine if indicated (see Box 12.5). If cervical spine injury is possible and airway protection is required, perform endotracheal intubation or cricothyrotomy while maintaining manual cervical spine immobilization.
3. Control bleeding with direct pressure.
   a. For intraoral bleeding, have the patient bite firmly on a gauze pad.
   b. For bleeding from the nose, squeeze and hold the nostrils together, use nasal packing, or deploy a Foley catheter (see Nasal Fracture and Epistaxis, later).
4. Treat shock (see Chapter 13).
5. Recover any completely avulsed teeth or other tissues, irrigate with normal saline solution, and transport in a saline-soaked gauze sponge.

DISORDERS
Lacerations
Facial lacerations may be complicated by damage to associated structures that requires specialized medical care.

Signs and Symptoms
* *Lacrimal drainage system:* injury confirmed if a probe inserted into the punctum at the medial canthus of the eye emerges from the laceration
* *Parotid duct:* injury suspected if there is buccal nerve paralysis or leakage from the wound when Stensen's duct is irrigated with saline solution or water
* *Facial nerve:* asymmetry when the patient moves the eyebrows, eyelids, and mouth

Treatment
1. Wash and irrigate wounds copiously with soap and clean water or sterile saline.
2. Remove any foreign debris and devitalized tissue
3. Local anesthesia and primary suture closure may be appropriate in the field for small, minimally contaminated lacerations (see Chapter 20).
4. Lacerations involving the salivary ducts, facial nerves, or complicated facial structures, such as the vermilion border of the lips, nasal alar rims, or auricular helical rims of the ears, should be repaired by experienced providers or cleaned and bandaged for delayed closure following evacuation.
5. Clean, simple, and uncontaminated facial wounds less than 6 hours old may be appropriate for skin glue or adhesive tape closure.

Mandibular Fracture
Signs and Symptoms
* Inability to occlude the teeth in a normal manner
* Sublingual hematoma

- Deformity, crepitus, mandibular mobility
- Restricted opening or deviation of the jaw when opening
- Pain elicited by placing one hand over each angle of the jaw and pressing inward

Midface (Le Fort) Fractures
Signs and Symptoms
- Tenderness, ecchymosis, and swelling over fracture site
- Le Fort I fracture—facial edema and mobility of the hard palate and upper teeth
- Le Fort II fracture—facial edema, telecanthus, subconjunctival hemorrhage, mobility of the maxilla at the nasofrontal suture, epistaxis, and possible cerebrospinal fluid rhinorrhea
- Le Fort III fracture—massive edema with facial elongation and flattening. An anterior open bite may be present because of posterior and inferior displacement of the facial skeleton. Movement of the entire upper dental arch or face on grasping the alveolar process and anterior teeth between the thumb and forefinger and rocking gently back and forth, epistaxis, and cerebrospinal fluid rhinorrhea.

Treatment of Mandibular or Midface Fracture
1. Elevate the patient's head to reduce bleeding and swelling.
2. Stabilize the site with bandages (Fig. 17.1).
3. Control epistaxis (see later).
4. Evacuate the patient immediately.

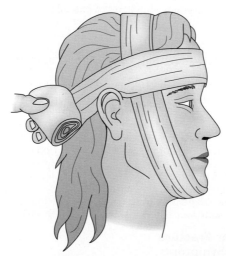

FIGURE 17.1   Barton Bandage. A simple bandage can be used to temporarily stabilize a jaw fracture.

5. Administer antibiotic prophylaxis with penicillin V or clindamycin for 5 to 7 days (see Appendix H).

Orbital Floor Fracture
Signs and Symptoms
- Periorbital edema, crepitus, ecchymosis, enophthalmos, and ocular injury can be present
- Diplopia, worsened with upward gaze
- Lowering of the globe or decreased upward gaze on the affected side secondary to entrapment of the inferior rectus muscle
- Decreased facial sensation

Treatment
1. Evacuate the patient for definitive management.
2. Avoid blowing the nose.
3. Administer antibiotic prophylaxis with amoxicillin-clavulanate or levofloxacin (see Appendix H).

Nasal Fracture and Epistaxis
Signs and Symptoms
- Swelling, tenderness, mobility, ecchymosis, or deformity of the nasal bones
- Evidence of septal hematoma (blue or purplish fluid-filled sac overlying the nasal septum)

Treatment
Treatment of epistaxis depends on whether the source is anterior or posterior.
1. If a septal hematoma is present, make a small incision through the mucosa and perichondrium to allow drainage. Pack the anterior nasal cavity (see later) to prevent accumulation of blood.
2. Treat anterior epistaxis.
   a. If bleeding cannot be controlled by firmly pinching the nostrils against the septum for a full 10 minutes, nasal packing may be necessary. Insert a piece of cotton or gauze soaked with a vasoconstricting agent, such as oxymetazoline hydrochloride 0.05% (Afrin) or phenylephrine hydrochloride (Neo-Synephrine), into the nose, and leave it in place for 5 to 10 minutes. Next, layer-pack petrolatum-impregnated gauze or strips of a nonadherent dressing into the nose so that both ends of the gauze remain outside the nasal cavity to lessen the likelihood that the patient might inadvertently aspirate the packing.
   b. To pack an adult's nasal cavity completely, at least 3 to 4 ft (approximately 1 m) of 0.6-cm ($\frac{1}{4}$ -inch) material is required to fill the nasal cavity and tamponade the bleeding site.
   c. Expandable packing materials, such as Weimert Epistaxis Packing, Epi-Max, Rapid Rhino, or Rhino Rocket balloon catheters, are available for treatment of anterior, posterior, or both anterior and posterior epistaxis (Fig. 17.2). They

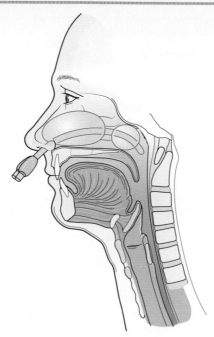

FIGURE 17.2 Commercially available nasal packing balloons are lightweight, inexpensive, and easy to deploy.

should be used only if compression and simple anterior packing with gauze fails to control bleeding. Once placed, nasal balloons should remain in place for 1 to 3 days. Although recent evidence has challenged the necessity for prophylactic antibiotics, consider therapy such as cephalexin, erythromycin, or amoxicillin, to prevent sinusitis and toxic shock syndrome (see Appendix H).
   d. A tampon or balloon tip from a Foley catheter can also be used as improvised packing.
3. Treat posterior epistaxis.
   a. Use a 14- to 16-French Foley catheter with a 30-mL balloon to tamponade the site. The catheter should be lubricated with either petrolatum or a water-based lubricant. Insert the catheter through the nasal cavity into the posterior pharynx. Next, inflate the balloon with 10 to 15 mL of water and gently draw it back into the posterior nasopharynx until resistance is met. Inflation should be done slowly and should be stopped if painful. Secure the catheter firmly to the patient's forehead with several strips of tape. Finally, pack the anterior nose in front of the catheter balloon with gauze as described earlier.

b. Alternatively, use a commercially available balloon catheter, such as the Epi-Max or Rapid Rhino, specifically designed to control both posterior and anterior epistaxis.

c. Consider administration of prophylactic antibiotics, such as cephalexin, erythromycin, or amoxicillin (see Appendix H).

d. Evacuate the patient.

Foreign Body in the Nose
Signs and Symptoms

- Pain, foul-smelling drainage, sometimes fever
- Skin extremely sensitive, possibly swollen with accumulation of mucus and blood

Treatment

A foreign body can be difficult to remove because of tissue sensitivity. Also, irritation in the nasal area causes swelling that traps the foreign object inside an accumulation of mucus and blood.

1. Attempt to visualize the object and extract it.
   a. Initially attempt to blow out of the nose while blocking the unaffected side.
   b. Instrumentation may be indicated and attempted in the wilderness.
   c. Do not proceed if you find the object moving deeper into the nostril or the patient is in extreme pain.
   d. If unable to remove safely, leave the object in place and prepare the patient for evacuation.
2. If the patient develops a fever, administer an antibiotic, such as cephalexin, erythromycin, or amoxicillin (see Appendix H).

18 Orthopedic Injuries, Splints, and Slings

PHYSICAL EXAMINATION AND FUNCTIONAL CONSIDERATIONS
JOINT FUNCTION

- Begin palpation of the long bones distally, and proceed across all joints.
- Palpable crepitus at the joint level mandates application of a splint.
- If the patient can cooperate, have him or her move every joint through an active range of motion (ROM). This exercise quickly focuses the examination on the injury's location.
- When this is not possible, undertake passive ROM of each joint, after palpating the joint for crepitus and swelling.
- If crepitus, swelling, deformity, or resistance to motion is noted, apply a splint.
- If a joint is dislocated, attempt reduction after completing the neurovascular examination.
- Reduction of the joint generally relieves much of the discomfort.
- After reduction, assess stability of the joint by careful, controlled ROM evaluation.
- Remember to perform serial neurovascular examinations (i.e., recheck status).
- A joint with an associated fracture or interposed soft tissue is frequently unstable after reduction. In such circumstances, take great care while applying the splint to prevent recurrent dislocation.
- Report to the definitive care physician the details of the reduction maneuver, including orientation of the pull, amount of force involved, sedation, residual instability of the joint, and prereduction and postreduction neurovascular status.

CIRCULATORY FUNCTION

- Injury to the major vessels supplying a limb can occur with penetrating or blunt trauma.
- A fracture can produce injury to vessels by direct laceration (rarely) or by stretching, which produces intimal flaps. These flaps can immediately occlude the distal blood flow or lead to delayed occlusion. For this reason, repeated examination of circulatory function is mandatory before and during transport.
- Assess color and warmth of the skin in the extremity distal to the injury. Distal pallor and asymmetric regional hypothermia may identify a vascular injury.

- In the upper extremity, the brachial, radial, and ulnar pulses should be palpated. In the lower extremity, the femoral, popliteal, posterior tibial, and deep peroneal pulses should be palpated. If blood loss and hypothermia make pulses difficult to assess, temperature and color of the distal extremity become keys to the diagnosis.
- Any suspected major arterial injury mandates immediate evacuation after splinting.

NERVE FUNCTION

- Nerve function may be impossible to assess in an unconscious or uncooperative patient.
- Whenever possible, it is important to establish the status of nerve function to the distal extremity after the patient's condition is stabilized.
- Periodically compare the initial findings with additional examinations during transport of the patient. Deteriorating neurologic findings guide the speed of evacuation and any ameliorating maneuvers, such as further fracture reduction or splint modification. These decisions may greatly affect patient outcome.
- Carefully document sensory examination of the peripheral nerves regarding light touch and pinprick.
- Assess muscle function by observing active function and grading the strength of each muscle group against resistance.

EVACUATION DECISIONS

See Box 18.1
- Musculoskeletal injuries that warrant immediate evacuation to a definitive care center include any suspected cervical, thoracic, lumbar, pelvic, or femur injury.
- A patient who has a suspected pelvic injury with instability, significant suspected blood loss, or injury to the sacral plexus should receive immediate emergency evacuation on a backboard (if possible) or modified immobilization (see Figs. 57.17 to 57.20).
- All open fractures require definitive debridement and care within 18 hours to prevent infection. Emergency evacuation is imperative.

BOX 18.1   Indications for Emergent Evacuation

Suspected spine injury
Suspected pelvic injury
Open fracture
Suspected compartment syndrome
Hip or knee dislocation
Vascular compromise to an extremity
Laceration with tendon or nerve injury
Uncertainty of severity of injury

BOX 18.2   Antibiotic Options

Intravenous Solutions
Cefazolin (Ancef) 1 g q6h and gentamicin (5 mg/kg) q24h or piperacillin with tazobactam (Zosyn) 3.375 g q6h

Intramuscular Injections
Ceftriaxone (Rocephin) 1 g q24h

Oral
Ciprofloxacin 750 mg q12h and cephalexin (Keflex) 500 mg q6h

Water Exposure
Ciprofloxacin 400 mg IV or 750 mg PO bid; or a sulfonamide and trimethoprim combination (Bactrim DS: 800 mg sulfamethoxazole and 160 mg trimethoprim) with either cefazolin (Ancef) 1 g IV q8h or cephalexin (Keflex) 500 mg PO q6h

Dirt or Barnyard Exposure
Add penicillin 20 million units IV daily or 500 mg PO q6h

If Penicillin Allergy
Use clindamycin 900 mg IV q8h or 450 mg PO q6h in place of penicillins and cephalexin (Keflex)

Alternatives
Erythromycin 500 mg PO q6h or amoxicillin with clavulanic acid 875 mg PO q12h

Bid, twice a day; *IV*, intravenously; *PO*, orally; *qid*, four times a day.

If evacuation time exceeds 8 hours, in addition to antibiotic administration and splinting, irrigation and debridement in the field should be attempted. Antibiotic options are listed in Box 18.2.

- A patient with a suspected compartment syndrome should be evacuated on an emergent basis.
- A joint dislocation involving the hip or knee warrants immediate evacuation, even if relocated, because of the associated risk for vascular injury or posttraumatic osteonecrosis of the femoral head (in the case of the hip).
- A laceration involving a tendon or nerve warrants prompt evacuation to a center where an experienced surgeon is available.
- In all but the most remote wilderness expeditions, arrangements should be made to promptly evacuate the patient when treatment or significance of the injury is uncertain.

SPECIAL CONSIDERATIONS WITH OPEN FRACTURE

- An injury that includes disruption of the skin and a broken bone is an open fracture and is at risk for bacterial contamination. Assume that any deep wound over a known fracture represents an open fracture. If soil or foreign body contamination is severe, the patient is at risk for osteomyelitis and sepsis.

- If medical care is less than 8 hours away and the bone (limb) is not severely angulated or malpositioned, treat the injury with a compression dressing, splint, and broad-spectrum antibiotic.
- If the delay will be more than 8 hours before definitive medical care, irrigation of the open wound is beneficial and may help prevent serious soft tissue and bone infection.
  - The water used for irrigation does not have to be sterile. Clean tap water or water disinfected for drinking can greatly diminish the bacterial burden.
  - Use a syringe from the medical kit as an irrigating tool (see Fig. 20.1).
  - Attach an 18-gauge needle (or irrigation tip) to the syringe.
  - Irrigate the wound copiously with the pressurized stream of water. For a large wound, more than a liter of water may be necessary.
- Once the wound has been cleaned and irrigated, cover it with a sterile compression dressing.
- Additives, such as povidone-iodine, hydrogen peroxide, and chlorhexidine, are ineffective and may even be harmful.
- Administer a broad-spectrum antibiotic (see Box 18.2) and splint the extremity. If evacuation time exceeds 8 hours, the incidence of osteomyelitis is high.

SPECIAL CONSIDERATIONS WITH AMPUTATION

- In the wilderness environment, the amputation patient requires immediate evacuation.
- Attempt to control hemorrhage by direct pressure. If a tourniquet is applied as a lifesaving measure, document the time and date of application and be prepared to sacrifice the limb. Check at reasonable intervals (e.g., once an hour) to see if pressure alone will control bleeding (see Chapter 12).
- Without cooling, an amputated part remains potentially viable for only 4 to 6 hours; with cooling, viability may be extended to 18 hours.
- Cleanse the amputated part with water, wrap it in a moistened sterile gauze or towel, place it in a plastic bag, and transport it on ice or snow, if available. Do not transport it in direct contact with ice or ice water.
- Make sure the amputated part accompanies the patient throughout the evacuation process.

SPECIAL CONSIDERATIONS WITH COMPARTMENT SYNDROME

A compartment syndrome exists when locally increased tissue pressure compromises circulation and neuromuscular function. In the wilderness setting, this most frequently occurs in association with a fracture or severe contusion. The lower leg and forearm are the most common sites for this syndrome because tight fasciae encase the muscle compartments in these regions and because these areas are frequently involved with fractures or severe contusions. A compartment syndrome can also occur in the thigh, hand, foot, and gluteal regions.

Signs and Symptoms
- Complaints by the conscious patient of severe pain that seem out of proportion to the injury
- Extremely tight feel to the muscle compartment, with applied pressure increasing the pain
- In the cooperative patient, decreased sensation to light touch and pinprick in the areas supplied by the nerve or nerves traversing the compartment, which is usually noted on the dorsum of the foot in the first web space, caused by pressure affecting the deep peroneal nerve in the anterior compartment of the leg
- Most reliable signs: pain, tightness to palpation, and pain on passive stretch
- Never wait for hypoesthesia, absence of a pulse, presence of pallor, or slow capillary refill to make the diagnosis. Even late in the course, there is usually a pulse and normal capillary refill (unless there is an underlying arterial injury)

Treatment
1. Expedite emergency evacuation. The patient must be definitively treated in the first 6 to 8 hours after onset of this condition to optimize return of function to the involved limb.
2. Avoid tight bandages, dressings, or splints that can exacerbate the condition.
3. Do not elevate the limb; try to keep it at the level of the heart. Elevation reduces mean arterial pressure in the limb, which can reduce blood flow.
4. Perform emergency fasciotomy to relieve the pressure, which, if untreated, can produce nerve and muscle cell death within 12 hours. An experienced physician or surgeon can perform limited fasciotomies in the field if evacuation will take more than 8 hours.
5. Antibiotics should be started (see Box 18.2) if a fasciotomy is performed in the field.

SPLINTING
Improvisation: General Guidelines
- When working with a complex improvised system, test your creation on an uninjured person (i.e., "work out the kinks") before you use it on the patient.
- Remember to include improvisation construction materials, including a knife, tape, parachute cord or line, safety pins, wire, and plastic cable ties, in your survival kit.
- Maintain a creative approach to obtaining improvisational materials. Much of the patient's gear can be harvested to provide necessary items. A backpack can usually be dismantled to obtain foam pads, straps, etc.

- Practice constructing certain items before you must do this in an actual rescue setting.
- Be sure to use adequate padding and check underneath both prefabricated and improvised splints frequently for skin irritation.
- Cover open wounds with sterile or the cleanest possible dressings.

Extremity Splints: Basic Principles

1. Splint the fracture before the patient is moved unless the patient's life is in immediate danger.
2. Make sure the splint incorporates the joints above and below the fracture. If possible, fashion the splint on the uninjured extremity and then transfer it to the injured one.
3. Skis, poles, canoe and kayak paddles, ice axes, and snow anchors can be used as improvised splints. Airbags used as flotation for kayaks and canoes can be converted into pneumatic splints for arm and ankle injuries. The Minicell or Ethafoam pillars found in most kayaks can be removed and carved into pieces to provide upper and lower extremity splints. A life jacket can be molded into a cylinder splint for knee immobilization or into a pillow splint for the ankle. The flexible aluminum stays found in internal-frame backpacks can be molded into an upper extremity splint. Other improvised splinting materials include sticks or tree limbs; rolled-up magazines, books, or newspapers; tent poles; and dirt-filled garbage bags or fanny packs.
4. Ideally a splint should immobilize the fractured bone in a functional position. In general, functional position means that the leg should be straight or slightly bent at the knee, the ankle and elbow bent at 90 degrees, the wrist straight, and the fingers flexed in a curve as if one were attempting to hold a can of soda or a baseball. The "soda can" position is appropriate for initial management and transport; however, for long-term splinting, apply a hand splint with the metacarpophalangeal (MCP) joints flexed at 90 degrees and the interphalangeal joints extended (the "intrinsic positive" position). This position places the collateral ligaments at maximum length and helps prevent joint contractures.
5. Secure the splint in place with strips of clothing, belts, duct tape, pieces of rope or webbing, pack straps, elasticized roller wraps, or gauze bandages.

Ensolite (Closed-Cell Foam) Pads

The era of Therm-a-Rest types of inflatable pads has rendered closed-cell foam pads increasingly scarce; however, closed-cell foam remains the ultimate padding for almost any improvised splint or rescue device. Even die-hard Therm-a-Rest fans should carry a small amount of closed-cell foam, which doubles as a lightweight, comfortable seat cushion. Unlike inflatable pads, Ensolite will not puncture and deflate.

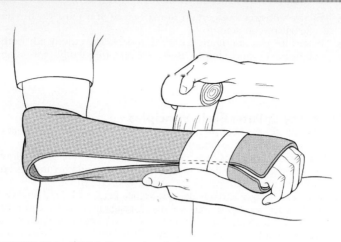

FIGURE 18.1   SAM Splint used to fashion a sugar-tong splint. For a distal radius fracture, the forearm should be placed in a neutral, not pronated, position.

- A Therm-a-Rest pad can be used as padding for a long-bone splint immobilizer (e.g., an improvised universal knee immobilizer).
- An inflatable pad can also be used to stabilize a pelvic fracture.
  - Wrap the deflated pad around the pelvis.
  - Secure the pad with tape and inflate the pad, thus creating an improvised pelvic sling.

SAM Splint

The versatile SAM Splint (Fig. 18.1) has filled the niche formerly occupied by military-style ladder splints and wire mesh splints. It is constructed of a thin sheet of malleable aluminum sandwiched between two thin layers of closed-cell foam, weighs approximately 128 g (4½ oz), and can be easily rolled into a tight cylinder. Initially the splint has no rigidity, but after structural U-shaped bends are placed along the axis of the splint, it becomes quite rigid.

- The SAM Splint(s) can be used for splinting virtually any long bone in the body (see Fig. 18.1).
- It can also be used for fabricating an improvised cervical collar (see Fig. 12.11).

Triangular Bandage

One of the most ubiquitous components of first-aid kits and one of the easiest to fashion through improvisation is the triangular bandage.

- Typically used to construct a sling and swath bandage for shoulder and arm immobilization, a good substitute for this bulky item

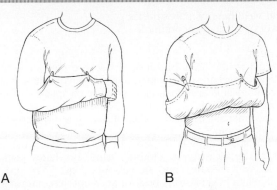

A   B

FIGURE 18.2   Techniques for pinning arm to shirt as an improvised sling. **A,** With long-sleeved shirt or jacket, the sleeved arm is simply pinned to the chest portion of the garment. **B,** With short-sleeved shirt, the bottom of the shirt is folded up over the injured arm and secured to the sleeve and upper shirt.

can be made with two or three safety pins. Pinning the shirtsleeve of the injured arm to the chest portion of the shirt effectively immobilizes the extremity against the body (Fig. 18.2A).

• If the patient is wearing a short-sleeved shirt, fold the bottom of the shirt up and over the arm to create a pouch. This can be pinned to the sleeve and chest section of the shirt to secure the arm (see Fig. 18.2B).

• Triangular bandages are useful for securing splints and constructing pressure wraps. Common items, such as socks, shirts, belts, pack straps, webbing, shoelaces, fanny packs, and underwear, can easily be used as substitutes.

DISORDERS
SPINE FRACTURES
Cervical, Thoracic, Lumbar, and Sacral Spine
Spinal cord injuries are rare but may result in long-term disability. Complete spinal immobilization in the wilderness setting may not always be practical but should always be considered if there is concern for possible spinal injury. Spinal stabilization is first accomplished by manual techniques, and then with mechanical devices (see Figs. 57.17 to 57.20).

Signs and Symptoms
• Complaints of or physical examination findings of midline neck or back pain
• Physical examination findings of midline neck or back deformity or bony step-off
• Inability to range the neck from side to side past 30 degrees because of pain

- Focal weakness or paresthesias
- Bowel or bladder incontinence

Treatment

1. Consider spinal immobilization for severe pain or tenderness, traumatic mechanism of injury, altered mental status, distracting injury, unreliable examination, neurologic complaints, head injury, or extremes of age.
2. Use commercial cervical collars if available for cervical spine immobilization.
3. Cervical spine immobilization can be improvised using towel rolls, backpack material, clothing, sandbags, fanny packs, SAM Splints, water bottles, and shovels (see Figs. 57.18 and 57.21).
4. A full-length backboard is best for accomplishing immobilization of the thoracolumbar spine.
5. Thoracolumbar immobilization can be improvised using commercial or improvised rescue litters and carriers (see Chapter 57).
6. Maintain spinal alignment during patient movement with "logrolling" and manual cervical spine immobilization.

UPPER EXTREMITY FRACTURES
Clavicle
A fracture of the clavicle generally occurs in the middle or lateral third of the bone and is typically associated with a direct blow or fall onto the lateral shoulder.

Signs and Symptoms
- Complaints of shoulder pain, which may be poorly localized and exacerbated by arm or shoulder motion
- Crepitus at the clavicle confirms the diagnosis; deformity
- Although rare, associated pneumothorax, because the cupola of the lung is punctured
- Shortness of breath and deep pain on inspiration
- Associated injury to the brachial plexus, axillary artery, or subclavian vessels

Treatment
1. Localize the pain by gentle palpation to identify the area of maximum tenderness.
2. Auscultate the chest for equal breath sounds if a stethoscope is available.
3. Perform a thorough neurovascular examination of the adjacent extremity.
4. Examine the skin carefully for disruption because of the subcutaneous location of the bone.
5. If there is a significant open wound, suspected pneumothorax, or an injury to a nerve or vascular structure, arrange for evacuation.
6. Most midclavicle fractures are improved by applying a sling or figure-8 type of support, easily improvised with a shirt jacket

or cravat. A figure-8 support works by pulling the shoulder girdle back, applying longitudinal traction to the clavicle so that the bony fragments are somewhat realigned. Figure-8 straps are poorly tolerated by some patients and, if applied too tightly, can cause nerve injury. Figure-8 supports may also worsen distal clavicle fractures and should not be used if a distal fracture is suspected. Usually a simple sling with swath is adequate.

7. Judicious use of ice or snow packs and analgesics should be used. Elevation may provide added relief during rest. Elevate the patient's upper body and head by 10 to 30 degrees when supine. This is a general rule for any shoulder injury. Supine positioning is generally poorly tolerated by patients after shoulder injuries.

Humerus

A fracture of the humeral shaft may be produced by a direct blow or torsional force on the arm. This fracture frequently occurs with a fall, rope accident, or skiing accident.

Signs and Symptoms

- Fracture of the proximal humerus, often caused by a high-velocity fall onto an abducted, externally rotated arm or by a direct blow to the anterior shoulder
  - Difficult to differentiate from a shoulder dislocation in the acute phase. If there is crepitus or if the upper arm is rotated while palpating the proximal humerus and they do not move as a unit, the humerus is fractured
  - Severe pain around the shoulder and with any arm motion
  - Anterior fullness in the proximal humerus, suggesting associated anterior humeral head dislocation
- Fracture of the distal humerus
  - More frequently extra-articular in children and intra-articular in adults, with the child generally sustaining a supracondylar fracture with an extension moment across the elbow in a fall from a height
  - Peak age of incidence 4 to 8 years, although this can also occur in an adult
  - Deformity, swelling, pain, and crepitus
- Radial nerve damage (rare unless the fracture occurs in the mid to distal one-third of the humerus)
  - The radial nerve courses around the posterior aspect of the humerus and is occasionally traumatized when the humeral shaft is injured
  - Numbness over the dorsum of the hand and inability to extend the wrist or fingers
  - Usually caused by contusion or traction injury to the nerve and not to complete disruption

Treatment

1. When a fracture of the humeral shaft is suspected, firmly apply an appropriate splint of fiberglass, wood, or other improvised

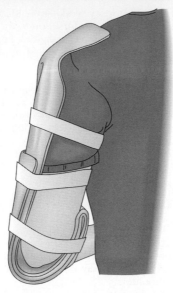

FIGURE 18.3 Humerus splint. Used in conjunction with a sling and swath, this splint adds extra support and protection for a fractured humerus.

material with an elastic bandage on the medial and lateral sides of the humerus. Construct the splint so that it reaches proximal to the level of the fracture (Fig. 18.3).
2. Have the patient use a sling and swath for comfort.
   a. With suspected proximal humeral injury, use the uninjured side as a reference and palpate the anterior aspect of the injured shoulder firmly while rotating the arm. Palpable crepitus with arm motion confirms the diagnosis. It is unlikely that a combined fracture and dislocation can be reduced in the field. Treat this as a fracture, with splinting of the extremity to the torso with a sling or a sling and swath.
   b. Arrange for urgent evacuation for any associated significant distal nerve or vascular injury.
3. For an adult with pain, crepitus, deformity, and swelling after a fall, apply a splint and immobilize the arm to the torso. Be sure to apply the splint with the elbow at 45 to 90 degrees of flexion, depending on the patient's comfort. A splint on the inner and outer surface of the arm that is molded to curve around the elbow provides satisfactory stabilization. Arrange for prompt evacuation if there is an open fracture or neurovascular deficit.
4. With radial nerve injury, there is a high incidence of spontaneous recovery of function. However, if the patient complains of arm pain associated with deformity and crepitus, carefully check the

sensory and motor function of the radial nerve as part of the overall neurovascular examination.

Radius
Signs and Symptoms
- Radial shaft fracture: usually a history of a fall with angular or axial loading of the forearm
  - Pain, deformity, and crepitus over the radial shaft after a fall or direct blow, with any arm motion exacerbating the pain
  - Possibly associated with dislocation of the distal radioulnar joint (Galeazzi fracture); tenderness, swelling, and deformity in the wrist
  - If associated with fracture of the ulna, possibly marked forearm instability or tenderness, crepitus, and deformity in the elbow and wrist
- Radial head fracture: generally, occurs in a young to middle-aged adult who falls onto an outstretched hand
  - Pain around the elbow with loss of full extension
  - Tenderness at the radial head on the lateral side of the elbow, and pain with passive rotation of the forearm
  - With a more severe, comminuted radial head fracture: pain and crepitus with attempts at motion; ROM severely limited
  - Frequently, hemarthrosis of the elbow
  - Swelling is noted as fullness posterior to the radial head and anterior to the tip of the olecranon.
- Fracture of the distal metaphyseal radius: generally associated with a fall onto the outstretched hand from a significant height
  - Obvious pain, "dinner fork deformity," and crepitus
  - Intra-articular distal radius fracture often associated with fracture of the ulnar styloid

Treatment
1. Carefully examine the wrist and elbow, looking for tenderness, swelling, deformity, and crepitus.
2. Once a shaft fracture of the radius or radius and ulna is suspected, splint the wrist, forearm, and elbow in the position of function.
3. For a radial head fracture, move the elbow through gentle ROM and then place it in a posterior splint at 90 degrees of flexion with neutral pronation and supination.
   a. On a prolonged expedition when definitive care cannot be reached, remove the splint at 5 days and perform intermittent active ROM exercises; then reapply the splint for comfort.
   b. With a nondisplaced or minimally displaced radial head fracture, early ROM prevents permanent loss of elbow motion.
   c. If hemarthrosis has occurred, proper equipment is available, and you are confident about the diagnosis, aspirate the hemarthrosis and instill 5 to 10 mL of lidocaine to facilitate pain relief. This must be done under sterile conditions by a skilled individual.

4. For a distal radius fracture with significant deformity at the wrist (Colles fracture), apply longitudinal traction after appropriate sedation (Fig. 18.4). In certain circumstances with a Colles fracture, simple longitudinal traction will not work because the fracture is locked dorsally. To reduce, reproduce the injury deforming force to unlock the fracture (Fig. 18.5). That is, increase the volar angulation (hyperextend the wrist) at the fracture site, then pull distal traction, reducing the distal fragment volarly with your thumb.
   a. Next, apply a splint that immobilizes the wrist and elbow. A U-shaped ("sugar-tong") splint, used in conjunction with a sling to limit rotation, is adequate for transport (see Fig. 18.1).
   b. With an open fracture, significant neurologic deficits, or abnormal circulatory examination, apply the splints promptly and initiate evacuation. Keep the limb elevated above the heart during transport to minimize swelling.

Ulna
Signs and Symptoms
- Ulna shaft fracture: when a patient attempts to brace a fall with the forearm
  - Most often associated with fracture of the radial shaft at the same level
  - When isolated, most often occurs because of a direct blow, the so-called nightstick fracture
  - Can be associated with dislocation of the radial head (Monteggia fracture), affecting elbow function
  - Pain, localized swelling, and crepitus
- Fracture of the proximal ulna (olecranon): result of a fall onto the posterior elbow or from an avulsion after violent asymmetric contraction of the triceps
  - Inability to extend the elbow actively against gravity if the triceps is dissociated from the forearm with a complete fracture of the olecranon
  - On initial examination: pain, significant swelling, and ecchymosis; palpable gap in the olecranon, with possible open fracture

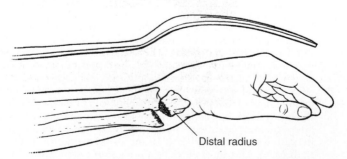

Distal radius

FIGURE 18.4   Colles fracture ("dinner fork deformity").

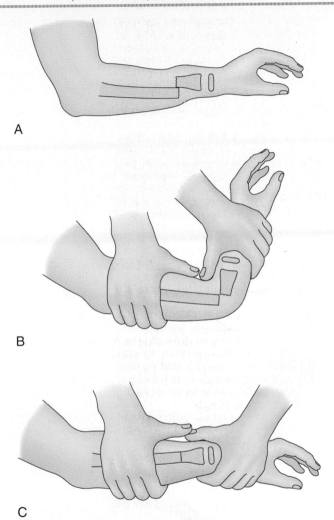

FIGURE 18.5 Technique for reduction of a complete fracture of the forearm. **A,** Initial fracture position. **B,** Hyperextended fracture to 100 degrees to disengage the fracture ends. **C,** Push with the thumb on the distal fragment to achieve reduction. (From Green N, Swiontkowski MF: *Skeletal trauma in children*, ed 2, vol 3, Philadelphia, 1998, WB Saunders.)

- With severe trauma, associated with intra-articular fracture of the distal humerus

Treatment

1. For ulna shaft fracture, apply a long-arm splint in the position of function. If the fracture is open, arrange for prompt evacuation.
2. For fracture of the proximal ulna, after the distal neurovascular examination and shoulder and wrist assessment, apply a splint in the position of function.
3. A posterior splint at 90 degrees usually works well. If there is an open fracture, absent pulse, severe swelling, or neurologic deficit, arrange for immediate evacuation.

Wrist and Hand
Signs and Symptoms

- Wrist fracture: history of significant rotational or high axial loading forces, such as those occurring with a fall onto the hand
  - Pain at first, then swelling of the wrist
  - Significant pain with any use of the hand or with rotation of the forearm
- Carpal bone fracture: precise diagnosis impossible without radiographs
  - Scaphoid most frequently fractured carpal bone
  - Diagnosis suspected if patient's area of maximum tenderness within the "anatomic snuffbox" (Fig. 18.6)

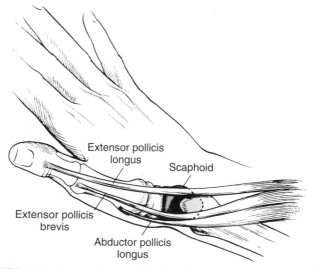

FIGURE 18.6 The scaphoid (navicular) bone sits in the "anatomic snuffbox" of the radial aspect of the wrist.

- Fracture of the hook of the hamate
  - Point of maximum tenderness at base of hypothenar eminence
  - History of using the hand to apply great force to an object with a handle, such as an axe or a hammer, and meeting great resistance

Treatment

1. Swelling can become severe. Remove all jewelry as soon as possible to prevent constriction as tissue swells.
2. Make a temporary hand splint with the hand in the position of function, with the wrist straight and the fingers flexed in a curve as if holding a beverage can.
3. Apply a long-term hand splint with the MCP joints flexed 90 degrees and the interphalangeal joints extended, creating the "intrinsic positive position."
4. This position places the collateral ligaments at maximum length and prevents later joint contracture. For an open fracture or one accompanied by median nerve dysfunction, arrange for prompt evacuation.
5. For carpal bone fracture/wrist dislocation, reduce the fracture by grasping the hand in a handshake fashion and pulling with axial traction. Apply a short-arm splint.
6. For suspected scaphoid fracture, if appropriate splinting materials are available, apply a thumb spica splint, immobilizing both the radius and the first metacarpal bone (thumb).
   a. Encourage the patient to follow up with an orthopedist as soon as practical.
   b. Lack of appropriate immobilization can result in nonunion and/or avascular necrosis, which can develop into severe osteoarthritis and chronic pain.
7. For fracture of the hook of the hamate bone, use a short-arm splint, which also suffices for other suspected carpal injuries, until definitive treatment can be obtained.
8. Wrist fractures with significant swelling or fractures that have not been anatomically reduced can induce traumatic carpal tunnel syndrome. If there is evidence of median nerve paresthesias, urgent carpal tunnel release may be essential.

Metacarpal
Signs and Symptoms

- Fracture of the metacarpal base or shaft: result of a crush injury or an axial load when a rock or other immovable object is struck; produces tenderness, crepitus, and deformity
- Fracture of the metacarpal neck: result of the same mechanism as for the metacarpal base or shaft
  - Fourth and fifth metacarpals most frequently involved
  - Occurs at the base of the knuckle and can be associated with significant rotational deformity
- Fracture of the base of the thumb metacarpal

- When an individual falls with an object grasped between the index finger and thumb (a common position with a ski pole)
- Difficult to differentiate from an ulnar collateral ligament injury because these injuries often occur simultaneously

Treatment
1. For fracture of the metacarpal base or shaft, apply a short-arm splint (e.g., gutter splint, volar splint, U-splint) extending to the proximal interphalangeal (PIP) joint.
2. For possible fracture of the metacarpal neck, check for rotation of the metacarpal by observing the orientation of the fingernails as the MCP and interphalangeal joints are flexed to 90 degrees.
   a. Make sure that the fingernails are parallel to one another and perpendicular to the orientation of the palm.
   b. Ensure that the terminal portions of each digit point to the scaphoid tubercle.
3. For fracture of the metacarpal neck, if malalignment or significant shortening is noted, attempt rotation and reduction with traction on the involved digit.
   a. For a fractured metacarpal shaft or neck, immobilize by applying an aluminum splint (or stick) to the volar surface and taping the involved digit to the adjacent digit with the MCP joint positioned at 45 to 90 degrees.
   b. If splinting material is available, apply a radial or ulnar gutter splint, with the MCP joint positioned at 45 to 90 degrees. The splint should extend to the end of the fingers.
4. For suspected fracture of the base of the thumb metacarpal, immobilize the thumb and wrist in a thumb spica splint.
5. For open metacarpal fracture, clean the wound, debride as needed, and give presumptive antibiotic therapy for 48 hours or until definitive care can be obtained (see Box 18.2).

Phalanx
Signs and Symptoms
- Fracture usually a result of a crush injury or when a digit is caught in a rope
- Angular rotational deformity and crepitus
- Without radiography, intra-articular fracture with subluxation or dislocation difficult to differentiate from interphalangeal joint dislocation

Treatment
1. Reduce the fracture by applying traction and correcting the deformity.
2. Immobilize the fracture by taping the injured digit to a volar splint.
3. Cleanse any nail bed fracture or crush site with soap, and then place a sterile dressing and protective volar splint. If the nail

bed contains a large or poorly approximated laceration, suture repair may be necessary to preserve future functional nail growth.

UPPER EXTREMITY DISLOCATIONS
Sternoclavicular Joint
Signs and Symptoms
- Generally injured by a fall onto an abducted shoulder
  - Direction of dislocation with the medial head of the clavicle anterior to the manubrium of the sternum
  - Direct blow to the sternum also possibly causes this injury, along with rib fracture(s)
- Pain in the sternum region, frequently accompanied by difficulty taking a deep breath
- With posterior dislocation, significant pressure placed on the esophagus and superior vena cava
  - Step-off between the sternum and medial head of the clavicle (compared with the uninjured side)
  - Difficulty swallowing and engorgement of facial veins, like that seen with superior vena cava obstruction syndrome

Treatment
1. Attempt reduction as soon as possible.
   a. Place a large roll of clothing or other firm objects between the scapulae, and position the patient on a firm surface.
   b. Apply sharp, firm pressure directed posteriorly to both shoulders.
   c. Repeat this maneuver several times with a larger object placed between the scapulae if reduction attempts are initially unsuccessful.
   d. After reduction, use a sling.
2. With a posterior dislocation, if the patient transcends into extremis, grasp the midshaft clavicle with a towel clip or pliers and forcefully pull it out of the thoracic cavity (Fig. 18.7).
3. Posterior dislocation mandates evacuation.

Acromioclavicular Joint Separation
Signs and Symptoms
- Injured by a blow on top of the shoulder
- First-degree injury (sprain of the acromioclavicular [AC] ligaments): to the capsule between the acromion and the clavicle; no superior migration of the clavicle seen
- Second-degree injury (complete tear of the AC ligaments and sprain of the coracoclavicular [CC] ligaments): complete capsular disruption, with the CC ligaments remaining intact; superior migration of the clavicle relative to the acromion of one-half the diameter of the clavicle
- Third-degree injury (tear of both the AC and CC ligaments): total disruption of the joint capsule and the CC ligaments, which allows superior migration of the clavicle of up to 2 cm

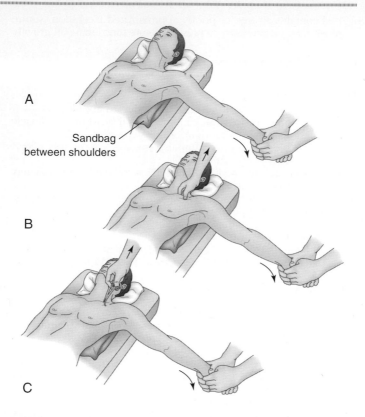

FIGURE 18.7 Posterior sternoclavicular dislocation. **A,** Place a sandbag between the shoulder blades. **B,** Attempt to pull the clavicle back into position. **C,** If necessary, grasp the clavicle with a towel clip or pliers to accomplish reduction.

(approximately 1 inch) (Fig. 18.8). It appears as if the clavicle is superiorly migrated, but the scapula (including the glenoid and humeral head) is depressed and the clavicle is in the normal position.

- Type IV is a tear of both the AC and CC ligaments with the distal clavicle displaced posteriorly into the trapezius muscle (surgical indication).
- Type V is a tear of both ligaments with the distal clavicle displaced superiorly into the muscle (surgical indication).
- Type VI is a tear of both ligaments with the distal clavicle displaced inferior to the coracoid process (surgical indication and extremely rare).
- Differentiating between type III and type IV to VI injuries: In

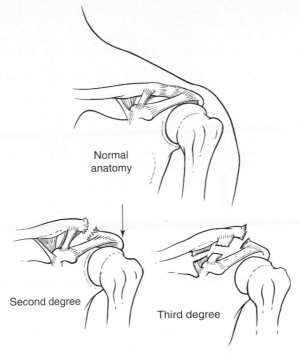

FIGURE 18.8 Acromioclavicular joint injury.

a type III, the distal clavicle is easily reducible with palpation, while in types IV to VI, the clavicle is not reducible.
- If a separation of type IV or greater is suspected, there is a high incidence of associated injuries (i.e., clavicular fractures, scapular fractures, pneumothorax).

Treatment
1. Because using the arm increases pain, place the arm on the affected side in a sling.
2. Evacuation is not mandatory if the individual can tolerate the discomfort associated with the injury. Always rule out more severe associated injuries, such as rib fractures and pneumothorax.
3. Apply ice packs and administer appropriate analgesics.
4. Elevate the upper torso to provide additional relief during rest.

Glenohumeral Joint (Shoulder) Dislocation
Signs and Symptoms
- Generally dislocated anteriorly, or anteriorly and inferiorly; mechanism of injury usually a blow to the arm in the abducted and externally rotated position (e.g., during "high-bracing" in

kayaking or other paddle sports, in which extreme abduction and external rotation occur)
- Recurrent anterior shoulder instability, seen in 30% to 50% of individuals and often easier to reduce than a first-time dislocation
- Holding the extremity away from the body, unable to bring the arm across the chest
  - Shoulder that appears square because of anterior, medial, and inferior displacement of the humeral head into a subcoracoid position
  - No crepitus unless there is an associated fracture
- Possible loss of sensation over the mid-deltoid region with axillary nerve injury in 20% of dislocations

Treatment

1. Do a thorough motor, sensory, and vascular examination of the involved extremity.
2. Carefully assess the axillary and musculocutaneous nerves because they are the nerves most often injured in this dislocation.
3. If within 30 to 60 minutes of definitive medical care, transport the patient with support for the dislocated joint.
4. If skilled individuals are present or if definitive medical care is distant, early reduction of the dislocation can greatly improve the patient's discomfort and enable the patient to function more actively during evacuation (Box 18.3).
   a. The key element is rapid initiation because the longer a shoulder remains dislocated, the more difficult the eventual reduction.
   b. Common to all methods of shoulder reduction are the following: relaxation of muscle spasm, reassurance of the patient, and a method of traction to pass the humeral head over the anterior edge of the glenoid.
   c. In some remote settings, it may be easier to apply a method of reduction that can be carried out with the patient either standing or sitting. This requires access to a flat, comfortable area on which to place the patient in the supine or prone position.
5. After any shoulder reduction, remember to monitor circulation and motor-sensory function to the wrist and hand.
6. Narcotic or benzodiazepine premedication may be helpful if muscle spasm has developed.
7. If the shoulder cannot be reduced after three vigorous attempts, arrange for evacuation. For a difficult reduction, consider administration of 15 to 20 mL of a local anesthetic into the shoulder joint. This injection should only be attempted in a sterile fashion by someone skilled at shoulder injection.
8. After relocation, to prevent a recurrent dislocation, splint the patient's arm across the chest with a sling or swath or by safety-pinning the sleeve of the arm across the chest. If circumstances require further limited use of the arm (e.g., ski pole

BOX 18.3   Reduction Techniques

Standing Method

- Have the patient bend forward at the waist while you support the chest with one hand.
- With the other hand, grasp the patient's wrist and apply steady downward traction and external rotation (Fig. 18.9).
- While maintaining traction, slowly flex the patient's shoulder by moving it in a cephalad direction until reduction is obtained.
- If two rescuers are available, one supports the patient at the chest and the other exerts countertraction and flexion at the arm (Fig. 18.10).
- To help with the reduction, apply scapular manipulation by adducting the inferior tip using thumb pressure and stabilizing the superior aspect of the scapula with the cephalad hand.

Sitting Method

- Perform the reduction with the patient sitting upright with the elbow on the affected side flexed at a 90-degree angle.
- Form an article of clothing into a 91-cm (3-foot) loop around the proximal forearm.
- Apply downward traction by placing your foot in the loop, freeing your hands to apply gentle rotation (usually slightly external), while maintaining elbow flexion.
- Have an assistant stand on the opposite side of the patient and maintain countertraction by placing his or her arms around the patient's chest, with hands in the axilla.

Supine and Prone Methods

- An alternative method is to have the patient lie prone so that the injured arm dangles free.
- A thick pad is placed under the injured shoulder.
- A 4.5- to 9-kg (10- to 20-lb) weight is attached to the wrist or forearm (the patient should not attempt to hold the weight).
- The weight is allowed to exert steady traction on the arm, using gravity to relocate the humeral head.
- The weight can be improvised from a stuff bag, helmet, or bucket filled with sand (Fig. 18.11).
- Another common method of reduction is linear traction along the axial line of the extremity while stabilizing the torso with a blanket or rope (Fig. 18.12).
- The patient lies supine, on the ground or a makeshift table.
- A sheet or padded belt or strapping can be tied around the caregiver's waist and the patient's bent forearm so that the caregiver (standing or kneeling) can lean back to apply traction, leaving his/her hands free to guide the head of the humerus back into position (Fig. 18.13).
- Padding is placed in the armpit and bend of the elbow to prevent pressure injury to sensitive nerves beneath the skin.

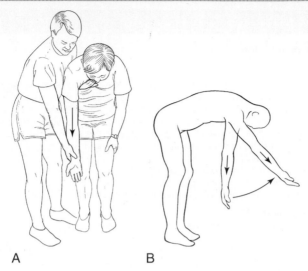

A   **B**

FIGURE 18.9 Technique for shoulder relocation with patient standing. Rescuer supports patient's chest with one hand (**A**) and pulls down and forward (**B**) with the other hand.

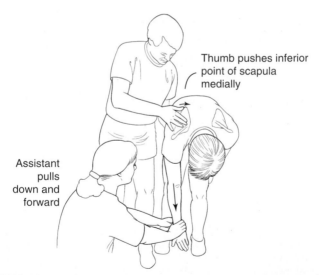

Thumb pushes inferior point of scapula medially

Assistant pulls down and forward

FIGURE 18.10 Scapular rotation is an assistive maneuver for any method used to reduce an anterior shoulder dislocation. If two rescuers are available, scapular rotation to assist the shoulder relocation can be performed while the second rescuer pulls the arm down and forward. The inferior tip of scapula is pushed medially.

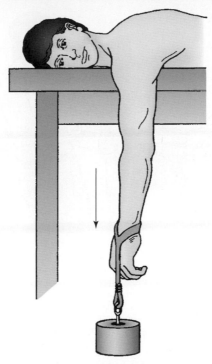

FIGURE 18.11 Stimson technique. (Redrawn from Rockwood CA, Green CA, editors: *Fractures in adults*, ed 6, vol 2, Philadelphia, 2001, Lippincott Williams & Wilkins, p 1305.)

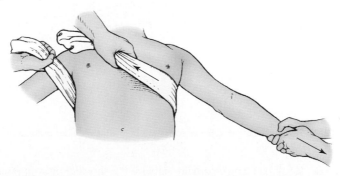

FIGURE 18.12 Traction and countertraction for dislocated shoulder reduction.

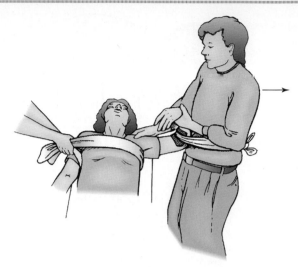

FIGURE 18.13   Repositioning a dislocated shoulder. Attached to the patient's forearm with a strap, rope, or sheet, the rescuer uses his body weight to apply traction, leaving his hands free to manipulate the patient's arm. A second rescuer applies countertraction, or the patient can be held motionless by fixing the chest sheet to a tree or ground stake. (From Auerbach PS: *Medicine for the outdoors: The essential guide to emergency medical procedures and first aid*, ed 6, Philadelphia, 2016, Elsevier.)

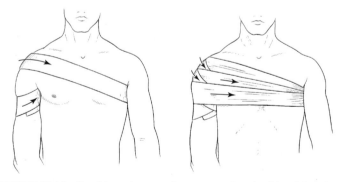

FIGURE 18.14   Shoulder spica wrap for support after shoulder dislocation.

use, kayak paddling), partially stabilize the shoulder by wrapping an elastic wrap around the torso and upper arm to limit abduction and external rotation (Fig. 18.14).
9. Any patient with a first-time dislocation or severe postreduction pain requires evacuation and formal evaluation.

Posterior Shoulder Dislocation
Signs and Symptoms
- Occurs in less than 5% of shoulder dislocations; caused by a direct blow to the anterior shoulder or may result from marked internal rotation associated with a grand mal seizure
- Significant pain and loss of shoulder motion, with external rotation often completely lost; greater ROM is more common than with anterior dislocation; diagnosis often missed owing to this motion and the lack of obvious deformity
- Using palpation, can usually detect posterior fullness not appreciated on the uninjured (comparison) side

Treatment
The reduction maneuver, aftercare, and indications for evacuation are like those for anterior dislocation.

Shoulder Fracture/Dislocation
Signs and Symptoms
- More common with a high-velocity accident (e.g., motor vehicle accident) or an older patient
- Crepitus may be noted over fracture site

Treatment
1. Do not reduce suspected fracture/dislocation in the field.
2. Treat this injury as a fracture, with splinting of the extremity to the torso with a sling or a sling and swath.

Elbow
Signs and Symptoms
- Occurs with hyperextension or axial loading from a fall onto the outstretched hand, generally posterior and lateral
- Signs obvious, with posterior deformity at the elbow and foreshortening of the forearm

Treatment
1. After careful examination of the distal sensory, motor, and circulatory status, perform reduction.
   a. With countertraction on the upper arm, apply linear traction with the elbow slightly flexed and the forearm in the original degree of pronation or supination (Fig. 18.15).
   b. Premedication with an opiate or benzodiazepine can be extremely helpful.
   c. Reduction (which can be a painful maneuver) leads to nearly complete relief of pain and restoration of normal surface anatomy.
2. After reduction, apply a posterior splint with the elbow in 90 degrees of flexion and the forearm in neutral position.
   a. Use a sling for comfort.
   b. If reduction is not successful after three vigorous attempts or if a nerve or vascular injury is suspected, apply a splint

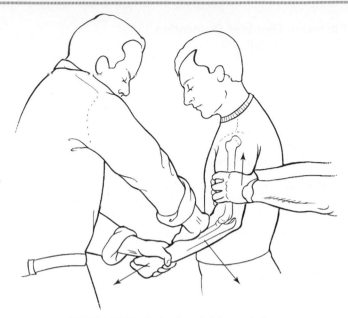

FIGURE 18.15   Reduction of dislocated elbow.

to the arm in the most comfortable position and initiate evacuation.

Wrist
Signs and Symptoms
- Frequently associated with carpal fracture(s)
- Generally produced by a fall onto the outstretched hand
- Severe pain, swelling, and deformity within the distal wrist
- Without radiograph, difficult to differentiate from a distal radius fracture

Treatment
1. Carefully assess distal neurovascular function, emphasizing median nerve function.
2. For wrist dislocation or fracture, perform a reduction maneuver.
3. Grasp the patient's hand as for a handshake, place countertraction on the upper arm, and apply linear traction. Note that significant force is required, and premedication, if available, may be extremely helpful.
4. If reduction is unsuccessful after three vigorous attempts or if there is median nerve dysfunction, arrange for evacuation.

5. Apply a short-arm (U or volar) splint if reduction is successful (see Fig. 18.1).
6. Elevate the arm as much as possible until the definitive care center can be reached.

Metacarpophalangeal Joint

Dislocation is rare and usually follows a crush injury, or occurs when a hand is caught in a rope. The site is usually dorsal, and it may be difficult to reduce in the field.

Signs and Symptoms
- Finger shortened, deviated to the ulnar side, and positioned in extension
- Metacarpal head possibly prominent in the palm
- The thumb MCP joint typically injured
- Injury to the ulnar collateral ligament of this joint ("skier's thumb") is a result of valgus stress, such as when an individual falls holding an object (e.g., pole) in the first web space

Treatment
Metacarpophalangeal Joint
1. Dorsal dislocation may be irreducible if the head of the metacarpal becomes trapped between the volar ligaments (Fig. 18.16).
2. Reduction depends on the degree of disruption of supporting structures, such as the volar plate and collateral ligaments. Thus,

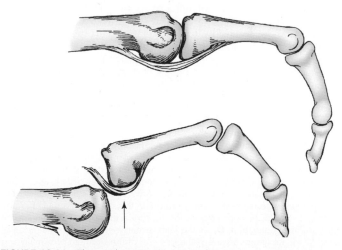

FIGURE 18.16   The single most important element preventing reduction in a complex metacarpophalangeal dislocation is interposition of the volar plate within the joint space. It must be extricated surgically. (From Rockwood CA Jr, Green DP, Bucholz RW, editors: *Rockwood and Green's fractures in adults,* ed 3, Philadelphia, 1991, JB Lippincott.)

this dislocation frequently requires open reduction in an operating room setting.

3. Most dorsal dislocations are easily reduced.
    a. First, the proximal phalanx is hyperextended 90 degrees on the metacarpal
    b. Then, the base of the proximal phalanx is pushed into flexion, maintaining contact always with the metacarpal head to prevent entrapment of the volar plate in the joint (see Fig. 18.16).
    c. Straight longitudinal traction is avoided.
    d. The wrist and interphalangeal joints are flexed to relax the flexor tendons.

4. The joint usually reduces easily with a palpable and audible clunk.

5. If reduction of a digital MCP joint dislocation is successful, apply a volar splint with the joint held in 90 degrees of flexion and interphalangeal joints in full extension.

6. If reduction is unsuccessful, splint the joint in the position of comfort and arrange for definitive treatment as soon as possible.

Thumb Metacarpophalangeal Joint

1. The thumb MCP joint is the most commonly injured.
2. Dislocations are reduced as already described.
3. Injury to the ulnar collateral ligament of this joint (skier's or gamekeeper's thumb) results from a valgus stress, as may occur when an individual falls holding an object in the first web space.
4. The patient complains of tenderness over the ulnar aspect of the MCP joint.
5. There may be instability to radial stress with the joint held in 30 degrees of flexion, an indication for surgical repair.
6. Often the adductor aponeurosis becomes interposed between the ligament and its bony attachment, resulting in a Stener lesion (Fig. 18.17).

FIGURE 18.17   Diagram of the displacement of the ulnar collateral ligament of the thumb metacarpophalangeal joint. **A,** Normal relationship, with the ulnar ligament covered by the adductor aponeurosis. **B,** With slight radial angulation, the proximal margin of the aponeurosis slides distally and leaves a portion of the ligament uncovered. **C,** With major radical angulation, the ulnar ligament ruptures at its distal insertion. In this degree of angulation, the aponeurosis has displaced distal to the rupture and permitted the ligament to escape from beneath it. **D,** As the joint is realigned, the proximal edge of the adductor aponeurosis sweeps the free end of the ligament proximally and farther away from its insertion. This is the Stener lesion. Unless surgically restored, the ulnar ligament will not heal properly and will be unstable to lateral stress. (Redrawn from Stener B: Skeletal injuries associated with rupture of the ulnar collateral ligament of the metacarpophalangeal joint of the thumb: A clinical and anatomical study, *Acta Chir Scand* 125:583, 1963.)

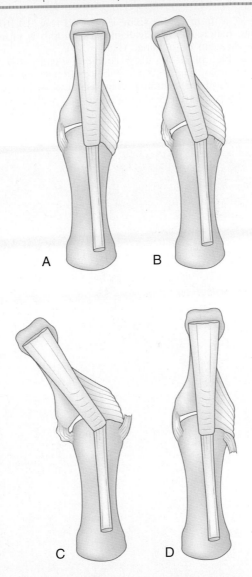

A

B

C

D

7. In the field, a thumb spica splint is applied (Fig. 18.18).
8. If splinting material is not available, the thumb is taped until definitive care can be obtained (Fig. 18.19).
9. When possible, place an ulnar collateral ligament tear in a thumb spica splint (Fig. 18.20). Instability often requires a lateral stress radiograph for definitive diagnosis and is an indication for surgical repair. Arrange for definitive care within 10 days of the injury.

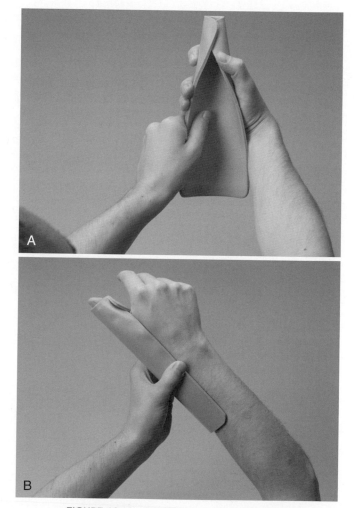

FIGURE 18.18   Padded aluminum thumb spica.

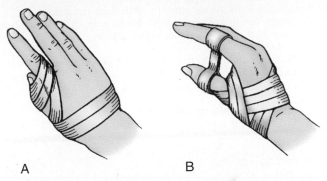

A   B

FIGURE 18.19   Taping the thumb for immobilization. **A,** The buddy-taping method. **B,** A thumb-lock. If possible, padding should be placed between the thumb and forefinger. (From Auerbach PS: *Medicine for the outdoors: The essential guide to emergency medical procedures and first aid*, ed 6, Philadelphia, 2016, Elsevier.)

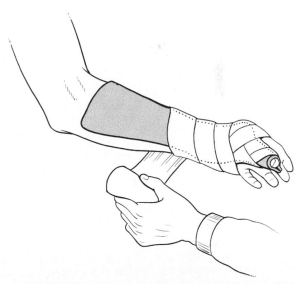

FIGURE 18.20   SAM Splint used to fashion a thumb splint.

10. For dorsal dislocation, attempt MCP joint reduction.
    a. Grasp the finger and apply longitudinal traction, moving from MCP joint extension into flexion ("up and over" the metacarpal head).
    b. Splint the thumb in the position of function (see Figs. 18.18 and 18.20).
11. Obtain orthopedic follow-up within 10 days.

Proximal Interphalangeal Joint

PIP joint dislocation is common and occurs with axial loading of a finger.

Signs and Symptoms

- Dislocation occurring when an individual attempts to catch an object or a finger becomes entangled in a rope or another piece of equipment
- Dislocation generally dorsal (middle phalanx in relationship to the proximal)

Treatment

1. Reduction of dorsal PIP dislocation is performed as described for dorsal MCP dislocation (Fig. 18.21).
2. Straight longitudinal traction is avoided to prevent entrapment of the volar plate into the joint.
3. After reduction, do the following:
    a. Tape the finger to an adjacent finger to avoid hyperextension and allow early motion (Fig. 18.22).
    b. Alternatively, apply a volar splint and tape the finger to the splint in slight flexion.
4. Initiate early motion of the joint to regain full extension.
5. Keep the distal interphalangeal (DIP) joint free for active ROM. The active ROM of the DIP encourages the lateral bands to stay dorsal and thus help prevent a boutonnière deformity. Be careful not to hyperextend the PIP, especially with significant swelling, to avoid serious dorsal wound breakdown.
6. With either volar or distal dislocation, arrange for definitive care as soon as possible.

Distal Interphalangeal Joint

The DIP joint is less frequently injured than the PIP joint.

Signs and Symptoms

- Volar dislocation or subluxation, resulting in disruption of the terminal extensor mechanism (mallet deformity)
- Occasionally, when an object is firmly grasped and then pulled away, rupture of the flexor profundus tendon ("jersey finger")
- DIP joint dislocation: active extension of the DIP joint absent
- Rupture of the flexor profundus tendon: active flexion of the DIP joint absent

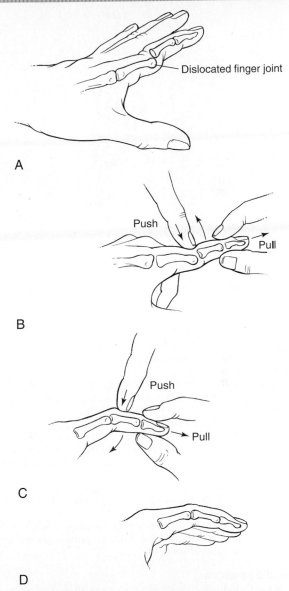

FIGURE 18.21 Traction method of joint reduction.

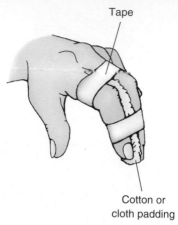

Tape

Cotton or
cloth padding

FIGURE 18.22   Buddy-taping method to immobilize a finger. (From Auerbach PS: *Medicine for the outdoors: The essential guide to emergency medical procedures and first aid*, ed 6, Philadelphia, 2015, Elsevier.)

Treatment

1. DIP joint reduction.
   a. Obtain reduction with traction; then examine the joint for full active extension.
   b. Splint the joint in 0 degrees of extension for 3 weeks.
   c. Radiographic examination must be performed to rule out an intra-articular fracture.
2. For rupture of the flexor profundus tendon, splint the digit in flexion and instruct the patient to see an upper extremity surgeon within 7 days.

Pelvis Fractures

In the wilderness setting, a pelvis fracture is generally associated with a fall from a significant height or a high-velocity skiing accident.

The key factor in pelvis fracture is identification of instability to the pelvic ring, which is associated with significant hemorrhage, neurologic injury, and mortality.

Bleeding associated with a pelvis injury is from cancellous bone at the fracture sites, retroperitoneal lumbar venous plexus injury, or—rarely—pelvic arterial injuries.

Signs and Symptoms

- On clinical examination, a simple fracture is an area of tenderness not associated with detectable instability.
- Diagnosis of an unstable pelvis fracture is based on instability of the pelvis associated with posterior pain, swelling, ecchymosis, and motion on examination.

- To palpate, place hands on each iliac crest. Press outward and then inward to determine whether the pelvis is unstable. An unstable pelvis "gives" with this type of compression or distraction force. This test should only be performed once to establish the diagnosis but not repeated, to prevent unnecessary neurovascular injury.
- In addition, look for leg-length discrepancy, which can be a sign of a vertically unstable pelvis fracture.
- Flank, gluteal, perianal, and scrotal swelling with ecchymosis are additional signs of an unstable pelvis fracture.
- Pelvic hemorrhage may occur rapidly, so identify the injury without delay. Monitor hemodynamic changes.
- Unstable fractures are associated with a high incidence of significant hemorrhage, neurologic injury, and mortality. Hemorrhage, gastrointestinal, genitourinary, and neurologic injuries contribute to mortality. An open pelvis fracture (displacement of the pelvic ring) has a mortality rate of up to 50%.
- Anterior–posterior compression injury presents as anterior instability, along with a palpable ramus fracture or gapping of the pubic symphysis ("diastasis").
- Pelvis fracture may be associated with bladder, prostate, and urethral injury.

Treatment

1. The key factor in initial management of a pelvis fracture is identification of instability to the pelvic ring. If you find this, arrange for immediate evacuation with the patient on a backboard, taking care to minimize leg and torso motion.
2. Be aware that the patient is usually most comfortable with the hips and knees in slight flexion. Pad the patient generously with blankets or sleeping bags.
3. Attempt to stabilize the pelvis:
   a. Use a SAM Sling, or improvise a similar device (Fig. 18.23).
   b. Wrap an inflatable mattress around the patient's hips and pelvis, securing it with tape or rolled elastic wrap, and then inflating to a firm, but not rigid, pressure (Fig. 18.24).
   c. If an inflatable mattress or SAM Sling is not available, tie a garment securely around the pelvis. A bedsheet or jacket wrapped snugly around the pelvis of an individual with a suspected unstable pelvic fracture may provide stability and accomplish adequate tamponade of bleeding from the fracture.
   d. A standard SAM Splint unrolled inside the jacket sling may increase an improvised sling's efficacy.
   e. The applied sling belt or similar contrivance should be left in place until definitive care is available.
4. Be aware that an unstable pelvis fracture can cause significant hemorrhage. If available, arrange for intravenous (IV) fluid volume replacement pending early blood product transfusion. If possible, start two 16-gauge IV catheters in the upper extremities. Do

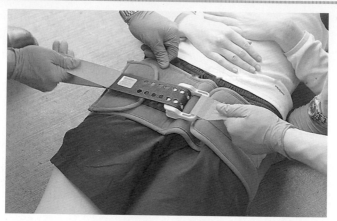

FIGURE 18.23   SAM Sling.

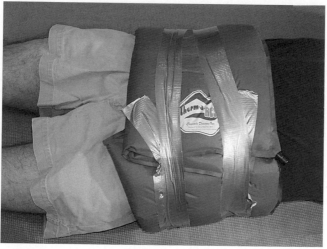

FIGURE 18.24   Pelvic sling improvised with inflatable sleeping bag and duct tape.

not use the lower extremities because if there is venous disruption in the pelvis, the fluid may extravasate.

LOWER EXTREMITY FRACTURES
Proximal Femur (Hip)
Most hip fractures occur in the femoral neck or intertrochanteric region.

Signs and Symptoms

- Pain around the proximal thigh
- With some proximal femur fractures, little local reaction in terms of swelling or deformity around the hip region to aid in diagnosis
- Significant pain from any movement of the affected limb
- Affected limb often noticeably shortened and externally rotated
- Patient can rapidly lose 2 units of blood into the proximal thigh

Treatment

1. After doing a careful sensory, motor, and circulatory examination, realign the limb into anatomic position.
2. Light traction with a Kendrick, Thomas, Sager, or improvised splint should be considered for transport. However, traction should be avoided if a pelvic fracture cannot be ruled out.
3. If a traction splint is not available, transport the patient on a backboard, with the limbs strapped together and padding placed between them.
4. Because evidence indicates that emergency treatment of a fracture of the femoral neck decreases the risk for posttraumatic necrosis, arrange for rapid evacuation of any patient in whom this injury is suspected.

Femoral Shaft

Fracture of the femoral shaft follows a fall from a significant height or results from a high-velocity injury.

Signs and Symptoms

- Crepitus and maximum deformity at mid-thigh
  - Severe pain and tenderness
  - Possible shortening of the injured extremity
- Often massive swelling

Treatment

1. This may be an open injury; remove the patient's clothing at the injured site to complete the examination. If you find an open wound, arrange for rapid evacuation.
2. Be aware that there may also be an associated femoral neck fracture.
3. After completing a neurovascular examination, place the limb in a commercial or improvised traction device. Box 18.4 lists general principles of traction; Box 18.5 outlines femoral traction systems and discusses the ankle hitch and rigid support; and Box 18.6 lists traction mechanisms, anchors, and the method for securing and padding. Several commercial traction splints are available, including the Hare, Klippel, Sager, Thomas, Trac 3, Reel, Slishman, and Kendrick. The Slishman and Kendrick

Text continued on p. 213

BOX 18.4   General Principles of Traction

Why Use Traction?
In the backcountry environment, traction is essential for two fundamental reasons:
1. A general inability to provide IV volume expansion
2. Prolonged transport time to definitive care. One primary
   purpose of femoral traction is to limit blood loss into the thigh.
   For a constant surface area, the volume of a sphere is greater
   than the volume of a cylinder. Pulling (via traction) the thigh
   compartment back into its natural cylindrical shape limits blood
   loss into the soft tissue. Enhanced patient comfort and
   decreased potential for neurovascular damage are important
   secondary benefits.

What Criteria Should Be Used to Evaluate a Traction System?
Consider five key design principles when evaluating a femoral traction
system:
1. Does the splint provide in-line traction, or does it incorrectly pull
   the patient's leg off to the side or needlessly plantar flex the
   patient's ankle?
2. Is the splint comfortable? Ask the patient how it feels.
3. Does the splint compromise neurologic or vascular function?
   Constantly check the patient's distal neurovascular function.
4. Is the splint durable, or will it break when subjected to backcountry stress? Try your traction design on an uninjured patient
   first.
5. Is the splint cumbersome? Many reasonable splint designs
   become so bulky and awkward that litter transport, technical
   rescue, or helicopter evacuation is impossible. For example, a
   full-length ski splint is not compatible with evacuation in certain
   small helicopters.

BOX 18.5   Femoral Traction Systems

Every femoral traction system has six components: ankle hitch, rigid
support, traction mechanism, proximal anchor, method for securing,
and padding. The ankle hitch and rigid support are outlined next.
Box 18.6 lists traction mechanisms, proximal anchoring, a method for
securing, and padding.

Ankle Hitch
Various techniques are used to anchor the distal extremity to the
splint. Many work well, but some are difficult to recall in an emergency.
Choose a technique that is easy to remember, and practice it.

Double-Runner System
This system is a very straightforward technique. Lay two short webbing
loops ("runners") over and under the ankle (Fig. 18.25A). Pass the
long loop sides through the short loop on both sides and adjust

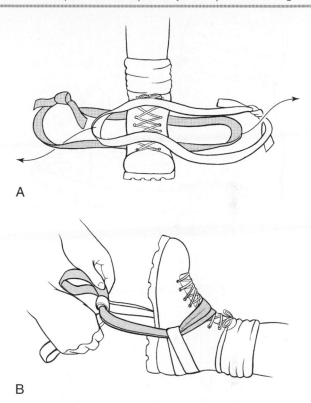

A

B

FIGURE 18.25   Double-runner ankle hitch.

BOX 18.5   Femoral Traction Systems—cont'd

(see Fig. 18.25B). This system is infinitely adjustable, enabling you to center the pull from any direction. Proper padding is essential, especially for a lengthy transport. Use the patient's boot to distribute the pressure over the foot and ankle, although this obscures visualization and palpation of the foot. You can leave the boot in place and cut out the toe section for observation.

Patient's Boot System

Use the patient's own boot as the hitch. Cut two holes into the sidewalls of the boot just above the midsole, in line with the ankle joint. Thread a piece of nylon webbing or a cravat through to complete the ankle hitch (Fig. 18.26). Because the boot is now functionally ruined, cut away the toe to allow direct neurovascular assessment.

Continued

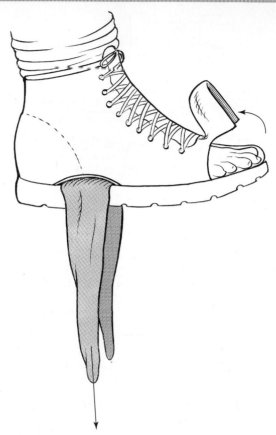

FIGURE 18.26 Traction using cut boot and cravat.

BOX 18.5 Femoral Traction Systems—cont'd

Buck's Traction
For extended transport, improvise Buck's traction using a closed-cell foam pad (Fig. 18.27). Duct tape stirrups are added to a small foam pad that is wrapped around the leg. The entire unit is wrapped with a securing bandage. This system helps distribute the force of the traction over a large surface area.

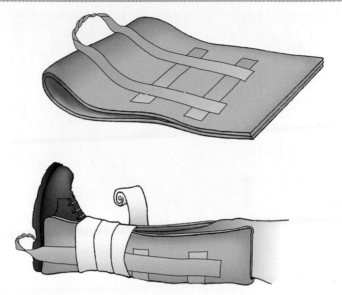

FIGURE 18.27   Buck's traction.

BOX 18.6   Traction Mechanisms

Historically the first traction mechanism is the Boy Scout-style "Spanish windlass." A windlass works, but it can be awkward to apply and is often not durable. The windlass can unwind if it is inadvertently jarred and can apply rotational forces to the leg. The amount of traction required is primarily a function of patient comfort. A general rule is to use 10% of body weight or 4.5 to 6.8 kg (10 to 15 lb) for the average patient. After traction is applied, always recheck distal neurovascular function (circulation, sensation, movement). An improvised traction system invariably relaxes during transport and should be rechecked for proper tension.

Cam Lock or Fastex Slider
This is a simple, effective system that uses straps that have Fastex-like sliders and are often used as waist belts or to strap items to packs. Alternatively, use a cam lock with nylon webbing. Attach the belt to the distal portion of the rigid support and then to the ankle hitch. Traction is easily applied by cinching the nylon webbing (Fig. 18.28).

Trucker's Hitch
Fashion a windlass using small-diameter line (parachute cord) and a standard trucker's hitch for additional mechanical advantage (Fig. 18.29). An adjustable tent pole allows traction to be applied by elongating the pole during manual traction.

Continued

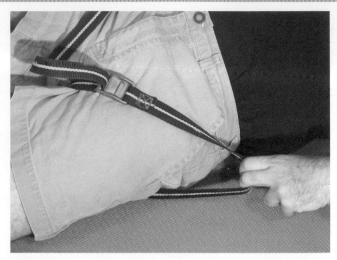

FIGURE 18.28 Proximal anchor using cam lock belt. The belt is applied as shown. The strap is adjusted loosely to allow the belt to ride up to the point of the hip. If the strap is improperly tightened, it can create pressure over the fracture, and moves the traction point to a less optimal distal position. Padding is helpful but not always necessary if the patient is wearing pants and the strap is properly adjusted.

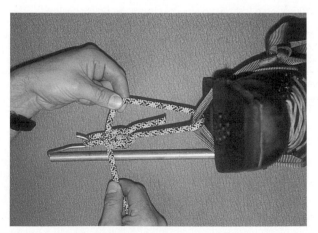

FIGURE 18.29 Tent pole traction with trucker's hitch. A bent tent stake is placed into the end of the tent pole as the distal traction anchor. A simple trucker's hitch is used to provide traction.

BOX 18.6   Traction Mechanisms—cont'd

Prusik Knot
This is useful with almost any system (see Fig. 18.37A). Prusik knots provide traction from rigid supports with few tie-on points (e.g., a canoe paddle shaft or a tent pole). The Prusik knot can be used to apply the traction (by sliding the knot distally) or simply as an attachment point for one of the traction mechanisms already mentioned.

Litter Traction
If no rigid support is available and a rigid litter (e.g., Stokes) is being used, apply traction from the rigid bar at the foot end of the litter. If this system is used, you must immobilize the patient on the litter with adequate countertraction, such as that using inguinal straps.

Proximal Anchor
The simplest proximal anchor uses a single ischial strap, which can be made from a piece of climbing webbing or a prefabricated strap, belt, or cam lock (Fig. 18.30). A cloth cravat can be used in a pinch. On the river, a life jacket can be used (Fig. 18.31), and when climbing, a climbing harness is ideal. The preferred system is a proximal ischial strap, but a padded medial support (analogous to a Sager Splint) also can be used. When using a medial traction system (Sager analog), generously pad the inguinal area. A folded SAM Splint attached to the proximal end of the rigid support works well.

Continued

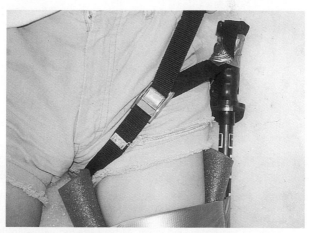

FIGURE 18.30   Proximal anchor using a cam-lock belt. The belt is applied as shown. A ski pole is used laterally as the rigid support. Duct tape is useful for securing components, and padding is helpful but not always necessary if the patient is wearing pants.

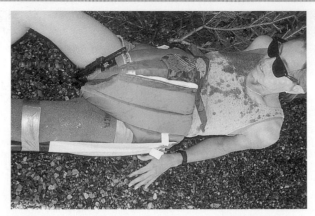

FIGURE 18.31   Life jacket proximal anchor. An inverted life jacket worn like a diaper forms a well-padded proximal anchor. A kayak paddle is rigged to the life jacket's side adjustment strap.

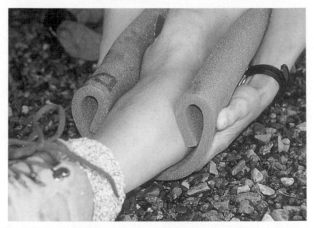

FIGURE 18.32   Folding Ensolite padding often provides better visualization of an extremity than does a circumferential wrap.

BOX 18.6   Traction Mechanisms—cont'd

Securing and Padding
All potential pressure points should be checked to ensure that they are adequately padded. An excellent padding system can be made by first covering the upper and lower parts of the leg with a folded length of Ensolite (Fig. 18.32). Folded Ensolite is preferred over the circumferential wrap because the folded system allows for visualization of the extremity. The patient will be more comfortable if femoral

BOX 18.6 Traction Mechanisms—cont'd

traction is applied with the knee in slight flexion (place padding beneath the knee during transport). The splint must be secured firmly to the leg. Almost any strap-like object will work, but a 10- to 15-cm (4- to 6-inch) elasticized (Ace) bandage wrapped circumferentially will provide a comfortable and secure union. Finally, the ankles or feet should be strapped or tied together to give the system additional stability. Tying the ankles together also protects the injured leg from external rotation and jarring during transport.

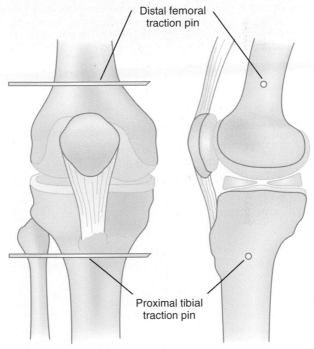

Distal femoral
traction pin

Proximal tibial
traction pin

FIGURE 18.33 Proper positioning of a distal femoral or proximal tibial traction (Steinmann) pin.

devices are well-suited for wilderness use because of their minimal weight, low volume, and portability.

4. In austere or disaster environments where definitive care is provided in resource-limited settings, it may be reasonable for a physician or surgeon with proper training to place a distal femoral or proximal tibial traction (Steinmann) pin under sterile conditions with local anesthesia (Fig. 18.33).

a. The femoral pin is the method of choice for acetabular or proximal femur fractures and is placed from medial to lateral, and proximal to the femoral epicondyle to avoid the neurovascular bundle.

b. The tibial traction pin is the method of choice for mid or distal femur fractures and is placed from lateral to medial, 2 cm (0.8 inch) posterior and 1 cm (0.4 inch) distal to the tibial tubercle to avoid the common peroneal nerve.

c. Once placed, up to 20% of the patient's body weight can be applied as traction to the pin.

Distal Femur and Patella

Fracture of the distal end of the femur is frequently intra-articular and occurs with high-velocity loading when the knee is flexed. With axial loading of the femur, the patella becomes the driving wedge and the femoral condyles are impacted.

Signs and Symptoms
- Crepitus, significant instability (not seen with patellar fracture)
- Possible patellar fracture or splitting of the distal femoral condyles
- With patellar fracture:
  - Injury often obvious on deep palpation
  - If complete fracture of the patella, extensor mechanism will not work and active knee extension will be absent
  - Injury often open because very little soft tissue overlies this sesamoid bone

Treatment
1. After initial examination of nerve and vessel function, realign the limb into an anatomic position.
2. Apply a splint to the realigned limb for transportation.
3. With an open wound in the region of the fracture or an abnormal nerve or vascular examination, arrange for immediate evacuation.

Rigid Support
This can be fabricated as a unilateral support, like the Sager traction splint or the Kendrick traction device, or as a bilateral support, such as the Thomas half-ring or the Hare traction splint. Unilateral supports tend to be easier to apply than bilateral support.

Double Ski Pole System
This is fashioned like a Thomas half-ring, with the interlocked pole straps slipped under the proximal thigh to form the ischial support. Some mountain guides carry a prefabricated, drilled ski pole section or aluminum bar that can be used to stabilize the distal end of this system (Fig. 18.34).

Single Ski Pole System
Use a single ski pole either between the legs, which is ideal for bilateral femoral fractures, or lateral to the injured leg. The ultimate

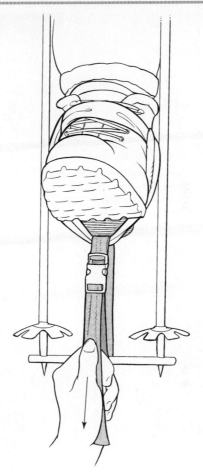

FIGURE 18.34 Double ski pole system with prefabricated crossbar and webbing belt traction. Prefabricated, drilled ski section is used to attach the ends of two ski poles. Traction is applied with a webbing belt and a sliding buckle.

rigid support is an adjustable telescoping ski pole used laterally. You can elongate the pole to the appropriate length for each patient, making the splint very compact for litter work or helicopter evacuation (Fig. 18.35).

Tent Pole System
Fit conventional sectioned tent poles together to create the ideal length for rigid support. Because of their flexibility, make sure the

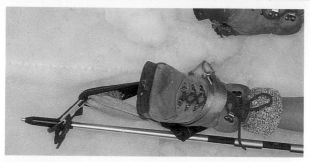

FIGURE 18.35 Single ski pole system. An adjustable telescoping ski pole is used as the rigid support. A stirrup is attached to a carabiner placed over the end of the pole. Traction is applied by elongating the ski pole while another rescuer provides manual traction on the patient's leg.

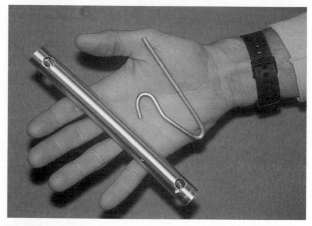

FIGURE 18.36 Prefabricated, drilled tent pole section, and bent stake, which serves as a distal traction anchor if a tent pole is used as the rigid support.

tent poles are well secured to the leg to prevent them from flexing out of position. Place a blanket pin or bent tent stake (Fig. 18.36) in the end of the pole to provide an anchor for the traction system. Alternatively, use a Prusik knot to secure the system to the end of the tent pole (Fig. 18.37).

Miscellaneous

You can use any suitable object, such as a canoe paddle, two ice axes taped together at the handles, or a straight tree limb, to fashion a rigid support. Although skis immediately come to mind as a suitable rigid component, they are often too cumbersome. Because of their length, skis may extend far beyond the patient's feet or

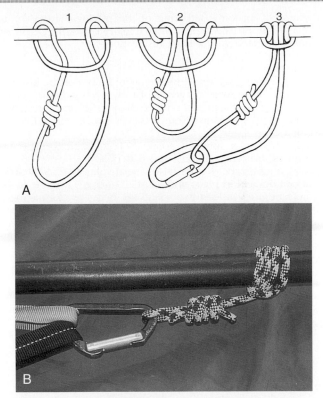

FIGURE 18.37   A, Prusik knot made from a small-diameter cord is used as an adjustable distal traction anchor. **B,** Two Prusik wraps are shown. Three or four wraps provide additional friction and security. If a Prusik knot slips, it can be easily taped in place.

require placement into the axilla, which is unnecessary and inhibits the patient's mobility (e.g., sitting up during transport). Prefabricated canvas pockets, available through the National Ski Patrol System, provide a ski tip and tail attachment grommet for use with the ski system.

Tibia and Fibula

Tibial shaft fracture is associated with fibular shaft fracture in 90% of cases. These fractures result from high-impact trauma. The tibial plateau can be fractured by a fall or jump from a height.

Signs and Symptoms

- Pain, swelling, and deformity obvious on initial examination
- With a tibial plateau fracture, hemarthrosis quickly noted with significant swelling around the knee

- Because of anatomic tethering of the popliteal artery by the fascia of the soleus complex, arterial injury is possible, especially when associated with a knee dislocation

Treatment

1. When this injury is suspected, the entire limb must be inspected for distal sensory, motor, and circulatory function before realignment. Check distal pulses and capillary refill and for signs of compartment syndrome. Neurovascular checks should be performed every hour.
2. Apply a posterior splint, U splint, or combination, made from fiberglass, plaster, or improvised materials.
3. Use a custom-made or improvised metal splint (e.g., SAM Splint) that can be held in place with elastic bandages or tape. If SAM Splints are used, at least two splints are necessary for the medial and lateral component, and preferably a third for the posterior section (Fig. 18.38). A foam sleeping pad stabilized with rigid tent poles, ski pole sections, wooden branches, etc., may also be used.
4. Always pad the leg sufficiently before splinting.
5. An air splint also provides adequate immobilization of the tibiofibular fracture.
6. Hold the ankle in neutral position.
7. Strap the injured leg to the noninjured leg to reduce rotational forces during transport.

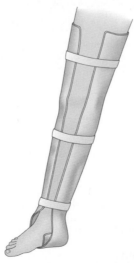

FIGURE 18.38 Lower leg and/or ankle splint. A sugar-tong splint can be used to immobilize fractures of the tibia, fibula, or ankle.

8. If materials are limited, fashion a crude splint by strapping the injured leg to the noninjured leg with a well-padded tree limb or walking stick placed between them for support.
9. Transport any patient with an unstable lower extremity fracture or dislocation with the limb elevated.

Ankle

The intra-articular distal tibia, medial malleolus, distal fibula, or any combination of these may be involved in an ankle fracture, generally produced by large torsional forces around a fixed foot. With the distal tibia, axial loading from a fall or jump also may be involved.

Signs and Symptoms

- Significant pain and swelling when the shoe is removed
- Crepitus and deformity possible

Treatment

1. Palpate along the medial and lateral malleoli to confirm the clinical suspicion.
2. After the shoe is removed to inspect the skin for open wounds, perform a neurovascular examination.
3. With rotational deformity in the ankle, realign the ankle with gentle traction before applying a posterior splint with the ankle in the neutral position.
4. Apply a U-shaped blanket roll or pillow splint.
5. During transport, elevate the limb above the level of the heart, with the patient supine on a backboard if possible.

Talus and Calcaneus

Signs and Symptoms

- Fracture of the calcaneus and talus during a fall or jump from a height when the patient lands on his or her feet
- With calcaneus fracture, significant heel pain, deformity, and crepitus immediately evident after the boot is removed
- Severe swelling within a couple of hours
- Examine patient for possible lumbar spine fractures
- With talus fracture, it may be impossible to differentiate clinically from ankle fracture:
  - Occurs when the foot is forced into maximum dorsiflexion
  - Tenderness and swelling distal to or at the level of the malleoli
- With ankle fracture, tenderness and deformity at the level of the malleoli
- Fractures of other tarsal bones, although exceedingly rare, defined by localizing the tenderness to a specific site

Treatment

1. Apply a short-leg splint with extra padding for all these fractures.
2. Elevate the limb during transportation.

3. If a talus fracture is suspected, expedite evacuation of the patient, because post-traumatic necrosis of the talar body is a common complication.

Metatarsal

Fracture at the base of a metatarsal often occurs in combination with a midfoot dislocation. Fractures frequently occur across the entire midfoot joint and are often associated with fractures at the bases of the second and fifth metatarsals. They usually occur with axial loading of the foot while it is in maximum plantar flexion.

Metatarsal shaft fractures occur with crush injuries and with falls or jumps from moderate heights. Midshaft metatarsal fracture also occurs as a stress, or so-called march, fracture. This injury is often the result of prolonged hiking or running.

Signs and Symptoms
- With metatarsal base fracture
  - Midfoot pain and swelling
  - Once the shoe is removed, there is crepitus and tenderness at the base of the metatarsal
  - Generally, overall alignment of the foot maintained, but instability is revealed with stressing the midfoot by stabilizing the heel and placing stress across the forefoot in the varus and valgus directions
- With metatarsal shaft fracture
  - Dull pain at the midshaft of a metatarsal (often the second or fifth) converted to more severe pain with associated crepitus by a jump from a log or rock
  - Tenderness usually localized

Treatment
1. For metatarsal base fracture, place the foot in a well-padded posterior splint and elevate.
2. Do not allow a patient with a suspected midfoot fracture/dislocation to ambulate because swelling will intensify and further injury to the midfoot may result. Beware of compartment syndrome with midfoot or Lisfranc fracture/dislocation.
3. For metatarsal shaft fracture, manage temporarily by having the patient wear a stiff-soled boot or orthotic insert. If fracture instability or extreme pain is present, apply a short-leg splint and allow no further weight bearing.

Phalanx

The great toe phalanx fracture is a significant problem functionally because of the necessary force placed on the great toe during the toe-off phase of weight bearing. A toe phalanx can be fractured by a crush injury or by having a heavy object drop onto the foot. This injury can be prevented using a hard-toed boot.

Signs and Symptoms
- Pain
- Ecchymosis
- Swelling

Treatment
1. Manage any phalanx fracture by taping the toe to an adjacent uninjured toe with cotton placed in between.
2. Be aware that a stiff-soled boot minimizes the discomfort accompanying weight bearing.

LOWER EXTREMITY DISLOCATIONS
Hip
Posterior hip dislocation is produced by axial loading of the femur with the limb in relative adduction. This injury occurs most commonly with the hip and knee flexed and force applied to the anterior knee or proximal leg. Dislocation may also occur when a large force is applied to the sole of the foot with the knee in extension.

Signs and Symptoms
- With posterior dislocation, severe pain around the hip
- Affected limb apparently shortened, adducted, and internally rotated, with any hip motion increasing the pain
- Not clinically possible to determine presence of an associated acetabular fracture
- With rare case of anterior dislocation, limb abducted and flexed and severely externally rotated. Anterior dislocation is generally produced by wide abduction of the hip from a significant force

Treatment
Place the patient in a supine position and perform a complete survey of all organ systems. Examine the distal limb carefully for associated fracture(s), and perform a careful sensory and motor examination. When the patient is any distance from definitive care, attempt closed reduction using one of the following techniques:
1. Captain Morgan technique (Fig. 18.39)
   a. Place the patient on a flat, hard surface.
   b. Provide analgesia with a narcotic, benzodiazepine, or both.
   c. Have an assistant stabilize the pelvis by placing both palms on the anterior iliac crests.
   d. The caregiver flexes the patient's hip and knee to 90 degrees. The caregiver then places their thigh under the calf of the flexed, dislocated hip.
   e. With one hand pressing downward on the ipsilateral ankle of the dislocated hip and the other hand lifting upward behind the ipsilateral knee of the dislocated hip, the caregiver plantarflexes their own ankle of the leg that is under the patient's thigh.
   f. This slow plantarflexion, along with the concomitant downward pressure distally and upward pressure proximally, allows

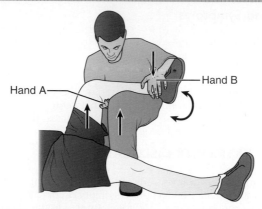

FIGURE 18.39 Captain Morgan technique for reducing a dislocated hip. (From Auerbach PS: *Medicine for the outdoors: The essential guide to first aid and medical emergencies,* ed 6, Philadelphia, 2016, Elsevier.)

the caregiver's thigh to be used as a fulcrum to facilitate the hip relocation
2. Alternatively, use the traction–countertraction technique
    a. Have an assistant stabilize the pelvis by placing both palms on the anterior iliac crests.
    b. Bend the patient's knee, and apply upward linear traction in line with the thigh (with an anterior dislocation) and with the hip flexed 30 degrees (with a posterior dislocation).
    c. If an assistant is available, try pulling a lateral force on the proximal thigh during longitudinal traction.
3. If unable to reduce the hip, expedite evacuation because a direct relationship exists between the time to reduction and the incidence of osteonecrosis of the femoral head.

Knee
The tibia may be dislocated in any of four directions relative to the distal femur. The most common direction is anterior (tibia anterior to the femur). This injury represents a true emergency because of the high incidence of associated vascular injury, which occurs because of tethering of the popliteal vessels along the posterior border of the tibia by the soleus fascia. Be aware of a spontaneously reduced knee dislocation. If there is complete rupture of the anterior and posterior cruciate ligaments, assume dislocation with spontaneous reduction until proven otherwise. These injuries may result in intimal tears of the popliteal artery and can lead to loss of the limb.

Signs and Symptoms
• Knee dislocation is obvious because of the amount of deformity involved

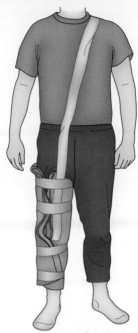

FIGURE 18.40 Functional knee and lower leg immobilizer. Wrap a sleeping pad around the lower leg from the mid-thigh to the foot. Fold the pad so the top of the leg is not included in the full splint. This provides better visualization of the extremity and leaves room for swelling. A full-length pad can be trimmed before rolling. A pair of suspenders can be fashioned if the patient is required or able to walk with assistance.

- Intimal flap tears of the popliteal artery, possibly producing delayed arterial thrombosis

Treatment

1. When this injury is suspected, perform a careful neurovascular screening examination. Intact distal pulses do not definitively rule out arterial injury.
2. After the initial examination, apply linear traction to the lower limb to reduce the knee. This is generally successful regardless of the direction of dislocation.
3. Immediate evacuation is indicated.
4. Emergency angiography may be indicated.
5. Apply a splint to the limb, and transport the patient on a backboard if possible. If the patient must walk with assistance, immobilize the knee with a splint and create suspenders to maintain splint position (Fig. 18.40).

6. Be vigilant for an arterial injury or compartment syndrome. If either is suspected, arrange for emergency evacuation.

Patella Dislocation

Because of the increased femorotibial angle in a female, patella dislocation is much more common in women. Generalized ligamentous laxity may predispose to this problem. Dislocation of the kneecap may result from a twisting injury or asymmetric quadriceps contraction during a fall.

Signs and Symptoms
- Pain
- Malposition of patella
- Large effusion in a spontaneously reduced patella dislocation

Treatment
1. The patella lies lateral to the articular distal femur. Although neurovascular injury rarely occurs in association with this injury, conduct a screening examination.
2. Reduce the patella by simply straightening the knee.
3. If this is not successful, apply gentle pressure to the patella to push it back up onto the distal femoral articular groove.
4. Apply a knee splint with the joint in extension. Encourage the patient to avoid weight bearing, but if this is not possible, be aware that further damage is unlikely.
5. Keep the patient's knee in extension until definitive care can be obtained (see Fig. 18.40).
6. Radiography is ultimately required to rule out osteochondral fracture, which is frequently associated with an acute injury.

Ankle
Signs and Symptoms
- Ankle dislocation is almost always accompanied by fracture(s) of one or both malleoli. This may involve the posterior malleolus from an avulsion fracture of the posterior talofibular ligament ("trimalleolar" fracture/dislocation)
- Swelling
- Pain
- Severe deformity

Treatment
1. Align the ankle joint by grasping the patient's posterior heel, applying traction with the knee bent (to relax the gastrocnemius–soleus complex), and bringing the foot into alignment with the distal tibia.
2. After this maneuver, reexamine the foot, dress any wounds, and apply a posterior splint or wrap splint (Fig. 18.41). Note that a U-shaped blanket roll or pillow splint can also be applied.
3. During transport, keep the limb elevated.
4. Use snow or ice to create cold compresses.

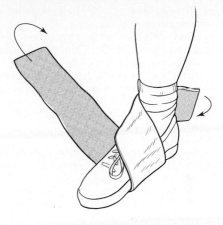

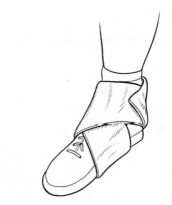

FIGURE 18.41   SAM Splint on ankle.

Hindfoot
Signs and Symptoms
Calcaneus dislocated medially or laterally relative to the talus, the latter being slightly more common

Treatment
1. Attempt a reduction if it will be more than 3 hours until the patient can be transported to a definitive care center.
2. If no other injuries are apparent, give the patient a sedative during reduction.
3. Medial dislocation is reduced more easily than lateral dislocation, in which the posterior tibial tendon frequently becomes displaced

onto the lateral neck of the talus, blocking the reduction. In either case, the maneuver is the same.

   a. Grasp the heel with the patient's knee flexed (relaxing the gastrocnemius–soleus complex), and apply linear traction to bring the heel over the ankle joint.

   b. Be aware that this maneuver is generally successful for medial dislocation, but lateral dislocation often requires open reduction.

4. After you attempt reduction, apply a posterior splint, a U-shaped blanket roll, or a pillow splint.

5. Make sure the limb is elevated.

6. Even if the reduction is successful, do not allow the patient to bear weight until definitive care is obtained.

Midfoot

Midfoot (Lisfranc) dislocation is generally associated with one or more fractures at the base of the metatarsals, usually the second and fifth metatarsals. Midfoot dislocation occurs with axial loading of the foot in maximal plantar flexion.

Signs and Symptoms

- Forefoot generally displaced laterally relative to the midfoot when the injury is initially unstable; more often, the foot is normally aligned
- Significant swelling with tenderness at the base of the second and fifth metatarsals
- Instability and crepitus, with dorsoplantar-oriented force frequent

Treatment

1. After the neurovascular examination, stress the forefoot by stabilizing the heel and applying a varus and valgus directed force. If the forefoot is unstable and associated with significant swelling, pain, or crepitus, consider a midfoot dislocation to be present.

2. Apply a short-leg (posterior or U-shaped) splint.

3. Elevate the foot during transport.

4. Do not allow the patient to bear weight.

Metatarsophalangeal and Interphalangeal Joints

Metatarsophalangeal joint dislocation of a toe is relatively uncommon but can occur in the great toe with moderate axial force. An injury of this type at the great toe may be associated with fracture of the metatarsal or phalanx; the dislocation is generally distal.

The lesser metatarsophalangeal joints are generally dislocated laterally or medially. The most common mechanism for this injury is striking unshod toes on immovable objects.

Signs and Symptoms

- Open fracture
- Pain

- Swelling
- Ecchymosis

Treatment

1. Because this may be an open fracture, perform a careful inspection of the foot.
2. Relocate the toe by applying linear traction with the patient supine and using the weight of the foot as countertraction.
3. Consider reduction of an interphalangeal joint by applying linear traction with gentle manipulation.
4. Once reduced, tape the injured toe to the adjacent toe for 1 to 3 weeks.
5. Have the patient wear a protective boot with a stiff sole and deep toe box.

FIREARM INJURY

The type and severity of wounds inflicted by a firearm depend on the amount of energy (a function of velocity) the bullet (projectile) has when leaving the firearm. The higher the velocity of the bullet, the greater the energy and potential for injury. Firearms with muzzle velocities greater than 762 m/s (2500 ft/s) are considered high velocity, 457.2 to 762 m/s (1500 to 2500 ft/s) medium velocity, and less than 457.2 m/s (1500 ft/s) low velocity.

The energy of a bullet may be transmitted to the tissue in part or total, depending on the surface area the bullet presents to the tissue. Bullets that yaw, expand, or fragment present more surface area than bullets that stay in one axis and maintain shape. Hunting ammunition is designed to expand on impact up to two or three times its diameter, resulting in a larger wound channel, greater tissue damage, and rapid incapacitation and death. In addition to direct tissue destruction by the deforming bullet, fragmentation may occur when a bullet strikes bone and sends bone and bullet fragments in different directions. These secondary missiles cause injuries within the body similar to those from the original bullet and may even exit the body to injure bystanders.

Other problems are explosions that occur within the firearm itself. These can cause burns or fragment types of injuries. When firearms are loaded with excessive amounts of powder or when the wrong powder is used in reloading bullets, the resultant detonation may cause the frame or cylinder of the firearm to explode. Obstruction of the barrel of the firearm by snow, mud, or other foreign material may cause an explosion.

Treatment

1. Follow the basic principles of trauma care and resuscitation concerning airway, breathing, circulation, control of bleeding, immobilization of the spine and fractured extremities, wound care, and stabilization of the patient for transport (see Chapter 12). Anticipate that a bullet may have ricocheted within the victim, and thereby injured structures and organs that are not in the direct path from entry to exit wounds.
2. Remove the weapon from the vicinity where you are giving medical care. Remove the ammunition and leave open the firing chamber.
3. Perform endotracheal intubation as soon as possible if the patient has a neck wound and expanding hematoma. If endotracheal intubation is not possible and the airway becomes

obstructed, perform a cricothyrotomy (see Chapters 10 and 12).

4. Provide immediate relief of a tension pneumothorax with a needle or tube thoracostomy, or occlusion of a sucking chest wound with petrolatum-impregnated gauze (see Chapter 15).

5. Control external bleeding by direct pressure and compression wraps.
   a. If bleeding from an extremity cannot be stopped by direct pressure, apply a tourniquet (see Chapter 12).
   b. Hemostatic agents are potentially useful products to stop bleeding that cannot be controlled by direct pressure or a tourniquet. When poured or packed into a wound, the granules or gauze combine with blood to induce a robust gel-like clot. Combat Gauze, which is kaolin-impregnated Kerlix gauze (the active agent is aluminum silicate), is the hemostatic dressing issued to the US military for combat use.

6. Treat for hemorrhagic shock, and take measures to prevent hypothermia (see Chapter 13).

7. Do not perform wide debridement of normal-appearing tissue.

8. Monitor the neurovascular status of an extremity wound; keep the extremity elevated to minimize swelling.

9. Remember that the path of the bullet cannot reliably be determined by connecting the suspected entrance and exit wounds.

10. Ultimate removal of the bullet or bullet fragments is not necessary unless the bullet is intravascular, intraarticular, or in contact with nerve tissue. It is certainly not necessary in the field.

11. Use forceps to remove from the skin any shotgun pellets that have minimal penetration.

12. For gunpowder burns, remove as much of the powder residue as possible with a scrub brush because gunpowder will tattoo the skin if left in place.

13. Aggressive intravenous (IV) fluid administration to maintain or reach normotension is discouraged in patients with penetrating injury in the field. Allowing the blood pressure to remain in the life-sustaining hypotensive range may prevent disruption of clots and dilution of clotting factors. Follow the most recent recommendations for fluid resuscitation for trauma-induced hemorrhage. Consider the use of tranexamic acid (see Chapter 12).

14. Administer broad-spectrum antibiotics that provide both aerobic and anaerobic coverage (e.g., cefotetan adult dose 2 g IV q12h or amoxicillin/clavulanate 875 mg/125 mg PO q8h if IV is not available).

ARROW OR SPEAR INJURY

Arrowheads used for hunting are designed to inflict injury by lacerating tissue and blood vessels, causing bleeding and shock. The force used to propel the arrow is usually measured in *draw weight*, which is the number of foot-pounds necessary to draw a 71.1-cm (28-inch) arrow to its full length. The higher the draw weight, the more powerful the bow and the deeper the penetration achieved by the same type of arrow. Spears are thrown and may impale people.

Treatment

1. Follow the same treatment principles of trauma care and resuscitation as for a firearm injury.
2. Irrigate lacerations inflicted by arrows or spears, and remove any foreign material. Close the wound primarily following the guidelines in Chapter 20.
3. The piercing arrow or spear lodged in a patient should be physically stabilized so that it remains as motionless as possible, and the object should be left in place during transport. Attempts to remove the weapon by pulling it out or pushing it through the wound may cause further injury. Cut the shaft, and leave about 8 to 10 cm (3 to 4 inches) protruding from the wound to make transport easier, if this can be accomplished with minimal disturbance. A large pair of paramedic-type shears can often cut through an arrow shaft.
4. Bolster and prop the portion of the weapon that remains in the wound with a stack of gauze pads or cloth and tape.
5. Administer broad-spectrum antibiotics that provide both aerobic and anaerobic coverage (e.g., cefotetan adult dose 2 g IV q12h or amoxicillin/clavulanate 875 mg/125 mg PO q8h if IV is not available).
6. Transfer the patient as rapidly as possible to a medical care facility for removal of the arrow or spear under controlled conditions.

FISHHOOK INJURY

Fishhooks have a curved barb or multiple curved barbs proximal to their tip. When force is applied to the hook, it penetrates deeper into tissue and the barb does not allow the hook to be backed out. Fishhooks can penetrate skin, muscle, and bone and may pierce the eye. Care must be taken in removing a fishhook so that further damage to underlying structures is avoided.

Treatment

1. Clean the skin surrounding the entry point with an antiseptic or with soap and water.
2. Remove the hook using one of the following techniques:
   a. Pass a string or shoelace through and around the bend of the hook; the hook can then be yanked from the skin while the shank of the hook is pressed toward the skin surface to disengage the barb (Fig. 19.1). Wear eye protection, and be certain that no one is in striking range of a flying hook.
   b. With a steady, firm motion, push the hook through the skin so that the barb completely appears. Cut off the barb or the shaft with a wire cutter or multipurpose tool, and pull the remainder of the hook back out of the skin (Fig. 19.2). When

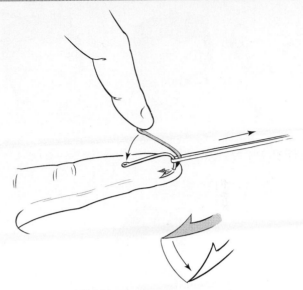

FIGURE 19.1   Fishhook Removal.

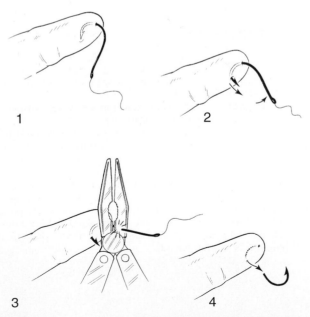

FIGURE 19.2   Removal of a fishhook that has penetrated a fingertip.

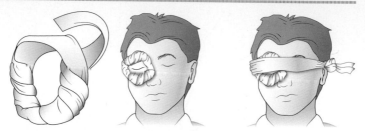

FIGURE 19.3   Bandage for the Injured Eye. A cravat or cloth is rolled and wrapped to make a doughnut-shaped shield, which is fixed in place over the eye.

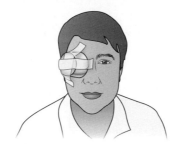

FIGURE 19.4   Using a cup to fashion an eye shield.

    cutting off the barb, take care to wear eye protection and look away during cutting.

3. Irrigate the wound with saline solution or water. Inspect the wound daily for signs of infection.

4. For a fishhook embedded in the eye or close enough to the eye that it cannot be removed without injury to the eye, leave it in place and first secure it with tape. Then, cover the eye with a sufficiently deep eye shield or paper/plastic cup cut to size, and transport the patient to an ophthalmologist for definitive care. Examples of such eye protection are shown in Fig. 19.3 (cravat) and Fig. 19.4 (cup). Do not apply a pressure patch.

5. If the eyeball is suspected to have been penetrated, administer an oral antibiotic as soon as possible to try to prevent end-ophthalmitis (see Chapter 32).

20 Lacerations, Abrasions, and Dressings

DEFINITION: LACERATION

Although sometimes distressing to view, a laceration is rarely life threatening. It is an injury to the integument and may overlie an occult injury such as a fracture or extend into the joint space.

General Treatment

The goals of wilderness wound management are to control bleeding, minimize infection, promote healing, and decrease the need for evacuation. To definitively manage a laceration, five specific steps should be followed: examination, anesthesia, cleaning and debridement, wound closure or packing, and bandaging (Box 20.1). If impermeable gloves and eye protection are available, use these to protect the rescuer from blood and other bodily fluids.

EXAMINATION

1. For an extremity injury, evaluate and keep a record of distal neurovascular function before administering local anesthesia.
   a. For wrist and hand lacerations, palpate the radial and ulnar pulses.
   b. Compare capillary refill, color, and temperature of each digit to the corresponding digit on the uninjured extremity.
   c. Assess sensation of the radial and ulnar aspects of each finger to sharp pain and two-point discrimination.
2. Explore the wound in a well-lighted environment to assess for tendon, muscle, or nerve injury; also look for foreign material. Test the motor function of each joint against resistance by isolating the joint and asking the patient to flex and extend the digit against resistance. A tendon that is 75% lacerated can still function, but its function may be decreased when it is offered resistance and is more painful during movement compared with the uninjured finger on the opposite hand.

ANESTHESIA

Topical Anesthesia

- Mix equal parts of 4% lidocaine, 0.1% epinephrine, and 0.5% tetracaine (LET). Soak a 2 × 2 inch sterile gauze pad with this mixture. Place the pad directly into and around the wound for 7 to 10 minutes. The maximum dose of the solution is 2 to 5 mL for adults.
- Use LET with caution on highly permeable tissue such as mucous membranes. Note that LET should be stored in a light-resistant container and is stable for 6 months when refrigerated and 4

BOX 20.1   First-Aid Supplies for Wound and Abrasion Care

Wound Management
10- to 15-mL irrigation syringe with an 18-gauge catheter tip
30 mL (1 fl oz) povidone–iodine solution USP 10% (Betadine)
Wound closure strips $\frac{1}{4}$ × 4 inches
Tincture of benzoin
Polysporin, mupirocin, bacitracin, or other antiseptic ointment
Tweezers
Sterile surgical gloves
4 × 4 inch sterile dressings
Nonadherent sterile dressing (Aquaphor, Xeroform, Adaptic, Telfa)
Elastic conforming bandage
Assorted adhesive bandages
Tape
Surgical stapler, suture material, and suturing supplies
2-octyl cyanoacrylate (Dermabond) or other tissue glue

Abrasion Management
First-aid cleansing pads, 2%–4% liquid lidocaine, viscous lidocaine
    jelly
Surgical scrub brush
Spenco 2nd Skin or other nonadherent dressing
Conforming woven bandage or nonwoven adhesive knit bandage
Aloe vera gel
Polysporin, mupirocin, bacitracin, or other antibiotic/antiseptic
    ointment
Tape

---

weeks stored at room temperature. It should be discarded if the solution becomes discolored or cloudy.

Local Anesthesia

1. Infiltrate the wound with 1% lidocaine (Xylocaine) or 0.25% bupivacaine (Marcaine) using a 25-gauge (or smaller) needle and syringe.
2. The adult dose of lidocaine should not exceed 4 mg/kg (28 mL of a 1% solution in a 70-kg [154-lb] adult).
3. Buffering lidocaine reduces the pain of local anesthetic infiltration. To buffer, add 1 mL of sodium bicarbonate (1 mEq/mL solution) to 10 mL 1% lidocaine. Once buffered, the shelf life of the product is greatly reduced; discard the solution after 24 hours.
4. Alternative anesthetic strategies include the following:
    a. Diphenhydramine (Benadryl) has anesthetic properties similar to, but less potent than, those of lidocaine. Dilute a 50-mg (1-mL) vial in a syringe with 4 mL normal saline (NS) solution to produce a 1% solution. Perform local infiltration as usual.

   b. Use NS solution alone as the injected agent. This may provide enough anesthesia to suture a small wound.
   c. Place ice directly over the wound to provide a short period of decreased pain sensation.

CLEANING AND DEBRIDEMENT

- Perform wound cleansing to remove as much bacteria, dirt, and damaged tissue as possible. The best method is to irrigate with a high-pressure liquid stream. See the following procedure.
- The method available to generate potable water (e.g., iodine tablets, mechanical filter, irradiation, boiling) is sufficient to generate water suitable for irrigation fluid for wound care.
- In addition to a vigorous soap-and-water scrub, use benzalkonium chloride to cleanse wounds inflicted by animals suspected of being rabid (see Chapters 42 and 43).

IRRIGATION METHOD

1. Draw the irrigation solution into a 10- to 15-mL syringe, and attach an 18-gauge catheter tip.
2. Hold the syringe so the catheter tip is 2.5 to 5 cm (1 to 2 inches) above the wound and perpendicular to the skin surface. Push down forcefully on the plunger while prying open the edges of the wound with your fingers, and squirt the solution into the wound (Fig. 20.1A). Be careful to avoid being splashed by the irrigant after it hits the skin. If you are not carrying a splash shield, such as ZeroWet, put on a pair of sunglasses or goggles to protect your eyes from the spray or place the catheter through the bottom of an upside-down plastic or Styrofoam cup.
3. Repeat this procedure until you have irrigated the wound with at least 100 mL per centimeter of wound length.
4. Remove any residual debris or devitalized tissue with a tweezers, scissors, knife, or any other sharp object. Any dirt left in a wound increases the likelihood of infection.
5. If the wound edges are macerated, crushed, or necrotic, perform sharp debridement.
6. Improvised wound irrigation can be performed with a puncturable container to hold water, such as a sandwich or garbage bag and a safety pin or 18-gauge needle. Fill the bag with irrigation solution and puncture the bottom of the bag with the safety pin. Enlarge the hole if necessary by puncturing it a second time. Hold the bag just above the wound and squeeze the top firmly to begin irrigating (see Fig. 20.1B). Understand that the pressure generated by this method is far less than that delivered by a syringe and catheter.

DEFINITIVE WOUND CARE

Lacerations that are not at high risk for infection can be safely closed in the backcountry. Time is a critical factor, however, and the longer closure is delayed, the more likely the wound is to become infected after it is closed. The period for safely closing a

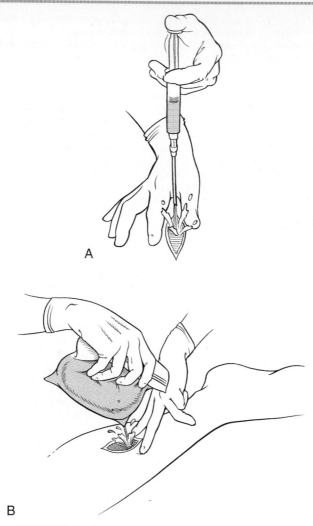

A

B

FIGURE 20.1   Wound Irrigation. A, Syringe. **B,** Plastic bag.

wound depends on its location. Lacerations on the extremity should ideally be closed within 8 hours of injury. Lacerations on the torso should be closed within 12 hours, whereas wounds on the face and scalp should be closed within 24 hours. Uncertain tetanus immunization status should be addressed as soon as possible upon return to civilization.

HIGH-RISK WOUNDS

High-risk wounds that should not be primarily closed in the backcountry include animal or human bites to the hand, wrist, or foot, over a major joint or underlying fracture, or through the cheek; deep puncture wounds; deep wounds on the hand or foot; wounds that contain a large amount of crushed or devitalized tissue; and wounds that are older than the periods described earlier. Wounds occurring in immunocompromised patients should be treated as high-risk wounds.

Treatment

1. Irrigate and debride the wound, and then pack it open with saline- or water-moistened gauze dressings.
2. Cover the packed wound with a conforming bandage, and splint the extremity in an elevated position.
3. Only if the wound is considered high risk, start the patient on an immediate course of oral antibiotic therapy. Options include amoxicillin/clavulanate 500 mg q6h; cephalexin 500 mg q6h; or penicillin 500 mg combined with dicloxacillin 500 mg q6h. For specific antibiotic recommendations for animal or human bites, see Chapter 42 and Appendix J.
4. Change the packing at least once a day.
5. The wound may be closed with sutures, staples, or tape after 72 hours if there is no sign of infection (delayed primary closure).

LOW-RISK WOUNDS

Treatment

Options for closing a wound in the backcountry include taping, suturing, stapling, gluing, and hair-tying.

1. *Wound taping:* Wound closure tape strips are stronger, longer, stickier, and more porous than are butterfly bandages.
   a. Achieve hemostasis, and dry the wound edges.
   b. Clip off hair near the wound with a scissors so that tape will adhere better. Hair farther from the wound edge can be closely clipped or lightly shaved. Avoid shaving hair directly adjacent to the wound edge because shaving abrades the skin and increases the potential for infection.
   c. Apply a thin layer of tincture of benzoin evenly along both sides of the wound, and allow it to dry (Fig. 20.2A) so that it is tacky, not slippery.
   d. Secure one-half of the tape to one side of the wound. Oppose the other wound edge with a finger while using the free end of the tape as a handle to help pull the wound closed (see Fig. 20.2B). Avoid squeezing the wound edges tightly together. They should just touch. Attach the other end of the tape to the skin.
   e. Allow the tape to overlap the wound edge by 2 to 3 cm ($\frac{3}{4}$ to $1\frac{1}{4}$ inches) on each side, and space the strips 2 to 3 mm apart to allow drainage.

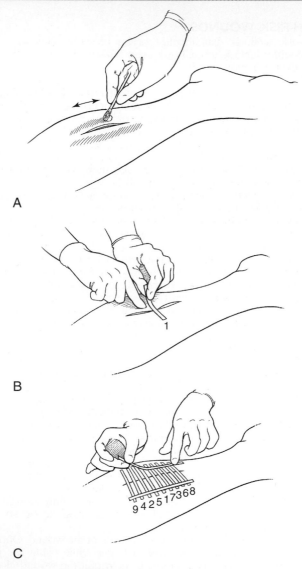

A

B

C

FIGURE 20.2 **A** to **C,** Wound taping.

   f. Place cross-stays of tape perpendicular to and over the tape ends to prevent them from peeling off (see Fig. 20.2C).
   g. Note that wound closure strips can be improvised from duct tape or other self-adhering tape. Cut 1-cm (½-inch) strips, and then punch tiny holes along the length of the tape with a safety pin to allow drainage.
2. *Improvised wound tape:* If no tape is available, glue strips of cloth or nylon from your clothes, pack, or tent to the skin with a "superglue."
   a. Cut 1-cm (½ -inch) strips of material, and then punch tiny holes along the length of the material with a safety pin to allow drainage.
   b. Place a drop of glue on the end of material only and hold it on the skin until it dries.
   c. Pull the wound closed, and glue the other end of the material to the skin on the other side of the wound.
   d. Avoid getting any glue in the wound. The glue is generally safe on intact skin but should not be used on the face.
   e. Expect the strips to fall off after about 3 days. The strips can be reapplied with fresh glue.
3. *Improvised tape/suture closure:* Another method of wound closure using tape, which may be more appropriate for a longer wound:
   a. Cut two strips of adhesive tape 2.5 cm (1 inch) longer than the wound.
   b. Fold a sufficient width of each strip of tape over lengthwise (sticky to sticky) to create a long, thin nonsticky edge on each piece (Fig. 20.3A).
   c. Enhance tape adherence to skin by applying a thin layer of benzoin to the skin on either side of the wound.
   d. Attach one strip of the tape on each side of the wound, 0.6 to 1.3 cm (¼ to ½ inch) from the wound, with the folded (nonsticky) edge toward the wound.
   e. Using a needle and thread, sew the folded edges together, cinching them tightly enough to bring the wound edges closer together (see Fig. 20.3B).
4. *Hair-tying a scalp laceration* (assumes the patient has enough hair):
   a. Take a piece of heavy suture material (0-silk works best), dental floss, sewing thread, or thin string, and lay it on top of and in the long axis of the wound (Fig. 20.4A).
   b. Twirl a few strands of hair on each side of the wound, and then cross them over the wound in opposite directions and pull tightly so that the force pulls the wound edges together.
   c. Have an assistant tie the strands of hair together with the material while you hold the wound closed. A square knot works best. Repeat this technique as many times as needed, along the length of the wound, to close the laceration (see Fig. 20.4B).
   d. If the tied knots will not hold, then pull the twirled strands of hair from opposite sides of the wound together and apply

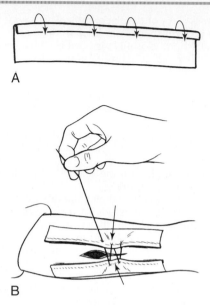

FIGURE 20.3 A and **B,** Improvised skin closure using tape and suture. (Redrawn from Auerbach PS: *Medicine for the outdoors: the essential guide to emergency medical procedures and first aid*, ed 6, Philadelphia, 2016, Elsevier.)

a drop of superglue to the intersection—this junction functions as would a knot.

5. *Gluing:* Dermabond (2-octyl cyanoacrylate) is a topical skin adhesive used to repair skin lacerations. It is packaged for a single-use application. Tissue glue is ideal for backcountry use because it precludes the need for topical anesthesia, is easy to use, reduces the risk for needlestick injury, and takes up less room in a backpack than does a conventional suture kit. When applied to the skin surface, tissue glue provides strong tissue support and peels off in 4 to 5 days without leaving evidence of its presence.

a. Irrigate the wound with copious amounts of disinfected water.

b. Control any bleeding with direct pressure.

c. Once hemostasis is obtained, approximate the wound edges using fingers or forceps. Dry the wound, or allow it to dry.

d. Paint the tissue glue over the apposed wound edges using a very light brushing motion of the applicator tip. Avoid excessive pressure of the applicator on the tissue because this could separate the skin edges and push glue into the wound. Apply multiple thin layers (at least three), allowing the glue to dry between each application (about 2 minutes).

e. Glue can be loosened from human skin with petrolatum jelly or removed from unwanted (nonhuman) surfaces with acetone.

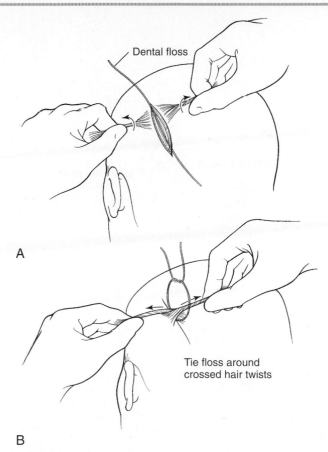

FIGURE 20.4 A and **B,** Scalp laceration closed using dental floss.

    f. Petroleum-based ointments and salves, including antibiotic ointments, should not be used on the wound after gluing because these substances can weaken the polymerized film and cause wound dehiscence.

6. *Skin staples:* Skin staples and sutures are best for large gaping cuts, wounds that are under tension or that cross a joint, or any other wounds that are difficult to keep closed with tape.

    a. Skin stapling is a relatively fast technique for closing wounds and is ideal for use in the wilderness, when evacuation to a medical facility is not readily available.

    b. Staples are as strong as sutures, produce less inflammatory response, and have less chance of seeding a wound infection.

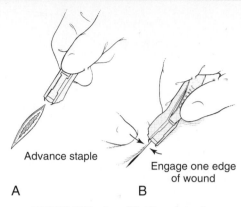

Advance staple

Engage one edge
of wound

A   **B**

FIGURE 20.5   A and **B,** Wound stapling.

   c. When used appropriately, staples yield an excellent cosmetic outcome.
   d. Staples should not be used on the feet, hands, or face or if the laceration extends into tendons or muscles.
   e. Staples are left in place for the same length of time as are sutures in similar anatomic sites.
   f. Staple removal requires a special device that is provided by each manufacturer.

STAPLING TECHNIQUE

Stapling devices have evolved significantly in the past several years. A good choice for backcountry use is the 3M Precise Disposable Skin Stapler with 25 staples.

1. Squeeze the stapler partway until it clicks and you feel resistance. The two points of the staple should now be protruding out from the stapler (Fig. 20.5A).
2. Grab one edge of the cut with one of the staples and use it as a hook to pull the wound closed. Use the index finger on your other hand to push the other wound edge inward until the wound edges just meet (see Fig. 20.5B). Hold the stapler upright at a 90-degree angle to the wound, and make sure that the stapler is positioned evenly over the cut so that it does not overlap one wound edge more than the other. Press the stapler firmly against the skin. Gently and evenly squeeze the stapler with your thumb to advance the staple into the tissue.
3. Once the staple is seated, relax thumb pressure fully on the stapler and back out the device to disengage it.

WOUND OINTMENT DRESSING AND BANDAGING

- The best dressing is one that does not stick to the wound. Representative dressings are Aquaphor, Xeroform, Adaptic, and Telfa.

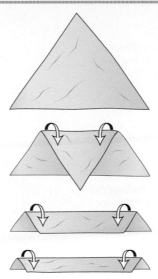

FIGURE 20.6   Making a Cravat From a Triangular Bandage. (Redrawn from Auerbach PS: *Medicine for the outdoors: the essential guide to emergency medical procedures and first aid*, ed. 6, Philadelphia, 2016, Elsevier.)

- Applying an antiseptic ointment such as bacitracin or mupirocin to the surface of the wound before bandaging may decrease the incidence of desiccation and harmful abrasion, and perhaps decreases infection risk. Honey applied topically on cutaneous wounds has been found to reduce infection and promote wound healing and is a reasonable substitute for a commercial ointment. The antimicrobial properties of honey are attributed to its hypertonicity, low pH, a thermolabile substance called inhibine, and enzymes such as catalase. Inhibines in honey include hydrogen peroxide, flavonoids, and phenolic acids.
- A bandage is a rolled gauze elastic wrap that secures a dressing in place. A triangular bandage, which is often used to create a sling, can be folded two to three times into a strap, called a cravat (Fig. 20.6). Cravat dressings are useful for applying pressure to a wound that is bleeding in order to promote hemostasis.
  - *Scalp bandaging:* Scalp wounds often require a dressing placed over hair, making adhesion very difficult. The dressing can be secured with a triangular bandage in a method that allows for considerable tension should pressure be necessary to stop bleeding (Fig. 20.7).
  - *Face and ear bandaging:* A wound to the face or the pinna of the ear may require a compression dressing. If so, gauze should be placed both anterior and posterior to the ear to allow it to maintain its natural curvature. A cravat is used to secure the dressing (see Fig. 23.13). This method may be

1. Drape a triangular bandage just over the eyes and fold the edge 1 inch under to form a hem. Allow the apex to drop over the back of the neck.

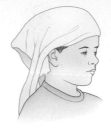

2. Cross the free ends over the back of the head and tie in a half-knot.

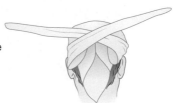

3. Bring the free ends to the front of the head and tie a complete knot. At the posterior aspect of the head, tuck the apex into the half-knot.

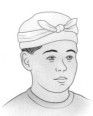

FIGURE 20.7   Scalp Bandaging. (Redrawn from Auerbach PS: *Medicine for the outdoors: the essential guide to emergency medical procedures and first aid*, ed. 6, Philadelphia, 2016, Elsevier.)

used for wounds anywhere along the side of the head or under the chin.

DEFINITION: ABRASION
An abrasion is an area of scraped or denuded skin that is often embedded with dirt, gravel, and other debris, which can result in scarring or infection.

General Treatment (See Box 20.1)
1. Apply a topical anesthetic, such as 2% to 4% lidocaine or viscous lidocaine jelly, over the wound and let it sit for 5 to 10 minutes, or wipe the area with a lidocaine-containing cleansing pad.
2. Vigorously scrub the abrasion with a surgical brush or cleansing pad until all foreign material is removed.

3. Use tweezers to pick out any embedded particles. Irrigate the abrasion with NS solution or water.
4. Apply a thin layer of topical antiseptic ointment, aloe vera gel, or honey to the abrasion.
5. Cover with a nonadherent protective dressing, and secure it in place with a bandage. Spenco 2nd Skin works well because it soothes and cools the wound while providing an ideal healing environment. The dressing can also be secured with a woven or nonwoven adhesive knit bandage and left in place for several days, as long as there is no sign of infection.

WOUND MYIASIS

Although maggots are often thought to be beneficial for necrotic wounds and used in maggot debridement therapy (MDT) to treat diabetic ulcers and other chronic wounds, there is no value in allowing naturally occurring, uncontrolled wound myiasis to persist, because this does not improve wound care and is more often detrimental. In a field setting, most wound myiasis is caused by the flies *Cochliomyia hominivorax*, *Chrysomyia bezziana*, or *Wohlfahrtia magnifica*. The maggots of these species are obligate parasites that eat live tissue, unlike the maggots used for MDT. In addition to destroying viable tissue, flies and larvae transmit bacteria that promote infection (including *Clostridium tetani*). Thus it is important to treat wound myiasis by applying larvicides and then irrigating with povidone–iodine solution (5% to 10% in saline or water) or applying ivermectin as a 10% topical solution. Alternatively, ivermectin may be administered as a single, oral dose of 200 mcg/kg body weight. Another effective method is to occlude the wound with petroleum-based ointment or dressings for at least 24 hours and then manually extract the larvae using forceps. If nothing else is available, irrigation with povidone–iodine solution in water at a concentration of approximately 5% to 10% will usually cause the maggots to flee the wound.

21 | Sprains and Strains

DEFINITIONS

A sprain is stretching or tearing of ligaments that attach one bone to another. Symptoms include tenderness at the site, swelling, ecchymosis, and pain with movement. Because these symptoms are also present with a fracture, it may be difficult to differentiate between the two.

A strain is injury to a muscle or its tendon. Strains often result from overexertion, or lifting and pulling a heavy object without using optimal body mechanics. Symptoms are initially the same as for sprains.

GENERAL TREATMENT

1. First-aid treatment for sprain and strain injuries is summarized by the acronym RISE (rehabilitation, ice, support, and elevation).
   a. *Rehabilitation:* Rehabilitation replaces the outdated advice to put the joint at rest. Instead, early mobility, light-touch weight bearing, and range of motion activities promote earlier recovery from a sprain.
   b. *Ice:* Ice reduces swelling and eases pain. Make sure to provide a layer of cloth between skin and ice to prevent freezing the underlying tissue. For ice or cold therapy to be effective, apply ice early and for up to 20 minutes at least three or four times a day for the first 72 hours after injury.
   c. *Support:* More helpful than compression is support of the injured tissues, ideally with an air splint type of device or with taping (see Chapter 23 for taping information).
   d. *Elevation:* Elevate the injured joint above the level of the heart as often as possible to reduce swelling.
2. Administer an oral nonsteroidal antiinflammatory drug (NSAID), such as ibuprofen 400 to 600 mg q6h, to reduce pain and inflammation.

DISORDERS
Ankle Sprain
Signs and Symptoms

- Ankle sprain: The most commonly injured ligaments (anterior and posterior talofibular and calcaneofibular ligaments) are on the lateral aspect of the joint (Fig. 21.1).
- A syndesmosis injury, or "high ankle sprain," may occur. Tenderness occurs over the anterior tibiofibular and deltoid ligaments.

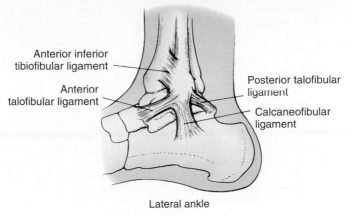

Lateral ankle

FIGURE 21.1 Ligament complexes of the ankle.

A positive squeeze test, in which pain radiates through the interosseous membrane with compression of the tibia against the fibula, exists. The fibula may be fractured. Symptoms of proximal fibular fracture include associated proximal fibular tenderness or crepitus.
- Differentiate ankle sprain from fracture (see Chapter 18).

Treatment
- Use RISE therapy
- If the patient can walk, tape the ankle for support (see Chapter 23)

Ruptured Achilles Tendon
This injury is generally caused by an eccentric stress, such as suddenly running hard from a standing position or trying to jump over an obstacle.

Signs and Symptoms
- An audible "pop," with a sensation similar to being kicked in the calf
- Difficulty plantar flexing the foot, although the plantaris muscle can plantar flex the foot as well. The only reliable sign is Thompson's test.
- Thompson's test: The patient is placed in a prone position with the foot hanging free. If there is no plantar flexion of the foot as the calf is squeezed, Thompson's test is positive.
- Swelling of the distal calf
- Sometimes, a palpable defect in the tendon 2 to 6 cm ($\frac{3}{4}$ to $2\frac{1}{2}$ inches) proximal to its insertion can be appreciated within

the first hour. After that, if there is significant bleeding, the defect can be more difficult to detect.

Treatment
1. If the tendon is strained and not completely torn or ruptured, follow RISE.
2. Have the patient gently stretch the tendon to keep it flexible, then gradually put weight on the foot, with walking as pain allows.
3. In-shoe, firm heel lifts should be used in both shoes. The goal of using a heel lift is to reduce the strain on the Achilles tendon while allowing the patient to remain mobile, and to permit the tendon to be less stretched and relaxed while healing slowly occurs. Because tendons have no blood supply, this healing typically requires weeks or months, and the tendon can easily be reinjured if it is stressed during this time.
4. If the Achilles tendon is ruptured, walking will be difficult. Splint the ankle in slight plantar flexion and evacuate the patient. Surgery is generally necessary to repair the torn tendon.
5. Use improvised crutches.

Patellofemoral Syndrome
Patellofemoral syndrome encompasses many diagnoses that are also known as "anterior knee pain." These can include anterior fat pad syndrome, plica syndrome, patellofemoral maltracking, patellar instability, and chondromalacia patellae.

Signs and Symptoms
- A dull, aching pain under the patella or in the center of the knee that is aggravated by climbing or descending a hill or by sitting for a long period with the knee bent
- Swollen knee
- Crepitus, often heard when knee is flexed and extended

Treatment
1. Apply ice, and allow the patient to rest.
2. Administer an NSAID, such as ibuprofen 400 to 600 mg q6h.
3. Place a wide supporting elastic band around the leg below the patella to help prevent pain during walking. This should not be overly tight.
4. Use two trekking or ski poles while hiking to help absorb impact and reduce pain.

Iliotibial Band Syndrome
This is irritation of the connective tissue along the outside of the thigh.

Signs and Symptoms
- Stinging pain along the outside of the knee aggravated by running downhill or jumping
- Pain reproduced by pressing on the outside of the upper knee

Treatment
1. Apply ice, and allow the patient to rest.
2. Administer an oral NSAID, such as ibuprofen 400 to 600 mg q6h.
3. Aggressive stretching.

Ligament Sprain
Twisting, rotating, hyperextending, or falling in an awkward position is more likely to produce a sprain injury to one of the major ligaments that support the knee than to create a fracture.

Terminology
- *ACL:* anterior cruciate ligament
- *PCL:* posterior cruciate ligament
- *MCL:* medial collateral ligament
- *LCL:* lateral collateral ligament

Signs and Symptoms
- An audible "pop" at the time of the injury is common with ACL injuries and less common with MCL and LCL injuries
- Immediate pain that soon becomes a dull ache
- Often marked swelling with joint effusion
- For a severe sprain, instability of the knee while walking or turning
- Severity based on percentage of ligament injured
  - *First-degree sprain:* pain but no instability when the knee is stressed
  - *Second-degree sprain:* pain and slight instability when the knee is stressed
  - *Third-degree sprain:* significant instability, often less pain when the knee is stressed than with lower-grade sprains. A third-degree sprain is a completely torn ligament.

Treatment
1. For first-degree sprain, use RISE. Walking can usually be resumed with little or no additional support.
2. For second-degree sprain, use RISE. Ensure that the patient wears a knee immobilizer while walking. This device should be cylindrical and extend from mid-thigh to mid-calf (see Chapter 18).
3. For third-degree sprain, as in #2, use improvised crutches or ski/trekking poles for additional support. If, after applying a knee immobilizer, the patient's knee still feels unstable and is prone to buckling with weight, evacuate the patient without allowing walking.

Knee Taping
For first- or second-degree sprains, the knee can be taped for added support while ambulating (see Chapter 23).

Torn Meniscus (Cartilage)

Menisci are crescent-shaped pieces of cartilage situated between the femur and tibia that act as shock absorbers for the knee. Partial or total tears of the meniscus often occur at the same time that ligaments are torn. They can also occur as isolated injuries with the following:

- Significant axial compression (big ski jump landing flat on skis)
- Squatting injuries (lifting up a heavy object from a squatting position or rotating/twisting while in the squatted position, especially in someone who may have an underlying ACL deficiency)

Signs and Symptoms

- Pain localized along the joint line after injury. Tenderness is usually medial, lateral, or posterior
- Catching, clicking, or locking of the knee
- Joint painfully locked in a partially flexed position
- Pain with squatting
- Mild swelling

Treatment

1. Apply ice and allow the patient to rest.
2. Administer an oral NSAID, such as ibuprofen 400 to 600 mg q6h.
3. If the knee feels unstable, apply a complete immobilizer.
4. If the patient has a locked knee, attempt to unlock it by positioning the patient with the leg hanging over the edge of a table or flat surface with the knee in approximately 90 degrees of flexion. After a period of relaxation, apply gentle longitudinal traction to the knee with internal and external rotation. Parenteral or oral pain medication and a muscle relaxant may facilitate the reduction. If the injury does not reduce easily, immobilize the knee and transport the patient.

Finger Sprain

Finger sprains are caused by overstretching and tearing of one or more ligaments involving the finger joints.

Signs and Symptoms

- Severe pain at the time of injury
- Often a feeling of popping or tearing inside one or more fingers
- Tenderness, swelling, and bruising of the finger
- Impaired use of the injured finger

Treatment

1. Use RISE.
2. Buddy-tape the injured finger to the adjacent finger as a natural splint. The second and third fingers, and fourth and fifth fingers, are always paired (see Chapter 23).

3. Administer an oral NSAID, such as ibuprofen 400 to 600 mg q6h.

Thumb Sprain
The thumb (ulnar collateral ligament) is frequently injured when placed in extreme extension or abduction, such as occurs when it is caught in the strap of a ski pole when falling. Taping can prevent reproducing the mechanism of injury, particularly when grasping an object (see Chapter 23).

Wrist Sprain
Wrist sprains generally occur during falls and initially can be difficult to distinguish from fractures.

Signs and Symptoms
• Pain and swelling at the wrist

Treatment
1. Use RISE.
2. Administer an oral NSAID, such as ibuprofen 400 to 600 mg q6h.
3. Although splinting is initially the most desirable treatment, there are two basic taping approaches that can be used, depending on the nature of the injury (see Chapters 18 and 23).

Plantar Fasciitis
Plantar fasciitis is inflammation of the fascia on the sole of the foot.

Signs and Symptoms
• Pain at the origin of the plantar fascia, which is located at the most anterior aspect of the heel pad
• Activities that stretch the plantar fascia elicit pain
• Pain is worst when first getting up in the morning or after resting

Treatment
1. Heel cord stretching 20 minutes twice a day.
2. Administer an oral NSAID, such as ibuprofen 400 to 600 mg q6h.
3. Wear an orthotic that cups the heel, has a soft spot under the tender area, and supports the arch.
4. Wear an ankle–foot splint at night while sleeping.

DEFINITION

"Hot spots" are produced by friction. If the rubbing continues unabated, a blister forms. After the blister is unroofed, an infection may develop.

DISORDERS

Hot Spots

Signs and Symptoms

Painful area of erythema before formation of a fluid-filled blister

Treatment

1. Cut an oval hole the size of the hot spot in the middle of a rectangular piece of moleskin or Molefoam. Center this over the affected area and secure it in place, making sure that the sticky surface is not on inflamed skin (Fig. 22.1). Reinforce adhesion of the moleskin or Molefoam with tape or a piece of nonwoven adhesive knit dressing.
2. If moleskin or Molefoam is not available, place a piece of tape over the hot spot, provided that it will not rub or slide. Moleskin may be improvised from the cuff of a sweatshirt or flannel shirt and Molefoam from a piece of padding from a backpack shoulder strap or hip belt. The improvised moleskin can be secured in place with cyanoacrylate "superglue," Dermabond, or other tissue glue.
3. Apply a Blist-O-Ban bandage or improvised friction relief bandage (Fig. 22.2) directly to the hot spot prior to emergence of a natural blister.

Blisters

Signs and Symptoms

- Blisters develop over predisposed hot spots. With continued abrasion, most blisters eventually rupture, predisposing to infection and painful ulceration.

Treatment

1. If the blister is small and still intact, do not puncture or drain it.
2. Place a piece of moleskin or Molefoam, with a hole cut out slightly larger than the blister, over the site. Make sure it is thick enough to keep footwear from rubbing against the blister (similar to hot spot treatment; see Fig. 22.1). Additional layers may be required. Secure this with tape.

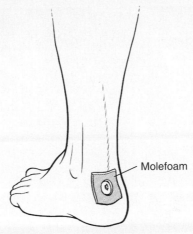

FIGURE 22.1   Hot spot treated with Molefoam.

3. If the blister is large but still intact, gently clean the skin, then aspirate fluid from the blister using a needle and syringe. Alternatively, the blister can be punctured with a clean needle or safety pin at its base and fluid massaged out.
4. Debride any dead, stiff, or necrotic skin using scissors.
5. Clean the area with an antiseptic or with soap and water.
6. Apply antiseptic ointment or aloe vera gel, and cover with a nonadherent dressing.
   a. An excellent dressing for a blister is Spenco 2nd Skin. Made from an inert, breathable gel of 4% polyethylene oxide and 96% water, it absorbs anything oozing from the wound, helps prevent infection, relieves pain, and reduces further friction. It comes packaged between two sheets of cellophane. First, remove the cellophane from the gooey side and place the dressing against the blister. Once it adheres to the skin surface, remove the cellophane from the outside surface. Secure the dressing in place with the adhesive knit bandage that comes with the product. Replace the entire dressing daily.
   b. Other excellent dressings for blisters are Spyroflex, Compeed's hydrocolloid dressing, and Elasto-Gel.
7. Place a piece of Molefoam, with a hole cut out slightly larger than the blister, around the site. Secure this with tape or a piece of nonwoven adhesive knit dressing. Benzoin applied to the skin around the blister site will help hold the Molefoam in place.
8. When supplies are limited, improvise by draining the fluid from the blister with a pin or knife and injecting a small amount of a superglue or benzoin into the evacuated space.
   a. Press the loose skin overlying the blister back in place, and cover the site with tape or a suitable dressing.

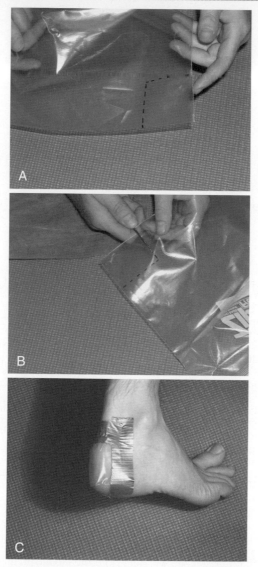

FIGURE 22.2 **A** to **C,** Blister dressing improvised with plastic sandwich bag.

b. Although this can initially be quite painful, it should allow the patient to continue hiking out of the wilderness.

Improvised Blister Management

- To dress a blister without moleskin, Molefoam, or other commercial blister dressing, improvise with a piece of duct tape. Duct tape's smooth outer surface provides protection from friction, while its adhesive side adheres strongly to skin.
- A sandwich bag can be used to improvise another type of blister dressing. It somewhat simulates the Blist-O-Ban bandage. The smooth, gliding surface of the bag helps to stop friction and reduce development of hot spots and blisters. Create this bandage by cutting off the corner of a sandwich bag, and apply a lubricant between the two surfaces. Secure the piece of bag to the blister site with tape or glue (see Fig. 22.2).
- One can improvise a blister dressing from a piece of gauze, antibacterial ointment, and water.
  - Moisten the gauze with water.
  - Squeeze out any excess water, then smear the ointment onto both sides of the gauze. Apply this to the blister.
- A small square of silk can be glued to the heel or other pressure point.
- Methyl acrylate–based glue can be used to repair skin fissures. Another method to treat a blister is as follows:
1. Cover the previously aspirated blister with paper tape cut to overlap the blister edge (Fig. 22.3). This very important step protects the blister roof from avulsion when the overlying tape is removed.
2. Cover the paper tape with benzoin adhesive and allow it to become tacky.
3. As a final layer, apply shaped adhesive tape such as Elastikon over the paper-taped blister (Fig. 22.4). Rounding the corners of the overlying adhesive tape will prevent it from peeling off. Blisters that recur under intact tape can be drained through the tape with a prepared safety pin.

Prevention

- Make sure that footwear fits properly. A shoe that is too tight causes pressure sores; one that is too loose leads to friction blisters.
- Wear a thin liner sock (synthetic materials like acrylic are better than cotton) under a heavier one. The liner will promote wicking of moisture, and friction will then occur between the socks instead of between footwear and skin.
- Dry feet regularly. The use of foot powder has not been scientifically proven to reduce blister formation.
- Keep toenails short and beveled downward to reduce the incidence of subungual hematomas. Before a big event, consider having a professional pedicure at least a week before the planned outing, allowing time for manipulations to the epidermis and

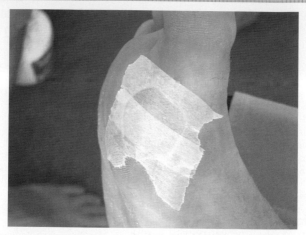

FIGURE 22.3 Paper tape covering of drained blister. (Courtesy Grant S. Lipman, MD.)

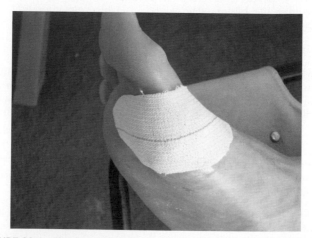

FIGURE 22.4 Elastikon tape layer over paper-taped blister. The elastic tape allows smooth application and contours to the foot. Note rounded corners to prevent peeling. (Courtesy Grant S. Lipman, MD.)

BOX 22.1   Personal Foot Care Kit

Safety pins
Alcohol swabs/squares
Benzoin swabs/squares
Spenco 2nd Skin burn pads (in resealable bag)
Lubricant (e.g., Hydropel)
Paper tape
10-cm (4-inch) Elastikon roll
Small roll of duct tape
Small scissors
18-gauge needle
Blist-O-Ban bandages

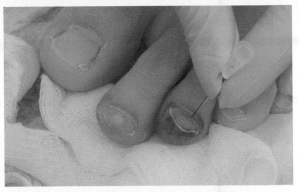

FIGURE 22.5   A subungual hematoma about to be drained with an 18-gauge hypodermic needle. (Courtesy Brandee Waite, MD.)

cuticles to heal, to prevent potential bacterial entry and infection on the trail.
- Carry a foot care kit (Box 22.1).
- Apply moleskin to sensitive areas where blisters typically occur before hot spots develop.
- Duct tape placed on the inner lining of shoes decreases friction between the sock and shoe.

Subungual Hematoma
Signs and Symptoms
Subungual hematoma is a collection of blood that develops underneath a fingernail or toenail. Large fluid collections cause pain.

Treatment
Subungual hematomas need be drained only if they cause pain.
1. Hold an 18-gauge needle perpendicular to the proximal nail bed over the area of greatest fullness (Fig. 22.5).

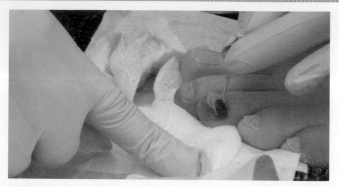

FIGURE 22.6   Moderate downward pressure applied to a rotating 18-gauge hypodermic needle will drill a hole and release the blood under a toenail. (Courtesy Brandee Waite, MD.)

2. With gentle downward pressure, hold the needle between the thumb and first finger. Twirl the needle back and forth between the thumb and finger to drill through the nail, releasing the hematoma (Fig. 22.6).
3. Another method is to heat one end of the wire of a paper clip and use this to burn a hole through the nail. The release of blood under pressure through the hole may be dramatic, causing it to squirt, so use appropriate universal precautions.

23 | Bandaging and Taping Techniques

TAPING

- In general, taping requires practice, but certain simple techniques can be easily mastered.
- Taping is most often used to treat mild to moderate sprains and strains, with the intent to maintain some functional capacity, such as weight bearing and lifting.
- Although taping offers dynamic support, it is not comparable to splinting, which is intended to immobilize an extremity.
- Athletic tape may be applied to skin, although it may lose adhesion if the body part is not shaved and tape adhesive not applied.
- Circumferential wrapping techniques should be used with considerable caution with acute injuries. Marked swelling may cause severe vascular constriction when tape encircles the extremity. Always monitor distal neurovascular status.
  Some keys to successful taping include the following:
- Avoid leaving any gaps in the tape because these will lead to blisters.
- Avoid excessive tension on tape strips that serve to fill these gaps.
- Apply tape in a manner that follows the skin contour to avoid wrinkles.
- Try to overlap a half-width on successive strips.

TYPES OF TAPE

- Athletic tape
  - Although the major advantage of athletic tape is versatility, its major disadvantage is the tendency of zinc oxide to lose adhesive properties with heat and moisture, resulting in loss of support when the patient sweats.
  - A variety of techniques are used to increase durability of athletic tape under these conditions, and are described later in this section.
- Elastic tape
  - Elastic tape (e.g., Elastikon) is cotton elastic cloth tape with a rubber-based adhesive. The elasticity of the tape allows greater flexibility and is particularly useful for large joints, such as knees or shoulders.
  - Self-adherent elastic wrap (e.g., Coban) functions like tape, but sticks only to itself. It is available in sterile and nonsterile styles, and in a variety of widths and colors.

SKIN PREPARATION

- Time spent on skin preparation increases longevity of tape adhesion and patient comfort.
- If tape is to be applied directly to the skin, the area is usually shaved to remove hair that may interfere with direct contact. Avoid creating small abrasions in the skin when shaving that can become sites of infection.
- Any abrasion should be covered with a thin layer of gauze or small adhesive bandage strip before taping.
- A variety of commercially available skin adhesives are available in aerosolized form.
  - These preparations use benzoin as the adhesive. One example is Tuf-Skin.
  - Skin adhesives are applied after the skin has been shaved and abrasions dressed.
  - In the wilderness environment, a small plastic bottle of tincture of benzoin is practical. It can be applied with a sterile applicator or gauze pad.
- If the area is not shaved, a foam underwrap or prewrap is used to protect body hair. Prewrap is generally supplied in 7.5-cm (3-inch) rolls.
- After applying a topical skin adherent such as Tuf-Skin, prewrap is applied over the part to be taped in a simple, continuous circular wrap.
- The prewrap is sufficiently self-adherent that it does not need to be taped down.
- When tape is applied over bony prominences, it can create tension on the skin surface that leads to blistering. Therefore, heel-and-lace pads and foam pads are used to provide greater comfort by relieving potential pressure points. Heel-and-lace pads are prefabricated pieces of white foam that are stuck together with petroleum jelly and then applied to the anterior and posterior aspects of the talus when the ankle is taped.
- Pads of foam can be cut to size to fit over painful areas that need to be taped, as in medial tibial stress syndrome, or they can be used for support in special cases, such as taping for patellar subluxation.

ANKLE TAPING

- The most common injury to the lower extremity while hiking is a sprained ankle.
- Pain and swelling linger for several days, and taping can help offer support if the patient is able to bear weight.
- Because most injuries occur to the lateral ligaments, taping supports the lateral surface by restricting inversion.
- Ankle taping uses anchor strips on the lower leg and foot, stirrups that run in a medial to lateral direction underneath the calcaneus, and support from either a figure-8 or heel-lock technique (Fig. 23.1).

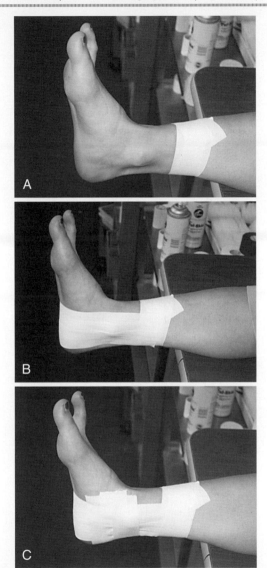

FIGURE 23.1   Ankle taping. **A,** (1) Ankle at 90 degrees; (2) apply anchors of 4-cm (1½-inch) tape at the lower leg and distal foot. **B,** (3) Apply three stirrups from medial to lateral in a slight fan-like projection. **C,** (4) Fill in gaps with horizontal strips.   *Continued*

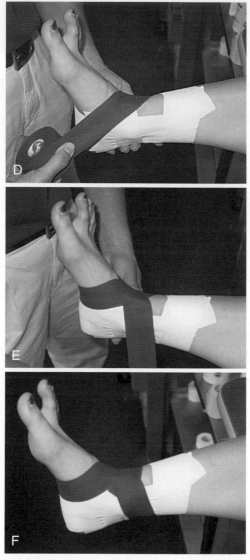

FIGURE 23.1, cont'd D, (5) Begin figure-8. Apply tape across the front of the ankle in a left-to-right direction. **E,** (6) Continue under the foot to the opposite side, and cross back over the top of the foot. **F,** (7) Complete by wrapping around the leg, and end at the anterior aspect of the ankle.

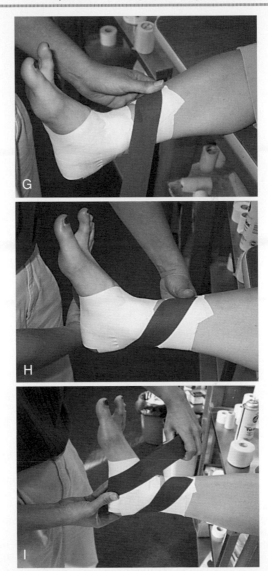

FIGURE 23.1, cont'd G, (8) Apply heel locks for both feet (omit if not familiar with this technique). Start in a left-to-right direction, and apply tape across the front of the joint. **H,** (9) Wrap around the heel (bottom margin of tape should be above the superior edge of the calcaneus) to form the first heel lock. **I,** (10) Continue under the foot to the opposite side, and cross back over the top of the foot. *Continued*

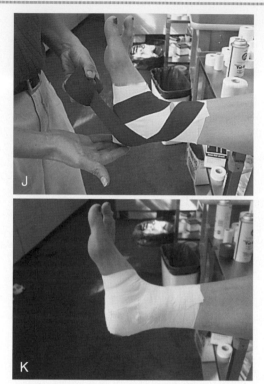

FIGURE 23.1, cont'd   J, (11) The tape is then brought back around the superior margin of the calcaneus and down and around the heel. **K,** (12) Finish by wrapping around the ankle. Repeat figure-8 or heel lock as desired.

- The heel lock requires expertise to perform, so most operators are initially more comfortable with the figure-8.
- Apply caution when taping any body part that is swollen.

TOE TAPING
- Taping toes that are sprained or fractured is simple and effective.
- This treatment involves buddy-taping to the adjacent toe with one or two pieces of tape to provide support. Fig. 23.2 demonstrates buddy-taping of fingers.
- A piece of gauze, cotton, or cloth can be placed between the toes to avoid skin breakdown.

LOWER LEG TAPING
- Medial tibial stress syndrome, commonly referred to as "shin splints," can be taped for support and comfort.

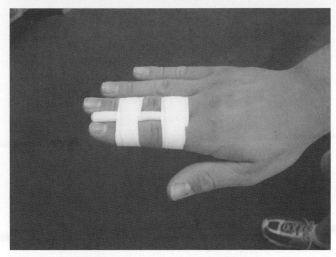

FIGURE 23.2   Buddy-taping of fingers.

- Tape is brought from a lateral to medial direction, and a small foam pad can be cut to cover the area of tenderness.
- Underwrap should be used over a foam pad to secure it in place (Fig. 23.3).

KNEE TAPING
- Underwrap should not be used because adequate traction to support the joint can be achieved only by taping directly to the skin.
- The patient's knee should be shaved 15 cm (6 inches) above and below the joint line.
- Standard athletic tape should not be used because it cannot provide enough support.
- The foundation is 7.5-cm (3-inch) elastic tape.
- Taping for injuries to the medial aspect of the knee is described in Fig. 23.4.

PATELLA TAPING
- Subluxation of the patella is exacerbated by the stress of walking long distances across uneven terrain.
- Incorporating a piece of foam into taping the knee can help relieve symptoms.
- As with all taping around the knee, underwrap should not be used (Fig. 23.5).

FINGER TAPING
Injuries to the fingers are common in a variety of outdoor settings. Both simple fractures and sprains can initially be treated by taping.

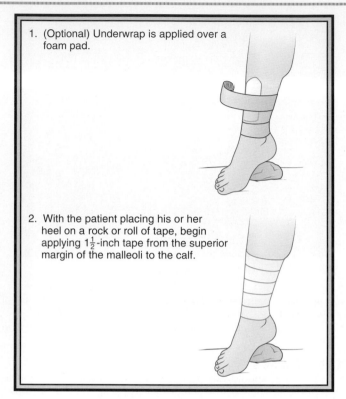

1. (Optional) Underwrap is applied over a foam pad.

2. With the patient placing his or her heel on a rock or roll of tape, begin applying $1\frac{1}{2}$-inch tape from the superior margin of the malleoli to the calf.

FIGURE 23.3 Lower leg taping.

- The most common scenarios involve fingers that are hyperextended or "jammed."
  - It is always best to splint or tape the finger in slight flexion to avoid further injury to the flexor apparatus.
  - Fingers are buddy-taped to the adjacent finger as a natural splint (see Fig. 23.2).
  - The second and third fingers, and fourth and fifth fingers, are always paired.
  - If the third and fourth fingers are paired, this makes injury to the second and fifth fingers more likely with subsequent activity.
  - A small piece of gauze, cotton, or cloth should be placed between the fingers to avoid blistering or pressure on a tender joint.
  - Strips of tape should be applied around fingers but not over the joints.

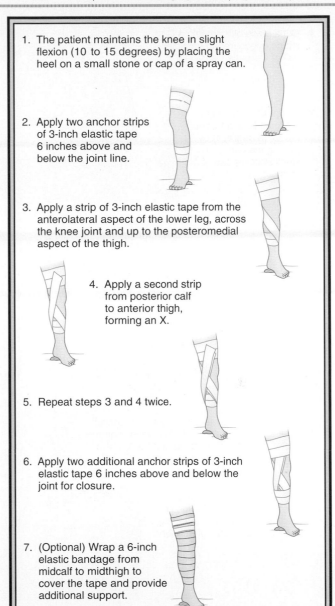

1. The patient maintains the knee in slight flexion (10 to 15 degrees) by placing the heel on a small stone or cap of a spray can.

2. Apply two anchor strips of 3-inch elastic tape 6 inches above and below the joint line.

3. Apply a strip of 3-inch elastic tape from the anterolateral aspect of the lower leg, across the knee joint and up to the posteromedial aspect of the thigh.

4. Apply a second strip from posterior calf to anterior thigh, forming an X.

5. Repeat steps 3 and 4 twice.

6. Apply two additional anchor strips of 3-inch elastic tape 6 inches above and below the joint for closure.

7. (Optional) Wrap a 6-inch elastic bandage from midcalf to midthigh to cover the tape and provide additional support.

FIGURE 23.4 Knee taping.

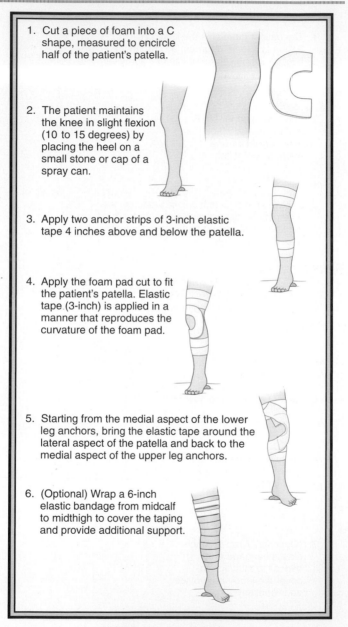

1. Cut a piece of foam into a C shape, measured to encircle half of the patient's patella.

2. The patient maintains the knee in slight flexion (10 to 15 degrees) by placing the heel on a small stone or cap of a spray can.

3. Apply two anchor strips of 3-inch elastic tape 4 inches above and below the patella.

4. Apply the foam pad cut to fit the patient's patella. Elastic tape (3-inch) is applied in a manner that reproduces the curvature of the foam pad.

5. Starting from the medial aspect of the lower leg anchors, bring the elastic tape around the lateral aspect of the patella and back to the medial aspect of the upper leg anchors.

6. (Optional) Wrap a 6-inch elastic bandage from midcalf to midthigh to cover the taping and provide additional support.

FIGURE 23.5 Patella taping.

- Although not as common, injuries to the extensor tendons can occur.
  - Typically these occur with hyperflexion, but they can also occur with hyperextension and axial loading.
  - Injuries in which the extensor mechanism is clearly disrupted should be treated with the finger taped in full extension.
  - A straight splint, such as a tongue blade or smooth stick, can be placed on the dorsal surface and the finger taped to it for additional extensor support (Fig. 23.6).
  - An injury to the fingers or hands should always be evaluated by a physician, who can determine whether radiographs are necessary.

THUMB TAPING
- The thumb is frequently injured when placed in extreme extension or abduction, such as occurs when it is caught in the strap of a ski pole when falling.
- Taping can prevent reproducing the mechanism of injury, particularly when grasping an object (Fig. 23.7).

WRIST TAPING
- Wrist sprains generally occur during falls and initially can be difficult to distinguish from fractures.
- Although splinting is initially the most desirable treatment, there are two basic taping approaches that can be used, depending on the nature of the injury.
- As with the finger, the most important factor is whether the injury occurred in hyperextension or hyperflexion.
- Anchors are placed around the palm and distal wrist, then support strips to prevent undesirable movements are placed on the palmar aspect for hyperextension injuries or the dorsal aspect for hyperflexion injuries (Fig. 23.8).

BANDAGING
Bandaging may be used to wrap and support an injury or help dress a wound. Many of the techniques described in the section on taping, such as figure-8 patterns, are used in bandaging.

Types of Bandages
- The type of bandage depends on its purpose.
- Elastic bandages (e.g., Ace wrap) come in a variety of widths and are used to wrap injuries such as sprains and strains. In the discussion of bandaging different parts of the body later in this chapter, the method for using an elastic bandage is described.
- These bandages generally come with separate clips or clips built into the bandage to secure it.
- Of note is the double-length 15-cm (6-inch) elastic bandage that is useful for wrapping large joints, such as the knee and shoulder.
- Bandaging wounds generally involves rolled gauze or cotton-based wraps that secure a dressing in place.

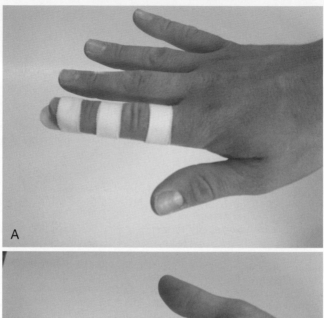

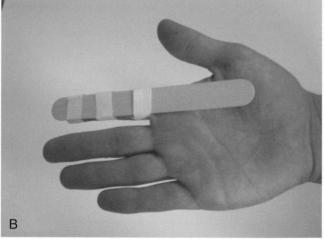

FIGURE 23.6   A and **B,** Extension taping of finger with small splint. Primarily used for extensor injuries.

- These wraps are more desirable than elastic bandages in wound care because they do not place as much tension on the wound dressing.
- A triangular bandage, which is often used to create a sling, can be folded two to three times into a strap, called a cravat.
- Cravat dressings are useful for applying pressure to a wound that is bleeding to promote hemostasis. When securing a wound

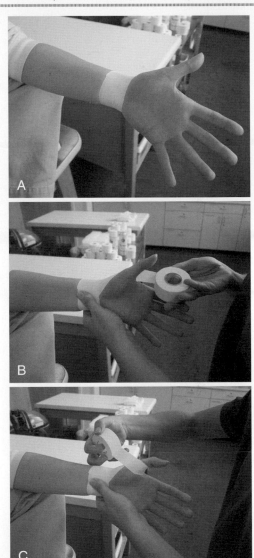

FIGURE 23.7 Thumb taping. **A,** Using 4-cm (1½-inch) athletic tape, wrap an anchor strip around the wrist. **B,** Using 2-cm (¾-inch) tape, start at the volar aspect and continue along the dorsal aspect of the thumb toward the first web space. **C,** Allow the patient to crimp the tape as it comes across the web space and continues around the base of the thumb.

Continued

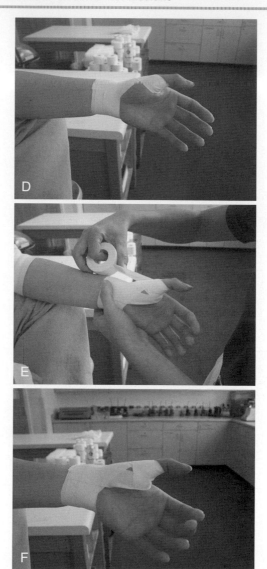

FIGURE 23.7, cont'd D, Bring the tape around to the volar aspect of the wrist, and tape at that point. To complete a thumb spica, apply several more strips in succession. To reinforce, rather than repeating a series of strips, continue as follows. **E,** Apply an anchor strip from volar to dorsal aspects of the wrist through the first web space (note crimping). **F,** Apply strip from the dorsal to volar aspect of the anchor strip.

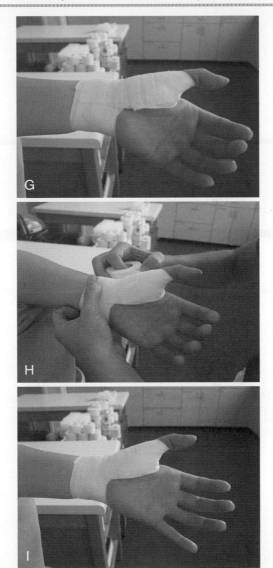

FIGURE 23.7, cont'd   G, Apply successive strips until at wrist. **H,** Add a finishing anchor strip through the first web space. **I,** Complete with an anchor strip.

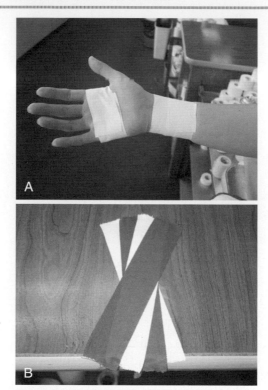

FIGURE 23.8 Wrist taping. **A,** With the hand wide open, apply one anchor across the palm of the hand and two to three anchors across the distal forearm. **B,** Measure out the distance between the two anchors, and construct a fan of three strips of varying angles on a smooth surface.

dressing, the same methods may be used, except that rolled gauze or cotton bandages should be substituted.
• If there is a special technique for wound care, it will be described separately.

Securing Bandages

Because bandages are not adhesive, they must be secured with tape or clips or by tying them to the body. Two techniques for tying off a bandage are as follows:

1. As you finish wrapping with a bandage, bend the free end backward over your fingers, creating a loop. Now double back around the body part, and tie the remaining free end to the loop to secure the bandage.

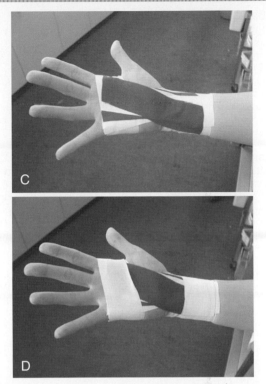

FIGURE 23.8, cont'd C, For hyperextension injuries, apply these support strips to the palmar aspect. For hyperflexion injuries, apply them to the dorsal aspect. **D,** Apply another set of anchors over the support strips.

2. As you finish wrapping, tear or cut the remaining portion of bandage lengthwise down the middle. Double back with one of the resulting strips, and tie off.

Ankle and Foot Bandaging

- Ankle bandaging with a 5- to 7.5-cm (2- to 3-inch) elastic wrap can be used to support a sprain. The bandage can be applied over a sock or directly to the skin.
- It is usually simplest to use a series of figure-8 wraps or, if preferred, a series of heel locks as described in the section on ankle taping.
- Anchors and stirrups are not used.
- When bandaging the foot, the same technique should be carried out to the metatarsophalangeal joint.
- Circumferentially bandaging the foot by itself will result in the bandage slipping, as opposed to bandaging the ankle as well.

Knee Bandaging

- A double-length, 15-cm (6-inch) elastic bandage can provide support to the knee. Ask the patient to hold the knee in slight flexion by placing their heel on a small stone or piece of wood (see Fig. 23.4).
- The elastic wrap is applied circumferentially from midquadriceps to midcalf (see Fig. 23.4).
- If using gauze to secure a dressing or a smaller elastic wrap, a series of figure-8 wraps can be applied, leaving the patella exposed.

Thigh and Groin Bandaging

- Quadriceps, hamstring, and hip adductor ("groin") strains can all be treated with an elastic bandage in a hip spica.
- The bandage is modified slightly for a groin strain (Fig. 23.9).
- Although the quadriceps and hamstring can be supported by wrapping only the leg with a 15-cm (6-inch) elastic bandage, the hip spica helps prevent slippage and provides additional support.

Wrist and Hand Bandaging

- Support to the wrist can be supplied by a 5- to 7.5-cm (2- to 3-inch) elastic wrap using a continuous technique (Fig. 23.10).
- This same technique can be used with gauze to secure a dressing to a wound that can occur when falling on an outstretched hand.
- A hand cravat bandage can be used for wounds that continue to bleed despite manual pressure.

Finger Bandaging

Finger wounds are generally easily treated with adhesive bandages.
   However, if size or degree of bleeding necessitates a larger dressing, then the following method may be used:
1. Fold a 2.5-cm (1-inch) rolled gauze back and forth over the tip of the finger to cover and cushion the wound (Fig. 23.11).
2. Next, wrap the gauze around the finger until the gauze is snug.
3. On the last turn around the finger, pull the gauze over the top of the hand so that it extends beyond the wrist.
4. Split this lengthwise; tie the ends around the wrist to secure the bandage.

Thumb Bandaging

Application of a bandage or dressing to the thumb usually involves a thumb spica, as described in the taping section. Rather than apply individual strips, the gauze or elastic bandage is looped continuously.

Shoulder Bandaging

- A shoulder spica is used to support shoulder sprains, strains, and subluxations (Fig. 23.12).
- A triangular bandage can be used to dress a shoulder wound.

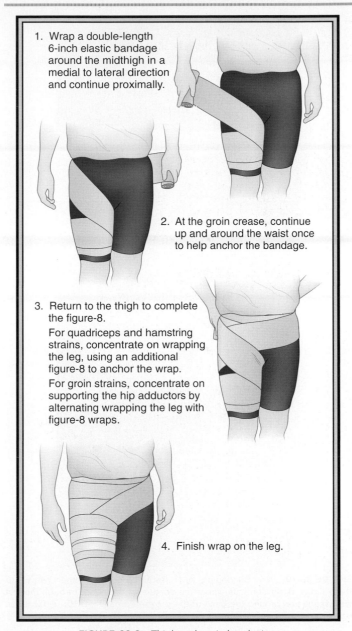

1. Wrap a double-length 6-inch elastic bandage around the midthigh in a medial to lateral direction and continue proximally.

2. At the groin crease, continue up and around the waist once to help anchor the bandage.

3. Return to the thigh to complete the figure-8.

   For quadriceps and hamstring strains, concentrate on wrapping the leg, using an additional figure-8 to anchor the wrap.

   For groin strains, concentrate on supporting the hip adductors by alternating wrapping the leg with figure-8 wraps.

4. Finish wrap on the leg.

FIGURE 23.9 Thigh and groin bandaging.

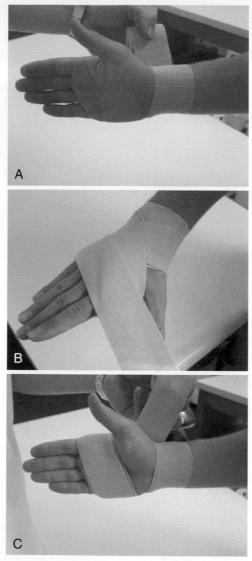

FIGURE 23.10   Wrist bandaging. **A,** (1) Begin by encircling the wrist two to three times. **B,** (2) Continue across the dorsum of the hand, through the first web space and around the base of the proximal phalanges. **C,** (3) Continue down and across the dorsum of the hand.

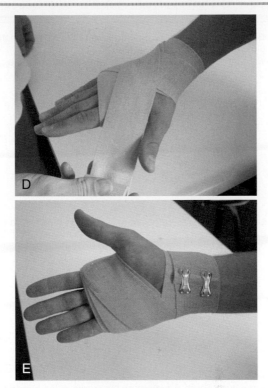

FIGURE 23.10, cont'd D, (4) Circle the wrist, and bring across the dorsum of the hand to form a figure-8. **E,** (5) Repeat, alternating figure-8 patterns on the dorsum of the hand, and secure at the wrist.

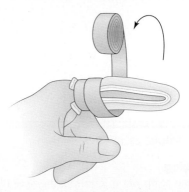

FIGURE 23.11 To begin a finger bandage, place layers of gauze over the fingertip. (Redrawn from Auerbach PS: *Medicine for the outdoors: The essential guide to emergency medical procedures and first aid*, ed 6, Philadelphia, 2016, Elsevier.)

1. Begin by encircling the midhumerus with a double-length 6-inch elastic bandage and continue proximally while wrapping. Once near the axilla, wrap over the acromio-clavicular joint and around the posterior thorax.

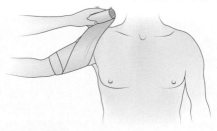

2. Continue under the opposite axilla, across the chest and bring down over the acromioclavicular joint and onto the upper arm.

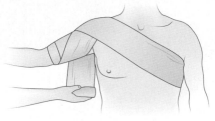

3. Repeat the figure-8 pattern as the length of the bandage allows and finish on the upper arm.

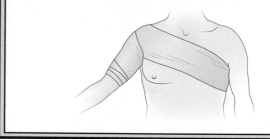

FIGURE 23.12   Shoulder bandaging.

Scalp Bandaging

- Wounds to the scalp often require a dressing placed over hair, making adhesion difficult.
- The dressing can be secured with a triangular bandage in a method that allows for considerable tension should pressure be necessary to stop bleeding (see Fig. 20.7).

Ear Bandaging

- A wound to the pinna may require a compression dressing.
- If so, gauze should be placed both anterior and posterior to the ear to allow it to maintain its natural curvature.
- A cravat is used to secure the dressing (Fig. 23.13).
- This method may be used for wounds anywhere along the side of the head or under the chin.

Eye Bandaging

- When bandaging an eye, a shield is placed over the eye socket to protect the globe, followed by application of a bandage over the shield.
- The shield may be constructed from commercially available sterile pads, foam, felt, stacked gauze, or a shirt or cravat fashioned into a doughnut shape (Fig. 23.14).

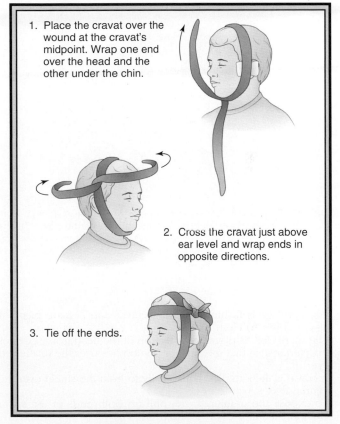

1. Place the cravat over the wound at the cravat's midpoint. Wrap one end over the head and the other under the chin.

2. Cross the cravat just above ear level and wrap ends in opposite directions.

3. Tie off the ends.

FIGURE 23.13   Ear bandaging.

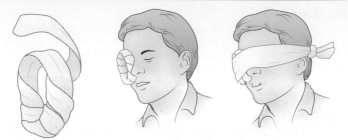

FIGURE 23.14 Bandage for the injured eye. A cravat or cloth is rolled and wrapped to make a doughnut-shaped shield, which is fixed in place over the eye. (Redrawn from Auerbach PS: *Medicine for the outdoors: The essential guide to emergency medical procedures and first aid*, ed 6, Philadelphia, 2016, Elsevier.)

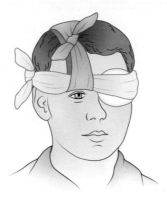

FIGURE 23.15 Holding an eye patch in place with a cravat. Hang a cloth strip over the uninjured eye. Hold the patch in place with the cravat. Tie the cloth strip to lift the cravat off the uninjured eye. (Redrawn from Auerbach PS: *Medicine for the outdoors: The essential guide to emergency medical procedures and first aid*, ed 6, Philadelphia, 2016, Elsevier.)

- The bandage is fashioned from a cravat and a spare piece of 38-cm (15-inch) cloth or shirt.
- The spare cloth is placed over the top of the head from posterior to anterior such that the anterior portion lies over the unaffected eye.
- A cravat is then applied horizontally to hold the shield over the injured eye.
- To expose the uninjured eye, pull up both ends of the spare cloth and tie at the top of the head (Fig. 23.15).

24

Pain Management

Effective pain management can dramatically enhance a rescue effort and minimize morbidity and mortality. Any health-care worker providing medical support to a backcountry trip or expedition should be adequately prepared to provide pain relief (Box 24.1).

FIRST CONTACT

Initial contact with a patient following a painful injury or illness should follow a basic plan of initial stabilization, assessment, and initiation of comfort measures (Fig. 24.1). Fundamental actions to stabilize and de-escalate an acute injury or pain event are as follows:

1. Create a safe and calm environment with clear leadership for pain treatment.
2. Clearly communicate reassurance, allay fears, and encourage calm and confidence.
3. After completing a primary survey to assess and manage life-threatening injuries, objectively assess the nociceptive pain generator (injury), functional status of the injured party, and expedition situation.

EVALUATION OF PAIN

The basis of the wilderness pain evaluation should include the following:

- Location of the pain
- Time of onset
- Precipitating or aggravating factors
- Frequency and duration
- Character
- Severity (i.e., scale of 1 to 10; 10 is worst pain ever experienced)
  Previous treatment (i.e., prior response to pain medications)
  Also determine the following:
- Past medical and surgical history (including history of substance abuse and/or dependence)
- Environmental exposures
- Diet and medications
- Associated symptoms (e.g., nausea, vomiting, fever, vertigo, dyspnea)
- Allergies to pain or anesthetic medications

BOX 24.1   Pain Management First-Aid Kit

Basics
Materials for splinting, protection, and compression wrapping of an
    injured extremity

Oral Medications
NSAIDs: acetaminophen, 500-mg tablets; ibuprofen, 200-mg
    tablets
Opioid: hydrocodone, 5-mg tablets, or other oral opioid
Antiemetic: ondansetron, 8-mg sublingual tablets;
    diphenhydramine, 25 mg
Anxiolytic: lorazepam, 1-mg tablets, or another benzodiazepine

Injectable Medications
Opioid: fentanyl, 0.05 mg/mL, 5-mL vial; morphine, 5 mg/mL, 5-mL
    vial
Opioid reversal: naloxone, two 0.4-mg ampules
Ketamine, 50 mg/mL, 10-mL vial
Benzodiazepine: lorazepam, 2 mg/mL, 4-mL vial

Topical Therapies
Capsaicin ointment, 0.1%, 2-g tube
Lidocaine ointment, 5%, 50 g or lidocaine patch, 5%
Diclofenac, 1% gel, 100 g, or 1.3% patch (Flector Patch)
Proparacaine hydrochloride 0.5% ophthalmic solution, 10-mL vial

Regional Anesthetics and Equipment
Extension tubing set and syringes, 10 mL, 20 mL, 30 mL
Block needles: 22-gauge blunt tip, 50 mm; 18- to 22-gauge Tuohy
    tip, 80 mm
1% and 2% Lidocaine with epinephrine, 20-mL vials
3% 2-Chloroprocaine, 30-mL vials
1% Ropivacaine, 30-mL vials
0.9% Normal saline, 10-mL vials

Acupuncture Materials
Auricular semipermanent (ASP) needles, stainless steel; box of 80
    needles with injectors

PRICE: Protection, Rest, Ice, Compression, and Elevation

Protection
- Stabilize the injured extremity
- Remove constricting garments
- Move into a position of maximum comfort

Rest
- Minimizes additional pain and inflammation.

Ice or Other Cold Application
- Apply cold source, such as an ice pack, or immerse in cold
  stream.

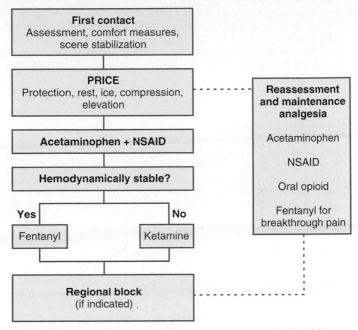

FIGURE 24.1 Summary approach for pain management in the wilderness.

- Can reduce inflammation and pain from an acute injury.
- Ice should be applied intermittently by alternating ice with no ice in 20-minute intervals to avoid the risks of decreased blood flow to the region.
- A towel or a similar material should be placed between the ice and skin, and tissue status closely monitored.

Compression
- Apply a close-fitting elastic bandage to reduce swelling and associated pain.
- The bandage should provide support, protection, and light compression that does not constrict blood flow.
- As an injury evolves and swelling increases, regular checks of the bandage and distal tissues should be done to prevent potentially harmful constriction.
- Care should be taken when using a nonelastic bandage that could result in overcompression with reduction of sufficient blood flow and potentially ischemia.

Elevation
- Reduce swelling by increasing venous return of blood and alleviating tissue edema.

- Left in the dependent position, extremity swelling increases after injury, potentially causing compression of the veins, which in turn leads to worsening bleeding, swelling, and pain.
- Further swelling may compress nerves and arteries (i.e., compartment syndrome), which will result in ischemia distal to the injury.
- If possible, the injured site should be maintained above the level of the heart.

Topical Anesthetics
- A local anesthetic may provide relief in a topical application before more invasive cleansing and debridement.
- The local anesthetic EMLA is a mixture of 2.5% lidocaine and prilocaine. After this cream is applied to intact skin under a nonabsorbent dressing for at least 45 minutes, an invasive procedure such as intravenous (IV) needle insertion may be more easily tolerated.
- Lidocaine gel can also be used for this purpose (Table 24.1).

LOCAL ANESTHETIC PHARMACOLOGY
Anesthetic Toxicity
- Infiltration into a highly vascular site such as around an intercostal nerve leads to more rapid escalation of anesthetic blood level than does injection into less vascular subcutaneous tissues.
- Use of an anesthetic/epinephrine mixture leads to slower absorption.
- As anesthetic toxicity levels are approached, common early symptoms include: circumoral numbness, tinnitus, and cephalgia.

Table 24.1   Comparable Anesthetic Dosages* for Peripheral Blocks and Local Infiltration

	DOSAGE (MG/KG)
Amide Anesthetics	
Lidocaine	5
Prilocaine	5
Etidocaine	4
Mepivacaine	5
Bupivacaine	2
Ester Anesthetics	
Procaine	5
Tetracaine	1–2
2-Chloroprocaine	5

*No epinephrine included.

- Central nervous system (CNS) toxicity in the form of seizures occurs at lower anesthetic blood levels than does cardiotoxicity, seen as ventricular arrhythmias and cardiovascular collapse.
- Anesthetic allergy per se is uncommon, with perhaps 99% of all adverse anesthetic reactions related to pharmacologic toxicity.

Anesthetic Infiltration Techniques and Nerve Blocks

- Soft tissue analgesia is accomplished with local injection of 1% lidocaine. Generally, the maximum injectable dose for lidocaine is 4 mg/kg.
- In larger wounds, injections proceed from an area previously anesthetized, to lessen discomfort from subsequent injections.
- Epinephrine may provide useful hemostasis, especially in head and scalp lacerations. Although recent literature supports the safe use of epinephrine added to local anesthetic injected in the distal extremities, continue to exercise caution with epinephrine in the nose, ears, and digits to avoid possible ischemic injury and subsequent necrosis.
- Many central and regional nerve blocks require special training, including a thorough knowledge of anatomy and management of potential complications, but several blocks can be appropriate in a wilderness setting if the provider is cautious and limits the amount of anesthetic injected.
- Make all infiltrations after aseptic preparation of the skin, whenever possible.

Digital Nerve Blocks

Anesthesia to the digits is easily accomplished with a low-volume field block to the medial and lateral aspects of the digit at the base of the respective phalanx (Fig. 24.2).
1. Approach the digital nerves from the dorsum of the hand or foot rather than from the palm or sole.
2. The dorsal digital nerves and proper digital nerves course along the medial and lateral aspects of the digits, approximately at the 10- and 2-o'clock and 4- and 8-o'clock positions, respectively.
3. A satisfactory digital nerve block is created by injecting 3 to 5 mL of lidocaine 0.5% to 1% with a 25-gauge or smaller-diameter needle to the medial and lateral aspects of the proximal digit.

Wrist Blocks

The entire hand may be anesthetized by blocking the nerves at the wrist. The radial nerve supplies the cutaneous branches of the dorsum of the hand and thumb and distally to the distal interphalangeal joints of the index, long, and radial aspect of the ring fingers (Figs. 24.3 and 24.4). Median nerve sensory distribution includes the palmar surface of the hand, ulnar aspect of the thumb, palmar aspect of the index finger, and long and radial portions of the ring finger. Median nerve innervation extends dorsally over

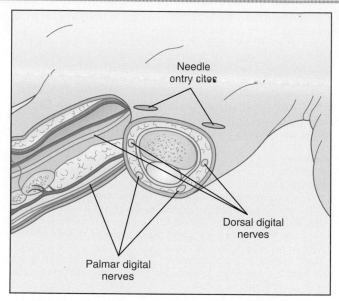

FIGURE 24.2   Digital nerve block. (Courtesy Bryan L. Frank.)

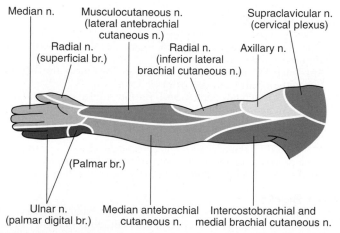

FIGURE 24.3   Ventral nerve distribution of the upper extremity. (From Brown D: *Atlas of regional anesthesia*, Philadelphia, 1999, Saunders. Illustration by Jo Ann Clifford.)

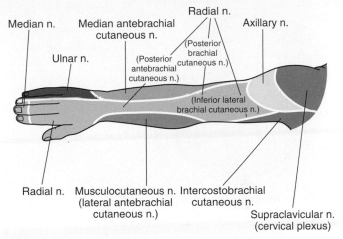

FIGURE 24.4 Dorsal nerve distribution of the arm. (From Brown D: *Atlas of regional anesthesia*, Philadelphia, 1999, Saunders. Illustration by Jo Ann Clifford.)

the index, long, and ring fingers to the distal interphalangeal joint. The ulnar nerve transmits sensation from the palmar and dorsal surfaces of the lateral hand, the fifth finger, and the ulnar half of the ring finger.

1. Using a 25- or 27-gauge needle, inject 2 to 4 mL of lidocaine 1% in the subcutaneous tissue overlying the radial artery. A superficial subcutaneous injection from this point and over the radial styloid anesthetizes cutaneous branches from the proximal forearm and extending into the hand.
2. Block the median nerve with 2 to 4 mL of lidocaine 1% just proximal to the palmar wrist crease between the tendons of the palmaris longus and the flexor carpi radialis muscles. Make the injection deep to the volar fascia.
3. If a paresthesia is elicited during the injection procedure (resulting from contact with the nerve), withdraw the needle slightly before completing the injection.
4. Block the ulnar nerve with 2 to 4 mL of lidocaine 1% injected just lateral to the ulnar artery, which is radial to the flexor carpi ulnaris tendon at the level of the ulnar styloid.

Axillary Nerve Block
Sites distal to the elbow can be blocked by placing local anesthetic near the musculocutaneous, median, radial, and ulnar nerves at the distal axilla, guided by the axillary artery pulse (Fig. 24.5).

1. Position the patient supine with shoulder abducted to 90 degrees and externally rotated, with the elbow flexed.

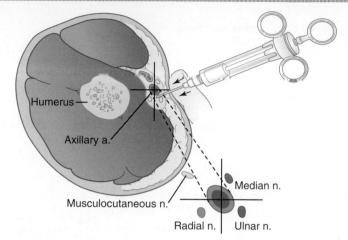

FIGURE 24.5 Axillary block. (From Brown D: *Atlas of regional anesthesia*, Philadelphia, 1999, Saunders. Illustration by Jo Ann Clifford.)

2. Stand or sit at the patient's side caudal to the arm, and identify the axillary pulse over the proximal humerus.
3. The site of entry is sterilized and local anesthesia injected locally before a blunt needle is placed. Blunt needles have a shorter bevel than do traditional hypodermic needles. These needles may be safer when performing nerve blocks, because they may be less likely to injure vascular and neural structures.
4. A 22-gauge blunt needle is then advanced superior to the pulse. The musculocutaneous nerve lies deep to the artery, and this is where 5 to 10 mL of local anesthetic is deposited.
5. Superficial to the musculocutaneous nerve and the pulse of the axillary artery is the median nerve, where an additional 5 to 10 mL of local anesthetic is deposited.
6. The needle is withdrawn to just under the surface of the skin and then redirected inferior (medial) and deep to the artery, where the radial nerve is located; another 5 to 10 mL of local anesthetic is deposited.
7. Finally, the needle is withdrawn to the depth of the axillary artery, where the ulnar nerve is located, and the remaining 5 to 10 mL of local anesthetic is deposited.

During this procedure, the patient may experience paresthesias, which can be used to verify the location of the needle. However, this is not necessary. If the axillary artery is entered, continue to advance the needle through the artery, and then aspirate to make sure that the needle is deep to the artery (not intravascular) before depositing the local anesthetic. If the artery is entered, direct pressure should be maintained over the site for 5 minutes after completion of the nerve block, to limit bleeding. If 0.25% to 0.5% bupivacaine

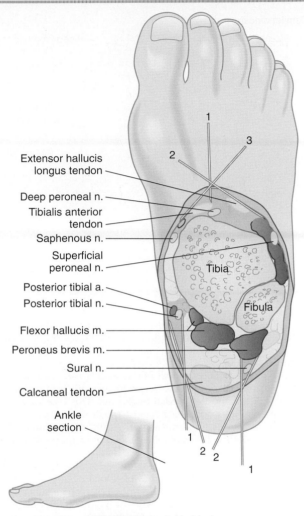

FIGURE 24.6   Ankle block.

without epinephrine is used, the block duration will be 4 to 6 hours; with the addition of epinephrine, it may be 8 to 12 hours. Potential complications include intravascular injection of local anesthetic and vascular or nerve injury.

Ankle Blocks

Anesthesia of the foot is easily accomplished with blocks of the sensory nerves at the ankle (Fig. 24.6).

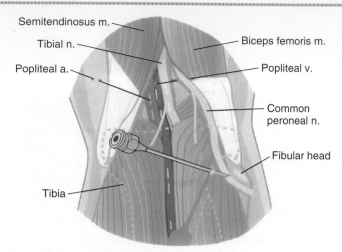

FIGURE 24.7 Common peroneal block. (From Waldman SD: *Atlas of interventional pain management*, Philadelphia, 2009, Saunders.)

1. Using a 25-gauge needle, block the deep peroneal nerve, which provides sensation between the great and second toes, with 5 mL of lidocaine 1% between the tendons of the tibialis anterior and the extensor hallucis longus at the level of the medial and lateral malleoli. The needle may be passed to the bone just lateral to the dorsalis pedis artery.
2. Inject the superficial peroneal nerve with 5 mL of lidocaine 1% with a superficial ring block between the injection of the deep peroneal nerve and the medial malleolus. This blocks sensation to the medial and dorsal aspects of the foot.
3. Inject the posterior tibial nerve with 5 mL of lidocaine 1% just posterior to the medial malleolus, adjacent to the posterior tibial artery.
4. Block the sural nerve, which provides sensation to the posterolateral foot, with a similar volume of lidocaine 1%, between the lateral malleolus and Achilles tendon, followed by a subcutaneous infiltration from this site and over the lateral malleolus.
5. Paresthesias are sought in these blocks and will increase the likelihood of success. Posterior tibial nerve distribution includes the heel and plantar foot surface. Follow paresthesias by a slight withdrawal of the needle before injection.

Common Peroneal Nerve Block

A common peroneal block may be helpful for distal tibia and ankle trauma (Figs. 24.7 and 24.8).

1. With the patient in a lateral position, the fibular head is identified.
2. A blunt-bevel needle is introduced just below the fibular head.

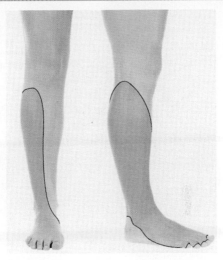

FIGURE 24.8   Distribution of the common peroneal nerve. (From Obrien MD: *Aids to the examination of the peripheral nervous system*, ed 4, United Kingdom, 2008, Saunders.)

3. A paresthesia can be elicited at a depth of 0.5 to 1 cm (0.2 to 0.4 inch), and then 5 mL of local anesthetic is deposited.

Femoral Nerve Block (Fig. 24.9)

The sensory distribution of the femoral nerve includes the anterior and medial thigh and knee as well as the medial lower leg in the saphenous nerve distribution (Fig. 24.10). A femoral nerve block can be used for a femur fracture.

1. With the patient supine, the inguinal ligament, anterior-superior iliac spine, pubic tubercle, and femoral pulse at the level of the inguinal ligament are identified.
2. A 4-inch, 22-gauge, blunt-bevel needle is entered through the skin 1 cm (0.4 inch) lateral to the femoral pulse and advanced in the anterior-posterior plane.
3. As the needle is advanced, a paresthesia may be elicited, although this is variable.
4. A total volume of 20 to 40 mL of local anesthetic is injected while redirecting the needle from the initial medial position adjacent to the femoral artery to a more lateral position, thereby achieving a field block.
5. The use of 0.25% bupivacaine will provide good analgesia; if motor block and anesthesia are necessary, 0.5% bupivacaine should be used.
6. Because this is a field block, it may be slower in onset than other nerve blocks.
7. The femoral artery is near the injection site, so arterial puncture

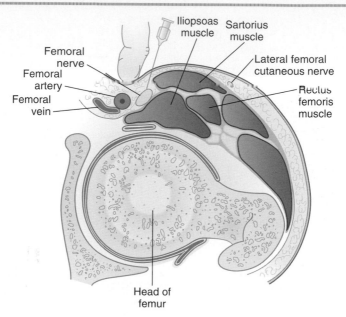

FIGURE 24.9 Femoral nerve block.

of the artery and intravascular injection are possible (see Fig. 24.9).

Trigger Point Injections

Pains from muscular spasm are readily identified. Palpation of the affected muscle group will localize sites of maximal tenderness, which are known as trigger points. Injecting 2 to 3 mL of local anesthetic will temporarily block pain and spasm. Care should be taken to avoid volumes greater than 15 mL of 0.5% bupivacaine, which is absorbed quickly from muscles.

PHARMACOLOGIC TREATMENT OF PAIN
Nonnarcotic Analgesics

Nonsteroidal antiinflammatory drugs (NSAIDs) have both analgesic and antiinflammatory properties. Common agents, such as ibuprofen and naproxen, are readily available and offer first-line treatment for various minor aches and pains (Table 24.2). They offer an inexpensive and effective means of treatment without concern about the possible adverse effects of opioids and are generally free from regulation in foreign countries. Ketorolac is a parenterally administered NSAID that can be used for moderate to severe pain (see Table 24.2). Recommended dosage is 60 mg intramuscularly (IM) or 30 mg IV q4-6h (every 4 to 6 hours). Use half this dose if

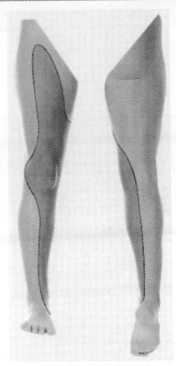

FIGURE 24.10   Distribution of the femoral nerve. (From Obrien MD: *Aids to the examination of the peripheral nervous system*, ed 4, United Kingdom, 2008, Saunders.)

the patient is older than 65 years or weighs less than 50 kg (110.2 lb). Oral dose is 10 mg.

Narcotic Analgesics

- Opiates are effective for moderate to severe pain.
- Oral administration remains the easiest form of delivery and may be accomplished with an isolated opiate (e.g., oxycodone) (see Table 24.2) or in combination with acetaminophen (e.g., Vicodin, Norco, Lortab, Percocet).
- Care should be taken to avoid consuming more than 4 g of acetaminophen in 24 hours, because hepatic toxicity may occur.
- IV administration of opioids reduces variability introduced by oral administration and decreases the time to onset of analgesia (Table 24.3).
- IV administration can be by intermittent injection or continuous infusion. Intermittent bolus injections in remote locations are more practical.
- IM administration of opioids is feasible in remote areas, but

drugs have variable absorption from different muscle groups.
- Subcutaneous administration of opioids may have similar efficacy as IM administration and is less painful. The dosing for subcutaneous administration is the same as IM.
- Manage nausea and vomiting with ondansetron (Zofran).
- For oversedation and opiate side effects, use naloxone judiciously in 40-mcg increments.

Table 24.2 Common Oral Analgesics: Dosage Recommendations for 70-kg (154-lb) Adults

DRUG	DOSAGE (MG)	INTERVAL (H)	RISKS AND PRECAUTIONS
Salicylates			
Acetylsalicylic acid	325–650	4–6	Gastrointestinal distress; inhibited platelet function; contraindicated in children with viral illness
Diflunisal	300–600	8–12	Similar to aspirin
Para-Aminophenol			
Acetaminophen	300–1000	4–6	Hepatic toxicity with overdose
Indoles			
Indomethacin	50	4–6	Similar to aspirin
Sulindac	50–75	4–6	Similar to aspirin
Ketorolac	10	4–6	Similar to aspirin; use for 5 days or less because of the potential for gastrointestinal bleeding
Propionic Acids			
Fenoprofen	400–600	4–6	Similar to aspirin
Ibuprofen	300–400	4–6	Similar to aspirin
Ketoprofen	25–50	6–8	Similar to aspirin
Dexketoprofen	25	8	Similar to aspirin, with less gastrointestinal distress
Naproxen	200–275	6–8	Similar to aspirin

Table 24.2   Common Oral Analgesics: Dosage Recommendations for 70-kg (154-lb) Adults—cont'd

DRUG	DOSAGE (MG)	INTERVAL (H)	RISKS AND PRECAUTIONS
Cyclooxygenase-2 Inhibitor			
Celecoxib	100–200	12–24	Gastrointestinal distress; skin rash
Narcotic Agonists (Oral)			
Codeine*	15–60, with a maximum of 360 mg per 24 h	4–6	Narcotic side effects; note the cumulative acetaminophen dosage
Hydrocodone*	5–10	4–6	Narcotic side effects; note the cumulative acetaminophen dosage
Hydromorphone	7.5	3–4	Narcotic side effects
Levorphanol	1–3	6–8	Narcotic side effects
Meperidine	300	2–3	Narcotic side effects
Methadone	2.5–150	4–12	Narcotic side effects
Morphine	30–60	3–4	Narcotic side effects
Oxycodone*	5–10	4–6	Narcotic side effects; note the cumulative acetaminophen dosage
	Extended release, 10	12	

*Codeine, hydrocodone, and oxycodone are manufactured as single drug preparations, and also commonly in combination with acetaminophen. Dosing provided is for the narcotic component only. Total daily acetaminophen administration should not exceed 4 g.

From Burnham T, Short RM, editors: *Drug facts and comparisons,* St Louis, 1999, Facts and Comparisons Inc; and Emermann CL, Spenetta J: Pain management in the emergency department. *Emerg Med Rep* 23:53, 2002.

Table 24.3　Common Parenteral Analgesics: Dosage Recommendations for 70-kg (154-lb) Adults

DRUG	DOSAGE (MG)	INTERVAL (H)	RISKS AND PRECAUTIONS
Narcotic Agonists			
Codeine	15–75 IM	4–6	Narcotic side effects
Fentanyl	50–100 mcg	0.5–1	Narcotic side effects; wide range of dosages
Hydromorphone	1–2 IM	3–4	Narcotic side effects; choose over morphine for a patient with hepatic impairment
Levorphanol	1–3	6–8	Narcotic side effects
Morphine	10–20 IM, 2.5 IV	3–5	Narcotic side effects
Meperidine	50–100 IM, 25–50 IV	2–4	Narcotic side effects; active metabolite accumulates in patients with renal impairment and may cause seizures
Oxymorphone	1	3–4	Narcotic side effects
Narcotic Agonists and Antagonists			
Buprenorphine	0.3–0.6 IM	6–8	May precipitate narcotic withdrawal
Butorphanol	2–4 IM	3–4	May precipitate narcotic withdrawal
Dezocine	5–20 IM, 5–10 IV	2–4	May precipitate narcotic withdrawal
Nalbuphine	10–20 IM, 1–5 IV	3–6	May precipitate narcotic withdrawal
Nonsteroidal Antiinflammatory Drug			
Ketorolac	15–30 IM/IV	4–6	Similar to aspirin

Table 24.3 Common Parenteral Analgesics: Dosage Recommendations for 70-kg (154-lb) Adults—cont'd			
DRUG	**DOSAGE (MG)**	**INTERVAL (H)**	**RISKS AND PRECAUTIONS**
Dissociative Analgesic and Anesthetic			
Ketamine	50–75 IM, 15–30 IV	2–4	Increased secretions, emergence reaction

IM, Intramuscularly; *IV,* intravenously.
From Burnham T, Short RM, editors: *Drug facts and comparisons,* St Louis, 1999, Facts and Comparisons Inc; and Emermann CL, Spenetta J: Pain management in the emergency department. *Emerg Med Rep* 23:53, 2002.

- Full-dose (0.4 mg) naloxone is still the appropriate treatment for respiratory depression.

Antineuropathic Drugs

The efficacy of antineuropathic agents is variable because of the complexity of the mechanisms present within neuropathic pain states. Anticonvulsants (particularly gabapentin) offer a safe and reasonably tolerated therapy for the pain of nerve injury. Although it is sedating at higher doses, gabapentin started at 300 mg q8h and then increased to 600 mg q8h over the course of several days is usually well tolerated. Sedation is the major side effect, so dose escalation is not advised if the patient receives benefit at lower doses or cannot tolerate higher doses.

ADDITIONAL AGENTS
Narcotic Agonist-Antagonist Combinations
- Drugs in this class include buprenorphine, butorphanol, and nalbuphine.
- In the wilderness setting, a drug that may be useful is transnasal butorphanol (Stadol NS).
  - The recommended dose for initial nasal administration is 1 mg (1 spray in *one* nostril).
  - Adherence to this dose reduces the incidence of drowsiness and dizziness. If adequate pain relief is not achieved within 60 to 90 minutes, an additional 1 mg dose may be given.
  - Stadol is rapid acting and offers good analgesia but can cause significant sedation and often considerable dysphoria.

Ketamine
Ketamine is a powerful dissociative anesthetic that, when used in a small parenteral dose, can provide profound analgesia. Ketamine is effective for all types of pain.
- Subdissociative doses of ketamine:
  - 0.1 to 0.3 mg/kg IV or IO

Table 24.4	Herbal and Botanical Analgesic Remedies				
BOTANICAL NAME	COMMON NAME	REPORTED USES	MECHANISM	ADMINISTRATION	SIDE EFFECTS
Aloe vera	Aloe	Burns and sunburn	Promotes wound healing	Topical	No topical toxicity, reported cathartic effect when taken orally
Arnica montana	Arnica	Myofascial pain and bruising	Flavonoids, carotenoids, volatile oils, possibly reduce production of inflammatory cytokines	Topical ointment, homeopathic, tea, tincture	Vagal inhibition, GI irritation headache, convulsions, cardiovascular collapse
Capsicum species	Red peppers	Skin and joint pain	Nociceptor desensitization	0.25%–0.75% capsaicin cream	GI upset if taken orally, skin irritation
Curcuma longa	Turmeric	Osteoarthritis	Possible COX-2, prostaglandin, leukotriene inhibitor	500 mg PO q6h to q12h	Rare GI upset
Erythroxylon coca	Cocaine	General pain	Topical anesthetic	Topical	Hyperactivity, seizures, coma, respiratory depression, cardiovascular collapse

Lavandula species	Lavender	Burns and other injuries in topical and aromatherapy form	Contains linalool and linalyl aldehyde, possible antispasmodic and analgesic effects, calming effects	Topical, food, extract, dried capsule	No known toxicity
Matricaria chamomilla	Chamomile	GI upset	Contains chamazulene, antihistamine	Extract, topical salves, tea, tincture	No known toxicity
Oenothera biennis	Evening primrose	Diabetic neuropathy, PMS, rheumatoid arthritis, mastalgia	Possibly reduces PGE and IL-1	2–4 g PO daily	May be associated with nocturnal seizures, birth complications
Origanum vulgare	Oregano	Rheumatic pain	Lack of evidence for analgesic properties	200 mg PO q6h or as strong tea 1 teaspoon in 250 mL water	Possibly unsafe in pregnancy; otherwise likely safe orally
Piper methysticum	Kava	General pain, anxiety	Possible GABA agonist, Possible COX-1 and MAO inhibition	100 mg of 70% standard extract q8h	May be hepatotoxic with long-term use, GI upset, headache

Continued

Table 24.4 Herbal and Botanical Analgesic Remedies—cont'd

BOTANICAL NAME	COMMON NAME	REPORTED USES	MECHANISM	ADMINISTRATION	SIDE EFFECTS
Plantago major	Plantain	Bites and stings, poison ivy discomfort, and toothache	Abrasions, stings, bites	Topically applied crushed leaves may have antihistamine effect	No known toxicity
Salix species	Willow	General pain	Contains salicin and other salicylate compounds, COX-1 and COX-2 inhibitor	250 mg PO daily	GI upset, allergy
Symphytum officinale	Comfrey	Bruises, dislocations, and sprains	Allantoin, antiinflammatory	Topical	Oral ingestion of its pyrrolizidine alkaloids has been associated with hepatotoxicity and/or carcinogenicity
Syzygium aromaticum	Clove	Topically for dental pain	Eugenol likely depresses sensory nerves by inhibiting prostaglandin synthesis	Topical	Generally safe, in high doses associated with lactic acidosis, hepatic dysfunction, mucosal irritation
Zingiber officinale	Ginger	Rheumatoid arthritis, osteoarthritis, and fibromyalgia	Antiinflammatory	250 mg PO q6h	No known toxicity

COX, Cyclooxygenase; GABA, γ-aminobutyric acid; GI, gastrointestinal; MOA, monoamine oxidase; PMS, premenstrual syndrome; PO, orally.

- 0.25 to 5 mg/kg IM
- 0.25 mg to 4 mg/kg intranasal with mucosal atomizer
- If needed, the dose may be repeated every 2 to 3 hours. Titration to effect or to the presence of side effects is imperative.
- Ketamine has emerged as a first-line agent for severely injured patients at risk of hemorrhagic shock or respiratory depression in emergency and austere settings.
- Psychomimetic effects (e.g., hallucinations, bad dreams) can be seen with higher doses (e.g., >1 mg/kg).
- A calm and quiet setting with minimal stimulation is the ideal setting for use.

Muscle Relaxants

Muscle relaxants may help relieve acute muscle spasms related to injury. Baclofen is a relatively potent muscle relaxer with γ-aminobutyric acid B receptor activity. However, sedation is a common side effect that may limit its usefulness. Carisoprodol (Soma), metaxalone (Skelaxin), and cyclobenzaprine (Flexeril) are generally less effective alternatives.

COMPLEMENTARY AND ALTERNATIVE MEDICINE THERAPIES

Acupuncture

Properly administered acupuncture should have a very low risk for morbidity and may be extremely effective in alleviating pain and possibly restoring function to an injured wilderness traveler.

- Sterile acupuncture needles are compact, lightweight, and easy to include in a daypack or first-aid kit.
- Integration of acupuncture into the care of wilderness trauma, pain, and illness may dramatically enhance patient comfort and facilitate extrication from a remote setting.
- Most acupuncture treatment requires substantial training to be responsibly integrated with conventional Western therapies. National and international standards of training have been established for Western-trained physicians who desire to incorporate acupuncture into their traditional medical practices.
- Physicians interested in learning acupuncture may contact the American Academy of Medical Acupuncture for information on training programs designed specifically for physicians that meet or exceed standards established by the World Health Organization.

Herbal/Botanical Remedies (Table 24.4)

Combinations of several herbs are often more effective than a single herb, and common formulas have been recorded worldwide for centuries. Appropriate application or prescription of botanical products rarely leads to toxicity or adverse reactions, although such are possible if botanicals are used excessively or carelessly.

25

Life-Threatening Emergencies (Rescue Breathing/CPR/Choking)

BASIC RESUSCITATION

The American Heart Association/American College of Cardiology consensus guidelines advocate a circulation, airway, and breathing (CAB) approach to basic life support. This strategy involves immediate initiation of chest compressions for unconscious patients without spontaneous or normal cardiorespiratory function. The logic for this paradigm shift is that there is likely ample oxygen present in the lungs and arterial system for several minutes following cardiac arrest to avoid ischemia if blood can reach the target organs. Thus, immediate circulation of blood via chest compressions is recommended to facilitate optimal oxygenation of the brain and other key organs sooner than the conventional airway-first approach.

Adult

The currently recommended sequence of adult basic life support performed by a health-care provider can be summarized as follows:

1. Check the patient for unresponsiveness. If the person is not responsive and not breathing or not breathing normally, call for help and return to the patient.
2. *C:* If the patient is still not breathing normally, coughing, or moving, check for a carotid pulse for no longer than 10 seconds. If no pulse is detected in 10 seconds, begin chest compressions. Push down in the center of the chest a distance of 5 cm (2 inches) 30 times. Pump hard and fast at the rate of at least 100 pumps/min, faster than once per second (Figs. 25.1 and 25.2).
3. *A:* Tilt the head back, and lift the chin.
4. *B:* Pinch nose and cover the mouth with yours, and blow until you see the chest rise. Give two breaths. Each breath should take 1 second. An improvised (CPR) barrier may be crafted from a glove (Fig. 25.3).
5. Continue with 30 pumps and two breaths until help arrives, then the rescuers should switch roles every five cycles, continuing at a ratio of 30: 2 to minimize fatigue. A brief resuscitation pause to assess for the presence of spontaneous pulses should be performed every 2 minutes.

Defibrillation

After 2 minutes of CPR, when accessible, an automated external defibrillator should be applied to evaluate for the presence of a cardiac rhythm that may respond to electrical therapy. This is rarely

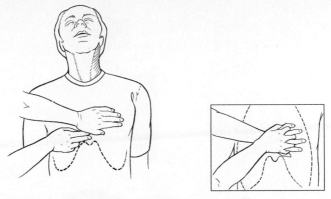

FIGURE 25.1   Hand position for chest compressions in cardiopulmonary resuscitation.

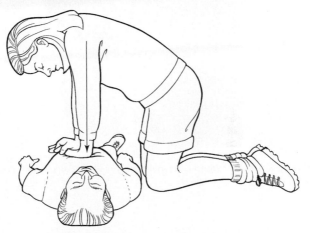

FIGURE 25.2   Chest compressions: adult.

an option in the wilderness environment. An acceptable, although infrequently successful, method of terminating a malignant tachyarrhythmia is the precordial thump. To perform a precordial thump, the patient's chest should be cleared of clothing to facilitate accurate assessment of anatomy. Next, one or two firm blows should be delivered to the middle to lower one-third of the sternum with a closed fist from a height of 20 to 25 cm (8 to 10 inches) above the chest. A central artery should again be palpated for a pulse. If unsuccessful after one attempt, the precordial thump approach should be abandoned and further life support initiated.

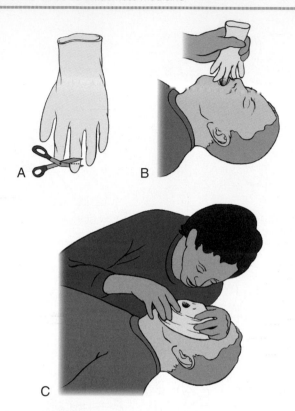

FIGURE 25.3 An improvised cardiopulmonary resuscitation barrier is created using a protective surgical glove.

Child and Infant

The guidelines are the same as for an adult with the following exceptions:

1. Chest compressions should attempt a depth of one-third of the depth of the chest (about 4 cm [1½ inches]).
2. See hand placement for children (Fig. 25.4) and infants (Fig. 25.5).
3. See rescue breathing for infants (Fig. 25.6).

There are certain situations in which resuscitation may be deferred in the wilderness environment. These include the following:

1. A situation in which resuscitation efforts would put rescuers at risk for significant morbidity or mortality

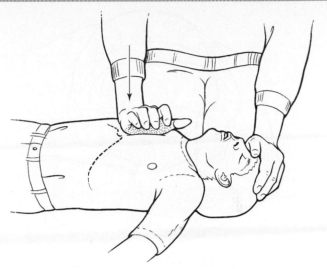

FIGURE 25.4   Chest compressions: child.

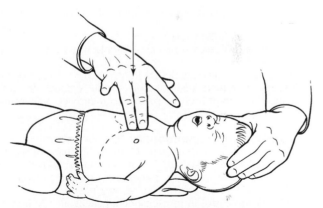

FIGURE 25.5   Chest compressions: infant.

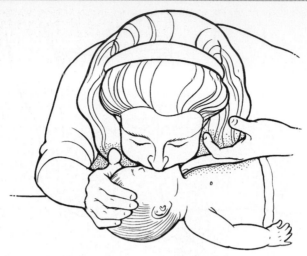

FIGURE 25.6   Rescue breathing: infant.

2. A patient with a core body temperature of less than 15°C (59°F)
3. A patient with a frozen chest wall
4. A patient who has been submersed in cold water for more than 60 minutes
5. A patient with an obvious lethal injury such as decapitation
6. A situation in which resuscitation would significantly delay evacuation of a hypothermic patient to controlled rewarming

When to Stop Cardiopulmonary Resuscitation
1. It is well established that after 15 to 30 minutes of CPR, if a patient does not respond, he or she probably never will. The exceptions have been patients who were profoundly hypothermic.
2. If CPR is not successful in resuscitating a patient after 30 minutes, and the patient is not profoundly hypothermic, then it is usually reasonable to discontinue CPR.
3. Current resuscitation guidelines provide recommendations for specific wilderness situations (Table 25.1).

CHOKING/OBSTRUCTED AIRWAY
Choking is a life-threatening emergency that occurs when something obstructs the patient's airway so that he or she cannot breathe.

Table 25.1   Considerations for Resuscitation of Cardiac Arrest Patients in Specific Wilderness Situations

WILDERNESS SITUATION	SPECIAL CONSIDERATIONS
Trauma	A jaw thrust, not a head tilt–chin lift maneuver, should be used to establish a patent airway for a patient with a mechanism of injury that could cause a cervical spine injury. Ventilation should be performed using a barrier device whenever possible, especially if the patient's face is bloody. Visible hemorrhage should be controlled with direct pressure and compressions to minimize blood loss.
Hypothermia	Wet garments should be removed if they can be replaced with dry insulating cover, ideally during early stages of the resuscitation efforts. As pulse and respirations may be very slow, check for both pulse and breathing for at least 60 sec before considering CPR. Consider prolonged resuscitation effort (>30 min) if it can serve as a bridge to a medical facility with active rewarming capabilities. See Figs. 3.2 and 3.3.
Avalanche burial	Resuscitation should not be conducted in a location with continued snow instability that could put care providers at risk. Decision to initiate resuscitation efforts must be tailored to person's burial time and injuries. Individuals without clear evidence of fatal trauma (e.g., decapitation) or frozen chest should receive resuscitation for burial times <35 min. See Figs. 3.2 and 3.3.
Drowning	Rescuers must take great care to avoid personal injury during the retrieval of a submerged or potentially drowned person. Use ABC (compressions without ventilation should not be used.) See Chapter 50 for further information about resuscitation in drowning injury.
Lightning strikes	Rescuers must take great care to avoid lightning strikes to themselves. Concomitant trauma to the head and spinal column is a common injury following lightning strike and should be assumed in all patients. See Chapter 9 for discussion of "reverse triage" (i.e., in a multiple casualty situation, treat first persons without signs of life) pertinent to a lightning strike situation.

ABC, Airway, breathing, and circulation; *CPR,* cardiopulmonary resuscitation.

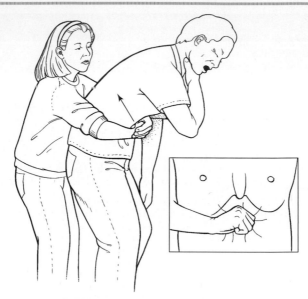

FIGURE 25.7　Heimlich maneuver: standing.

Signs and Symptoms

- Suddenly agitated
- Clutching the throat, especially while eating
- Inability to speak
- Cyanosis

Treatment

1. For a choking adult or child, perform the Heimlich maneuver:
   a. Stand behind the patient, and wrap your arms around the patient's waist.
   b. Make a fist with one of your hands, and place it just above the patient's navel and below the rib cage, with the thumb side against the abdomen.
   c. Grasp your fist with the other hand, and pull your hands forcefully toward you, into the patient's abdomen and slightly upward with a quick thrust.
   d. If unsuccessful, repeat the procedure to achieve a total of four or five thrusts (Fig. 25.7).
2. If the adult or child becomes unconscious, do the following:
   a. Lay the patient on his or her back, and attempt rescue breathing.
   b. If rescue breathing is unsuccessful because of an airway obstruction, perform the Heimlich maneuver while kneeling down and straddling the patient's thighs. Use the heel of the hand instead of a fist (Fig. 25.8).

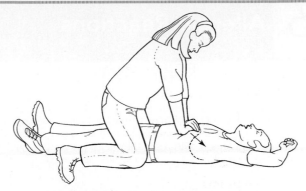

FIGURE 25.8   Heimlich maneuver: supine.

    c. If still unsuccessful, sweep the mouth with one or two fingers to try to remove any foreign material.

    d. Continue to perform the Heimlich maneuver, and periodically attempt rescue breathing.

    e. If multiple attempts at clearing the airway and ventilating the patient are unsuccessful, perform a cricothyrotomy.

3. For a choking infant (younger than 1 year), do the following:

    a. If the infant is coughing and appears to be getting sufficient air, do not interfere with his or her attempts to cough the obstruction out of the airway.

    b. If the infant cannot cough, cry, or get sufficient air, lay him or her face down, supported by and straddling your forearm, while resting your forearm on your thigh. Support the infant's head by grasping under the chin and holding onto the jaw. Make sure the infant's head is lower than the rest of the body.

    c. Using the heel of your free hand, give up to five firm back blows between the infant's shoulder blades.

    d. If the obstruction is not cleared, place your free hand on the infant's back, holding the back and head so that they are sandwiched between both of your arms.

    e. Carefully support the trunk and head while flipping the infant over to a supine position. Support the infant on your thigh, keeping the infant's head lower than the rest of the body. Give five quick, downward chest thrusts with two fingertips positioned over the infant's lower breastbone 1.3 cm ($\frac{1}{2}$ inch) below the nipples.

    f. Look into the infant's mouth for a foreign object, and try to remove it.

    g. If the infant becomes unconscious, try mouth-to-mouth rescue breathing. If you are unsuccessful at getting air into the infant's lungs, repeat Steps a through e until you have removed the object or the child has started to breathe on his or her own.

26 | Allergic Reactions

ANAPHYLAXIS

Anaphylaxis is a serious allergic reaction typically rapid in onset and may cause death. Anaphylaxis can present with obvious skin signs and symptoms, or it may present as unexplained shock. The goals are early recognition and treatment with epinephrine to prevent progression to life-threatening respiratory and/or cardiovascular collapse.

Signs and Symptoms
- Urticaria (hives), diffuse erythematous rash, and soft tissue edema are present in up to 90% of patients
- Wheezing, stridor, cough, chest tightness, hoarseness, dyspnea
- Dysphagia, nausea and vomiting, diarrhea, abdominal pain
- Hypotension and tachycardia (shock)
- Seizures
- Edema involving the face, lips, tongue, pharynx, and larynx, producing an obstructed airway and respiratory arrest
- Cardiovascular collapse with shock can occur rapidly, without any other antecedent symptoms.
- In general, the more immediate the reaction after exposure to the inciting antigen, the more severe the degree of anaphylaxis.
- Most anaphylactic reactions occur within 5 minutes to 2 hours after exposure to an inciting agent. The median time interval between onset of symptoms and respiratory or cardiac arrest is 5 minutes in medication-induced anaphylaxis, 15 minutes in stinging insect venom–induced anaphylaxis, and 30 minutes in food-induced anaphylaxis.

Treatment
1. In the event of anaphylactic shock, immediately administer epinephrine in the field.
   a. Epinephrine 1:1000 (1 mg/mL solution) should be injected intramuscularly into the mid–anterolateral thigh (vastus lateralis muscle). Subcutaneous administration results in slower absorption and is less reliable. The dose for an adult is 0.3 to 0.5 mL (0.3 to 0.5 mg), and for a child it is 0.01 mL/kg (0.1 mg/kg), not to exceed a total dose of 0.3 mL (0.3 mg). Repeat in 5 to 15 minutes if relief is not complete.
   b. Epinephrine is available in a spring-loaded injectable cartridge that facilitates self-administration (EpiPen 0.3 mg [Figs. 26.1 and 26.2], Auvi-Q 0.3 mg, or Adrenaclick 0.3 mg per dose adult dose). A child who weighs less than 30 kg (66 lb) should be injected with an EpiPen Jr 0.15 mg, Adrenaclick 0.15 mg, or Auvi-Q 0.15 mg per dose.

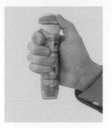

1. Flip open the yellow cap of the EpiPen or the green cap of the EpiPen Jr Auto-Injector carrier tube.

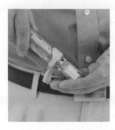

2. Remove the EpiPen or EpiPen Jr Auto-Injector by tipping and sliding it out of the carrier tube.

FIGURE 26.1 Steps to remove the auto-injector from the carrier tube. (Image courtesy Dey Pharma, L.P., Basking Ridge, New Jersey).

   c. If the reaction is life threatening and if the patient does not respond to intramuscular epinephrine, administer epinephrine intravenously. Mix 0.1 mL (0.1 mg) of 1:1000 aqueous epinephrine in 10 mL of normal saline (final dilution, 1:100,000) and infuse over 10 minutes. In an infant or child, the starting dose is 0.1 mcg/kg/min up to a maximum of 1.5 mcg/kg/min. This solution can also be injected through the venous plexus under the tongue if an intravenous line cannot be established.
   d. There are no absolute contraindications to the use of epinephrine in the treatment of anaphylaxis, but caution is advised when treating a person older than age 50 years because epinephrine can produce cardiac ischemia and arrhythmias. The risk for death or serious disability from hypoxic encephalopathy as a result of inadequately treated anaphylaxis almost always outweighs other concerns.
   e. In a refractory case in which the individual is not responsive to epinephrine (e.g., an individual on a β-blocker medication), administer glucagon 1 to 2 mg (adult dose) or 20 to 30 mcg/kg to a maximum of 1 mg (pediatric dose) intravenously over 5 minutes, or intramuscularly. Rapid administration of glucagon can induce vomiting; therefore protect the airway, for example, by placing the patient in the lateral recumbent ("rescue") position, if there is drowsiness or obtundation.

1. Grasp unit with the orange tip pointing downward.
2. Form fist around the unit (orange tip down).

3. With your other hand, pull off the blue safety release.

4. Hold orange tip near outer thigh.

DO NOT INJECT INTO BUTTOCK.

5. Swing and **firmly push** against outer thigh until it clicks so that unit is perpendicular (at 90° angle) to the thigh.

(Auto-Injector is designed to work through clothing.)

6. Hold firmly against thigh for approximately 10 seconds to deliver drug. (The injection is now complete. The window on auto-injector will be obscured.)

7. Remove unit from thigh (the orange needle cover will extend to cover needle) and massage injection area for 10 seconds.

8. Call 911 and seek immediate medical attention.

9. Take the used auto-injector with you to the hospital emergency room.

Note: Most of the liquid (about 85%) stays in the auto-injector and cannot be reused. However, you have received the correct dose of the medication if the orange needle tip is extended and the window is obscured. Trainer label has blue background color. Blue background labeled trainer contains no needle and no drug.

FIGURE 26.2 How to use the auto-injector. (Image courtesy Dey Pharma, L.P., Basking Ridge, New Jersey).

2. Place the individual in the Trendelenburg position, although this is of limited utility to support the blood pressure during shock.
3. Obtain and maintain the airway, administering oxygen as needed.
4. Administer an antihistamine such as diphenhydramine (Benadryl) 50 mg orally (PO) q4-6h (every 4 to 6 hours) for an adult; for children give 1 mg/kg PO q4-6h.
5. Consider adding a histamine2 receptor antagonist ("H2 blocker"), such as cimetidine 400 to 800 mg PO.
6. Treat bronchospasm and wheezing with albuterol via a handheld, metered-dose inhaler with a spacer (adult dose: 200 to 400 mcg [4 to 8 full inhalations, depending on the preparation] q15-20 min as needed [prn]).
7. Administer a corticosteroid. If intravenous (IV) access is available, administer 125 mg methylprednisolone or 15 mg dexamethasone. If therapy is initiated orally, administer prednisone, 60 to 100 mg for adults and 2 mg/kg for children. Oral dexamethasone 8 to 16 mg adult dose and 0.15 to 0.6 mg/kg for children may also be used as an alternative to prednisone.
8. If a stinger remains embedded after an insect sting, remove it by the most rapid means possible. This may be by scraping or by grasping and pulling.
9. Note that in severe cases, endotracheal intubation may be necessary. Be sure to visualize the vocal cords with a rigid laryngoscope because of the distortion caused by laryngeal edema. If an airway cannot be obtained immediately, perform a cricothyrotomy (see Chapter 10); for a child under 12 years of age, perform a needle cricothyrotomy or tracheotomy if oral intubation is not successful. If field endotracheal intubation is contemplated as a possibility, carry a bougie for assistance with a difficult-to-visualize opening through the vocal cords.
10. After treatment, be prepared to transport the patient immediately for medical evaluation, because an anaphylactic reaction can recur as the effects of the epinephrine diminish.
11. If the reaction is limited to only pruritus and urticaria with no wheezing or facial swelling, administer antihistamines (see earlier) alone.

ALLERGIC RHINITIS
Signs and Symptoms
- Sneezing, nasal congestion, rhinorrhea
- Pruritus of the nose and eyes; dark, puffy circles under eyes
- Coughing, wheezing
- Urticaria (hives)
- Nasal mucosa pale blue and edematous, or erythematous

Treatment
1. Nasal corticosteroids are the gold standard of treatment for allergic rhinitis. Several preparations are available; all are equally effective. These are shown in Table 26.1.

Table 26.1 Intranasal Corticosteroids

GENERIC NAME	TRADE NAME	RECOMMENDED DOSE (EACH NOSTRIL)	AMOUNT PER SPRAY (MCG)	MINIMUM AGE (YEARS)
Beclomethasone	Beconase AQ	1–2 sprays bid	42	6
Budesonide	Rhinocort Aqua	1–4 sprays daily	32	6
Flunisolide	Nasarel	2 sprays bid	29	6
Fluticasone propionate	Flonase	1–2 sprays daily	50	4
Fluticasone furoate	Veramyst	1–2 sprays daily	27.5	2
Mometasone	Nasonex	1–2 sprays daily	50	2
Triamcinolone	Nasacort AQ	1–2 sprays daily	55	2
Ciclesonide	Omnaris	1–2 sprays daily	50	6

All preparations are aqueous based.
bid, Twice daily.

Table 26.2 Newer-Generation Antihistamines

CHEMICAL NAME	TRADE NAME	Dosages		MINIMUM AGE
		ADULT	CHILDREN (<12 YEARS)	
Cetirizine	Zyrtec	10 mg daily	2.5–10 mg daily	6 months
Levocetirizine	Xyzal	5 mg daily	1.25–2.5 mg daily	6 months
Loratadine	Claritin	10 mg daily	2.5–10 mg daily	2 years
Desloratadine	Clarinex	5 mg daily	1.0–2.5 mg daily	6 months

Table 26.2 Newer-Generation Antihistamines—cont'd				
		Dosages		
CHEMICAL NAME	TRADE NAME	ADULT	CHILDREN (<12 YEARS)	MINIMUM AGE
Fexofenadine	Allegra	60 mg bid to 180 mg daily	30 mg bid	2 years
Azelastine	Astepro	2 sprays per nostril bid	1 spray per nostril bid	6 years
Olopatadine	Patanase	2 sprays per nostril bid	1 spray per nostril bid	6 years

bid, Twice daily.

2. For more immediate relief of symptoms, administer an oral newer generation H1 receptor antagonist ("H1 blocker") antihistamine (may be in combination with nasal corticosteroids). These are shown in Table 26.2.
3. In some individuals, addition of a decongestant, such as pseudoephedrine (Sudafed) 60 mg PO q4-6h, to the antihistamine may be helpful. Topical vasoconstrictors may be used briefly, not to exceed 3 to 5 consecutive days to avoid rhinitis medicamentosa.
4. Leukotriene receptor antagonists (LTRAs) are approved for use in allergic rhinitis. Montelukast and zafirlukast are examples of oral LTRAs. The dose of montelukast for adults and adolescents 15 years of age and older is 10 mg at bedtime. Pediatric dose is 5 mg and 4 mg at bedtime for ages 6 to 14 years and 6 months to 5 years, respectively.
5. Other drugs that may be helpful are cromolyn sodium (one spray each nostril q6-8h) to relieve sneezing, itching, and rhinorrhea, but not nasal congestion; and the anticholinergic ipratropium for rhinorrhea. The recommended dose of ipratropium is 1 to 2 sprays in each nostril 2 to 4 times per day.

CARDIAC EMERGENCIES
Acute Coronary Syndromes (Unstable Angina and Acute Myocardial Infarction)
Signs and Symptoms
- Chest pain that is often described as pressure, heaviness, tightness, or crushing or squeezing sensation and located in the center of the chest. The pain may be poorly localized or of a sharp, stabbing nature. It may radiate into the neck, jaw, or shoulders or down the inner aspect of the arms (left more frequent than right). Sometimes there is only mild chest pain, a burning sensation in the lower chest or upper abdomen, or a feeling of indigestion.
- Diaphoresis, eructation, nausea, vomiting, anxiety, or dyspnea may be present.
- Pain is often preceded or exacerbated by physical exertion.

Treatment
1. The patient should discontinue all exertion.
2. Administer oxygen 2 to 4 L/min by nasal cannula if the patient appears cyanotic or has respiratory distress.
3. Administer aspirin 325 mg orally (PO) if the patient is not allergic and does not have any serious contraindication.
4. If pain continues and the patient is judged to have normal blood pressure, administer nitroglycerin 0.4 mg sublingually (the patient should be lying down before nitrate administration). If pain persists, repeat this dose every 5 minutes for three doses. Nitrates should be withheld if the patient is suspected of being hypotensive (systolic blood pressure lower than 90 mm Hg) or has ingested erectile dysfunction drugs in the past 24 hours. In the absence of a blood pressure cuff, hypotension can be recognized by the inability to palpate a strong radial pulse in the wrist or dorsalis pedis pulse in the foot.
5. If no allergy or bleeding predisposition and if available, consider giving a dose of low molecular weight heparin (e.g., enoxaparin 1 mg/kg maximum 150 mg subcutaneously.) (Box 27.1.)
6. Evacuate the patient immediately to the closest medical facility with the patient exerting as little as possible.

Heart Failure
Many of the signs and symptoms of congestive heart failure are similar to those of high-altitude pulmonary edema (HAPE). and a

---

BOX 27.1   Contraindications/Cautions for Administration of Enoxaparin

- Hypersensitivity to enoxaparin
- Hypersensitivity to pork products
- Major active bleeding
- Thrombocytopenia by history
- Hemophilia
- Thrombocytopenic purpura
- Contraindicated if recent surgery/trauma
- Caution if history of gastrointestinal (GI) ulcer/bleed
- Caution if uncontrolled hypertension
- Contraindicated if history of hemorrhagic stroke

---

thorough history (and/or information from portable ultrasonography) is critical to supporting clinical diagnosis.

Signs and Symptoms
- Dyspnea, which is often worsened by exertion or lying flat (orthopnea)
- Tachycardia, tachypnea
- Fatigue
- Paroxysmal nocturnal dyspnea
- Peripheral edema
- Jugular venous distention
- Pulmonary rales and wheezes
- Cyanosis and diaphoresis

Treatment
1. Keep the patient sitting up, unless he or she is more comfortable lying on his or her back.
2. Administer 100% oxygen by face mask.
3. Administer nitroglycerin sublingually at a dose of 0.4 mg every 5 minutes for three doses (the patient should be lying down before nitrate administration). Nitrates should be withheld if the patient is suspected of being hypotensive (systolic blood pressure lower than 90 mm Hg). In the absence of a blood pressure cuff, hypotension can be recognized by the inability to palpate a strong radial pulse in the wrist or dorsalis pedis pulse in the foot.
4. Give furosemide 20 to 40 mg intravenously (IV), intramuscularly (IM), or PO; if the patient takes daily diuretics, give a dose equal to double the usual daily dose.
5. Treat wheezing with albuterol via a handheld, metered-dose inhaler with a spacer (adult dose 200 to 400 mcg [2 to 8 inhalations, depending on the preparation] every 15 to 20 minutes (as needed).
6. Evacuate the patient immediately to the closest medical facility with the patient exerting as little as possible.

PULMONARY EMERGENCIES
Pulmonary Embolism

A pulmonary embolus is a blood clot that has embolized to the pulmonary circulation. The most common sources of the embolus are the deep veins of the pelvis or legs. Predisposing factors to pulmonary embolism include dehydration, periods of prolonged rest in a single position (sitting in a plane or in a car), recent surgery, pregnancy, cancer, cigarette smoking, and medications (e.g., birth control pills).

Signs and Symptoms
- Sudden, sharp chest pain that is often pleuritic
- Dyspnea
- Cough (occasionally with hemoptysis)
- Tachypnea and tachycardia
- If the clot is large, the patient may become hypotensive and cyanotic and die rapidly

Treatment
1. Administer 100% oxygen by face mask.
2. Give enoxaparin (Lovenox) 1 mg/kg subcutaneously q12h (maximum dose 150 mg) if there are no contraindications (see Box 27.1).
3. Immediately evacuate patient to the closest medical facility.

Asthma

Generally, most people know that they are prone to asthma attacks; however, first-time episodes may occur in persons exposed to cold, emotional stress, or exertion or during an allergic reaction.

Signs and Symptoms
- Dyspnea
- Wheezing
- Cough
- Prolongation of the expiratory phase of breathing
- Use of accessory muscles of inspiration (neck muscles are most prominent)
- In severe cases, wheezing may diminish because the bronchioles become so "tight" that there is not enough air movement to create the abnormal sounds and the patient will appear cyanotic.

Treatment
1. Administer 100% oxygen by face mask.
2. Administer an inhaled bronchodilator, such as albuterol, via a handheld, metered-dose inhaler with a spacer (adult dose 200 to 400 mcg q2-6 h prn).
3. Administer diphenhydramine 50 mg IV, IM, or PO if the attack is associated with an acute allergic reaction.

4. Administer a corticosteroid (prednisone 60 to 100 mg PO for adults and 2 mg/kg/day for children).
5. In severe cases, intubation and assisted ventilation may be necessary.
6. A person with asthma who is in severe distress or who does not have rapid and marked improvement with medication should be transported rapidly to the nearest medical facility.

Pneumonia
Signs and Symptoms
- Cough that may be productive of green or yellowish sputum
- Fever and shaking chills
- Chest pain that may be pleuritic
- Dyspnea, tachypnea, and tachycardia may be present

Treatment
1. Administer oxygen by nasal cannula to maintain SaO_2 greater than 90%.
2. Administer a broad-spectrum antibiotic. Excellent choices include the following:
   a. Azithromycin (Zithromax) 500 mg daily for 7 to 10 days (pediatric dose 10 mg/kg first dose, then 5 mg/kg/day for 4 days, with maximum dose 500 mg)
   b. Levofloxacin (Levaquin) 750 mg/day for 7 to 10 days (should only be used in children who are skeletally mature: pediatric dose 8 to 10 mg/kg/day, with maximum dose 500 mg)
   c. Amoxicillin/clavulanate (Augmentin) 500 to 875 mg bid for 7 to 10 days (pediatric dose 90 mg/kg/day in two divided doses)
   d. Erythromycin 250 to 500 mg q6h for 7 to 10 days (pediatric dose 30 to 50 mg/kg/day in four divided doses, with maximum dose 2 g/day)
3. Evacuate any patient with presumed pneumonia who demonstrates profound dehydration, is in sustained respiratory distress, shows signs of hypoxia, or has comorbid illnesses (e.g., diabetes, chronic obstructive pulmonary disease).

STROKE

Stroke is a disease process that disrupts vascular blood flow to a distinct part(s) of the brain. Although the causes of strokes are diverse, ranging from cardiac emboli to rupture of a congenital aneurysm, there are two major mechanisms of brain injury: (1) ischemia caused by vessel occlusion and (2) hemorrhage caused by vessel rupture. Eighty to 85% of all strokes are ischemic. Effective treatment for one stroke type may be disastrous when applied to the other type. A patient in the backcountry suspected of having a stroke should be transported immediately to the nearest medical facility because the anatomic location of the lesion and mechanism of the stroke must be known before effective treatment can be given. Ischemic (thrombotic) strokes can be effectively treated in many cases with intravenous (IV) tissue plasminogen activator (t-PA) if symptoms have been present for less than 12 hours. Mechanical clot removal and intraarterial t-PA may be effective in reversing stroke manifestations up to 8 hours after symptom onset. Stroke therapies and protocols are in evolution, so the time recommendations for effectiveness of interventions will likely change.

A review of the patient's demographics and past medical history may suggest the cause of the stroke. A 30-year-old, otherwise healthy patient with a stroke-like syndrome is more likely to have a hemorrhagic stroke. A 65-year-old patient with a history of hypertension, coronary artery disease, and diabetes is more likely to have a thrombotic stroke. Stroke in a patient with underlying atrial fibrillation suggests a cardioembolic source. Stroke in an individual with previous transient ischemic attack (TIA)–like symptoms suggests a thrombotic cause.

Signs and Symptoms

Any or all the following signs and symptoms may be present:

- Patient may be alert, drowsy, lethargic, obtunded, or comatose
- Visual field deficit or gaze preference
- Sudden onset of unilateral weakness and numbness
- Unilateral facial motor weakness (facial droop)
- Dysarthria and/or aphasia
- Sudden onset of dizziness, vertigo, diplopia, and ataxia
- Sudden onset of severe headache ("the worst headache of my life")

Treatment

1. Maintain an adequate airway, and administer oxygen.
2. Dehydration should be corrected with IV normal saline.
3. Assess the patient for hypoglycemia, and give dextrose if indicated (see later). Otherwise, dextrose-containing solutions should be avoided.
4. Consider aspirin (75 to 325 mg by mouth [PO] or 300- to 600-mg suppository) if timely evacuation is unlikely.
5. Keep the patient's head and torso slightly elevated (at least 30 degrees).
6. Transport the patient immediately to the closest medical facility. Continuously assess the patient's airway and level of consciousness because the condition can worsen dramatically during transport.

TRANSIENT ISCHEMIC ATTACK

A TIA is a neurologic deficit resembling a stroke that resolves within 24 hours (although most resolve within 30 minutes) and is most commonly associated with thrombotic stroke. Signs, symptoms, and treatment are the same as for stroke. Patients suspected of having a TIA should be evacuated for more detailed medical evaluation to reduce the risk of having a stroke.

SEIZURE

Seizure can result from head injury, heat illness, infection, hyponatremia, hypoglycemia, stroke, epilepsy, drugs, and other causes.

Signs and Symptoms

- A generalized (grand mal) seizure begins abruptly (there may be an aura) with loss of consciousness as the patient suddenly becomes rigid, with trunk and extremities extended, and falls to the ground. As the rigid (tonic) phase of the seizure subsides, there is increasing coarse trembling that evolves into rhythmic (clonic) jerking of the trunk and extremities. The eyes may deviate to one side, there is difficulty breathing, and occasionally there is loss of bladder and/or bowel control and tongue biting.
- Most seizures last only 1 or 2 minutes.
- After most seizures, the patient will be confused or combative ("postictal") for a period (10 to 30 minutes) and then slowly return to normal.

Treatment

1. Protect the patient from injury during the seizure. This may be done with cushions, sleeping bag, or by moving hard objects away from the patient.
2. If possible, the patient should be turned to one side to reduce the risk for aspiration should vomiting occur.
3. Do not attempt to place a bite block or any object between the teeth or into the mouth.

4. Do not give the patient anything orally until they are awake and lucid.
5. If the patient is suffering from hypoglycemia, administer sugar as soon as possible.
   a. If the patient is conscious and able to swallow, give them something containing sugar to drink or eat. This could be fruit juice, a banana, candy, or a nondiet soft drink. As soon as the patient feels better, have him or her eat a meal to avoid a recurrence.
   b. If the patient is unconscious, place tiny amounts of sugar granules, cake icing, or Glutose paste (one tube contains 25 g [0.9 oz] glucose) under the patient's tongue, where it will be passively swallowed and absorbed.
   c. If available, administer one to three vials of IV 50% dextrose (D_{50}) in water while completing the circulation, airway, and breathing (CAB) approach to resuscitation. In a child younger than 8 years of age, give 2 to 4 mL/kg of 25% dextrose (D_{25}) or even 5 mL/kg of 10% dextrose (D_{10}) in water. As an alternative in a patient for whom you cannot quickly obtain IV access, give 1 to 2 mg of glucagon intramuscularly (IM) or subcutaneously. This dose may be repeated as needed.
6. If the patient has continuous seizure activity for 10 minutes or more, or two or more seizures that occur without full recovery of consciousness between the attacks (status epilepticus), do the following:
   a. Administer 100% oxygen.
   b. Protect and if necessary, secure the airway; endotracheal intubation may be indicated.
   c. Check for head and other injuries. Maintain cervical spine precautions as indicated.
   d. Administer IV dextrose as per earlier dosing.
   e. Anticonvulsant drugs
      • Diazepam (5 to 10 mg IV at 5 mg/min or less every 5 to 10 min to a maximum of 30 mg).
      • Rectal diazepam (10 to 20 mg) or buccal midazolam (10 mg, which may be repeated once) after 10 min if IV access is impossible.

If status epilepticus persists, consider other anticonvulsant drugs:
• Lorazepam (4 mg at 2 mg/min IV every 10 to 15 min to a maximum of 8 mg)
• Phenytoin (adult dose 10 to 20 mg/kg IV, not exceeding 50 mg/min)
• Phenobarbital (adult dose 10 to 20 mg/kg IV to a maximum of 30 mg/kg, not exceeding 60 mg/min)
• Valproate (adult dose 15 to 45 mg/kg IV, not exceeding 6 mg/kg/min)
• The potential adverse effects of anticonvulsant drugs include hypotension, cardiac dysrhythmias, and cardiorespiratory arrest.

HEADACHE

Headaches stem from innumerable causes, including tension and stress, migraine, dehydration, altitude illness, alcohol hangover, carbon monoxide poisoning, brain tumor, stroke, aneurysm, intracranial hemorrhage, fever, flu, meningitis and other infectious diseases, high blood pressure, sinus infection, and dental problems. Going "cold turkey" without caffeine during a backpacking trip, especially if you regularly drink more than three cups of coffee a day, can precipitate a headache (Box 28.1).

Tension Headache (Stress or Muscle Contraction Headache)

This is the most common type of headache and affects people of all ages. The pain is related to continuous contractions of the muscles of the head and neck. Tension headaches have gradual onset and worsen as the day progresses.

Signs and Symptoms

- The headache is typically bilateral and often described as tight or vise-like, especially in the back of the head and neck.
- The pain is not made worse by walking, climbing, or performing physical activity.
- Sensitivity to light may occur, but nausea and vomiting are usually not present.
- Pain can last from 30 minutes to 7 days.

Treatment

1. Loosen any tight-fitting pack straps or hat, and adjust the person's pack so that it rides comfortably.

BOX 28.1   Headaches—"When to Worry"

Some headaches may signal a life-threatening illness. Someone with any of the following symptoms should seek medical attention as soon as possible:

- The headache is the worst of one's life and began suddenly and severely (aneurysmal [subarachnoid] or intracranial bleeding).
- The headache is associated with extremity numbness or weakness, diplopia, visual field deficit, unilateral facial paralysis, or ataxia (stroke).
- The headache is associated with an altered level of consciousness, aphasia, dysarthria, or ataxia (stroke, intracranial infection).
- There is fever, stiff neck, or rash (meningitis).
- The headache grows steadily worse over time (mass lesion, bleeding, infection).
- There is repetitive or projectile vomiting (mass lesion, bleeding, infection).

2. Administer a nonsteroidal antiinflammatory drug (NSAID), such as ibuprofen 400 mg PO q6h, or acetaminophen 1 g PO q6h as needed (prn).

Migraine Headache
Signs and Symptoms
- Throbbing, recurrent headaches that typically involve one side of the head
- Nausea and vomiting are common
- Photosensitivity
- Walking or physical exertion makes the pain worse
- About 15% of individuals with migraine headaches experience an aura (flashing lights, distorted shapes and colors, blurred vision, or other visual apparitions) before the onset of the headache.

Treatment
1. Place patient in a quiet and dark environment.
2. Administer an NSAID such as ibuprofen 400 mg PO q6h, or acetaminophen 1 g PO q6h prn.
3. Administer an antiemetic along with oral or IV hydration
   a. metoclopramide (5 to 10 mg PO every 6 hours)
   b. ondansetron (4 to 8 mg PO every 8 hours)
   c. prochlorperazine (10 mg PO every 6 hours)
   d. prochlorperazine suppository (10 to 25 mg, with a daily maximum of 50 mg)
4. Caffeine-containing beverages such as coffee may help relieve symptoms, especially if taken early during the migraine.
5. Consider administering sumatriptan succinate (Imitrex) 6 mg subcutaneously by autoinjector or 25 mg PO, or as a 5- or 20-mg nasal spray. Doses may be repeated in 1 hour if not effective to a total of 12 mg subcutaneously, 200 mg PO, or 40 mg nasally in 1 day.
6. Prevent a recurrent attack:
   a. Maintain adequate sleep and minimize alterations of the sleep-wake cycle.
   b. Keep regular mealtimes.
   c. Avoid dehydration.
   d. Utilize trigger management (e.g., avoid red wine and chocolate; avoid exposure to loud noises and prolonged sunlight).

Cluster Headache
Signs and Symptoms
- Headache is unilateral, severe, and brief, lasting 30 to 90 minutes.
- Eye redness and tearing, nasal congestion, rhinorrhea, and eyelid edema are often present.
- Attacks may occur multiple times daily and are usually not associated with nausea or vomiting.

Treatment

1. Oxygen by face mask at 8 to 10 L/min may be helpful.
2. Administer an NSAID, such as ibuprofen 400 mg PO q6h, or acetaminophen 1 g PO q6h prn.
3. Migraine treatments (see earlier) have been shown to help some patients.

Meningitis

CNS infection requires a pragmatic approach when one is far from help. Differentiating between bacterial and viral meningitis is difficult. Bacterial meningitis may be fatal if not treated promptly and properly.

Signs and Symptoms

- Severe headache and photophobia
- Fever
- Neck stiffness and pain with neck flexion or straight leg raising
- Nausea and vomiting
- Mental status changes or focal neurologic signs may occur. Confusion may be the sole presenting complaint, especially in older adults.
- Skin rash comprised of petechiae and purpura (consider meningococcal meningitis).

Treatment

1. Evacuate the patient immediately to the nearest medical center.
2. Administer empiric antibiotics for common pathogens based on patient age (Table 28.1).
3. Administer dexamethasone (0.4 mg/kg IV) 15 to 20 minutes before the first dose of antibiotics and then every 6 hours.

Dehydration Headache

Headache can be a symptom of dehydration.

Signs and Symptoms

- The pain is felt on both sides of the head.
- The pain is usually made worse when the patient stands from a lying position.

Treatment

1. Administer at least 1 to 2 L (1 to 2 qt) of oral rehydration solution. If an electrolyte-supplemented liquid is not available, then water is acceptable.
2. Administer an NSAID, such as ibuprofen 400 mg PO q6h, or acetaminophen 1 g PO q6h prn.

Bell's Palsy

Bell's palsy involves paralysis of the facial muscles innervated by the seventh (facial) nerve. Bell's palsy is rapidly progressive, with maximum weakness present within 24 to 48 hours.

Table 28.1 Recommended Empirical Antimicrobial Therapy for Suspected Bacterial Meningitis Based on Age

AGE	COMMON BACTERIAL PATHOGENS	ANTIMICROBIAL THERAPY
<1 month	*Streptococcus agalactiae, Escherichia coli, Listeria monocytogenes*	Ampicillin, 100 mg/kg, *plus* cefotaxime, 50 mg/kg every 6 h *or* Ampicillin, 100 mg/kg, *plus* an aminoglycoside (gentamicin, 2.5 mg/kg, *or* tobramycin, 2.5 mg/kg) every 8 h
1–23 months	*Streptococcus pneumoniae, Neisseria meningitidis, S. agalactiae, Haemophilus influenzae, E. coli*	Vancomycin, 15 mg/kg IV every 6 h (maximum daily dose of 4 g), *plus* cefotaxime, 100 mg/kg IV, followed by 200–300 mg/kg/day in four divided doses (maximum daily dose of 12 g), *or* ceftriaxone, 50 mg/kg IV every 12 h (maximum daily dose of 4 g)
2–50 years	*N. meningitidis, S. pneumoniae*	• *Children:* Vancomycin, 15 mg/kg every 6 h, *plus* ceftriaxone, 75–100 mg/kg every 12–24 h, or cefotaxime, 75–100 mg/kg every 6–8 h • *Adults:* Vancomycin, 15 mg/kg every 8 h, *plus* ceftriaxone, 2 g every 12 h, or cefotaxime, 2 g every 4 h
>50 years	*S. pneumoniae, N. meningitidis, L. monocytogenes,* aerobic gram-negative bacilli	Vancomycin, 15 mg/kg every 8 h, *plus* ampicillin, 2 g every 4 h, *plus* ceftriaxone, 2 g every 12 h, *or* cefotaxime 2 g every 4–6 h

Signs and Symptoms

- Nearly 50% of patients experience pain in the mastoid region behind the ear when symptoms are first noted.
- Weakness and/or paralysis of the muscles (upper and lower) of one side of the face. It is important to differentiate Bell's

palsy from a stroke. Bell's palsy should cause weakness on one side of the face, including the forehead. A stroke will not produce weakness of the forehead (the patient will still be able to wrinkle his or her forehead when looking upward).

- Taste may be reduced or lost on the anterior two-thirds of the tongue on the same side as the facial weakness.

Treatment
1. Administer prednisone 60 to 80 mg/day PO for 7 days.
2. Use of antiviral therapy is controversial because of limited evidence. Current recommendations suggest valacyclovir 1 gm PO three times daily for 1 week for moderate to severe dysfunction: obvious weakness, no forehead movement, asymmetric mouth with maximum effort, and incomplete closure of the eye.
3. The patient should wear an eye patch to protect the eye.
4. Lacri-Lube or another eye lubricant should be applied every 3 to 4 hours.

SLEEP
Problems sleeping are common in wilderness settings, often from a combination of changing time zones, physical discomfort, anxiety or depression, and disrupted daily routine (e.g., long watches at sea, predawn starts on climbs, precarious bivouac sites). At high altitude, hypoxia causes disrupted sleep patterns, irregular breathing, and episodes of sleep apnea.

Signs and Symptoms
- Exhaustion
- Poor judgment
- Mild confusion
- Seizures in persons with a low seizure threshold
- Sleepwalking
- Jerking episodes
- Fitful sleep

Sleep Management
1. Ensure adequate sleep duration (7 to 8 hours at a stretch for adults; 9 to 11 hours for children).
2. Ensure that sleeping accommodations are as comfortable as possible. A pillow, warm headgear, dry night clothes, and earplugs can be helpful.
3. Avoid sedatives unless they are necessary. Recognize repeated early-morning awakening as a possible feature of emotional depression.
4. Avoid caffeine, if possible, for 6 hours or more before attempting to sleep.

Diabetes Emergencies

DEFINITIONS AND CHARACTERISTICS

Diabetes is the most common endocrine disease. Acute complications include hypoglycemia, diabetic ketoacidosis (DKA), and hyperglycemic hyperosmolar state (HHS). Long-term complications include disorders of the microvasculature, cardiovascular system, eyes, kidneys, skin, and nerves. Type 1 diabetes is characterized by destruction of pancreatic beta cells, leading to absolute insulin deficiency. Type 2 diabetes, the most common type, is characterized by variable degrees of insulin deficiency and resistance. Although diet and oral hypoglycemic medications are initially used to control type 2 diabetes, many individuals lose beta cell function over time and require insulin for glucose control.

Ensuring that insulin does not freeze and glucose testing equipment works properly is important for diabetic individuals in the wilderness. Strategies to ensure that insulin does not freeze include carrying the medication inside a pouch that is worn around the neck next to the body and keeping insulin in the sleeping bag at night. Carrying glucose monitoring equipment next to the skin may prevent the problems associated with battery malfunction at cold temperatures.

Accurate blood glucose measurement under extreme conditions is paramount for safe travel in the wilderness. Studies of blood glucose meters at high altitude (above 4000 m [13,123 ft]) have yielded conflicting data regarding accuracy and reliability. Both overestimation and underestimation of blood glucose level have been reported for all types of glucose meters. Glucose meters using the oxygen-insensitive enzyme glucose dehydrogenase (GDH) may perform better at high altitude than those using the enzyme glucose oxidase. High glucose levels seem to be misreported to a greater extent at altitude than are low to normal glucose levels. At altitudes above 5000 m (16,404 ft), the Accu-Chek Compact Plus GDH-based blood glucose meter was found to be most accurate when compared to standard reference glucose solutions, independent of the glucose solution used. The Accu-Chek Compact Plus also received an excellent rating by Consumer Reports for its reliability. FreeStyle Lite, FreeStyle Freedom Lite, and Accu-Chek Aviva also performed well with devices and strips purchased through regular distribution channels. Because of the variability of blood glucose meters in extreme environments, it is prudent to rely on one's clinical assessment and not just the blood glucose meter reading when evaluating a patient for hypoglycemia.

Diabetics should wear appropriate medical alert identification, such as bracelets or necklaces, in case assistance is necessary and they are not able to communicate. If a diabetic becomes confused, weak, or unconscious, he or she may be suffering from insulin-induced hypoglycemia or lapsing into a diabetic coma.

DISORDERS
Hypoglycemia

If a diabetic takes too much insulin or another glucose-lowering agent, fails to eat sufficient carbohydrate to match the exogenous drug administered, or exercises at a greatly increased rate, a rapid drop in blood glucose level can occur. Another factor contributing to hypoglycemia in the exercising individual with insulin-dependent diabetes is increased exogenous insulin mobilization from subcutaneous tissue because of increased blood flow. It is important for insulin-dependent diabetic patients to administer their dose of subcutaneous insulin before exercise in a location away from exercising muscle. They should avoid injections into the arms and legs, instead using the abdomen or back of the neck. Insulin absorption is fastest and most consistent when it is injected into the abdomen.

Another measure to prevent exercise-associated hypoglycemia is to reduce the dose of insulin that will be in effect during exercise. The best strategy for a type 1 diabetic patient is to monitor blood glucose level before, during, and after exercise to predict changes, and adjust insulin doses accordingly. This means that before a wilderness trip, the diabetic patient should exercise daily at a level of physical activity similar to that anticipated on the wilderness trip and consume similar types of food that will be ingested on the trip, so that adjustments in insulin dosing can be better predicted.

Signs and Symptoms

- Altered level of consciousness, such as confusion, behavioral changes, nervousness, belligerence, syncope, headache, seizures, unconsciousness, or coma
- Shakiness, hunger, weakness, tremor, diaphoresis ("cold sweats"), pallor, abdominal pain, ataxia, slurred speech, palpitations, tachycardia, hypothermia
- Minimal to absent prodrome; patient may become unarousable without warning

Treatment

1. If possible, obtain a blood glucose reading before initiating therapy.
2. Disable insulin pump if applicable.
3. If the patient is still conscious and able to swallow without choking, give the person something containing sugar to drink or eat as soon as possible. This could be sugar, fruit juice,

a banana, candy, or a nondiet soft drink. As soon as the patient feels better, have him or her eat a meal to avoid a recurrence.

4. If the patient is unconscious:
   a. Place tiny amounts of sugar granules, cake icing, oral glucose gel (one tube of Glutose 15 contains 15 g glucose), or other sugar source under the patient's tongue, or between the cheek and an inserted tongue blade, where it can be passively swallowed and absorbed.
   b. If intravenous (IV) access can be established, administer 1 to 2 ampules of dextrose (25 g of 50% glucose [dextrose] in each ampule) while attending to the circulation, airway, and breathing (CAB) approach to resuscitation. In a child younger than 8 years of age, administer an initial bolus of dextrose, 0.25 g/kg of body weight. This is usually achieved with 2.5 mL/kg of 10% dextrose solution, because extravasation out of a vein of higher concentrations of glucose will lead to severe tissue damage. The bolus should be administered slowly (2 to 3 mL/min), regardless of age.
   c. As an alternative in a patient for whom you cannot quickly obtain IV access, administer 1 to 2 mg of glucagon (see further for administration instructions) for adults and 0.5 mg for children weighing less than 20 kg (44 lb) intramuscularly, subcutaneously, or intranasally. Patients usually regain consciousness within 5 to 20 minutes of receiving glucagon, although it may be followed by marked nausea or vomiting. This dose may be repeated after 15 minutes if necessary. Glucagon kits should be checked regularly and replaced when they are beyond the expiration date.

5. The blood glucose level should be checked after 15 to 20 minutes to ensure that the glucose level has increased to a safe level (>100 mg/dL) before continuing with the physical activity. The person should be closely watched for evidence of recurrent symptoms.

Glucagon Administration Instructions (GlucaGen HypoKit)

1. Remove the seal from the bottle of glucagon.
2. Remove the needle protector from the syringe, and inject the entire contents into the bottle of glucagon.
3. Swirl bottle gently until glucagon dissolves completely.
4. Using the same syringe, hold bottle upside down and, making sure the needle tip remains in solution, gently withdraw all of the solution.
5. Cleanse an injection site on a buttock, arm, or thigh with the alcohol swab or, using a mucosal atomizer, give intranasally.
6. Insert the needle into the muscle under the cleansed injection site, and inject all (or one-half for children weighing less than 20 kg [44 lb]) of the glucagon solution.

7. Remove the needle, and apply light pressure at the injection site.
8. Provide supportive care, including airway management, aspiration and seizure precautions, administration of oxygen, and treatment of shock.

Diabetic Ketoacidosis

DKA is an acute, life threatening complication of diabetes. DKA mainly occurs in patients with type 1 diabetes, although some patients with type 2 diabetes develop DKA under certain circumstances (severe infection or other illness). In DKA, blood glucose levels become dangerously high (>250 mg/dL). The blood becomes acidotic as the byproducts of metabolism (ketones) accumulate, dehydration occurs, and body chemistry falls out of balance (decreased pH). DKA usually evolves over a 24-hour period.

Signs and Symptoms

- History of recent polydipsia, polyuria, polyphagia, blurred vision, weakness, weight loss, nausea, vomiting, and abdominal pain
- Early symptoms: polyuria, polydipsia, nausea, and vomiting
- Later symptoms: tachycardia, tachypnea with Kussmaul respirations (deep, rapid breathing), hyperventilation, and possibly fruity odor (similar to the odor of nail polish remover) on the breath because of exhaled acetone
- Abdominal pain, especially in children
- Signs of volume depletion (dry mucous membranes, absence of sweating, decreased skin turgor, orthostatic hypotension)
- Eventually: confusion, combativeness, or coma with signs of profound dehydration
- Possibly hyperthermia or hypothermia if sepsis is present

Treatment

1. If unsure whether the patient has hyperglycemia or hypoglycemia, assume it is hypoglycemia and administer glucose.
2. Treatment of DKA in the field is challenging because of the necessity for fluid, electrolyte, and insulin replacement and the need for frequent electrolyte monitoring. If the patient can drink, encourage him or her to consume large quantities of unsweetened fluids. The average fluid loss in DKA is 3 to 6 L.
3. If available, initially administer IV NS solution (2 L over 2 hours in adults and 10 to 20 mL/kg in children). Fluid resuscitation alone may help considerably in lowering hyperglycemia and begin to correct the metabolic abnormalities.
4. Provide supportive care, including airway management, oxygen administration, and shock treatment, while transporting the patient to a medical center.
5. If insulin is available and glucose levels can be closely monitored in the field, consider administering insulin as an IV infusion at a rate of 0.1 unit/kg/hr until the measured glucose level is less than 250 mg/dL (13.9 mmol/L).

6. Subcutaneous insulin therapy may also be used and is most effective with rapid-acting insulin analogs (insulin lispro and aspart) if the patient is not in shock. Administer subcutaneous insulin as an initial injection of 0.3 units/kg followed by 0.1 units/kg every hour until the serum glucose level is less than 250 mg/dL (13.9 mmol/L). During treatment, blood glucose should be measured at least every hour. The subcutaneous administration of insulin lispro and aspart has an onset of action within 10 to 20 minutes and reaches a peak insulin concentration within 30 to 90 minutes. These time intervals are significantly shorter than those observed with subcutaneous regular insulin, which has an onset of action of 1 to 2 hours and reaches a peak effect at 2 to 4 hours.

Hyperglycemic Hyperosmolar State

In HHS there is little or no ketoacid accumulation, serum glucose concentration frequently exceeds 1000 mg/dL, and neurologic abnormalities are frequently present. HHS develops more insidiously than does DKA, with polyuria, polydipsia, and weight loss often present for several days before the patient becomes markedly ill.

Signs and Symptoms

- Extreme dehydration, hyperosmolarity, and altered level of consciousness (including depressed sensorium that can be as severe as obtundation and seizures)
- Fever, thirst, polyuria, oliguria
- Orthostatic or nonpostural hypotension, tachycardia

Treatment

1. The average fluid loss in HHS is 8 to 10 L, largely as a result of the glucose-driven osmotic diuresis. If the patient can drink, encourage him or her to consume large quantities of unsweetened fluids.
2. If intravenous access is available, administer NS solution. In the absence of cardiac compromise, saline is infused at a rate of 10 to 15 mL/kg lean body weight per hour (about 1000 mL/hr in an average-sized person) during the first few hours, with a maximum of 50 mL/kg in the first 4 hours.
3. After an initial infusion of saline to increase insulin responsiveness by lowering the plasma osmolality, consider administering insulin as described earlier for DKA.
4. Transport the patient emergently to a medical facility.

AIR TRAVEL AND DIABETES MEDICATIONS AND SYRINGES

Under current air travel regulations, individuals carrying insulin and syringes should notify the security officer that they have diabetes and are carrying diabetes-related supplies. The following are allowed through the checkpoint once they have been screened:

- Insulin and insulin-loaded dispensing products (vials, jet injectors, and preloaded syringes)
- Unlimited number of unused syringes when accompanied by insulin or other injectable medication
- Lancets, blood glucose meters, alcohol swabs
- Insulin pump and insulin pump supplies
- Glucagon emergency kit

FOOT CARE

While not an emergency, foot care for diabetics is very important because peripheral neuropathy predisposes to pressure ulcers of the feet. Persons with diabetes should avoid prolonged traumatic weight-bearing exercise, monitor their feet meticulously with inspections of all surfaces once a day, be certain to wear properly fitted footwear that is well insulated and warm, and address any sign of inflammation, blistering, or infection.

In the wilderness, genitourinary tract disorders are common, and urinary tract infections (UTIs) constitute the majority of complaints. Also included in this chapter are pyelonephritis, urethritis, epididymitis, prostatitis, testicular torsion, urinary tract obstruction, and acute urinary retention. Gynecologic infections and emergencies are discussed in Chapter 31.

URINARY TRACT INFECTION
- UTIs are more common in women.
- The incidence increases in postmenopausal women and women with histories of recent frequent sexual intercourse.
- In women, the primary cause of UTI is invasion of the urinary tract by bacteria that have ascended the urethra from the introitus.
- Most of these infections are caused by gram-negative aerobic bacteria, most often *Escherichia coli.*
- UTIs are rare entities in men younger than 50 years.
- Despite the difference in prevalence, symptoms in men and women are similar.
- Infection of the urinary tract in a male is often associated with prostatic enlargement or infection.

Lower UTI (Uncomplicated UTI)
Signs and Symptoms
- Bladder irritation (dysuria, frequency, urgency, hesitancy)
- Hematuria

  Confirmation of the diagnosis by examination of urine is typically impossible in the wilderness. Other genitourinary processes that may be associated with or mimic UTI include the following:
- Pyelonephritis associated with chills and fever
- Urethritis (more probable in sexually active persons with multiple or new partners)
- Chlamydial or gonococcal cervicitis (often associated with cervical discharge)
- Vaginal infection (associated with vaginal discharge, external irritation, or pain with intercourse)
- Ureterolithiasis (dysuria with flank pain, restlessness, and costovertebral angle [CVA] tenderness suggests urinary tract stone[s])
- Prostatitis

Treatment
1. Perform a physical examination, including determination of temperature, abdominal examination, and assessment for CVA tenderness.

2. Perform a pelvic (bimanual) examination in a woman whose symptoms are associated with pelvic pain or vaginal bleeding. Although a formal pelvic examination using a speculum with the individual in a lithotomy position is virtually impossible in the wilderness, a simple bimanual examination might identify an adnexal or uterine process (e.g., ectopic pregnancy, pelvic inflammatory disease). Perform a pregnancy test.
3. Give oral antibiotic therapy using one of the following:
   a. Trimethoprim/sulfamethoxazole one double-strength (DS, 160/800 mg) tablet bid for 3 days
   b. Ciprofloxacin 500 mg bid for 3 days
   c. Nitrofurantoin 100 mg bid for 5 days is a safe option for pregnant women
   d. Fosfomycin 3 g one dose
4. If symptoms persist after standard therapy:
   a. Consider a resistant organism.
   b. In a male, consider a relapse caused by prostatitis.
5. In addition to the antibiotic therapy, provide pain relief for dysuria by administering phenazopyridine (a urinary anesthetic) 200 mg PO tid for a maximum of 2 days. Warn the patient that the urine (and possibly contact lenses) will turn orange.

Pyelonephritis
Pyelonephritis is an infection of the upper urinary tract (kidney), most often caused by ascending infection from the lower urinary tract.

Signs and Symptoms
- Fever greater than 38.9°C (102° F), chills, CVA tenderness
- Symptoms of lower UTI
- Malaise, abdominal pain

Treatment
1. Administer an oral antibiotic if the patient is nonpregnant and immunocompetent and can tolerate oral medication.
   - Reasonable antibiotic choices include ciprofloxacin 500 mg bid or levofloxacin 750 mg daily for 10 to 14 days.
2. For a severely ill, immunocompromised, or pregnant patient, initiate therapy with a parenteral antibiotic such as a third-generation cephalosporin (ceftriaxone 1 g IM or IV daily).
3. When a high fever is present:
   - Routinely administer acetaminophen 500 mg q4h or ibuprofen 600 mg q6h to make the patient more comfortable.
   - If the fever persists, consider the possibility of a resistant organism, UTI, or abscess.
4. Arrange for evacuation of immunocompromised or pregnant patients, when protracted vomiting makes oral therapy impossible, or when generalized toxicity (volume depletion, fever greater than 38.9° C [102° F] or marked CVA tenderness) is present.

5. Instruct patients to seek medical follow-up on return, even if symptoms resolve fully.

Urinary Stones
Signs and Symptoms
- Location of pain depends on the site of stone impaction, but most patients complain of flank pain
  - Pain may radiate to the groin as the stone migrates distally
  - Consider other causes for pain: acute aortic dissection, back strain, or herniated lumbar disk
- Nausea and vomiting
- Restlessness and inability to lie still
- CVA tenderness
- Absence of peritoneal signs; if these develop, they indicate a possible intraperitoneal process (e.g., appendicitis)
- Absence of fever unless an associated UTI is present (which may develop in an obstructed ureter)
- Gross hematuria possible, but microscopic hematuria is more likely

Treatment
1. Consider evacuation for severe nausea and vomiting (inadequate oral intake), fever (suggestive of an infection proximal to the obstruction), or the presence of an intraperitoneal process.
2. Arrange for adequate hydration. Administer an antiinflammatory medication such as ketorolac (Toradol) 60 mg IM or 30 mg IV q8h, or an oral nonsteroidal antiinflammatory drug (NSAID) such as ibuprofen 600 mg q6h, to reduce the pain of renal colic. NSAIDs may be used in addition to narcotic analgesia.
3. Administer a narcotic analgesic if needed.
   - Use an oral narcotic combination drug such as hydrocodone bitartrate 5 mg with acetaminophen 325 mg, one or two tablets q4–6h.
   - For more severe pain, administer a parenteral narcotic such as morphine sulfate 2 to 5 mg IV q5min, titrated for pain relief. Make sure to monitor the patient for excessive sedation manifested by hypoventilation, and have naloxone 0.4 mg IV available for emergency administration.
4. For additional narcotic analgesic options, see Chapter 24.
5. Administer an antiemetic drug (ondansetron 4–8 mg oral dissolving tablet q6h) if nausea and vomiting develop.
6. Consider tamsulosin 0.4 mg once daily, an alpha adrenergic blocker, which may augment stone passage. Be aware that systemic effects may cause hypotension and dizziness so the patient should be advised to sit or stand slowly or with assistance after supine position.
7. Encourage the patient to seek medical follow-up even if symptoms resolve fully.
8. Although not usually practical in the wilderness, filtering the urine for stones is helpful for diagnosis.

Acute Scrotal Pain

When palpation of the scrotum, including the testes, epididymis, and cord structures, reveals no abnormality or tenderness, consider referred pain as a possible consequence of renal, ureteral, or prostatic disease.

Epididymitis

Epididymitis is abrupt inflammation of the epididymis that spreads rapidly and can appear as generalized inflammation of the entire hemiscrotum (Fig. 30.1). The differential diagnosis includes torsion of the testis, acute orchitis, or tumor of the testis with hemorrhage or hydrocele. Most cases of epididymitis in young men are caused by *Chlamydia trachomatis*. At any age, UTI caused by gram-negative rods can spread to the epididymis.

Signs and Symptoms

- Acute scrotal pain in men older than age 20 years (infectious epididymitis)
- Testicular torsion in men (usually) younger than age 30 years
- Gradual (over days) onset of pain
- Dysuria or urethral discharge
- Normal urinalysis in torsion, but pyuria in epididymitis (if urinalysis can be done)
- Fever possible
- Recent history of a UTI
- Tenderness and swelling localized to one epididymis (usually at the superior pole of the testis)
- Prehn's sign: relief of pain when elevating the testis (suggestive of epididymitis rather than torsion)

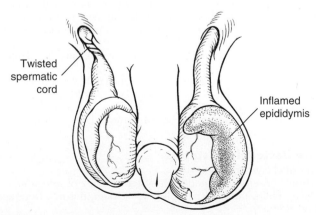

Twisted spermatic cord

Inflamed epididymis

FIGURE 30.1   Testicular disorders: twisted (torsed) spermatic cord and inflamed epididymis.

Treatment

1. Administer an antibiotic that covers *Neisseria gonorrhoeae* and *C. trachomatis*.
   Azithromycin 1 g PO in a single dose, or
   Doxycycline, 100 mg PO bid for 7 days
2. Allow the patient to rest supine with the scrotum elevated.
3. Administer analgesic medication.
4. Arrange for the patient to wear men's supportive briefs or an athletic supporter to offer pain relief if the patient is expected to ambulate.
5. Be aware that relief after therapy usually occurs within 24 hours.
6. Inform the patient that induration and edema in the region of the epididymis may persist for 6 to 8 weeks.

Testicular Torsion

Signs and Symptoms

- Rare in males older than 30 years
- May or may not occur during physical exertion
- Nausea and vomiting
- No preceding urethral discharge or fever
- Testis that rides high in the upper part of the scrotum
- Relief of pain when the affected testis is elevated (Prehn's sign) is suggestive of epididymitis rather than torsion, but this is not absolute (see Fig. 30.1)

Treatment

1. Be aware that testicular torsion of the spermatic cord requires surgical intervention. Therefore consider immediate evacuation if this diagnosis is suspected.
2. Attempt manual correction.
   a. Torsion most often occurs with the anterior portion of the testis rotating from its lateral aspect to its medial aspect.
   b. To correct the torsion manually, attempt to turn the right testis clockwise and the left testis counterclockwise, when viewed from above.
   c. Be aware that extreme tenderness may make manual correction difficult.
   d. Relief of pain suggests that torsion has been corrected.
3. Advise the patient that evaluation by a urologist is indicated after successful detorsion.
4. Be aware that if the torsion is not corrected, loss of the affected testis is likely.

Acute Bacterial Prostatitis

Signs and Symptoms

- Abrupt onset, associated with systemic signs of infection
- Fever, chills, perineal pain, low back pain, dysuria, frequency, and urgency

- Hematuria possible
- Tender, swollen ("boggy") prostate on palpation during rectal examination
- Resultant acute urinary retention

Treatment
1. Initiate oral antibiotic treatment with a fluoroquinolone, such as ciprofloxacin 500 mg bid or levofloxacin 500 mg daily.
2. Alternatively, administer trimethoprim/sulfamethoxazole one 160/800 mg (DS) tablet PO bid.
3. Continue therapy for at least 28 days.
4. If urinary retention is present, catheterization or suprapubic aspiration may be necessary.
5. Arrange for "bed rest" if conditions permit.

Urethritis
Urethritis in females is very difficult to distinguish from lower UTI, but if a female patient is treated for lower UTI and symptoms do not improve, consider the diagnosis. Lower UTI is infrequent in males, so dysuria in a male should prompt consideration of urethritis. Male urethritis is typically a sexually transmitted infection. In both sexes it is most often caused by *C. trachomatis.*

Signs and Symptoms
- In males, urethral discharge (mucopurulent with chlamydial and frankly purulent with gonococcal urethritis), dysuria, meatal pruritus
- Flank or abdominal pain, fever, or hematuria is not usually found; if present, another cause is suggested

Treatment
1. Administer an antibiotic that covers *N. gonorrhoeae* and *C. trachomatis:*
   a. Ceftriaxone 250 mg IM in a single dose plus
   b. Azithromycin 1 g PO in a single dose or doxycycline 100 mg PO bid for 7 days.
2. Notify any current sexual partners of the patient, and treat them with an appropriate regimen.

Acute Urinary Retention
Signs and Symptoms
- Principal symptoms are bladder distention and pain that may mimic an acute abdomen.
- Overflow incontinence
- Dribbling and hesitancy
- On examination:
  - Prostatic enlargement in men
  - Lower midline abdominal tenderness and distention

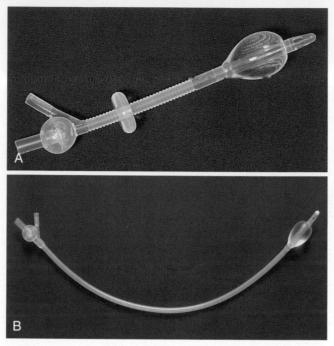

FIGURE 30.2 **A,** OPTION-*vf* (female) catheter. **B,** OPTION-*vm* (male) catheter.

Treatment

1. Tamsulosin 0.4 mg daily is a third-generation α-blocker that may provide some relief by promoting bladder neck and prostatic urethral relaxation.
2. Bladder decompression should be initially attempted with a standard Foley catheter.
3. In men with prostatic hypertrophy, passage of the catheter may be challenging, and a large catheter or coudé catheter should be used if a standard Foley catheter cannot be passed.
4. Instrumentation of the urethra with hemostats or dilators is dangerous and should not be attempted in the field.
5. OPTION-*vf* (Fig. 30.2A) and OPTION-*vm* (see Fig. 30.2B) catheters are valved urinary catheters that eliminate the need for urine drainage bags and connecting tubes normally required with Foley catheters. These catheters incorporate a manually activated valve at the end of the catheter that allows the patient to store urine in the bladder and to mimic normal voiding behavior. The catheters may be used with a continuous drainage adapter when appropriate so that a bag may be placed and urination rate and volume assessed.

31 | Gynecologic and Obstetric Emergencies

PATTERNS OF MENSTRUAL BLEEDING
- Normal cycle: every 28 ± 5 days with a duration of 3 to 6 days
- Normal menstrual flow: 80 mL or three to five pads or tampons per day with a duration of 3 to 5 days
- Menorrhagia: excessive flow
- Metrorrhagia: continuous duration or with no identifiable pattern
- Menometrorrhagia: increased quantity and duration
- Hypermenorrhea: increased quantity
- Intermenstrual spotting: small amounts of vaginal bleeding that may occur before or after menstruation or midcycle

VAGINAL BLEEDING ASSOCIATED WITH PREGNANCY
Ectopic Pregnancy
Ectopic pregnancy is a medical emergency that requires prompt evacuation of the patient to a surgical facility.

History
- Any history of prior ectopic pregnancy, salpingitis, pelvic inflammatory disease (PID), tubal surgery, or use of fertility agent or intrauterine device (IUD) should increase clinical suspicion.
- Prior bilateral tubal ligation does not exclude the diagnosis.
- History is usually suggestive of early pregnancy and includes nausea, amenorrhea, and breast tenderness.
- A prior seemingly normal or abnormal menstrual period is also possible.

Signs and Symptoms
- An ectopic pregnancy may rupture as early as 5 weeks' gestation but most commonly ruptures after 7 weeks' gestation.
- Most women will become symptomatic before 12 weeks' gestation.
- Ectopic rupture is generally preceded by abnormal vaginal bleeding and unilateral lower abdominal pain.
- A triad exists of vaginal bleeding, adnexal mass, and lower abdominal pain that is usually unilateral and may radiate to the shoulder.
- Cervical motion tenderness may be present on pelvic examination.
- Dizziness, syncope, and unstable vital signs may be present if blood loss is substantial.
- Rebound tenderness and rigidity are signs of rupture.

- Any patient with positive pregnancy test results and lower abdominal pain, usually unilateral, should be assumed to have an ectopic pregnancy until proven otherwise.
- Urine pregnancy test
  - This test is currently sensitive enough to detect levels of urinary β-human chorionic gonadotropin (β-hCG) as low as 10 milliunits/mL from the 3rd to 4th week after the first day of the last menstrual period.
  - This test should be included in remote expedition medical supplies. To ensure adequate performance of the test, use a test with an internal reference.

Treatment

1. Immediate evacuation
2. Treat for shock (see Chapter 13)

Spontaneous Abortion (Miscarriage)

Early pregnancy loss before 20 weeks' gestation

Types

Threatened

- Closed internal cervical os on pelvic examination
- Progressive bleeding and cramping
- Occurs in 25% of normal pregnancies
- 50% progress to termination, regardless of management

Inevitable

- Cervix dilated on pelvic examination
- Product of conception (POC) not yet passed, despite vaginal bleeding

Incomplete

- Dilated cervical os with partial passage of POC
- Accompanied by increased bleeding and persistent pain

Complete

- Diagnosis based on pathologic examination of all POC and cannot be made in the wilderness
- A presumed complete abortion is handled as an incomplete abortion.

Missed

- Closed internal os despite retained POC
- May lead to subsequent infection and hemorrhage if uterine contents not evacuated

Septic

- Associated with lower abdominal pain, tenderness, and fever
- Endometritis or parametritis after a spontaneous or therapeutic abortion
- Can lead to septic shock

Signs and Symptoms
- History suggestive of early pregnancy, including late or missed period and breast tenderness
- Positive urine pregnancy test results with above signs and symptoms
- Spontaneous abortion presents as abnormal vaginal bleeding, followed by uterine cramping.
- Bleeding can vary from dark red spotting to bright red clots.
- Consistency may be gritty, with passage of POC.
- Cervix may be dilated or closed.

Treatment
1. Unless a pre-trip ultrasound examination has verified an intrauterine pregnancy, immediately evacuate the patient to rule out ectopic pregnancy.
2. Keep the patient at "bed rest" if possible.
3. Direct all field treatment to volume replacement.
4. Evacuation of uterus to prevent further hemorrhage or infection will be necessary once transported to medical facility.
5. Treatment of septic abortion will involve broad-spectrum intravenous antibiotics (see Appendix H).
6. Treat for shock until evacuated (see Chapter 13).
7. Under wilderness conditions, control of significant maternal hemorrhage accompanying miscarriage may be difficult. Once the uterus is empty, uterine involution, spontaneous or aided by uterine massage, is usually sufficient to impede bleeding from the implantation site. In the absence of the ability to perform curettage, treatment with methylergonovine, 0.2 mg PO or IM, can enhance uterine contractions, accelerate expulsion of POC, and promote uterine involution to maintain hemostasis while plans are being made for patient evacuation. Methylergonovine should not be used in persons with hypertensive disorders or vascular disease unless the benefits outweigh the risks of generalized vasoconstriction. As an alternative, carboprost tromethamine 250 mcg IM, or misoprostol 400 to 600 mcg PO, sublingually, or vaginally, can be administered to stop uterine bleeding with less risk for cardiovascular compromise.

Placenta Previa
Painless vaginal bleeding secondary to placental implantation at the lower uterine segment. Placental implantation may completely obscure the cervical os or just rim the edge of the internal os.

History
- Suggestive of pregnancy (see earlier)
- History of painless bleeding
- Endometrial trauma or uterine surgery are both risk factors

Signs and Symptoms
- Definitive diagnosis impossible in the field
- Positive urine pregnancy test

- Painless vaginal bleeding (spotting to bright-red blood with clots)
- May lead to uterine contractions
- Can occur as early as 20 weeks' gestation

Treatment
1. Keep the patient at "bed rest" if possible
2. Volume replacement if indicated
3. Immediate evacuation
4. Vaginal/pelvic and/or rectal examination contraindicated

Placental Abruption
- Rupture of the placenta from the wall of the uterus
- Separation partial to complete
- History of painful bleeding in late pregnancy or after trauma

History
- History suggestive of pregnancy (see earlier)
- Most common in the third trimester of pregnancy
- Vaginal bleeding usually accompanied by pain
- History of trauma, maternal hypertension, cocaine abuse, or advanced maternal age should warrant suspicion

Signs and Symptoms
- Definitive diagnosis impossible in the field
- Positive pregnancy test results
- Vaginal bleeding. In some cases, the hemorrhage is concealed internally, and vaginal bleeding is minimal.
- Lower abdominal pain
- Uterine tenderness
- Uterine contractions

Treatment
1. Keep the patient at "bed rest" if possible.
2. Volume replacement if indicated
3. Immediate evacuation
4. Vaginal/pelvic and/or rectal examination contraindicated

Bleeding Not Associated With Pregnancy
Abnormal Uterine Bleeding in a Nonpregnant Woman
Abnormal bleeding that occurs in a nonpregnant woman is referred to as dysfunctional uterine bleeding (DUB).
- Includes bleeding between normal menstrual cycles, change in normal pattern of menstrual cycle, increased or decreased amount of menstrual bleeding
- Consider systemic or structural processes:
  - Complications of pregnancy: threatened, incomplete, or spontaneous abortion; ectopic or molar pregnancy
  - Infectious: vaginitis, cervicitis, PID
  - Coagulopathy

- Medications: estrogen, tamoxifen, nonsteroidal antiinflammatories (NSAIDs), warfarin, oral contraceptives, tricyclic antidepressants, and major tranquilizers
- Systemic illness: hepatic, thyroid, and adrenal dysfunction
- Polycystic ovary syndrome and other endocrinopathies
- Anatomic lesions: fibroids, polyps, ovarian cysts, endometriosis, endometrial hyperplasia, neoplasm
- IUD
- Vaginal or pelvic trauma
- Often associated with:
  - Intense exercise
  - Low-calorie diet
  - Rapid weight loss
  - Increased psychologic stress
- Common in perimenopausal women
- Common in adolescence secondary to immaturity of the hypothalamic-pituitary-ovarian axis

Treatment

1. Perform a urine pregnancy test to rule out pregnancy.
2. For women without contraindications to estrogen or progestin, hormonal therapy with either estrogen or progestin or a combined hormonal preparation may be used to stabilize the endometrial lining.
3. One option is to take an OC pill containing 30 to 35 mcg of ethinyl estradiol every 4 to 6 hours until bleeding is under control, and then continue taking one tablet a day until the 21 active pills are finished.
4. In perimenopausal women with irregular bleeding, a low-dose OC containing 20 mcg ethinyl estradiol may be tried.
5. Other options include conjugated estrogen or medroxyprogesterone acetate (Table 31.1).

Table 31.1 Medications for the Medical Kit for Women*†		
INDICATION	**MEDICATION**	**DOSAGE**
Dysmenorrhea	Ibuprofen	200 mg PO 3 tabs q6–8h
Headache/pain/fever	Acetaminophen	325–650 mg PO q6h; max 3 g/24 hr
Nausea and vomiting	Promethazine (tablet or suppository)	12.5–25 mg PO or per rectum q4–6h prn for nausea
	Ondansetron ODT (orally dissolving tablet)	4–8 mg SL (under the tongue) q6–12h prn for nausea

Continued

Table 31.1   Medications for the Medical Kit for Women—cont'd

INDICATION	MEDICATION	DOSAGE
Urinary tract infection	Nitrofurantoin	100 mg PO BID for 5 days
	Ciprofloxacin	250–500 mg PO BID for 3 days (for pyelonephritis, 500 mg BID for 7–14 days)
	Trimethoprim-sulfamethoxazole	160 mg/800 mg PO BID for 3–5 days
Pyelonephritis: Nitrofurantoin does not have appropriate renal penetration and thus should not be used. Other antibiotics listed can be used for an extended length of treatment (7–14 days) when pyelonephritis is clinically suspected.		
Urinary analgesic	Pyridium	200 mg PO TID for 2 days prn for burning
Yeast vaginitis	Miconazole cream or suppository	One applicator qhs for 1–7 days
	Fluconazole	150 mg PO single dose
Bacterial vaginosis	Metronidazole tablets	500 mg PO BID for 7 days
	Tinidazole	1 g PO qd for 5 days
		2 g PO qd for 2 days
	Metronidazole vaginal gel/clindamycin vaginal cream	One applicator qhs for 3–7 days
Menstrual regulation or breakthrough bleeding	Oral contraceptive pills	1 qd
	Conjugated estrogen	2.5 mg PO qd
	Medroxyprogesterone acetate	5–10 mg PO qd (for abnormal uterine bleeding, duration is 5–10 days starting day 16 or 21 of menstrual cycle)
Nutritional supplements	Ferrous sulfate	325 mg PO qd-TID
	Calcium carbonate	1000–1250 mg PO qd
	Multivitamin	1 PO qd

*These recommendations are in addition to the ones recommended for a general medical kit in Chapter 61.

†Suggested medications or equivalent depending on tolerance, allergy history, and patient preferences.

BID, Twice daily; *PO,* by mouth; *prn,* as needed; *q,* every; *qd,* daily; *qhs,* at bedtime; *TID,* three times daily.

6. Bleeding is typically controlled within 12 to 36 hours.
7. Side effects such as nausea, headache, fluid retention, and depression sometimes occur.
8. After completion of the oral contraceptive pills (i.e., after 7 days), expect significant withdrawal bleeding.
9. A nonsteroidal antiinflammatory agent may be used for pain management.
10. If abdominal or pelvic pain develops or if heavy bleeding persists, arrange for immediate evacuation of the patient. It is highly unusual for the bleeding to progress to massive hemorrhage.
11. Note that any patient with DUB in the field should seek definitive follow-up as soon as is practical.

VAGINAL DISCHARGE
Normal vaginal discharge is usually odorless, nonirritating, and white to transparent.

Bacterial Vaginosis
This is a non–sexually transmitted disease, usually with a polymicrobial cause. Pathogens include *Gardnerella vaginalis, Bacteroides non-fragilis, Mobiluncus, Peptococcus,* and *Mycoplasma hominis.*

Signs and Symptoms
- Copious amounts of thin gray or yellow discharge
- Malodorous fishy odor due to release of amines
- Minimal to no vulvar irritation

Treatment
1. Metronidazole 2 g PO single dose. Single-dose oral treatment is practical in the wilderness setting.
2. Metronidazole 500 mg PO q12h for 7 days or 0.75% vaginal gel once daily for 5 days is more effective.
3. Metronidazole 250 mg PO q8h for 7 days in second and third trimester of pregnancy. Avoid in the first trimester of pregnancy.
4. Alternatively, use tinidazole 1 g PO daily for 5 days or 2 g PO daily for 2 days.
5. Clindamycin 300 mg PO q12h for 7 days or 2% vaginal gel once daily for 7 days can also be used as an alternative.

Candida Vulvovaginitis
Candida albicans is the most common pathogen, responsible for 80% to 90% cases.

Signs and Symptoms
- Thick, white vaginal discharge
- Odorless
- Vulvar itching or burning
- Dysuria and dyspareunia

Treatment
1. Fluconazole (Diflucan) 150 mg single oral dose
2. Alternatives: azole derivatives (clotrimazole, miconazole, butoconazole, tioconazole, or terconazole) available as intravaginal creams, tablets, and suppositories; treatment of at least 3 days has been found to have lower immediate recurrence rates (e.g., clotrimazole, 200 mg intravaginally for 3 days or 100 mg for 7 days)
3. Prophylactic suppressive therapy with clotrimazole 500-mg vaginal tablet weekly or fluconazole 100-mg oral tablet weekly

Trichomonas Vaginitis
This is a sexually transmitted disease caused by *Trichomonas vaginalis*.

Signs and Symptoms
- Copious and adherent, frothy discharge that is yellowish gray or green
- Malodorous if mixed with bacterial vaginosis
- Severe pruritus
- Intense vulvovaginal erythema
- "Strawberry cervix": petechial lesions of the cervix
- Dysuria and dyspareunia

Treatment
1. Metronidazole 2 g as a single oral dose or 500 mg q12h for 7 days. Alternatively, tinidazole 2 g as a single oral dose may be used. Avoid in the first trimester of pregnancy. Metronidazole 0.75% vaginal gel is not appropriate for treatment.
2. Take with plenty of water and avoid alcohol to minimize gastrointestinal side effects.
3. Treat partner simultaneously.

GONORRHEA/CHLAMYDIA
This sexually transmitted disease causes a concomitant infection that warrants treatment of both *Neisseria gonorrhoeae* and *Chlamydia trachomatis* simultaneously.

Signs and Symptoms
- Gonorrhea is usually accompanied by urinary frequency, dysuria, and vaginal discharge.
- *Chlamydia* infection is often asymptomatic.
- Definitive diagnosis requires special cultures not available in the wilderness.

Treatment
1. Ceftriaxone 125 mg IM single dose, with azithromycin 1 g single oral dose
2. Alternatively, administer ceftriaxone 125 mg IM single dose, with doxycycline 100 mg PO q12h for 7 days.

PAIN: VULVAR/VAGINAL
Vulvovaginal Abscess and Cellulitis/Bartholin's Abscess

This usually results from polymicrobial infection and duct obstruction of Bartholin's gland. The causative organisms include *Neisseria gonorrhoeae* and *Chlamydia trachomatis*.

Signs and Symptoms
- Severe localized vulvar pain and tenderness just lateral to the posterior vaginal introitus
- Unilateral vulvar erythema and edema
- Tender, fluctuant palpable mass lateral to the posterior introitus

Treatment
1. Perform incision and drainage if adequate equipment is available.
2. Make the incision over the medial aspect of the mucosa, at the point of maximal fluctuance.
3. Insert a hemostat through the mucosal incision, and spread the tips into the deeper tissue. Ensure that there is entrance into a true cavity.
4. Irrigate with a syringe-and-catheter technique.
5. Apply gauze packing to maintain drainage for 24 to 48 hours.
6. With evidence of cellulitis, administer cephalexin (see Appendix H) until resolved.
7. If the availability of water and conditions permit, arrange for a sitz bath daily.
8. Change the dressing once to twice daily until the wound is well healed without drainage.
9. Recurrence is common after simple incision and drainage, warranting follow-up treatment on return.

HERPES SIMPLEX VIRUSES (HSV-1 AND HSV-2)
Signs and Symptoms
- Prodrome of hyperesthesia and localized pain preceding eruption of multiple vesicles
- Vesicles coalesce into ulcerations
- Initial outbreak may be accompanied by fever and malaise

Treatment
1. Acyclovir 200 mg orally five times daily (or 400 mg orally three times daily) for 7 to 10 days in patients with an initial outbreak
2. Acyclovir shortens the ulcerative phase.

PAIN: PELVIC/LOWER ABDOMINAL
Pelvic Inflammatory Disease

PID is a syndrome caused by pathogens ascending from the lower genital tract to the fallopian tubes and adjacent structures.

Risk Factors

- Other sexually transmitted diseases
- Previous episode of PID
- Multiple sexual partners
- IUD placement
- Immunocompromised

Signs and Symptoms

- Fever, vaginal discharge, unilateral or bilateral lower abdominal pain
- Yellowish endocervical discharge on pelvic examination accompanied by cervical motion tenderness

Treatment

1. Differential diagnosis includes appendicitis, septic abortion, pyelonephritis, as well as other entities in this category.
2. Pregnancy test to rule out ectopic pregnancy
3. If available, test for gonorrhea and chlamydia infection.
4. For severe symptoms, treat with doxycycline 100 mg PO q12h for 14 days and metronidazole 500 mg PO q12h for 14 days PLUS one of the following:
   a. Ceftriaxone 250 mg IM single dose OR
   b. Ofloxacin 400 mg PO q12h for 14 days OR
   c. Levofloxacin 500 mg PO once daily for 14 days
5. Evacuate immediately if there are positive pregnancy test results, adnexal mass, peritoneal signs, toxic appearance, presence of an IUD, or fever greater than 102.2° F (39° C).

Ectopic

See Ectopic Pregnancy, earlier.

Mittelschmerz

Pain associated with ovulation

Signs and Symptoms

- Sudden onset of right lower quadrant (RLQ) or left lower quadrant (LLQ) abdominal pain occurring mid-cycle (between days 12 and 16) in a reproductive woman at the time of ovulation
- The presentation is not associated with marked gastrointestinal, genitourinary, or systemic symptoms.
- Symptoms usually last less than 8 hours.
- Not associated with vaginal bleeding or spotting
- Associated with mild referred pain and rebound tenderness
- Pelvic examination to rule out PID (often less adnexal tenderness than with PID)
- Negative urine pregnancy test results and urinalysis
- Consider appendicitis if pain is right-sided.

Treatment

1. Non-narcotic analgesic for pain relief

Ovarian Torsion

This may be complete or incomplete. It may occur during pregnancy, involving the corpus luteum and resulting in adnexal torsion.

Signs and Symptoms

- RLQ or LLQ pain that is sharp, localized, and sudden in onset
- Pain is usually intermittent and may be accompanied by low-grade fever, nausea, and vomiting.
- Unilateral adnexal tenderness, which may or may not be accompanied by a palpable mass
- Consider appendicitis if pain is right-sided.
- Negative or positive pregnancy test results, depending on the cause of the torsion

Treatment

1. Immediate evacuation
2. Surgery once transported to a medical facility

Ovarian Cyst

- Rupture usually occurs after ovarian torsion or trauma
- May involve hemorrhage

History

Onset of symptoms may occur shortly after intercourse or exercise

Signs and Symptoms

- Sudden onset, unilateral sharp pain
- May or may not be accompanied by rebound tenderness
- Enlarging adnexal mass is ominous for hemorrhage
- May spontaneously resolve
- Consider appendicitis if pain is right-sided
- Negative or positive pregnancy test results, depending on type of ovarian cyst

Treatment

1. Immediate evacuation to surgical facility if symptoms persist
2. If hemorrhage is suspected, direct field treatment to volume replacement.
3. Treat for shock, if indicated (see Chapter 13).

EMERGENCY WILDERNESS CHILDBIRTH

General Considerations

- To the extent possible, a clean, comfortable, and quiet site should be prepared for the delivery. Clean and sterile supplies and medications, if available, should be collected and inventoried. Otherwise, clean towels, clothing, bedding, soap, and water should be made readily accessible.
- Any pregnancy with a fundal height at or above the umbilicus should be considered potentially viable.

- If in the early stages of labor with rupture of membranes but no strong, regular contractions, oral fluids and small meals should be encouraged. Only small sips of clear fluids are recommended when strong contractions begin.
- Fetal position should be assessed by palpation of the pregnancy and location of the fetal head and buttock to anticipate a nonvertex delivery.
- Digital examination of the cervix should be avoided in the wilderness unless sterility can be ensured, because of risk for infection.
- By necessity and practicality, delivery in the wilderness should avoid excessive interventions (e.g., repeated cervical examination, artificial rupture of membranes, augmentation of uterine contractions, manual cervical dilation) because they increase fetal and maternal risk.

Vertex Delivery (Fig. 31.1)

1. When the perineum begins to distend, instruct the woman to bear down with each contraction.
2. Support the perineum between the rectum and introitus, using your index finger and thumb.
3. Control delivery of the head, keeping it in flexion until it clears the symphysis pubis.
4. Once the head is cleared, ask the woman to stop pushing.
5. Exert steady inward and upward pressure at the perineum, against the chin with countertraction on the occiput. Allow for controlled extension of the head.
6. Once delivered, the head will automatically rotate laterally to align itself with the shoulders.
7. Suction the nose and mouth, using gauze or a cloth if a suction bulb is not available.
8. Palpate the fetal neck for a nuchal cord. If present, undo the nuchal cord by slipping it over the fetal head. The cord may also be clamped twice and cut if a nuchal cord cannot be reduced.
9. Instruct the woman to resume bearing down steadily, and cup both sides of the fetal head.
10. Apply gentle downward pressure on the head, until the anterior shoulder is visible.
11. Apply upward traction, until the posterior shoulder is delivered. The rest of the body will quickly follow.
12. Hold the baby below the perineum. Towel dry, and suction the oropharynx.
13. Clamp or tie the umbilical cord twice, and sever between the clamps or ties.
14. After a wilderness delivery, administer a broad-spectrum antibiotic to the mother for 24 to 48 hours (see Appendix H).
15. If the mother is Rh negative and the baby's blood type is Rh positive or unknown, administer Rh immune globulin, 300 mcg IM, to the mother.

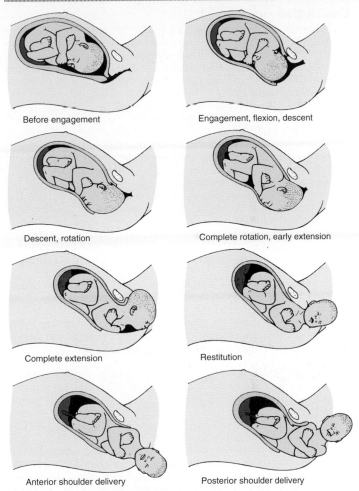

Before engagement

Engagement, flexion, descent

Descent, rotation

Complete rotation, early extension

Complete extension

Restitution

Anterior shoulder delivery

Posterior shoulder delivery

FIGURE 31.1   Cardinal Movements in Labor. The *cardinal movements* refer to changes in the position of the fetal head during its passage through the birth canal. Because of the asymmetry of the shape of both the fetal head and the maternal bony pelvis, such rotations are required for the fetus to successfully negotiate the birth canal. (From Kilpatrick S, Garrison E. Normal labor and delivery. In Gabbe SG, Niebyl JR, Simpson JL, et al. *Obstetrics: normal and problem pregnancies,* ed 7, Philadelphia, 2017, Elsevier.)

Breech Delivery (Fig. 31.2)

Because most wilderness deliveries will be "unexpected" and more likely to be premature, the baby also will more likely be in a breech lie. Under the best of circumstances, delivery of a breech carries a threefold to fourfold greater risk than a vertex presentation for morbidity resulting from prematurity, congenital abnormalities, and trauma at delivery.

1. Breech babies come in many forms: frank breech (hips flexed, knees extended, buttocks presenting); complete breech (both hips and both knees flexed, buttocks and feet presenting); incomplete breech (one hip flexed, one hip partially extended, both knees flexed, buttocks and feet presenting); and footling breech (hips and knees extended, feet presenting).
2. The approach in a wilderness setting demands patience. No effort should be made to deliver a breech baby until the presenting part is visible at the introitus and the cervix is completely dilated.
3. Membranes should not be artificially ruptured in breech presentations.
4. When the cervix is completely dilated, the woman is instructed to push.
5. Regardless of the type of breech presentation, the safest course is to allow the body to be extruded to at least the level of the umbilicus by maternal efforts alone.
6. A baby in a frank or complete breech lie should have the posterior leg delivered by gently grasping the thigh and flexing the leg at the knee as it is rotated medially and toward the introitus.
7. The baby should then be rotated to the sacrum anterior position, then another 45 degrees in the same direction to facilitate delivery of the other leg using the technique described for the first leg.
8. The legs and buttocks can be wrapped in a clean towel to provide a firmer grip and decrease trauma to the baby.
9. The delivery from this point is the same as for footling breech presentation. The upper legs should be grasped on each side with the index fingers crossing the infant's pelvic girdle and both thumbs positioned just above the crease of the buttocks.
10. Using gentle side-to-side rotational motion over an arc of 90 degrees outward and downward, traction should be applied while the mother pushes, until the upper portion of a scapula is visible at the introitus.
11. With the baby's body rotated 45 degrees toward the opposite side, the arm is delivered by flexion and medial rotation across the chest.
12. The baby is rotated to the opposite side in the same position, and the other arm is then delivered.
13. If assistants are present, the woman should be helped into the McRoberts position, with hyperflexion at the hips to maximize the space between the symphysis and the sacrum.

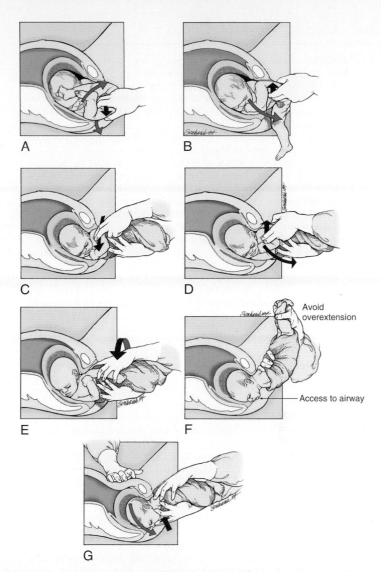

FIGURE 31.2 Management of vaginal breech delivery. After spontaneous expulsion to the umbilicus, external rotation of each thigh **(A)** combined with opposite rotation of the fetal pelvis results in flexion of the knee and delivery of each leg **(B)**. When the scapulae appear under the symphysis, the operator reaches over the left shoulder, sweeps the arm across the chest **(C)**, and delivers the arm **(D)**. **E**, Gentle rotation of the shoulder girdle facilitates delivery of the right arm. Following delivery of the arms, the fetus is wrapped in a towel for control and is slightly elevated. The fetal face and airway may be visible over the perineum. **F**, Excessive elevation of the trunk is avoided. **G**, Cephalic flexion is maintained by pressure *(arrow)* on the fetal maxilla, *not* the mandible. Often, delivery of the head is easily accomplished with continued expulsive forces from above and gentle downward traction. (From Lanni SM, Gherman R, Gonik B. Malpresentations. In Gabbe SG, Niebyl JR, Simpson JL, et al. *Obstetrics: normal and problem pregnancies*, ed 7, Philadelphia, 2017, Elsevier.)

14. Maintaining the baby in the same plane as the vagina, the birth attendant reaches palm up between the baby's legs and into the vagina, supporting the baby's entire body on the forearm while placing the second and fourth fingers over the infant's maxillae and placing the middle finger into the mouth or on the chin.
15. The other hand is positioned over the infant's upper back so that the fingers are overlying each shoulder.
16. If there is sufficient room, the middle fingers can be applied to the fetal occiput. Then with the woman pushing, the baby's head is flexed downward, completing the delivery.
17. Firm suprapubic pressure can help to maintain the head in flexion. During this final stage the baby's body should not be elevated more than 45 degrees above the plane of the vagina to avoid hyperextension of the head.
18. If the fetal head cannot be delivered because the cervix is incompletely dilated, the cervix can be cut at the 2 and 10 o'clock positions (Dührssen incisions) to provide sufficient room to complete the delivery.
19. Once delivered, if the baby breathes and cries spontaneously or with minimal stimulation, cutting the umbilical cord can be delayed while the baby is dried. This allows some of the blood retained in the placenta from umbilical vein compression (common with breech deliveries) to return to the baby.
20. If the baby is clearly depressed, the umbilical cord should be immediately clamped and cut and neonatal resuscitation begun.

Delivery of the Placenta
1. Place the heel of your hand just above the symphysis to hold the uterus in place.
2. Apply fundal pressure with the tips of the same hand.
3. Simultaneously apply steady downward traction on the umbilical cord with the other hand. Do not use excessive traction.
4. A gush of blood and lengthening of the cord signify placental separation.
5. Once separated, rotate the placenta several times as it passes through the introitus.
6. Massage the uterus to promote contraction.
7. Assess for lacerations to the perineum and repair accordingly with polyglactin 910 (Vicryl) sutures.
8. Apply pressure to control small amounts of bleeding.
9. Place ice packs to the perineum for the first 12 to 24 hours.

Breastfeeding
1. During the first 24 hours after delivery, feed every 2 to 3 hours, 5 minutes on each breast, alternating the first breast.
2. As milk production is established over the next 2 to 3 days, advance the feeding schedule to 10- to 15-minute periods on each breast 8 to 12 times per day.

3. Have the mother drink at least 2 L of fluids each day, increase caloric intake, and consume foods rich in calcium.
4. For engorgement, apply cool compresses after nursing, wear a nursing bra, and use acetaminophen for pain.
5. For mastitis, administer a course of antibiotics (e.g., dicloxacillin 500 mg or cephalexin 500 mg four times daily) for 10 to 14 days. In an appropriate circumstance, suspect methicillin-resistant *Staphylococcus aureus*.

Preeclampsia

The diagnosis is based in the field based on hypertension (140 mm Hg systolic or 90 mm Hg diastolic measured on two separate occasions 6 or more hours apart; severe preeclampsia is defined by the values of 160 mm Hg systolic or 110 mm Hg diastolic), decreased urine output, persistent epigastric pain, shortness of breath, and seizures (eclampsia). With any sign or suggestion of preeclampsia, including peripheral edema, visual disturbances, severe headache, irritability, epigastric or right upper quadrant pain, or persistent nausea and vomiting, it is best to seek prompt evacuation.

EMERGENCY CONTRACEPTION

Emergency contraception is defined as a method of contraception that women can use after unprotected intercourse or contraceptive failure to prevent pregnancy.

1. Two doses of levonorgestrel (Plan B) taken at one time within 120 hours of unprotected intercourse
2. Two doses of estrogen-progestin combination oral contraceptive pills taken 12 hours apart within 72 hours of unprotected intercourse:
   a. Levonorgestrel (Plan B) 1 tablet
   b. Ovrette 20 tablets
   c. Alesse 5 pink tablets
   d. Lo/Ovral 4 white tablets
   e. Nordette 4 orange tablets
   f. Levlen 4 orange tablets
   g. Levora 4 white tablets
   h. Seasonale 4 pink tablets
   i. Tri-Levlen 4 yellow tablets
   j. Triphasil 4 yellow tablets
   k. Trivora 4 pink tablets

IMMUNIZATIONS DURING PREGNANCY

See Table 31.2.

MEDICATIONS DURING PREGNANCY

The Food and Drug Administration has developed a set of guidelines to categorize drugs with regard to developmental toxicity and adverse fetal outcome (Box 31.1). Medication use during pregnancy and lactation is guided by these recommendations (Table 31.3).

Table 31.2 CDC Recommendations for Vaccination During Pregnancy

Vaccination of Pregnant Women Is Recommended

Hepatitis B	Recombinant or plasma-derived	Recommended for women at risk of infection.
Influenza	Inactivated whole virus or subunit	All women who are pregnant in the second and third trimesters during the flu season (Northern Hemisphere: October to May; Southern Hemisphere: April to September; tropics: year round) and women at high risk for pulmonary complications regardless of trimester.
Diphtheria-tetanus	Toxoid	If indicated, such as lack of primary series, or no booster within past 10 years.
Diphtheria-tetanus-pertussis (TDaP)	Toxoid-acellular	TDaP should be given during each pregnancy, preferably during the third trimester at 27–36 weeks to maximize maternal antibody response and passive antibody transfer to infant. However, it may be given at any time.
Hepatitis A	Inactivated virus	Data on safety in pregnancy are not available. Because hepatitis A vaccine is produced from inactivated hepatitis A virus, theoretical risk of vaccination should be weighed against risk of disease. Consider immune globulin rather than vaccine.

Pregnancy Is a Precaution, and Under Normal Circumstances Vaccination Should Be Deferred; Vaccine Should Only Be Given When Benefits Outweigh Risks

Japanese encephalitis	Inactivated virus	Data on safety in pregnancy are not available. Pregnant women who must travel to an area where risk is high should be vaccinated when theoretical risks are outweighed by risk of disease.

Meningococcal meningitis	Polysaccharide	Meningococcal conjugate vaccine (MCV4) is preferred for adults. However, there are no data on safety and immunogenicity in pregnant women. Polyvalent meningococcal meningitis vaccine (MPSV4) can be administered during pregnancy if the woman is entering an epidemic area. Indications for prophylaxis are not altered by pregnancy; vaccine recommended in unusual outbreak situations.
Pneumococcal	Polysaccharide	Safety of pneumococcal (PPV23) vaccine during the first trimester has not been evaluated, although no adverse events have been reported after inadvertent vaccination during pregnancy. Women with chronic diseases, smokers, and immunosuppressed women should consider vaccination.
Polio, inactivated	Inactivated virus	Indicated for susceptible pregnant women traveling in endemic areas or in other high-risk situations.
Rabies	Inactivated virus	Indications for postexposure prophylaxis not altered by pregnancy. If risk of exposure to rabies is substantial, preexposure prophylaxis may also be indicated.
Typhoid (ViCPS)	Polysaccharide	If indicated for travel to endemic areas.
Typhoid (Ty21a)	Live bacterial	Data on safety in pregnancy are not available; theoretical risk because live-attenuated.
Yellow fever	Live attenuated virus	Use caution. Safety of yellow fever vaccination in pregnancy has not been studied in a large prospective trial. Pregnant women who must travel to areas where risk of yellow fever infection is high should be vaccinated and their infants should be monitored after birth for evidence of congenital infect on and other possible adverse effects resulting from yellow fever vaccination. Pregnancy may interfere with the immune response to yellow fever vaccine. Consider serologic testing to document a protective immune response to the vaccine. Avoid in breastfeeding mothers unless travel to high endemic region is unavoidable.*

Continued

Table 31.2 CDC Recommendations for Vaccination During Pregnancy—cont'd

Pregnancy Is a Contraindication to Vaccination; Vaccine Should Not Be Administered to Pregnant Women

Tuberculosis (BCG)	Attenuated mycobacterial	Contraindicated because of theoretical risk of disseminated disease. Skin testing for tuberculosis exposure before and after travel is preferable when risk of possible exposure is high.
Measles-mumps-rubella	Live attenuated virus	Contraindicated. Vaccination of susceptible women should be part of postpartum care. Unvaccinated women should delay travel to countries where measles is endemic until after delivery. Unvaccinated pregnant women with a documented exposure to measles should receive immunoglobulin within 6 days to prevent illness.
Human papillomavirus	Recombinant quadrivalent	Contraindicated. Vaccine has not been causally associated with adverse outcomes of pregnancy. However, additional information is needed for further recommendations.
Varicella	Live attenuated virus	Contraindicated. Vaccination of susceptible women should be considered postpartum. Unvaccinated pregnant women should consider postponing travel until after delivery, when the vaccine can be given safely.

Vaccine/Immunobiologic

		Use
Immune globulins, pooled or hyperimmune	Immune globulin or specific globulin preparations	If indicated for preexposure or postexposure use. No known risk to fetus.

Adapted from Vaccines and immunizations: guidelines for vaccinating pregnant women; and Travel and other vaccines, CDC health information for international travel: cdc.gov/vaccines/pubs/preg-guide.htm.

*See Brunette GW, editor: *CDC health information for international travel 2016*, New York, 2016, Oxford University Press.

Table 31.3 Medication Use During Pregnancy and Lactation

MEDICATION	CATEGORY	ISSUES DURING PREGNANCY	ISSUES DURING LACTATION
Analgesics/Antipyretics			
		Try nonpharmaceutical methods, such as rest, ice, heat, massage, first to treat pain	
Acetaminophen	B	Safe in low doses short term	Compatible
Aspirin	C/D	Avoid first and last trimester. Has been associated with premature closure of ductus arteriosus and excessive bleeding. Low-dose aspirin (60–80 mg) may be used for preeclampsia.	Use caution
Nonsteroidal antiinflammatory (ibuprofen, naproxen)	B/D	Should not be used in first and last trimesters owing to effects on premature closure of ductus arteriosus and effects on clotting. Not teratogenic.	Compatible
Codeine	C/D	Use cautiously as may cause respiratory depression and withdrawal symptoms in fetus if used near term.	Compatible
Hydrocodone	C/D	Use cautiously as may cause respiratory depression in infant if used near term.	Use caution
Antibiotics for URI, UTI, GI, Skin, Other			
		Use antibiotics only if strong evidence of bacterial infection.	
Amoxicillin, amoxicillin + clavulanic acid (Augmentin), amoxicillin + sulbactam (Unasyn)	B	Safe. Use for treatment of otitis media, sinusitis, streptococcal pharyngitis.	Safe

Continued

Table 31.3 Medication Use During Pregnancy and Lactation—cont'd

MEDICATION	CATEGORY	ISSUES DURING PREGNANCY	ISSUES DURING LACTATION
Azithromycin	B	Safe. Use for bronchitis, pneumonia, gastroenteritis (Campylobacter, Shigella, Salmonella, Escherichia coli).	Use caution
Cephalosporins	B	Safe. Use for otitis, streptococcal infections, sinusitis, pharyngitis.	Use caution Can be used to treat mastitis
Clindamycin PO or Clindamycin vaginal cream	B	Safe. Use for bacterial vaginosis orally or locally in second or third trimester; avoid in first trimester.	Compatible
Ciprofloxacin, other quinolones	C	Controversial. Sometimes used short term in severe infections and/or long term in life-threatening infections (e.g., anthrax). May be used if potential benefit justifies risk to fetus.	Compatible
Dicloxacillin	B	Safe. Use for skin infections.	Safe Used to treat mastitis
Doxycycline, tetracycline	D	May cause permanent discoloration of the teeth during tooth development, including the last half of pregnancy, infancy, and childhood until 8 years of age.	Avoid
Erythromycin (base or state)	B	Safe. Use for bacterial causes of URI.	Compatible
Nitrofurantoin	B	Drug of choice for UTI in pregnancy	Use caution
Penicillin	B	Safe.	Safe

Sulfonamides	B/D	Safe. However, not recommended in third trimester owing to risk for hyperbilirubinemia and kernicterus.	Avoid
Trimethoprim	C	Avoid	Use caution
Gastrointestinal			
Antidiarrheal		*Replacing fluid losses is key.*	
Atropine sulfate diphenoxylate hydrochloride (Lomotil)	C	Use only if severe symptoms	Avoid
Loperamide (Imodium)	C	Use only if severe symptoms	Compatible
Nausea/Vomiting, Esophageal Reflux		*Encourage supportive measures first rather than medications: crackers upon arising, frequent small meals, protein meal at bedtime.*	
Antacids	B	May use sparingly for symptoms as needed	Safe
Bismuth subsalicylate (Pepto Bismol)	C/D	Avoid because it contains bismuth and salicylate	Use caution
Cimetidine, ranitidine, omeprazole	B/C	Safe. Study during the first trimester found it is not associated with an increase in congenital malformations.	Use caution
Ondansetron (Zofran)	B	Use for hyperemesis gravidarum	Use caution
Metoclopramide (Reglan)	B	Safe in small doses	Use caution
Dimenhydrinate (Dramamine)	B	Safe for severe nausea	Use caution

Continued

Table 31.3 Medication Use During Pregnancy and Lactation—cont'd

MEDICATION	CATEGORY	ISSUES DURING PREGNANCY	ISSUES DURING LACTATION
Prochlorperazine (Compazine)	C	Often clinically used for nausea and vomiting of pregnancy despite class rating.	Avoid
Promethazine (Phenergan)	C	Often clinically used for nausea and vomiting of pregnancy despite class rating.	Avoid
Acupressure (Sea-Bands)		Safe	Safe
Emetrol (fluid replacement)	B	Safe. Oral solution.	Safe
Ginger	C	Safe	Use caution
Meclizine	B	Safe for treatment of severe nausea and vomiting.	Compatible
Pyridoxine (B₆)	A	Safe. Used for nausea.	Compatible
Constipation		*Increase fiber and fluid in diet first.*	
Bisacodyl	C	Safe to use occasionally	Use caution
Milk of magnesia	B	Safe in small amounts	Safe
Psyllium hydrophilic mucilloid	C	Safe	Compatible
Hemorrhoids		Increase fiber and fluid in diet	
Anusol HC suppositories	C	Safe	Use caution

Antihistamines and Related Respiratory

URI, Congestion, Cough

Symptomatic treatment: steam, rest, fluids.

Chlorpheniramine	B	Use cautiously for severe symptoms.	Use caution
Cetirizine (Zyrtec)	B	Safe. Nonsedating but use cautiously.	Use caution
Diphenhydramine (Benadryl)	B	Safe. Use cautiously.	Use caution
Loratadine (Claritin)	B	Safe. Nonsedating but use cautiously.	Compatible
Dextromethorphan	C	Probably safe. Use in small amounts.	Compatible
Guaifenesin	C	Probably safe. Use only if needed.	Use caution
Pseudoephedrine (Sudafed)	C	Avoid in first trimester. Use cautiously.	Compatible
Saline nasal spray	A	Safe	Safe

Topical Nasal Decongestants

Oxymetazoline (Afrin)	C	Safe. Do not use for more than 3 days.	Safe

Asthma, Allergy

Inhaled bronchodilators (Albuterol)	C	Safe for use of wheezing during pregnancy	Unknown
Inhaled steroids (Fluticasone)	C	Use if indicated	Safe
Nasal steroids (Fluticasone)	C	Use if indicated	Safe

Continued

Table 31.3   Medication Use During Pregnancy and Lactation—cont'd

MEDICATION	CATEGORY	ISSUES DURING PREGNANCY	ISSUES DURING LACTATION
Antimalarials			
Artemether-lumefantrine (Coartem)	C	Used in second and third trimesters for treatment of severe malaria	Use caution. Excreted in breast milk. Infant still needs own chemoprophylaxis.
Mefloquine (Lariam)	C	Avoid during first trimester unless unavoidable travel to high-risk area. Safe in second and third trimesters for high-risk travel.	Use caution. Excreted in breast milk. Infant still needs chemoprophylaxis.
Chloroquine	C	Avoid in first trimester unless traveling to high-risk area	Use caution. Excreted in milk in small amounts. Infant still needs chemoprophylaxis.
Atovaquone, proguanil (Malarone)	C	Avoid in first trimester	Use caution. Safe if infant is >1 kg (24 lb) or if benefit for mother outweighs possible risk.
Doxycycline	D	Contraindicated for malaria prophylaxis. May be considered for treatment of severe infections.	Avoid
Primaquine	C	Do not administer during pregnancy because of the possibility the fetus may be G6PD deficient. If a causal cure with primaquine is indicated, continue to suppress with chloroquine (or other chemoprophylaxis) until delivery.	Use caution
Proguanil	C	Not associated with teratogenicity. Not effective as a single agent.	Use caution

OCULAR PROCEDURES
Examination of Vision
Any patient with ocular complaints should have his or her vision evaluated in each eye separately.
1. Have the patient cover one eye and read any fine print available. (Persons older than age 40 may require reading glasses or use a pinhole occluder to correct for refractive difficulties if glasses are not available.) A Snellen chart may be improvised by asking the patient to read letters or numbers from a card held 14 inches away.
2. If the patient is unable to read print, try to determine the level of visual acuity (count fingers, hand motion, light perception, no light perception).

Examination of Pupils
Examine the pupils for size, equality, shape, and reaction to light.
- Approximately 10% of the population has pupils of unequal size (anisocoria).
- If light is shined in either eye, both pupils should constrict equally (consensual response). If one pupil is seen to be dilated compared with the other when a penlight is rapidly alternated from one eye to the other, this may indicate retinal or optic nerve dysfunction.
- An irregularly shaped, tapered "teardrop pupil" suggests ocular penetration.
- When evaluating a red or painful eye, a significant difference in size between pupils may provide a clue to diagnose iritis (constricted) or glaucoma (dilated).
- Although somewhat rare, mid-dilation is noted in pupillary block/angle-closure glaucoma. Look for a mid-dilated pupil (5 to 7 mm), with pain and severe decreased vision in one eye. These patients tend to be farsighted and older than 50 years.
- A widely dilated, nonreactive pupil is suggestive of contact with medicine (e.g., scopolamine patch) or a cerebral aneurysm. If increased intracranial pressure is causing anisocoria, the patient will be obtunded or comatose.

Estimation of Anterior Chamber Depth (i.e., Rule Out Narrow Angle, a Contributing Factor to Glaucoma)
Shine a small flashlight obliquely from the temporal side of the eye (Fig. 32.1A).

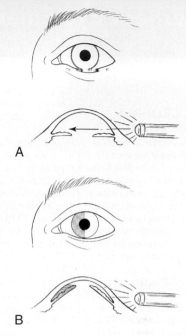

FIGURE 32.1   Estimating depth of anterior chamber.

- If the nasal iris is well illuminated, it suggests a normal anterior chamber.
- If the nasal iris lies in shadow, it suggests a shallow anterior chamber (narrow angle) (see Fig. 32.1B).
- This may be a difficult test to interpret. It is helpful to compare one eye with the other, or the patient's eye with that of another person.
- A history of being farsighted should raise suspicion; narrow angles accompany hyperopia and small anterior chambers (usually these individuals wear thick glasses that magnify their eyes on direct inspection).

Extraocular Muscle Testing
- Have the patient follow a flashlight or finger through the extremes of gaze in six directions. Ask if the patient sees one image or two images.
- Double vision in any field of gaze may represent extraocular muscle palsy.
- Fourth cranial nerve palsies tend to occur after head trauma and are generally benign. The patient will have vertical diplopia.

- Patients with sixth cranial nerve palsy will have horizontal diplopia.
- When both eyes have lateral gaze limitation, this is a sign of increased intracranial pressure.
- With a third cranial nerve palsy, the eye will be turned down and out. The patient may not complain of diplopia because of ptosis. If the same pupil is dilated, this is assumed to be from a posterior communicating aneurysm until proven otherwise. Evacuate the patient immediately.
- Grossly limited extraocular motion (EOM) with proptosis suggests acute orbital inflammation or retrobulbar hemorrhage. Retrobulbar hemorrhage is usually accompanied by periorbital ecchymosis and subconjunctival hemorrhage following trauma.
- If the eye appears sunken within the orbit and the patient exhibits limited upward gaze, suspect a blow-out fracture of the orbital floor. Fracture of the orbital floor with entrapment of the inferior rectus muscle causes vertical diplopia with limited gaze both up and down. Fracture of the medial orbital wall with entrapment of the medial rectus muscle causes horizontal diplopia and limited gaze both medially and laterally.

Visual Field Testing
1. Ask the patient to cover one eye completely and look directly at your opposing eye from a distance of about 1 m (3.3 ft).
2. Place your fingers outside the patient's field of peripheral vision and slowly move them centrally.
3. Ask the patient to inform you when he or she can see your fingers. The patient's fields are generally normal when they correspond with those of the examiner.

Upper Eyelid Eversion
1. Place the end of a cotton-tipped applicator horizontally above the tarsal plate while you pull the eyelashes and the lid margin down and out (Fig. 32.2A).
2. Flip the lid up to evert it. Hold the everted lid in position by pressing the lashes against the superior orbital rim (see Fig. 32.2B).

Fluorescein Examination
1. Use fluorescein staining to evaluate any red or painful eye.
2. Wet the fluorescein strip with a drop of saline (artificial tears) or a drop of topical anesthetic.
3. When examining an eye with a possible infection, always use a separate fluorescein strip for each eye to avoid cross contamination.
4. Next, apply the wetted strip to the inside of the patient's lower lid.
5. Ask the patient to blink, which will spread the fluorescein over the surface of the eye. Areas of corneal disruption stain brilliant green.

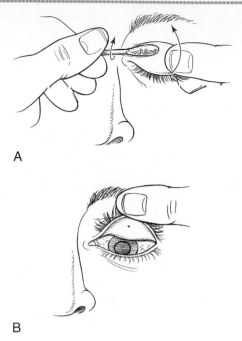

FIGURE 32.2 Upper eyelid eversion.

6. Use a small blue filter placed over a penlight, which works best in a dark setting.
7. Outside during the day, simple sunlight often causes any significant corneal lesion to fluoresce.
8. Fluorescein permanently stains soft contact lenses, so instruct patients to remove these lenses before the fluorescein examination and leave them out for several hours after the examination.
9. If there is concern regarding a penetrating injury, fluorescein can be used to paint the area of concern. Observe if fluorescein dilutes by pinpoint leak of aqueous fluid (a positive Seidel test indicates an open globe).

Eye Patching
- A pressure patch to hold the eyelid closed and thereby facilitate healing of a corneal defect may also provide some pain relief. Protect the injured eye from bright light. Using a patch for healing is not always necessary, but may be a personal preference.
- A (light) pressure patch is indicated in many common eye emergencies and whenever the surface of the cornea has been

injured, especially with a large corneal defect. The patient will be more comfortable; however, pressure patching probably does not speed up corneal healing.

- Small corneal defects usually heal rapidly without patching.
- Do not use patching when the corneal epithelial defect is secondary to an infection (e.g., conjunctivitis, corneal ulcer) or if injury was caused by or contaminated with organic matter.
- Use caution if the patient is a contact lens wearer, especially extended-wear lenses, which contribute to increased risk for infection.
- Never apply a pressure patch to an eye after a penetrating injury. After eye penetration or trauma, tape a protective cup (e.g., padded drinking cup) over the eye or fashion a cloth "donut" from a cravat or other cloth to avoid placing pressure on the eye or inflicting any further trauma during evacuation.
- "Plano" (noncorrective) soft contact lenses are often used by ophthalmologists for patching corneal lesions. These might be considered if available.

Equipment

Two gauze eye patches (gauze 2 × 2 inch or commercial patches)
1-inch (2.5-cm) tape
Antibiotic ointment
Mydriatic-cycloplegic eye drops

Procedure

1. Before patching a corneal abrasion, apply both a drop or two of a mydriatic-cycloplegic solution and a thin ribbon of antibiotic-antiseptic ointment.
   a. The cycloplegic relaxes ciliary muscle spasm that accompanies corneal abrasion.
   b. Check the patient for a narrow anterior chamber before instilling the drops (see Estimation of Anterior Chamber Depth, earlier), although this is usually not realistic in the field.
2. Use antibiotic ointment for prophylaxis, although corneal abrasions rarely become infected.
3. For the patch to be effective, you must put it on just tightly enough to keep the eyelid shut. Do not put undue pressure on the eye.
4. Use two patches.
   a. Double the first patch by folding vertically, and place it over the closed lid. If a second patch is not available, this patch can be held in place with a single piece of tape.
   b. Put the unfolded second patch over the first folded patch.
5. Prepare the skin near the eye with tincture of benzoin (if available) to help the tape adhere. Be careful to keep benzoin out of the eye.
6. Place the tape diagonally from the center of the forehead to the cheekbone. Make sure the tape completely covers the patch

to minimize slippage but does not extend onto the angle of the mandible.

7. Remove the patch every 24 hours so that the eye can be reexamined and the patch changed. Using a clean patch every 24 hours helps to prevent infection.

8. Instruct the patient with an eye patch to rest the uninjured eye. Discourage reading because rapid involuntary movement of the patched eye occurs.

Locating a Displaced Contact Lens

Soft contact lens wearers may occasionally have one of their lenses become displaced, causing blurred vision and a foreign body sensation. Once the lens is displaced, it may be difficult to locate.

1. The conjunctival fornix of the lower lid is easily examined by distracting the lens from the globe with gentle downward finger pressure applied to the lower lid.

2. If the contact lens has been displaced into the superior conjunctival fornix (usually the case), it may be more difficult to locate.

3. If visual inspection with a penlight and a handheld magnifying lens is not successful in finding the lens, gentle digital massage over the closed upper lid directed toward the medial canthus often results in the contact lens emerging at that location. Several minutes of massage may be required. A few drops of artificial tears, and topical anesthetic if available, often facilitate the process.

4. If this maneuver is unproductive, the eye may be anesthetized with a drop of topical anesthetic, the upper lid distracted from the globe with upward finger pressure, and the fornix swept with a moistened cotton-tipped applicator.

5. Alternatively, using a paper clip opened to a right angle to create a simple retractor, evert the eyelid after proparacaine (or other topical anesthetic) instillation, and then lift the edge of the tarsus with the rounded edge of the paper clip.

6. If the lens is not the last and can be discarded, it can often be easily located with fluorescein. Commonly, the missing contact lens will not be there, even in the presence of a persistent foreign body sensation.

DISORDERS

Sudden Loss of Vision in White, "Quiet" Eye

Acute and significant visual loss is an emergency. The common causes of acute visual loss are listed in Box 32.1.

Each of these conditions requires immediate evacuation and definitive follow-up. However, giant cell or temporal arteritis (a type of arteritic anterior ischemic optic neuropathy) requires immediate field treatment to avoid bilateral loss of vision.

Giant Cell (Temporal) Arteritis
Signs and Symptoms
- Rapid, painless vision loss
- Rare in persons younger than age 50

> **BOX 32.1** Differential Diagnosis of Acute Loss of Vision in White, "Quiet" Eye
>
> Retinal detachment
> Central retinal artery occlusion (giant cell/temporal arteritis)
> Anterior ischemic optic neuropathy
> Optic neuritis
> Central retinal vein occlusion
> Arteritic anterior ischemic optic neuropathy
> Vitreous hemorrhage
> High-altitude retinal hemorrhage

- Associated with temporal headache
- Jaw claudication
- Low-grade fever
- History of associated weight loss
- History of polymyalgia rheumatica
- Transient visual obscurations
- Usually affects one eye first, then the second eye within hours to days

Treatment
1. Because this disease can cause significant visual loss in the absence of effective treatment, initiate care immediately with a high-dose corticosteroid (e.g., prednisone, 80 to 100 mg/day PO).
2. Evacuate the patient so that a high-dose steroid can be administered intravenously.
3. When treated, symptoms often improve within 1 to 3 days. However, steroids are typically continued for many weeks.

Red Eye (Fig. 32.3 and Box 32.2)
Acute Angle-Closure Glaucoma
Acute angle-closure glaucoma results from a sudden rise in intraocular pressure (IOP). Patients at risk include elders and farsighted individuals.

Signs and Symptoms
- Acute onset of severe pain and blurred vision
- A red eye, often with the pupil slightly dilated and a "steamy" (edematous) cornea
- The affected eye often feels appreciably harder than the unaffected eye (palpate through the lid gently and with extreme caution).
- Symptoms beginning in low light
- Possible nausea, vomiting, and generalized head pain
- Person may complain of colored halos around lights
- May be intermittent

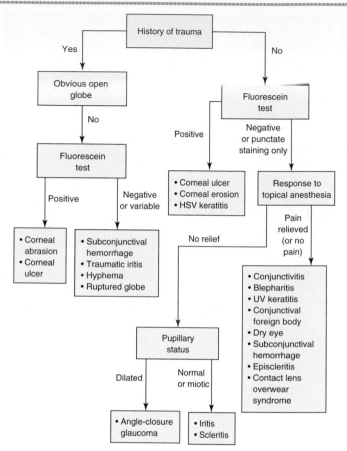

FIGURE 32.3 Algorithm showing wilderness diagnostic procedure for the acute red eye. *HSV,* Herpes simplex virus; *UV,* ultraviolet.

Treatment

1. Instill timolol 0.5% (Timoptic), 1 drop bid (caution if patient has asthma, chronic obstructive pulmonary disease, or history of heart block).
2. Instill pilocarpine 2% (Pilocar), 1 drop q15min × 4, then qid.
3. Administer acetazolamide 250 mg PO qid.
4. Arrange for immediate evacuation for emergency ocular surgery (laser iridotomy).
5. The other eye is also at risk; it is prudent to treat this eye with pilocarpine bid, prophylactically.

BOX 32.2 Differential Diagnosis of the Acute Red Eye

Obvious open globe
Corneal abrasion
Corneal ulcer
Subconjunctival hemorrhage
Traumatic iritis
Hyphema
Occult open globe
Herpes simplex virus keratitis
Corneal erosion
Acute angle-closure glaucoma
Iritis
Scleritis
Conjunctivitis
Blepharitis
Ultraviolet keratitis
Episcleritis
Conjunctival foreign body
Dry eye
Contact lens overwear syndrome

Corneal Abrasion
Signs and Symptoms
- Intense pain localized to the cornea after an injurious event
- Conjunctival erythema
- Pain is relieved with a drop of topical anesthetic (topical anesthetic not to be used repeatedly because it increases risk for infection and prolongs wound healing).
  - Identification of a corneal lesion sometimes made using visible light but often enhanced by fluorescein staining (see section "Ocular Procedures," earlier)

Treatment
1. Apply a topical antibiotic solution. A solution is preferable to an ointment when the patient is expected to remain active. If the patient is sleeping or if the eye is patched, an ointment has slightly greater duration of effect.
2. If the abrasion is extensive (>30% of the corneal surface) or painful, add a mydriatic-cycloplegic agent to the regimen.
3. Instruct the patient to avoid activity requiring frequent active eye movement.
4. Determine whether to patch (see Ocular Procedures, earlier).
5. Be aware that many small (<3 mm) abrasions resolve as quickly with or without corneal (eye) patching.
6. Base the decision to patch the eye on abrasion size and comfort (many patients with severe corneal defects feel more comfortable after patching).

7. NOTE: Do not patch if patient is a contact lens wearer or the corneal epithelial defect was caused by or contaminated with organic matter.
8. If the eye is not patched, apply cool compresses over the eye after the topical antibiotic to soothe the area.
9. Alternatively, a soft contact patch lens (e.g., plano or plus 0.5 to plus one correction) instilled with topical ketorolac (Acular) 0.5% ophthalmic solution is very comfortable, and antibiotic drops can be delivered through the lens.
10. Administer an oral analgesic or antiinflammatory drug to provide symptomatic relief.
11. A corneal abrasion typically resolves within 24 to 48 hours, although a large abrasion may take longer. Evacuate promptly any patient with a corneal lesion that does not resolve within 4 days or that is progressing (enlarging or becoming more painful).

Corneal Erosion
This occurs when a small portion of corneal epithelium is torn as the eyelid opens, usually in a person with a prior history of corneal abrasion (can occur months to years after initial injury). The cause of recurrent corneal erosion is failure of complete bonding of the healing corneal epithelium to its basement membrane.

Signs and Symptoms
- Acute ocular pain, photophobia, and tearing, often occurring at the time of awakening, when the eyes are first opened
- Typically, bright fluorescein staining of the erosion, but with the erosion sometimes healing before the examination, revealing a normal cornea; erosions often recur

Treatment
1. Apply antibiotic ointment to the eye (above lower eyelid) before patching.
2. Apply the cycloplegic drug one time only.
3. Patch the affected eye for 12 hours, then remove the patch to inspect the eye. If total resolution has not occurred, replace the patch for another 12 hours.
4. Use a lubricating ointment at night (e.g., Lacrilube, Refresh PM, or similar).
5. If hypertonic ophthalmic saline solution is not available, instill artificial tears four to eight times per day.
6. If the patient with corneal erosion does not respond to treatment, encourage evacuation.

Contact Lens–Related Corneal Abrasion
A lens-related corneal abrasion is at high risk for transformation into a corneal ulcer.

Signs and Symptoms
Same as for other corneal abrasions

Treatment
- Discontinue contact lens wear.
- Do not patch.
- Apply a fluoroquinolone antibiotic solution (e.g., gatifloxacin [Zymar] or moxifloxacin [Vigamox] ophthalmic solution, 1 to 2 drops q2–4h for 5 to 7 days).

Corneal Ulcer
Ulceration usually occurs after an injury or in a soft contact lens wearer. Soft contact lenses allow pathogens to adhere to the corneal surface, creating deposits of organisms that can invade the stroma. This is especially true if the soft lens is worn continuously.

Signs and Symptoms
- Red, painful eye
- A white or gray spot (white cell infiltrate) on the cornea visible without fluorescein
- Photophobia
- Decreased visual acuity in the affected eye
- Discharge may or may not be present

Treatment
1. Instill gatifloxacin 0.5% ophthalmic solution 1 drop q15 min for 6 hours, then 1 drop q30 min, continued during the evacuation. If gatifloxacin or another quinolone is not available, use another ocular antibiotic. These may have reduced efficacy.
2. *Pseudomonas* infection is not uncommon as a serious complication of overnight soft contact lens wear. Consider adding tobramycin drop for drop to the quinolone with a 5-minute interval between drops.
3. Apply a cycloplegic agent.
4. Do not patch the eye.
5. Do not wear contact lenses.
6. Administer an analgesic as needed.
7. Be aware that immediate ophthalmologic consultation is required for appropriate cultures and antimicrobial treatment. Do not withhold antibiotics pending evacuation.

Corneal Foreign Body
Signs and Symptoms
- Pain, irritation, tearing, redness, and a sensation of "something in the eye"
- Sometimes visualized with the naked eye, often enhanced with fluorescein staining (highlighting any corneal damage)

Treatment
1. A foreign body can often be removed by simple irrigation with a copious amount of the cleanest water available (disinfected drinking water).
2. If simple irrigation is unsuccessful and the foreign body can be visualized, use a moistened cotton swab to gently brush away

the foreign body. The corneal epithelium can be easily damaged by forceful or repetitive use of this technique. Do not blindly sweep in hopes of success.

3. After removal of the foreign body, instill topical antibiotic drops. You may apply an eye patch if there is an epithelial defect.
4. Apply a cool compress to ease discomfort.
5. Inform the patient that the foreign body sensation will return after the anesthetic wears off.
6. If the foreign body is metallic, a rust ring may develop. This is not dangerous and can be removed later by an ophthalmologist.
7. If the foreign body cannot be easily removed or if signs and symptoms (pain, irritation, redness) persist for more than a day after removal, initiate evacuation.

Conjunctivitis ("Pink Eye")

The specific determination of the cause for conjunctivitis can be difficult in the field. Many presentations are viral (e.g., adenovirus) or allergic. Fortunately, most cases are self-limited or are bacterial and respond to an antibiotic. Visual acuity should always be checked, even though conjunctivitis typically does not cause a change. Any deterioration is cause for concern and potential evacuation.

Acute Bacterial Conjunctivitis
Signs and Symptoms
- Hyperemia of the conjunctiva
- Irritation and tearing
- Eyelids that stick together during sleep
- Purulent discharge

Treatment
1. Apply topical antibiotic solution 1 to 2 drops q2–6h for at least 5 to 7 days.
2. If the infection progresses (increasing symptoms) despite antibiotic therapy, arrange for evacuation.
3. If corneal opacification is noted (e.g., corneal ulcer, more common in a soft contact lens wearer), arrange for evacuation.
4. Do not patch the eye.

Viral Conjunctivitis (Acute Follicular Conjunctivitis)
Signs and Symptoms
- Redness of the conjunctiva
- Tearing (with scant or no purulent discharge)
- Possible history of upper respiratory infection or contact with person with red eye
- Generally involves one eye, then progresses to other eye several days later
- Tender preauricular lymph nodes
- Redness and edema of the eyelids

Treatment

1. Consider instilling a topical antibiotic (because specific diagnosis is difficult in the field), 1 to 2 drops q2–6h for at least 5 to 7 days.
2. Administer artificial tears for relief, with or without vasoconstrictive drops qid for 1 to 2 days.
3. Apply cool compresses for symptomatic relief. Be careful not to cross-contaminate the uninvolved eye.
4. Be diligent about hand washing; avoid sharing towels to prevent spread to others.
5. Be aware that viral conjunctivitis may last 2 weeks.
6. Evacuate the patient if the condition is not resolving or if any corneal opacification is noted.
7. Do not patch the eye.
8. Do not apply steroids in the field, because of the risk for herpes simplex virus infection exacerbation.

Chemical Conjunctivitis and Chemical Injury to the Cornea

Chemical conjunctivitis may be caused by any irritant (e.g., sunscreen, insect repellent, hand sanitizer, stove fuel) accidentally introduced into the eye. Caustic substances may cause more serious burns affecting the cornea. Alkali and acid burns are true emergencies.

Signs and Symptoms

- Immediate pain, tearing, and irritation
- Redness of the conjunctiva
- Loss of vascularity (e.g., "whitening") of the conjunctiva is an ominous sign

Treatment

1. Instill a topical anesthetic.
2. Irrigate the eye with a copious amount of the cleanest water available immediately. In most cases, 1 to 2 L (1 to 2 qt) of irrigant is sufficient. However, for an alkali burn, use at least 3 L (3 qt) or 30 minutes of continuous irrigation.
3. If the injury was from an acid or alkali, transport the patient rapidly to definitive care. If possible, continue irrigation during transport.
4. Instill a cycloplegic to reduce ciliary spasm.
5. Instill antibiotic ophthalmic ointment.
6. Cool compresses may provide relief. Be careful not to cross contaminate the uninvolved eye.
7. Evacuate any patient with a corneal burn associated with corneal opacification or significant defect on fluorescein staining.

Allergic Conjunctivitis
Signs and Symptoms

- Itching and tearing (without purulent discharge)
- At times, swelling and redness of the conjunctivae

Treatment

1. Instill vasoconstrictive drops (e.g., 0.3% pheniramine maleate plus 0.025% naphazoline ophthalmic solution [Naphcon-A]) up to qid for 1 to 2 days.
2. Consider topical ketorolac (Acular) 0.5% ophthalmic solution, 1 drop q6–12h, for 1 to 2 days.
3. A topical antihistamine (e.g., ketotifen or pheniramine maleate) can also be very helpful.
4. Apply cool compresses.
5. May administer an oral antihistamine to relieve itching.

Herpes Simplex Viral Keratitis

Ocular herpes can result from sexually transmitted herpes simplex virus (HSV-2). However, it is usually caused by HSV-1, the virus responsible for cold sores.

Signs and Symptoms

- Symptoms mimicking those of corneal abrasion
  - Red eye
  - Pain, photophobia, tearing, foreign body sensation
  - Decreased vision
- History of previous episode
- In early herpetic infection, only small punctate lesions or a single vesicle on the cornea may be seen.
- Over time, typical dendritic (branching) pattern of corneal involvement becoming apparent on fluorescein staining
- Typically unilateral

Treatment

1. If available, instill a topical antiviral agent (trifluridine [Viroptic] 1% ophthalmic solution) q2h while the patient is awake until the corneal epithelium has healed. Instill this agent qid for 1 week.
2. Apply a fluoroquinolone antibiotic solution (e.g., gatifloxacin [Zymar] 0.5% or moxifloxacin [Vigamox] 0.5% ophthalmic solution, 1 to 2 drops qid) until patient is evaluated. This is in case of misdiagnosis or secondary bacterial infection.
3. Evacuate the patient.

Infection of the Eyelid
Blepharitis
Signs and Symptoms

- Itching and burning of the eyelids, often with crusting around the eyes on awakening
- Red eyelid margins are crusted and thickened
- Occasionally injected conjunctivae

Treatment

1. Gently scrub the eyelid margins with baby shampoo bid using a washcloth or cotton-tipped applicator.
2. Apply warm compresses for 15 to 20 minutes tid to qid.

3. Instill artificial tears for associated mild ocular irritation or dry eyes four to eight times a day.
4. Apply antibiotic ointment qid to the eyelid margin for 1 week, then qhs for 1 more week.

Hordeolum

Hordeolum is a common infection in a gland of the eyelid. A small hordeolum that forms an external pustule and points toward the skin is called a *stye*.

Signs and Symptoms

- Localized pain, swelling, and redness of the eyelid, often associated with a purulent discharge
- Infection pointing to either the skin or to the conjunctival side of the lid

Treatment

1. Apply warm compresses for 15 to 20 minutes several times per day.
2. Gently scrub the eyelid with soap and water several times per day.
3. Apply a topical antibiotic such as erythromycin ophthalmic solution q4–6h for 7 to 10 days.
4. If cellulitis is present, administer a systemic antibiotic for 7 to 10 days.
5. If the upper and lower lids are involved and there is orbital extension (i.e., extraocular movement limitation), it is an emergency and requires immediate evacuation.
6. Perform incision and drainage only if there is an identifiable pointing lesion and no response to conservative treatment.

Chalazion
Signs and Symptoms

- Noninflamed, nontender mass in the upper or lower lid
- May follow a hordeolum
- Usually points toward the conjunctival side of the lid

Treatment

1. Apply warm compresses.
2. Note that incision and curettage are often necessary if the condition persists (this should only be done by an ophthalmologist).

Periocular Inflammation (Box 32.3)
Preseptal Cellulitis
Signs and Symptoms

- Tenderness and redness of the eyelid, often associated with fever
- Consider using pen to outline the area of erythema for gauging clinical progression.
- Unlike orbital cellulitis, no pain with eye movement or restriction of extraocular movement
- Inability to open the eye because of marked eyelid edema

BOX 32.3   Differential Diagnosis of Acute Periocular Inflammation

Preseptal cellulitis
Orbital cellulitis
Dacryocystitis
Orbital pseudotumor
Insect envenomation

- Appearance resembling and easily confused with an allergic eyelid reaction or insect bite
- With an allergic or inflammatory process, usually itching without tenderness
- If eyelid is forced open, vision will usually be normal.

Treatment
1. Administer levofloxacin 500 mg PO bid for 7 to 10 days.
2. Alternatively, administer ciprofloxacin 750 PO bid for 7 to 10 days. Gatifloxacin or moxifloxacin may be used.
3. Alternatively, administer cephalexin 500 mg PO tid to qid for 7 to 10 days.
4. Apply warm compresses to the inflamed region qid.
5. Reexamine q2h initially.
6. Consider evacuation for any patient with the following conditions:
   - Toxic appearance
   - Decreased EOM
   - Afferent pupillary defect (Marcus Gunn pupil)
   - Significantly decreased vision
   - Child younger than age 5 years
   - No improvement or any worsening after 2 to 3 days of oral antibiotics

Orbital Cellulitis
Pathogens that cause orbital cellulitis include *Staphylococcus* and *Streptococcus* species, *Haemophilus influenzae* (common in children), *Bacteroides*, and various gram-negative rods (especially after trauma).

Signs and Symptoms
- Red eye, blurred vision, diplopia, headache, fever, eyelid edema
- Erythema, warmth, and tenderness over the affected area
- Conjunctival chemosis and injection
- Restricted ocular motility and pain developing on attempted ocular motion
- Possible coexisting meningitis
- Decreased vision
- Afferent pupillary defect (Marcus Gunn pupil)
- Often associated with ethmoid sinusitis

Treatment
1. Evacuate the patient immediately. These patients require surgery.
2. Administer ceftriaxone 1 to 2 g IV q12h.
3. Although oral antibiotics are considered suboptimal for this condition, a reasonable regimen initiated during transport might include any of the following:
   a. Levofloxacin 500 mg bid
   b. Ciprofloxacin 750 mg bid
   c. Absent these drugs, a second- or third-generation oral cephalosporin (e.g., cefpodoxime, or amoxicillin/clavulanate) could be used.

Dacryocystitis (Inflammation of the Lacrimal Sac)
Signs and Symptoms
- Pain, redness, and swelling over the lacrimal sac (innermost aspect of lower eyelid)
- Mucoid or purulent discharge expressed from the nasolacrimal punctum when pressure is applied

Treatment
1. Administer ciprofloxacin 750 mg bid for 7 to 10 days.
2. Be aware that topical antibiotics are minimally effective.
3. Apply warm compresses.
4. Administer pain medication as needed.
5. Do not attempt to drain by puncture or incision and drainage.

Episcleritis
Signs and Symptoms
- Normal vision
- Localized inflammation and dilation of the episcleral vessels
- Little discomfort or discharge
- Often in only one sector of the eye
- Caused by irritants or is idiopathic
- Often a history of prior similar episodes

Treatment
1. If irritation exists, use artificial tears or instill 0.3% pheniramine maleate plus 0.025% naphazoline ophthalmic solution (Naphcon-A) up to qid.
2. Consider topical ketorolac (Acular) 0.5% ophthalmic solution, 1 drop q6–12h.
3. Ibuprofen 400 mg PO tid may be beneficial.

Iritis
Iritis may result from a specific cause (e.g., infection, trauma, overexposure to ultraviolet [UV] light) or may occur independently.

Signs and Symptoms
- Moderate to severe pain that does not respond to topical anesthesia

- Photophobia
- Blurred vision
- Pupil of the involved eye constricted and less reactive
- Redness surrounding the cornea; ciliary vessels running through the sclera beneath the conjunctivae becoming injected, causing a purplish area of injection around the cornea ("ciliary injection")

Treatment

1. Address any specific cause.
2. Instill a mydriatic-cycloplegic agent to reduce pain and ciliary spasm and prevent synechiae.
3. Avoid topical steroids in the field (risk for herpes simplex virus infection exacerbation).
4. Ibuprofen 400 mg PO tid may be beneficial.
5. Evacuate the patient if the condition persists or progresses. Iritis associated with UV photokeratitis or corneal abrasion is usually self-limited.

Ultraviolet Photokeratitis (Snowblindness)

UV-induced photokeratitis represents corneal damage. Intense exposure to UV light may cause a corneal burn in 1 hour, although symptoms may not become apparent for 6 to 12 hours.

Signs and Symptoms

- Pain, although there is typically a 6- to 12-hour symptom-free interval just after exposure
- Severe gritty sensation in the eyes
- Photophobia
- Tearing
- Marked conjunctival erythema and chemosis
- Eyelid edema
- Ciliary injection with iritis
- Usually bilateral
- On fluorescein staining, a horizontal band-like uptake that corresponds with the shielding effect of the squinting eyelids

Treatment

1. Spontaneous healing generally occurs in 24 hours. However, take steps to minimize pain and disability.
2. Remove contact lenses.
3. Instill a single dose of a topical anesthetic to help control pain during the examination. Do not use the anesthetic more than once because prolonged use can impair corneal reepithelialization.
4. Consider administering a topical NSAID solution (ketorolac [Acular] 0.5% ophthalmic solution) 1 drop q6–12h.
5. Apply an antibiotic solution. If a pressure patch is used, apply topical antibiotic ointment before patching.
6. Administer an NSAID such as ibuprofen to control symptoms.

7. Administer a systemic narcotic analgesic, if necessary.
8. Apply cold compresses to provide some relief.
9. If needed, instill a mydriatic-cycloplegic agent to reduce pain associated with ciliary spasm.
10. Note that topical steroids are not recommended because of the potential for delayed epithelial healing.
11. Patch the affected eye for 12 hours, and then remove the patch to inspect the eye. If total resolution has not occurred, replace the patch for another 12 hours.

Prevention
1. Wear sunglasses that block more than 99% of UV type B light.
2. Add side shields to sunglasses to prevent reflected UV light from striking the cornea.
3. Always carry spare sunglasses.
4. Create a makeshift shield by cutting narrow horizontal slits in a piece of cardboard, foam padding, or duct tape and securing this over the eyes.

Subconjunctival Hemorrhage
This condition is usually caused by local trauma, coughing, or straining.

Signs and Symptoms
- Usually asymptomatic
- Blood seen underneath the conjunctivae, often localized to one sector of the eye
- After trauma, it is critical to consider the presence of a conjunctival lesion or a ruptured globe, especially if bulging hemorrhage exists along with a teardrop pupil and/or hyphema.

Treatment
1. In general, no treatment is required.
2. Reassure the patient.
3. Administer artificial teardrops qid to relieve mild ocular irritation.
4. Subconjunctival hemorrhage usually resolves spontaneously in 1 to 2 weeks.
5. If the condition does not resolve or recurs, seek ophthalmologic care.

Hyphema
Hyphema usually results from a blunt injury to the eye, resulting in hemorrhage into the anterior chamber.

Signs and Symptoms
- Meniscus or layering of blood along the lower anterior chamber (in front of the iris) after the patient has been upright for 5 to 10 minutes

- Decreased vision and eye pain
- Lethargy, nausea, and vomiting possible as a result of acutely increased IOP

Treatment
1. Allow the patient to rest in an upright (e.g., sitting) position.
2. Avoid activity and rest the eyes.
3. Place shield over eye; do not patch.
4. Instill an intermediate- to long-acting mydriatic-cycloplegic agent.
5. Consider acetazolamide 250 PO qid if available.
6. Do not give aspirin or NSAIDs.
7. If the hyphema is large, arrange for immediate evacuation. A small hyphema may be better treated with rest, avoiding high physical exertion, and jostling associated with evacuation.
8. History of sickle cell trait or disease worsens the prognosis and so evacuation of the patient is recommended.

Retrobulbar Hemorrhage
- Grossly limited EOM with proptosis suggests acute orbital inflammation or retrobulbar hemorrhage.
- Retrobulbar hemorrhage is usually accompanied by periorbital ecchymosis and subconjunctival hemorrhage following trauma.
- This is an emergency, so the patient should be evacuated immediately. If evacuation is impossible and evolving orbital compartment syndrome is suspected, consider lateral canthotomy (Fig. 32.4).

Ruptured Globe
Signs and Symptoms
- History of significant trauma or projectile injury
- Reduced vision, pain (see Examination of Vision, earlier)
- Pupil appears distorted and teardrop shaped, pointing toward the rupture.
- An abnormal anterior chamber (either shallow or deep compared with the contralateral eye)
- Significant conjunctival hemorrhage or with dark specks of uveal tissue underneath
- Limited EOM
- Hyphema

Treatment
1. Do not press on the eye.
2. Plan for evacuation.
3. Elevate the patient's head to decrease IOP.
4. Cover the eye with a cup or improvised shield to avoid any pressure on the globe.
5. Avoid any activities (including further ocular examination) that may cause the patient to blink excessively or to strain.

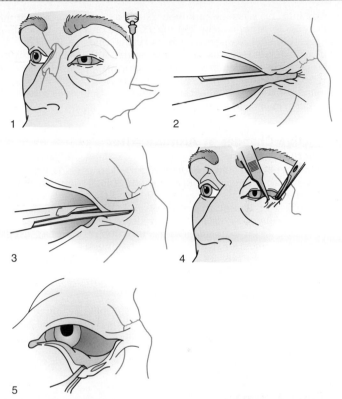

FIGURE 32.4   Lateral canthotomy and inferior cantholysis are indicated for casualties that manifest with orbital hemorrhage and evolving orbital compartment syndrome. **Step 1,** Infiltrate the lateral canthal area with a local anesthetic (e.g., 2% lidocaine with epinephrine), and use tetracaine drops in the eye for topical anesthesia. **Step 2,** Place a mosquito clamp on the lateral canthus that extends horizontally toward the orbital rim for a distance of 1 cm (0.4 inch). Leave it in place for 30 seconds to assist with hemostasis. **Step 3,** Remove the clamp, and use a pair of fine (e.g., Stevens) scissors to divide the lateral canthal tissues along the line created by the clamp. This completes the lateral canthotomy. **Step 4,** Next, use the scissors to cut the inferior crus of the lateral canthal ligament. Position the scissors perpendicular to the canthotomy incision that was made in Step 3 (i.e., not along the lid margin), and cut the ligament. This completes the inferior lateral cantholysis. **Step 5,** The completed lateral canthotomy and cantholysis are shown. These procedures allow the orbital tissues to move forward slightly, and they help to relieve the pressure in the orbital compartment.

6. Administer a systemic antibiotic such as levofloxacin 500 mg PO bid or ciprofloxacin 750 mg PO bid, or a third-generation injectable cephalosporin, such as ceftriaxone 1 g IV q12h.

7. If an extended evacuation is necessary and a small puncture wound can be identified, consider applying a drop or two of superglue to the wound. Although this is a radical maneuver, uninterrupted loss of aqueous or vitreous would otherwise result in permanent blindness.

Refractive Changes at Altitude After Refractive Surgery

- Acute hyperopic shift has been reported in persons who have had radial keratotomy (RK) and then experienced altitude exposure.
- The effect of altitude exposure on post-RK eyes is most likely caused by hypoxia rather than by decreased pressure.
- Breathing a normoxic-inspired gas mix does not protect against the development of hypoxic corneal changes.
- The effect of the post-RK hyperopic shift seen at altitude depends on the postoperative refractive state (undercorrected patients may actually have their vision improve) and the accommodative abilities of the individual.
- Individuals who have undergone RK and plan to undertake an altitude exposure of 2743 m (9000 ft) or higher while mountaineering should bring multiple eyeglasses with increasing plus lens power.
- Reports have noted mild myopic shifts at altitude in some individuals after LASIK.

Wilderness Eye Kit

See Appendix I.

Ear, Nose, and Throat Emergencies

EPISTAXIS

- Epistaxis is a common problem in travelers; reduced humidity in airplanes, cold climates, and high-altitude environments can produce drying and erosion of the nasal mucosa.
- Other major causes include infections, inflammatory rhinitis, inhaled medications, mucosal breakdown caused by infiltration by malignancy or granulomatous disease, and nasal trauma.
- Daily applications of a small quantity of petroleum jelly (Vaseline) or antiseptic ointment (e.g., bacitracin or mupirocin) to the septum can help to keep the nasal mucosa moist.
- Although most cases of epistaxis are minor, some present life-threatening emergencies.
- Ninety percent of nosebleeds are anterior, and exhibit unilateral, steady, nonmassive bleeding. Ten percent are posterior and may present with massive bleeding.
- A posterior source of the bleeding should be considered when epistaxis is bilateral, brisk, and not controlled with pinching the nostrils or with an anterior nasal pack.

Treatment

1. The existing clot should be completely cleared, usually by having the patient blow his or her nose.
2. One or two sprays of a topical nasal vasoconstrictor (e.g., oxymetazoline [Afrin] or phenylephrine [Neo-Synephrine]) should be inhaled into the affected nostril.
3. The patient should be kept sitting (i.e., keeping the head elevated and still).
4. The patient should be instructed to grasp and pinch his or her entire nose, maintaining continuous pressure against the septum for at least 15 minutes. If this maneuver does not control the bleeding, nasal packing may be required.
5. Anterior epistaxis nasal pack
   a. Soak a piece of cotton or gauze with a vasoconstrictor, such as oxymetazoline nasal spray, and insert it into the nose, leaving it in place for 5 to 10 minutes.
   b. Petroleum jelly–impregnated gauze or strips of a nonadherent dressing can then be packed into the nose so that both ends of the gauze remain outside the nasal cavity (Fig. 33.1). This prevents the patient from inadvertently aspirating the nasal packing.
   c. Complete packing of the nasal cavity of an adult patient requires a minimum of 1 m (3.3 ft) of packing to fill the

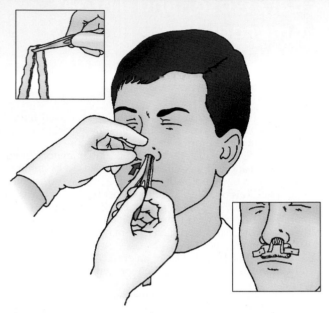

FIGURE 33.1 Anterior epistaxis from one side of the nasal cavity can be treated using nasal packing soaked in a vasoconstrictor. Petroleum jelly–impregnated gauze or strips of nonadherent dressing can be packed in the nose so that both ends of the gauze remain outside the nasal cavity.

nasal cavity and tamponade the bleeding site. When placing the gauze, it should be started as far posteriorly as is possible.

d. Expandable packing material, such as Weimert Epistaxis Packing, Merocel nasal tampon, Rapid Rhino, or the Rhino Rocket, is available commercially. The packing material can be lubricated with K-Y jelly or water before insertion. A tampon or balloon tip from a Foley catheter can also be used as improvised packing.

e. Anterior nasal packing blocks sinus drainage and predisposes to sinusitis. Prophylactic antibiotics (see Sinusitis, later) are sometimes recommended until the pack is removed in 48 to 72 hours.

6. Posterior epistaxis nasal pack
   a. If the bleeding site is located posteriorly, use a 14- to 16-French Foley catheter with a 30-mL balloon to tamponade the site (Fig. 33.2).
   b. Prelubricate the catheter with either petroleum jelly (Vaseline), clear or white antiseptic ointment, or a water-based lubricant.

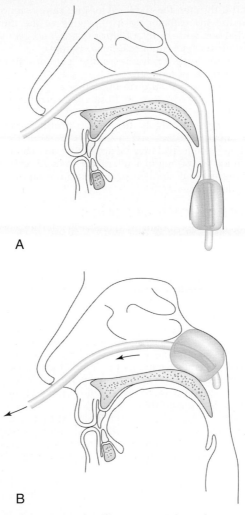

FIGURE 33.2   Posterior nasal packing using a Foley catheter. Insert a Foley catheter into the nose, and gently pass it back until it enters the back of the throat **(A)**. After the tip of the catheter is in the patient's throat, carefully inflate the balloon with 15 mL of air or water from a syringe. Inflation should be done slowly and should be stopped if painful. After the balloon is inflated, gently pull the catheter back out until resistance is met **(B)**.

    c. Insert it through the nasal cavity into the posterior pharynx. Visualize the catheter tip in the back of the throat. Inflate the balloon with 15 mL of air or water, and gently withdraw the catheter back until resistance is met.

    d. Secure the catheter firmly to the patient's forehead with several strips of tape.

    e. Avoid intense pressure on the nares.

    f. Pack the anterior nose in front of the catheter balloon as described earlier.

    g. Administer an antibiotic to provide prophylaxis for sinusitis (see later).

7. Topical tranexamic acid may be applied to an anterior nosebleed in a solution of 100 mg in 1 mL saline sprayed with an atomizer or 500 mg in 5 mL applied to a nasal tampon and placed on the bleeding mucosa.

ESOPHAGEAL FOREIGN BODIES

- Esophageal foreign bodies may cause significant morbidity.
- Respiratory compromise caused by tracheal compression or by aspiration of secretions can occur.
- Mediastinitis, pleural effusion, pneumothorax, and abscess may be seen with perforations of the esophagus from sharp objects or pressure necrosis caused by large objects.
- The use of a Foley balloon-tipped catheter passed beyond an obstruction and removed with gentle traction can be an effective method for removing a blunt esophageal foreign body. Associated complications include laryngospasm, epistaxis, pain, esophageal perforation, and tracheal aspiration of the dislodged foreign body. Uncooperative patients or sharp objects that completely obstruct the esophagus restrict use of this technique, which is recommended only in extreme wilderness settings or when endoscopy is not available.
  - Lubricate a 12- to 16-French Foley catheter, and place it orally into the esophagus while the patient is seated.
  - After placing the patient in the Trendelenburg position, pass the catheter beyond the foreign body and inflate the balloon with water.
  - Withdraw the catheter with steady traction until the foreign body can be removed from the hypopharynx or is expelled by coughing.
  - Take care to avoid lodging the foreign body in the nasopharynx.
  - Any significant impedance to withdrawal should terminate the attempt.

FOREIGN BODY IN THE EAR
Signs and Symptoms
- Patient may experience significant discomfort.
- Nausea or vomiting may occur if a live insect is in the ear canal.
- Patient may complain of a sense of fullness in the affected ear.

- Associated hearing loss may occur.
- Bleeding may occur either from direct trauma or the patient's attempts to remove the foreign body.
- Insects can injure the tympanic membrane or external canal.
- Erythema and swelling of the canal or a foul-smelling discharge may develop over time.

Treatment

1. The insect should be killed before removal. Instill one of the following:
   a. Lidocaine (2%)
   b. Alcohol
   c. Mineral oil
2. Irrigation is the simplest method of foreign body removal.
   a. Do not irrigate if the tympanic membrane is perforated.
   b. An ordinary 20- to 60-mL syringe with an irrigation tip or catheter may be used for irrigation.
   c. Use clean, tepid water (i.e., disinfected for drinking).
3. Sometimes the object can be easily extracted with forceps.
4. Avoid pushing the object in deeper.
5. Analgesics should be given if indicated.
6. Following removal, inspect the external canal.
7. If evidence of infection or abrasion is noted, administer a combination antibiotic and steroid otic suspension (e.g., neomycin and polymyxin B and hydrocortisone otic suspension [Cortisporin], or ciprofloxacin with hydrocortisone [Cipro HC]), four to five times per day for 2 to 3 days.

OTITIS MEDIA

Signs and Symptoms

In the wilderness, otoscopic examination is usually not possible. Diagnosis is based on clinical symptoms, including one or more of the following:

- Otalgia
- Otorrhea (less common)
- Fever (not required for the diagnosis)
- Associated upper respiratory infection
- Decreased hearing
- Nausea and vomiting

Treatment

Mild otitis may be managed with a short period of observation without specific treatment. Failure to improve within 48 to 72 hours should prompt initiation of antibiotic therapy.

Treatment is directed toward *Pneumococcus* and *Moraxella*. Less common causes are *Haemophilus influenzae*, *Mycoplasma* species, viruses, and other bacteria. Sterile effusions occur in approximately 20% of cases.

The antibiotic of choice is amoxicillin 500 mg PO q12h or 250 mg q8h or amoxicillin/clavulanate potassium (Augmentin)

500 mg PO q8h for 5 to 7 days (in adults). An alternative is azithromycin (Zithromax) 500 mg as a single dose on day 1, followed by 250 mg once daily on days 2 through 5. Perforation of the tympanic membrane may complicate otitis media. Treatment is essentially as described earlier. Appropriate follow-up is indicated following perforation. Perforations generally heal within a few weeks without complications.

OTITIS EXTERNA
See Chapter 55.

SINUSITIS
Signs and Symptoms
Common complaints include the following:
- Nasal congestion
- Purulent nasal discharge
- Facial pain (may be increased by leaning forward or with any head movement)
- Facial tenderness to palpation
- Retro-orbital pain (if the ethmoid sinus is involved)
- Headache
- Concomitant or preceding upper respiratory infection
- Maxillary tooth discomfort
- Decreased sense of smell
- Cough
- Fever may be present.

Treatment
1. Encourage hydration to promote sinus drainage.
2. Nasal vasoconstrictors (e.g., oxymetazoline) may provide relief during initial management. These should not be used for longer than 5 days to avoid a rebound phenomenon.
3. Warm facial compresses may provide symptomatic relief.
4. Decongestants and nonsteroidal antiinflammatory drugs may be useful in reducing secretions (avoid antihistamines).
5. In severe cases, a short course of oral prednisone may be considered to alleviate inflammation that contributes to pain.
6. Analgesic medication may be necessary.
7. The organisms most commonly implicated in bacterial sinusitis are *H. influenzae* and *Streptococcus pneumoniae* (in adults).
8. A higher incidence exists of anaerobic organisms (e.g., *Bacteroides*, *Peptostreptococcus*, and *Fusobacterium* species are seen in chronic sinusitis).
9. Specific antibiotic treatment if symptoms have persisted for a week or are clearly worsening involves the following:
   a. Amoxicillin 500 mg PO q8h for 10 to 14 days
   b. Trimethoprim/sulfamethoxazole (Bactrim, Septra) 1 tab (double strength) PO q12h for 10 to 14 days
   c. Amoxicillin/clavulanate (Augmentin) 500 mg PO q12h for 10 to 14 days

    d. Azithromycin (Zithromax) 500 mg as a single dose on day 1, followed by 250 mg once daily on days 2 through 5

    e. Doxycycline 100 mg PO q12h for 10 to 14 days

10. For worsening or severe toxicity (e.g., lethargy, vomiting, high fever), or if symptoms do not improve with antibiotics, seek urgent follow-up.

The most common dental emergencies result from inflammation, infection, or trauma.

TOOTHACHE (PULPITIS)

The common toothache is caused by inflammation of the dental pulp and is often associated with dental caries.

Signs and Symptoms

- Pain, which may be severe, intermittent, and difficult to localize. Pain often radiates to the eye or ear region.
- Pain that is often made worse by hot or cold foods or liquids.
- A carious lesion in the painful tooth is occasionally sensitive to percussion or palpation.

Treatment

1. If the offending carious lesion can be localized, first apply a piece of cotton soaked with eugenol (oil of cloves).
2. Place a temporary filling material, such as Cavit or zinc oxide-eugenol (ZOE) cement (intermediate restorative material [IRM]) into the lesion to protect the nerve. Softened candle wax can be used if necessary as a temporary filling material.
3. Administer a nonsteroidal antiinflammatory drug (NSAID) (e.g., ibuprofen 400 to 800 mg PO q6h prn).
4. If the episode of pain lasts longer, indicating a moderate pulpitis, fill the lesion as described earlier and give the patient a non-narcotic analgesic.
5. For severe pulpitis with continuous and severe pain, administer a local anesthetic and then evacuate the patient. You can achieve a nerve block with bupivacaine 2% with 1:200,000 epinephrine (Marcaine), which lasts for about 8 hours and does not produce central nervous system depression. Large doses of narcotics may not provide pain relief and can compromise the patient's ability to participate in evacuation.
6. In extraordinary circumstances, locate the offending tooth, expose the pulp, remove the inflamed tissue with a barbed hook, and cover the lesion with temporary filling material.

PERIAPICAL OSTEITIS

Inflammation of the supporting structures at the root of a tooth.

Signs and Symptoms
- Constant, often throbbing tooth pain
- Tooth is sensitive to tapping. Area over the apex of the tooth is tender to palpation, but there is no obvious swelling.
- Patient can usually localize the pain.

Treatment
1. Administer a NSAID.
2. Place a strip of leather, webbing, or something similar between the teeth on the nonpainful side to prevent occlusion of the offending tooth.
3. The patient should be kept on a soft diet.

CRACKED TOOTH
Signs and Symptoms
- The patient feels a sharp pain when chewing certain foods.
- The tooth feels weak or hurts only when the patient bites on something hard.

Treatment
1. Avoid chewing on the affected side.
2. See a dentist as soon as possible.

TEMPOROMANDIBULAR DISORDERS
Myofascial Pain and Dysfunction
Participants in wilderness activities are exposed to many of the risk factors for myofascial pain and dysfunction (stress-associated grinding of the teeth, increased jaw function from eating jerky and other dried foods).

Signs and Symptoms
- Pain in the muscles of mastication, which is usually unilateral and increases with chewing
- Headache or earache
- Intermittent clicking of the temporomandibular joint (TMJ)
- Limitation of jaw movement
- Change in bite
- Tenderness of the jaw muscles or TMJ to palpation
- Inability to open the mouth wide or deviation of the chin to one side on opening

Treatment
1. Rest the muscles (soft diet and control of tooth clenching and grinding habits).
2. Apply moist heat.
3. Place a soft material, such as a folded piece of gauze, between the front teeth to keep the teeth from touching.
4. Administer an analgesic.

Mandibular Dislocation

Dislocation of the mandible and inability to close the mouth can result from external trauma or sudden wide opening of the mouth, as occurs with yawning. If there is a history of trauma, a condylar fracture should be suspected.

Signs and Symptoms
- Inability to completely open or close the mouth.
- Pain at the TMJ.

Treatment
1. Place the rescuer's thumbs on the patient's lower molars and move the mandible down, then posteriorly, and then up. The thumbs should be padded to prevent bites as the jaw pops back into its socket.
2. Alternatively, rest the rescuer's palms on the mandible and wrap the fingers along the occlusal surface of the mandibular teeth. Rock the hands posteriorly and down, sliding the mandibular condyle back into the TMJ.
3. If muscle spasm is severe, sedation might be necessary.
4. After reduction of the mandible, the patient must avoid opening the mouth wide.

INFECTIONS
Aphthous Ulcers
Signs and Symptoms
- Painful oral mucosa lesions that are round, superficial, and have a red halo.
- The patient usually gives a history of similar ulcerations.
- The lesions typically last 10 to 14 days.

Treatment
1. Apply a topical steroid (fluocinonide 0.05%) mixed with oral benzocaine 20% over each ulcer six to eight times per day. Do not mix the medications until you are ready to apply them, and do not rub the mixture into the lesions.
2. Other options include premixed preparations, such as triamcinolone (Kenalog) in oral benzocaine 20%.
3. Tincture of benzoin or a topical anesthetic (viscous lidocaine 2%) can be applied to the dried surface of the ulcer before meals and at bedtime.

Viral Infections
Herpes labialis (cold sore, fever blister) is the most common oral viral infection. Use of sun-blocking agents on the lips helps to prevent herpes labialis.

Signs and Symptoms
- Prodrome of tingling or paresthesia in the area.

- Yellow fluid-filled vesicles that rupture to leave ragged ulcers on the lip, palate, tongue, and buccal mucosa.
- Primary herpetic gingivostomatitis is characterized by a thin zone of red, painful gingiva just next to the teeth. Sore throat, lymphadenopathy, and low-grade fever are also present.

Treatment

1. Administer valacyclovir (Valtrex) 2 g PO q12h for 1 day as soon as the patient becomes aware of a prodromal "tingle" or paresthesia.
2. For herpetic gingivostomatitis, use soothing mouth rinses, such as warm saline or a mixture of equal amounts of diphenhydramine (Benadryl) elixir (12.5 mg/5 mL), kaolin/pectin (Kaopectate), and viscous lidocaine 2%. Rinse with 5 mL q2h and expectorate.

Apical Abscess and Cellulitis

Signs and Symptoms

- Dental pain associated with swelling and fluctuance in the gum line at the base of the tooth; swelling is much more common on facial side than on the lingual side.
- Pain caused by percussion of the offending tooth.
- No sensitivity to hot or cold in the affected tooth.

Treatment

1. Incision and drainage is the treatment of choice (Fig. 34.1).
   a. Infiltrate the area with a local anesthetic. Adequate anesthesia may also be obtained by applying cold (ice or snow) to the area to be incised.
   b. Make an incision at the point of maximum fluctuance down to bone in one swift movement.
   c. Spread the incision with a hemostat or knife handle.
   d. Place a T-shaped drain into the wound. Drain material can be improvised from a piece of surgical glove or gauze dressing.
2. Administer warm saline rinses q2h and an analgesic as needed for pain.
3. If incision and drainage cannot be performed, administer an oral antibiotic such as penicillin or erythromycin (see Appendix H).
4. Evacuate the patient and seek dental care because this condition often requires dental extraction and antibiotics.

Pericoronitis

Pericoronitis is an infection of the gingival flap around a partially erupted tooth. The most common site is the mandibular third molar.

Signs and Symptoms

- May mimic streptococcal pharyngitis or tonsillitis
- Pain at the site of infection
- Trismus

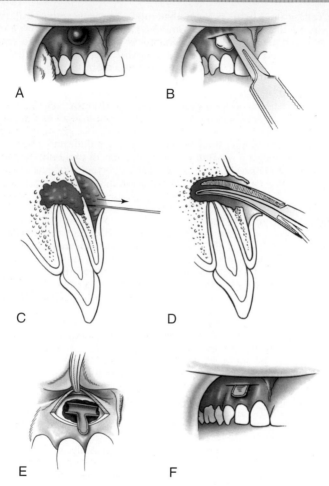

FIGURE 34.1 Apical dental abscess. **(A)** Abscess. **(B)** Incision. **(C)** Release of pus. **(D)** Open cavity. **(E)** Drain placement. **(F)** Drain in place.

Treatment

1. Initiate field treatment, which consists of curettage of the area around the tooth and under the flap. In the absence of proper dental instruments, use a small curved hemostat.
2. Irrigate the space under the flap with disinfected water.
3. Begin warm saline rinses q2h and administer an oral antibiotic such as penicillin or erythromycin (see Appendix H).

Deep Fascial Space Infection

Apical infection occasionally spreads beyond the local area to the canine, buccal, and masticator spaces and to the floor of the mouth.

Signs and Symptoms

- Trismus.
- Fever and sepsis.
- Swelling is minimal because of the overlying muscle mass.
- Submandibular space infection (Ludwig's angina) that produces elevation of the tongue and brawny, painful edema of the submandibular area.
- Continued swelling that restricts neck motion and produces dysphonia, odynophagia, and drooling; possible progression to acute airway obstruction and asphyxia.
- Mediastinitis and cavernous sinus venous thrombosis.

Treatment

1. Be aware that airway management with early intubation or cricothyroidotomy may be necessary.
2. Administer an intravenous antibiotic (penicillin, 2 million units) or oral antibiotic (penicillin, 1000 mg) if intravenous therapy is not available.
3. Evacuate the patient immediately to the nearest medical facility.

TRAUMA

See Table 34.1 for dental trauma definitions.

Uncomplicated Crown Fracture

Signs and Symptoms

- Fractured tooth but no pulp tissue visible
- Possible sensitivity to cold or heat

Treatment

1. Smooth any sharp edges with a fingernail file or cover with wax.
2. If thermal sensitivity is severe, apply ZOE B&T cement (zinc oxide–eugenol with polymer reinforcement), IRM, Cavit, or softened candle wax to the fractured crown.

Uncomplicated Crown-Root Fracture

Signs and Symptoms

Similar to uncomplicated crown fracture except that the fracture is nearly vertical, leaving a small, chisel-shaped fragment attached only by the palatal gingiva

Treatment

1. Treatment is the same as for an uncomplicated crown fracture.
2. Remove the mobile fragment to make the patient more comfortable.

Table 34.1	Dental Trauma	
CONDITION	**SIGNS AND SYMPTOMS**	**TREATMENT**
Concussion	Fully rigid tooth but has sustained trauma	Observation only
Subluxation	Loose tooth but in correct position	Splint
Extrusive luxation	Loose or rigid tooth displaced outward from occlusal surface	Pad contralateral occlusal surface, analgesia, dental follow-up
Lateral luxation	Loose or rigid tooth displaced laterally	Local anesthesia, reduction to anatomic position
Intrusive luxation	Loose or rigid tooth displaced inward from occlusal surface	Analgesia, dental follow-up
Avulsion	Tooth completely missing from alveolar socket	Locate missing tooth and rinse it in water or saline but do not scrub. Replace in socket if possible and splint. If unable to replace, transport in saline or saliva and evacuate to immediate dental care.
Fracture	Irregular surface with exposed dentin or pulp	File rough edges. Cover exposed dentin or pulp with Cavit, zinc oxide-eugenol cements, or warm wax.

Complicated Crown Fracture
Signs and Symptoms
- Tooth fractured
- Pulp exposed

Treatment
1. Stop the bleeding by placing a moistened tea bag into the socket or next to the bleeding gum.
2. Cap the exposed area with IRM, Cavit, or softened candle wax.

Complicated Crown-Root Fracture
Signs and Symptoms
Obliquely fractured tooth resulting in pulp exposure and a mobile fragment attached to the palatal gingiva

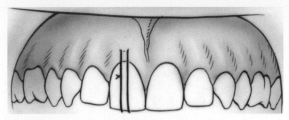

FIGURE 34.2   Suture used to stabilize a loosened or avulsed tooth.

Treatment
1. Remove the mobile fragment.
2. Cap the exposed area with IRM or Cavit.

Root Fracture
Signs and Symptoms
Slight to severe malposition of the crown

Treatment
1. Reposition the tooth as precisely as possible and splint the tooth by suturing it to the gum (Fig. 34.2).
2. If the coronal fragment cannot be stabilized and you are days away from a medical facility, remove the mobile fragment. Do not attempt to extract the apical fragment.

Extrusive Luxation
Signs and Symptoms
Tooth that is partially displaced outward from the occlusal surface and is commonly mobile.

Treatment
1. Reposition the tooth with gentle steady pressure, allowing time to displace the blood that has collected into the apical region of the socket.
2. Observe the patient's occlusion as a guide to proper reduction. If the patient bites and contacts only the injured tooth, further positioning is necessary.
3. If the patient is unable to close the occlusal surface normally, place soft padding on the contralateral occlusal surface for comfort.

Lateral Luxation
Signs and Symptoms
- Tooth displaced and commonly immobile because the apex is locked into its new position in the alveolar bone
- High metallic tone on percussion

Treatment
1. Use one finger to guide the apex gently down and back while another finger repositions the crown (Fig. 34.3). The

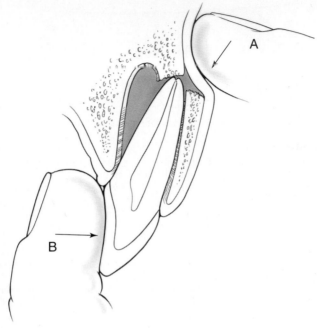

FIGURE 34.3 Reduction of lateral luxation. Use one finger **(A)** to guide the apex gently down and back while another finger **(B)** repositions the crown. (Modified from Andreasen JO, Andreasen FM: *Essentials of traumatic injuries to the teeth*, Copenhagen, 1990, Munksgaard.)

    tooth may snap back into place and be stable or may require splinting.
2. Use a suture to splint the tooth in place (see Fig. 34.2).

Total Avulsion
If a tooth is totally avulsed from the bone, it may be salvageable if replaced within 30 to 60 minutes.

Signs and Symptoms
- Tooth no longer attached to the bone
- Bleeding in the socket site

Treatment
1. Clean the debris off the tooth by rinsing gently (do not scrub) with either saline solution or milk. Handle the tooth only by the crown.
2. Remove any clotted blood from the socket with gentle irrigation and suction.

3. Gently replace the tooth in the socket with slow steady pressure.
4. Splint or suture the tooth into place.
5. If the tooth cannot be replaced immediately, store it in balanced Hank's solution, tissue culture medium, physiologic saline solution, white milk, or saliva in that order of preference.
6. Relieve bleeding by placing a moistened tea bag into the socket that is bleeding.
7. Do not replace children's primary (nonadult) teeth as this can cause complications with adult tooth eruption and alignment.

DENTAL FIRST-AID KIT

Items necessary to manage dental emergencies can be added to a wilderness first-aid kit without a large sacrifice of space or weight.

- Cavit is a temporary filling. Squeeze a small amount of the material from the tube and place it in the tooth. Wet a dental packing instrument or cotton-tipped applicator or toothpick to prevent sticking and pack the Cavit well, then remove any excess. Have the patient bite to displace material that would interfere with occlusion. The filling material will set in a few minutes after contact with saliva.
- Zinc oxide-eugenol cements consist of a liquid and a powder. Start with two drops of the liquid and begin mixing in the powder. Keep adding powder to make a consistency that is not sticky yet will hold together. Dip the instruments in some powder to keep the mixture from sticking. Insert and shape the filling material as explained earlier.
- For longer expeditions, include the following:
  - No. 151 universal extraction forceps
  - Straight elevator
  - Mouth mirror
  - Orthodontic wax
  - Dental floss
  - Dental syringe
  - 30-gauge needles
  - Anesthetic cartridges (bupivacaine 2% with 1:200,000 epinephrine [Marcaine] for long-term pain relief)

Mental Health

Psychiatric problems can emerge or worsen in response to the demands of wilderness experiences. Even in the absence of psychiatric disease, travel produces some level of stress in everyone. Psychodynamic issues develop in most groups and threaten to derail those without a plan to deal with them. Management of emotional problems in the wilderness, including the use of psychotropic medications, both in people who have preexisting psychologic difficulties and in those who develop new emotional problems in the wilderness, is outlined in this chapter.

Modern interpersonal theory suggests that most healthy adults manage stress by flexibly using different coping styles but that all adults develop an inflexible coping style under extreme stress. Individuals vary with regard to the magnitude of stress they can endure before innately settling into one of these styles, which they developed in infancy as a response to caregivers. The key to successfully intervening once one of these coping styles becomes inflexible is to challenge the core belief rather than reinforce it, respond to the core belief and not the behavior displayed, and avoid reinforcing the coping style.

- Moving toward others:
  - Typically, individuals with this coping style are highly emotionally expressive and may display "clinginess" and extreme dependence on others.
  - Core beliefs:
    - I am incompetent.
    - Group leaders and caregivers are unreliable and unlikely to meet my needs.
  - Strategy to intervene:
    - Avoid rejecting or isolating the person or coddling and overprotecting him or her.
    - Encourage competence (e.g., assign easily achievable duties).
    - Remain calm and accessible.
- Moving away from others:
  - Individuals distance themselves from others and appear aloof and self-sufficient.
  - Core beliefs:
    - I must appear superior to others.
    - Group leaders and caregivers will not care for me, so I must be self-sufficient.

- Strategy to intervene:
  - Avoid ignoring the person. Instead, make it clear that the person is cared for, valued, and missed when he or she isolates himself or herself from the group.
- Moving against others:
  - Individuals appear intimidating and act confrontationally.
  - Core beliefs:
    - I must be in control.
    - Group leaders and caregivers are frightening and unpredictable.
  - Strategy to intervene:
    - Avoid appearing to be frightened or intimidated.
    - Avoid reacting defensively/aggressively.
    - Stay calm and assertive (not aggressive) and project confidence.

ANXIETY
Signs and Symptoms
- Excessive worrying out of proportion to the situation, with preoccupying concerns and fears
- Increased heart rate, blood pressure, and respirations, sweaty palms
- Nausea and diarrhea, muscular tension
- Extreme: "fight or flight" with a dramatic increase in physical manifestations; altered memory

Treatment
1. Provide ample reassurance.
2. Suggest and support constructive behaviors.
3. Build rapport.
4. Listen uncritically.
5. Administer lorazepam 0.5 to 2 mg PO bid for severe symptoms.

PHOBIA (SUCH AS FEAR OF HEIGHTS OR SNAKES)
Treatment
1. Consider alternate routes of travel.
2. Reassure or distract the person.
3. Administer lorazepam 0.5 to 2 mg PO bid for extreme symptoms (use caution if sedation or diminished motor coordination poses a danger to self or others).

PANIC ATTACK
Signs and Symptoms
- Typically lasts 10 to 30 minutes
- With or without obvious cause or trigger
- Sensation of pounding heart, chest pain, nausea, dizziness, numbness, chills, hot flushes, shortness of breath
- Hyperventilation, sweating, trembling
- Desire to flee

- Fear of dying, having a heart attack, going crazy, or losing control

Treatment
1. Carefully evaluate to identify physical cause.
2. Do not leave the person alone but do not crowd the person.
3. Administer lorazepam 0.5 to 2 mg PO bid for severe symptoms.

OBSESSIVE-COMPULSIVE DISORDER
Obsessions and compulsions of a person with obsessive-compulsive disorder (OCD) are usually seen as irrational by the person who is experiencing them, but at the same time he or she feels helpless to stop them. Frank disclosure by a participant to a wilderness group about his or her OCD symptoms can diminish the group's anxieties about the person's odd behaviors and make the afflicted person less likely to be isolated by the group.

DEPRESSION (WITH OR WITHOUT MANIA)
Symptoms
- Feelings of sadness, uselessness, low self-esteem
- Failure to believe that the situation will improve
- Difficulty sleeping
- Diminished appetite, low energy, failure to concentrate
- Social withdrawal and lack of enjoyment
- Diminished sexual drive
- Crying for no apparent reason; emotional outbursts
- Psychosis
- Suicidal ideation

A wilderness traveler who has been divorced, widowed, or fired from his or her job shortly before the trip may be at higher risk for suicide. A family history of suicide or a history of suicidal behavior increases suicide risk. If there is a concern that someone might be suicidal, then he or she should be asked about suicidal thinking in a straightforward and concerned manner. Asking about suicide does not increase suicide risk. If the suicide potential is judged to be significant, then the person must be watched closely. People who are delirious or psychotic can suddenly become impulsively suicidal in the middle of their confusion and frenzy. Suicidal individuals should be evacuated.

MANIA
During the early part of the manic phase of bipolar disorder, sometimes known as *hypomania*, the person may exhibit positive behavior, productivity, hard work, high energy, and expansive thinking. However, as the person becomes manic, he or she may exhibit the following:
- Rapid, pressured speech that is difficult to interpret
- Lack of sleep
- Excessive gregarious behavior

- Hypersexual behavior
- Impaired judgment in all matters, including financial and social risk taking
- Feeling of superhuman powers
- Failure to listen to reason

Treatment
1. Administer respiradone 2 to 3 mg daily or olanzapine 10 mg daily.
2. Avoid confrontation.
3. Protect the patient from hurting himself or herself or others.
4. Remove all weapons from an available status.
5. Arrange for urgent evacuation.

Considerations for the Person Taking Lithium for Depression
- Keep the person well hydrated to avoid lithium toxicity.
- If lithium toxicity (symptoms: tremulousness, seizures) is suspected, stop the medication, enforce hydration, and seek evacuation.

SCHIZOPHRENIA
Signs and Symptoms
- Inability to perceive reality rationally
- Delusions (false beliefs not based in reality)
- Hallucinations (sensory perceptions with a sensory stimulus)
- Awkward behavior and emotional personal distancing
- Flat affect
- Jumbled thoughts

Treatment
For Florid Psychosis
1. Consider increase in prescribed antipsychotic medications.
2. Administer ketamine 0.5 mg/kg IM or intranasally, haloperidol 0.5 to 5 mg PO bid or lorazepam 2 to 4 mg PO bid.
3. Keep the patient from hurting himself or herself or others.
4. Arrange for emergent evacuation.
5. Consider other causes for the behavior: head injury, illicit drugs, brain tumor, metabolic disturbance, and heat-related illness.

For Acute Dystonia (Painful Involuntary Muscle Contractions) From Antipsychotic Medications
- Administer diphenhydramine 25 to 50 mg IM, IV, or PO q6h.

ORGANIC MENTAL DISORDERS
Delirium is a medical emergency and is often associated with a fluctuating level of consciousness. Confusion and disorientation are hallmarks; hallucinations may be present. Causes include the following:

- High-altitude cerebral edema
- Acute hypoxia
- Hypoglycemia
- Dehydration
- Head injury
- Heat-related illness
- Meningitis
- Encephalitis
- Metabolic abnormality (e.g., hyponatremia, hypercalcemia)
- Drug or alcohol intoxication or withdrawal

SUBSTANCE ABUSE DISORDERS

People who abuse illicit drugs or alcohol should not be on wilderness adventures; they are a hazard to themselves and others. Some people may be unaware of the depth of their substance abuse problem until they start to experience physical or psychologic withdrawal. Cocaine, methamphetamine, or narcotic abusers will not experience life-threatening withdrawal, but their symptoms can be extremely uncomfortable and disabling. Withdrawal from substances such as cocaine (i.e., "crashing") is associated with extreme irritability and fatigue. Aches and pains that are typical of influenza are seen in association with withdrawal from narcotics. Withdrawal symptoms may last several days.

Alcohol and benzodiazepine withdrawal are medical emergencies.

Signs and Symptoms
- Increased heart rate and blood pressure
- Seizures and delirium tremens
- Psychosis

Treatment
1. Administer lorazepam 0.5 to 4 mg PO or IM/IV titrated in increments to stabilize symptoms and vital signs.
2. Alcohol can be used to treat alcohol withdrawal symptoms, titrated as above.
3. Arrange for emergent evacuation.

POSTTRAUMATIC STRESS DISORDER

Posttraumatic stress disorder (PTSD) occurs after someone has experienced an event that involved injury or death or the threat of same. It can also occur following an extreme emotional or physical stress, witnessing a catastrophe, or other profoundly emotional or disruptive occurrence. It is not uncommon in soldiers after combat or persons who have responded to disasters or witnessed immense suffering. PTSD is commonly defined as lasting 30 days or more after the inciting event(s).

Symptoms
- Reliving the event, including "flashbacks," nightmares, upsetting memories, and periods of emotional disturbance when reminded

of an event. Images and memories may be suppressed for a period of time. There may be fear provoked by the thought of encountering situations similar to what caused the PTSD and seeming loss of bravery or blunted compassion.

- Disruption of the activities of daily living, manifested by avoidance behaviors. This includes apathy, a feeling of detachment, blunted or flat affect resembling depression, lack of joy and enthusiasm for activities, and failure to appreciate a purpose in what one is doing. In some circumstances, mood may become labile. Anger is not uncommon.
- Difficulty concentrating and becoming hypervigilant or fearful in situations that resemble the cause of the PTSD. Persons may startle easily, have periods of anger or sadness, feel generally unsettled, and suffer from poor sleep. It becomes difficult for them to make decisions.
- If a person has been witness to a catastrophic or horrible event, he or she may feel "survivor guilt." In addition, there may be elements of emotional shock, grief, resentment, helplessness, and hopelessness. There may also be frank depression, alcohol or drug abuse, severe anxiety, and panic attacks.
- Physical symptoms include headaches, easy startling, tachycardia, loss of appetite, loss of sex drive, and muscle aches.

Treatment

1. Persons who have experienced a traumatic event should share emotional support, eat and sleep properly, rest when fatigued, and maintain communications with friends and family.
2. Available evidence indicates that psychologic debriefing is not associated with benefits and may in fact complicate recovery after a disaster. Debriefing, which usually involves some review of the disaster, may increase physiologic hyperreactivity, increase the coding of traumatic memories, and promote rumination about the tragedy; debriefing can thus interfere with more adaptive and natural healing mechanisms (e.g., avoiding thinking about the trauma). If debriefing is used, it should be voluntary, involve clinical assessment, and be performed only by experienced and well-trained individuals.
3. Anxiolytic drugs are not recommended for the treatment of acute PTSD and have been associated with an increased incidence of PTSD.
4. Cognitive therapy may be useful to understand the root cause and achieve desensitization. It is very important after a traumatic event to allow a sufficient period of time for the individual to achieve rest, regain a normal menu and pace of activities, and not be compelled to explain their experiences to persons who might not understand.
5. Find outlets for mood swings. Use forms of expression to work through or even purge thoughts of sadness and disappointment.
6. Support groups may be helpful to some patients, but attendance should be voluntary.

36 Global Humanitarian Relief and Disaster Medicine

Wilderness medicine practitioners are ideally suited for international humanitarian and disaster medicine. Different types of events require unique and common considerations for preparation and practice, as well as for personal health, safety, and recovery. These events and episodes include armed conflict, population displacement, natural disasters, disease epidemics, sexual violence and mental illness, famine and malnutrition, and neglected diseases.

In order to be an effective responder, one needs to understand the capabilities, usual roles, and limitations of agencies and actors. These include the affected population, national government and local groups, the United Nations, foreign governments, the Red Cross (and equivalents), nongovernmental organizations (NGOs), religious or faith-based organizations, private corporations, donor agencies, academic institutions, ministries of health, the World Health Organization, and volunteer medical groups.

CATEGORIES OF DISASTER AND COMPLEX HUMANITARIAN EMERGENCIES WITH FAR-REACHING NEGATIVE IMPACT

- Rapid-onset natural disasters (e.g., floods, earthquakes, tropical storms, volcanic eruptions)
- Slow-onset natural disasters (e.g., drought, famine, desertification)
- Complex humanitarian emergencies (e.g., war)
- Epidemics (e.g., cholera, Ebola virus disease)
- Sudden large population movements
- Technologic disasters (e.g., pollution, spillage, explosion, fire)

NEEDS IN HUMANITARIAN CRISES

1. Water. Each individual should have, on average, 15 L/day of clean water for drinking, cooking, and personal hygiene. Water-gathering points should be within 500 m (1640 ft) of each household, with individuals queuing for no longer than 15 minutes and able to fill a 20-L container in 3 minutes or less.
2. Sanitation. A maximum of 20 people should use each toilet. Toilets should be segregated by gender. Toilets should be no more than 50 m (164 ft) from homes. Security concerns should be taken into account.
3. Food and nutrition. Each person should be provided with at least 2100 Kcal/d. Micronutrients, such as vitamin A, should be

provided to populations exhibiting symptoms of or at risk for deficiency. Whenever possible, local food sources should be used.
4. Shelter, security, and site planning. Adequate shelter, essential nonfood items, and security for displaced persons should be provided. Temporary shelters should provide a minimum of 3.5 m² of covered space per person. These arrangements should ensure adequate access to essential needs and keep families and social networks intact. Culturally acceptable nonfood items include the following:
   a. Clothing
   b. Bedding
   c. Pots
   d. Plates
   e. Utensils
   f. Soap
   g. Burial materials
   h. Lighting

HEALTH CARE IN THE EMERGENCY PHASE

Health care needs include acute, epidemic, and chronic trauma and medical illnesses, and malnutrition. One should anticipate being able to treat surgical disease, mental health disorders, obstetric conditions, and chronic diseases.
1. Control of communicable diseases and epidemics
   a. Measles
   b. Typhus
   c. Cholera and other infectious diarrheal diseases
   d. Meningococcal meningitis
   e. Relapsing fever
   f. Typhoid fever
   g. Respiratory illnesses
   h. Influenza
   i. Hepatitis A and E
   j. Leishmaniasis
   k. Malaria
   l. Scabies
   m. Hemorrhagic fevers
   n. Plague
   o. Japanese encephalitis
   p. Whooping cough
   q. Tetanus
   r. Poliomyelitis
   s. Conjunctivitis
   t. Guinea worm
2. Mass vaccination campaigns for such diseases as measles and tetanus
3. Public health surveillance to collect demographic, mortality, morbidity, needs, and program activity data

PRINCIPLES OF HEALTH ASSESSMENT IN DISASTERS AND CRISES

The objective of a health-related humanitarian intervention during the acute phase of an emergency is to reduce the number of deaths and to stabilize the population's health situation. A rapid health assessment (RHA) protocol should be followed.

The following are the main methods employed in any RHA:
- Review of existing information
- Interviews
- Observation
- Rapid surveys

Key questions to be answered by the RHA are as follows:
- Is there an emergency?
- What are the type, impact, and possible evolution of the emergency?
- What is the most severely affected geographic area and catchment population?
- What is the main health problem(s)?
- What is the existing response capacity?
- What are the critical information gaps for follow-up assessments?
- What are the priority actions for immediate response?
- What are the resources needed to implement the priority actions?

FUNDAMENTAL HUMANITARIAN PRINCIPLES

- *Humanity.* Humanitarian assistance is provided without discrimination to prevent and alleviate suffering wherever it is found.
- *Impartiality.* Humanitarian assistance makes no discrimination as to nationality, race, religious beliefs, class, or political opinions. It gives priority to the most urgent cases of distress.
- *Neutrality.* Humanitarian assistance may not take sides in hostilities or engage at any time in controversies of a political, racial, religious, or ideological nature.
- *Independence.* Humanitarian assistance must always maintain its autonomy by resisting any interference capable of diverting it from the course of action laid down by the requirements of humanity, impartiality, and neutrality.
- *Voluntary.* Humanitarian assistance is not prompted in any manner by desire for personal, political, or financial gain.

PROFESSIONAL CHARACTERISTICS OF THE AID WORKER

- Highest level of clinical skills
- Types of providers: emergency medicine, pediatrics, infectious diseases, obstetrics and gynecology, surgery, family and community medicine, mental health
- Knowledge of tropical medicine

- Team approach attitude and ability to work with others
- Humility
- Prior professional experience in resource-poor settings
- Communication skills, including the ability to speak a foreign language, particularly a knowledge of key phrases
- Alliance with language interpreters
- Keeping availability up to date
- Management and leadership capacities
- Appropriate behavior and cultural sensitivity; excellent bedside manner

HOW TO PREPARE FOR A MISSION

Prepare to

- Keep personal affairs in good order prior to the mission
- Deliver medical care in a crisis that might involve hundreds to thousands of patients
- Live, work, and thrive in austere conditions
- Manage trauma victims
- Manage infectious diseases, common pediatric illnesses, obstetrics and gynecology, and chronic diseases
- Manage public health emergencies predicted to occur in a postdisaster or humanitarian crisis setting
- Work outside of one's skill set, both medical and nonmedical
- Deal with death
- Recognize personal stress and posttraumatic stress disorder

AFTER RETURNING FROM A MISSION

- Do not expect friends and family to understand the stresses undergone by responders
- Rely on professional psychosocial support
- Anticipate reverse culture shock
- Plan "down time"
- Take time off before leaving on the next mission
- Do not become financially dependent on humanitarian work
- Seek medical care for posttravel illnesses

SUGGESTED PACKING LIST
Documents

Passport* (plus copy).
Visa* (plus copy)
Immunization card* (plus copy)
Air ticket* (plus copy)
Letter of invitation by NGO*
Medical evacuation insurance card* (plus copy)
Health insurance card*
Trip cancellation insurance*
International calling card*
Driver's license (consider an international driver's license)*

---

*These items should be packed in your carry-on bag.

ATM/credit cards (may not work)*
Cash (generally US currency, but check with contacts)*
Copy of medical school diploma
Copy of medical license
Curriculum vitae and/or resume
Hospital identification badge
Business cards
Extra passport photos
Address/contact list* (see below)

Gifts to Bring Your Team
Chocolate
Cheese
Newspapers
Movies
Comfort foods (relevant to the cultures of teammates)
Coffee
Gift packages for your teammates from their families sent to you
    before departure

Address or Contact List*
Field supervisor and local contacts
Arrival and airport contacts
Local embassy
Family and friends
Lost ATM or credit card reporting
Medical evacuation company
Health insurance company
Local airline office
Travel agent

Gear
Money belt*
Day pack
Alarm clock (that runs on batteries)
Headlamps or flashlights*
Mosquito net
Sunglasses
Sleep sack
Rain protection
Duct tape
Swiss Army knife (not for carry-on)
Sewing kit
Earplugs
Pocket tissues (toilet paper)*
Baby wipes
Luggage locks (for hotel, not flight)
Quick-dry travel towel
Flip-flops or shower sandals
Bandana or scarf

Travel clothesline
Laundry detergent
Sink stopper
Zip-lock bags
Water purifier or disinfection tablets
Phrasebook
Travel guide*
Stethoscope
White coat, surgical scrubs (where applicable)
Pocket medical references

Electronics

Laptop and power cord*
Electrical adapters and converter*
Surge protector
Flash drive*
Unlocked cell phone and charger*
Music player and charger*
Camera and memory cards*
Other cables and adapters
Handheld calculator
Extra batteries

First-Aid Kit

Sunscreen
Insect repellent
Antimalarial prophylaxis
Human immunodeficiency virus (HIV) postexposure prophylaxis
Alcohol-based hand sanitizer
Traveler's diarrhea antibiotic(s)
Antidiarrheal
Laxative
Acetaminophen or ibuprofen
Decongestant
Antihistamine
Albuterol inhaler
Prednisone
Fluconazole
Bacitracin ointment
Antiemetic
Vitamins
Oral contraceptive and emergency contraceptive
Condoms
Adhesive bandages
Blister dressings
Alcohol wipes
Cloth tape
Wound closure strips
Safety pins
Tweezers

Spare eyeglasses or contact lenses
Sunglasses
Sutures and needle driver
Nitrile gloves

Toiletries
Toothbrush and toothpaste
Dental floss
Shampoo and soap
Comb and brush
Razor and shaving cream
Deodorant
Contact lens kit
Eyeglasses (and spare)
Sunscreen
Makeup
Mirror
Lotions and creams
Lip balm
Tampons
Facecloth
Prescription medicines*

Extras
Notebook, journal, and pens
Photos from home
Gum, candy, and protein bars
Instant coffee packages and teabags
Magazines and novels
Playing cards and games
Textbooks and equipment donations

Snake and Other Reptile Bites

DEFINITIONS AND CHARACTERISTICS

Two main families of venomous snakes indigenous to the United States are Crotalidae (pit vipers) and Elapidae (coral snakes). Most snakebites are caused by the pit vipers, so called because of a depression, or pit, in the maxillary bone. Rattlesnakes (see Plate 7), the cottonmouth (water moccasin) snake (see Plate 8), and the copperhead snake (see Plate 9) are members of the pit viper family. The major snakes of medical importance outside of North America are the cobras, mambas, kraits, coral snakes, Australian elapids, sea snakes, vipers, rattlesnakes, asps, and colubrids (rear-fanged snakes). The fastest pit viper can crawl at a maximum speed of approximately 4.8 km/hr (3 mph). The speed of a pit viper's strike has been clocked at 2.4 m/sec (8 ft/sec); the snake can reach distances of approximately half its body length.

Identifying characteristics of pit vipers include the following (Fig. 37.1):

- Depression, or pit, in the maxillary bone, located midway between and below the level of the eye and the nostril on each side of the head
- Vertical elliptic pupils ("cat's eye")
- Triangular head distinct from the remainder of the body
- Single row of subcaudal scutes, or scales
- May have rattles on the tail
- One or two fangs on each side of the head

Two members of the coral snake family, Elapidae, are found in the United States: the western coral snake *(Micruroides euryxanthus)* (see Plate 10), found in Arizona and New Mexico, and the eastern coral snake *(Micrurus fulvius)* (see Plate 11), distributed from coastal North Carolina through the Gulf states to western Texas. The elapids differ from pit vipers in having very short fangs, round pupils, and subcaudal scales in a double row. Because many nonpoisonous mimics occur in coral snake territory, the rule of thumb for identifying a venomous species is that red bands bordered by yellow or white indicate a venomous reptile, whereas red bands bordered by black indicate a nonvenomous reptile. This rule applies to all coral snakes native to the United States but does not apply to species found south of Mexico City and in other non-US countries. A few essentially harmless, rear-fanged colubrid snakes in the United States, such as the night snake and lyre snake, possess elliptic pupils but lack facial pits.

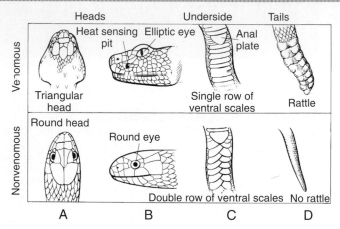

FIGURE 37.1 Identification of venomous pit vipers. **A,** Triangular head. **B,** Elliptic eye; heat-sensing facial pits on sides of head near nostrils. **C,** Single row of ventral scales leading up to anal plate. **D,** Rattles on tail (baby rattlesnakes have only "buttons" but are still quite venomous).

PIT VIPER ENVENOMATION

The clinical presentation of pit viper envenomation is quite variable and depends on the circumstances of the bite. Important factors include the species, size, and health of the snake; age and health of the victim; the circumstances that led to the bite; number of bites and their anatomic locations; and quality of the care rendered to the victim, in both the field and the hospital. Most bites occur to the lower extremities, followed by an upper extremity; they often coincide with the victim's intentional interaction with the snake (e.g., tormenting or attempting to capture the animal or handling a captive specimen). Most bites occur around dawn or dusk and during warmer months, when snakes and people are more active outdoors. About 75% to 80% of pit viper bites result in envenomation. Approximately 35% of snakebites result in mild envenomation, 25% moderate, and 10% to 15% severe. Observe the patient closely for signs and symptoms.

Signs and Symptoms

- *Common:* local burning pain immediately after the bite, weakness, nausea and vomiting, paresthesias, pain, fang marks, swelling and edema (usually within 5 minutes), faintness, dizziness
- *Less common:* ecchymosis, fasciculations, hypotension, bullae, necrosis, thirst, increased salivation, unconsciousness, blurred vision, increased respiratory rate
- Without treatment
  - May have rapidly progressing edema that can involve an entire extremity within 1 hour if envenomation is severe (Table 37.1)

Table 37.1	Grades of Envenomation
ENVENOMATION	**CHARACTERISTICS**
None	Fang marks but no local or systemic reactions
Minimal	Fang marks, local swelling and pain, but no systemic reactions
Moderate	Fang marks and swelling progressing beyond the site of the bite; systemic signs and symptoms such as nausea, vomiting, paresthesias, or hypotension
Severe	Fang marks present with marked swelling of the extremity, subcutaneous ecchymosis, severe symptoms including manifestations of coagulopathy

- More often spreads slowly, over 6 to 12 hours
- Edema that is soft, pitting, and limited to subcutaneous tissues
- Hemorrhagic blebs and bullae developing at the site of the bite within hours to days.
- Paresthesias of the scalp, face, and lips along with periorbital muscle fasciculations, indicating that a significant envenomation has occurred
  - Patient may complain of a rubbery or metallic taste in the mouth
  - General symptoms: weakness, sweating, nausea, faintness
- Hemorrhage manifested as skin petechiae, epistaxis, hematemesis, melena, hemoptysis, and blindness; pulmonary edema possible
- With some Mohave Desert rattlesnakes, bites produce neuro-muscular blockade, leading to respiratory paralysis in the absence of a significant local tissue reaction. Paralysis initially appears as cranial nerve deficits (hoarseness, difficulty swallowing, ptosis) and progresses to involve the diaphragm.

Treatment

1. Direct treatment at reducing venom effects, minimizing tissue damage, and preventing complicated sequelae.
2. Provide out-of-hospital management.
   a. Avoid panic. Instruct the patient to back out of the snake's striking range, which is approximately the length of the snake.
   b. Attempts to secure or kill the snake are not recommended because of the risk for additional bites to the patient or rescuer and because precious time can be lost. Absolute identification of the snake is not necessary for treatment. However, if the snake has been killed and plans are made to transport it, do not handle it directly; arrange to transport it in a closed container. Handle the snake using a stick that is longer than the snake. A severed snake head may envenom

for 20 to 60 minutes after decapitation. If a photograph of the snake can be taken from a safe distance, this can be used for identification.

   c. Immobilize the bitten extremity by splinting as if for a fracture. Keep the limb well padded at heart level (neither elevated nor lowered) in a position of function. Measure the bitten limb's circumference at two or more sites every 15 minutes, and mark areas of redness and swelling with a pen.

   d. Obtain medical assistance. Arrange for the patient, with minimal exertion, to be transported to the nearest medical facility.

   e. Encourage the patient to drink liquids to maintain adequate hydration.

   f. Treat pain (IV, IM, or SC opioids preferred if available).

   g. Remove any tight clothing or jewelry from involved extremities and anticipate swelling.

3. The pressure immobilization technique (see later for coral snakebite treatment) is not routinely recommended. If it is employed, the bandage should not be removed until antivenom is ready to be infused (if patient is asymptomatic) or is infusing (if patient is symptomatic) because of a potential bolus venom release after its removal. This technique may be considered in high-risk cases. High risk for potentially severe envenomation may include cases that involve large snakes, particularly venomous snakes, or when there is a history of prolonged fang contact. Risks for poor outcome may be higher in patients with previous venomous snakebites (treated or not) and in those who experience delays to medical care and antivenom administration.

4. Several old and scientifically unproven remedies are no longer recommended for snakebite (Box 37.1).

   a. Application of a tourniquet is no longer advised. An arterial-occlusive tourniquet represents a decision to sacrifice a limb to minimize systemic symptoms and save a life but has not been proven effective and may be harmful. A lympho-occlusive (a pressure of ≈20 mm Hg) constriction band applied proximal to the bite has been suggested but never proven to be helpful.

BOX 37.1   Treatments to Avoid in Pit Viper and Coral Snakebites

- Cutting and/or suctioning of the wound
- Ice
- NSAIDs
- Prophylactic antibiotics
- Prophylactic fasciotomy
- Routine use of blood products
- Shock therapy (electricity)
- Steroids (except for allergic phenomena)
- Tourniquets

NSAID, Nonsteroidal antiinflammatory drug.

If this method is chosen, take care to allow arterial inflow to the affected limb.

b. Incision and suction of the bite wound by mouth is not recommended.

c. Incision of the bite site across fang marks is not recommended.

d. Use of a negative-pressure device to extract venom is not recommended. The Extractor was claimed to remove a clinically significant amount of venom if applied over the bite site within 3 minutes of the bite and left in place for 30 to 60 minutes. However, it may also promote local necrosis in the pattern of the applied suction, and studies discourage its use.

e. Electroshock therapy can be dangerous to patients and has no proven value in managing bites by venomous snakes.

f. Immersion cryotherapy is not recommended because freezing or vasoconstricting already compromised tissues may contribute to necrosis. Local application of ice to the bite wound as a first-aid measure is not recommended.

5. Antivenom use in the field can be recommended only when a qualified physician is on the scene and when all equipment (including definitive airway management equipment) and drugs are available to manage a potential anaphylactic/anaphylactoid reaction to the serum. Backpacking the extensive equipment and drugs necessary to administer intravenous antivenom is cumbersome, and severe anaphylaxis must be anticipated. The currently recommended antivenom product for pit viper envenomations in North America, CroFab, poses a lesser risk for severe allergic reactions and may prove to be safe enough for field use, but it is not yet recommended for out-of-hospital use.

6. Hospital management of snakebite is beyond the scope of this book. *Auerbach's Wilderness Medicine*, 7th ed., or the local poison control center (1-800-222-1222) can be consulted.

7. Prophylactic antibiotics are unnecessary in most cases. If infection occurs, the initial antibiotic choice should be broad so as to cover gram-positive and gram-negative bacteria, aerobes, and anaerobes; it should be further guided by wound cultures and sensitivities.

8. Upon arrival at a medical facility, caregivers should ensure that the patient is adequately immunized against tetanus.

CORAL SNAKE ENVENOMATION

In the United States, bites by the eastern coral snakes (*M. fulvius*) tend to be more severe than those by Texas coral snakes (*M. fulvius tenere*), and both are significantly more dangerous than those of Sonoran coral snakes (*M. euryxanthus*). Because they have a less efficient venom delivery system, coral snakes effectively envenom only 40% of their victims. Following envenomation, the earliest symptoms may be nausea and vomiting, followed by

headache, abdominal pain, diaphoresis, and pallor. Severe envenomation results in predominantly neurotoxic sequelae.

Signs and Symptoms
- Little or no pain and no local edema or necrosis; fang marks
  may be difficult to see; venom is primarily neurotoxic.
- Within 90 minutes of envenomation, weak or numb feeling in
  bitten extremity.
- Several hours later, systemic symptoms appear, including tremors,
  drowsiness or euphoria, and marked salivation; systemic signs
  and symptoms may be delayed as long as 13 hours after significant
  bites and can then progress rapidly.
- After 5 to 10 hours, slurred speech and diplopia develop as
  cranial nerve palsies evolve.
  - Bulbar paralysis: manifested as dysphagia and dyspnea.
  - Total flaccid paralysis is possible.
- Paresthesias and muscle fasciculations common at the site of
  the bite.
- Flaccid paralysis, respiratory failure.
- Nausea and vomiting, weakness, dizziness, difficulty breathing.
- Less common: local edema, diplopia, dyspnea, diaphoresis,
  myalgia, confusion.
- Death is extremely rare.

Treatment
1. Apply the pressure immobilization technique. This technique
   (Fig. 37.2) has been used successfully to manage certain elapid
   snakebites and funnel-web spider bites in Australia as well as
   marine envenomations. The efficacy of the technique depends
   on collapsing small superficial lymphatic and venous vessels to
   retard venom uptake and distribution. Possible disadvantages
   include increased local tissue damage in crotalid bites because
   of the necrotizing effect of the venom if it remains localized to
   certain sites over time. Therefore it is not recommended for use
   with crotalid bites but might on rare occasion be considered
   when the deleterious local effects must be balanced against the
   life-threatening situation that would follow the systemic distribution of venom. This technique may be considered in high-risk
   cases. High risk for potentially severe envenomation may include
   cases that involve large snakes, particularly venomous snakes,
   or when there is a history of prolonged fang contact. Risks for
   poor outcome may be higher in patients with previous venomous
   snakebites (treated or not) and in those who experience delays
   to medical care and antivenom administration.
   a. To apply the pressure immobilization technique for venom
      sequestration, if the bite location permits, place a cloth or
      gauze pad (6 to 8 cm [2.4 to 3.1 inches] in size and 6 to
      8 cm by 2 cm [0.8 inch] thick) directly over the area and
      hold it firmly in place with a circumferential bandage 15 to
      18 cm (5.9 to 7 inches) wide applied at lymphatic-venous

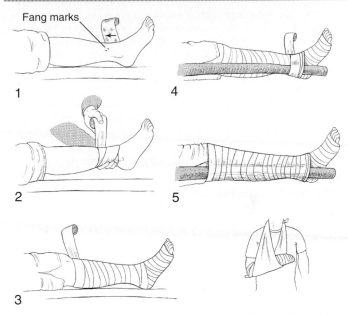

FIGURE 37.2 Australian pressure immobilization technique. This technique has proved effective in the management of elapid and sea snake envenomations. Its efficacy in viperid (true viper) bites has yet to be evaluated clinically.

occlusive pressure. If such a cloth or gauze pad is not available, the circumferential bandage may be used alone. Take care not to occlude the arterial circulation, as determined by the detection of arterial pulsations and proper capillary refill.

   b. Splint the limb and do not release the bandage until after the patient has been transported to definitive medical care or after 24 hours. Take care to check frequently that swelling beneath the bandage has not compromised the arterial circulation.

2. Note that because it is difficult to ascertain early whether envenomation by a coral snake has occurred, treatment and observation are mandatory. Early treatment with antivenom is advised in any suspected bite with envenomation because the onset of signs and symptoms can be delayed. Therefore transport the bitten patient to a medical facility where antivenom therapy can be administered.

3. North American Coral Snake Antivenom is effective against envenomations by the eastern coral snake (*M. fulvius*) and Texas coral snake (*M. fulvius tenere*). The single existing lot had expired in 2008, but it is tested and expiration is extended annually at the request of the US Food and Drug Administration

(FDA). For assistance with a suspected envenomation or current information about antivenom availability, contact a local snakebite specialist or the poison control center at 1-800-222-1222 or online at http://www.poisoncentertampa.org/antivenin/coral-snake-antivenin.aspx.

4 Monitor the patient's airway for swelling and difficulty breathing and swallowing.

5. Control pain with judicious titration of opiates (if available).

6. Avoid ineffective treatments that may cause the patient harm and delay transportation to definitive care (see Box 37.1).

ENVENOMATION BY NON–NORTH AMERICAN SNAKES
Signs and Symptoms

- For elapids (cobras, mambas, kraits, Australian venomous snakes, coral snakes):
  - *Local:* findings absent or minimal, significant pain with some species, regional lymphadenopathy and necrosis with some species, edema with some species
  - *Systemic:* neurotoxicity (cranial nerve dysfunction, ptosis, dysphonia, blurred vision, altered mental status, peripheral weakness and paralysis, respiratory failure) with delayed (up to 10 hours) onset possible, hypersalivation, diaphoresis, cardiovascular failure, coagulopathy, myonecrosis, renal failure
  - Eye exposure to venom from any of the spitting cobras or ringhals: immediate burning pain and tearing, which may lead to corneal ulceration, uveitis, and permanent blindness
- For sea snakes:
  - *Local:* trivial tissue damage, fang marks difficult to identify, fangs or teeth may be left in wound
  - *Systemic:* neurotoxicity (cranial nerve dysfunction, peripheral weakness and paralysis, respiratory failure), hypersalivation, dysphagia, dysarthria, trismus, muscle spasm, myotoxicity with resulting muscle pain and tenderness, rhabdomyolysis, myoglobinemia, myoglobinuria, hyperkalemia
- For vipers and pit vipers:
  - *Local:* pain, soft tissue swelling, regional lymphadenopathy, ecchymosis, bloody exudate from fang marks, hemorrhagic bullae; early absence of findings does not rule out significant envenomation; local necrosis possibly significant
  - *Systemic:* any organ system can potentially be involved; cardiovascular toxicity (hypotension, pulmonary edema), neurotoxicity (cranial nerve dysfunction, peripheral weakness) with some species, hemorrhagic diathesis, renal failure, altered taste sensation, headache, diarrhea, vomiting, fever, abdominal pain, hypotension
- For burrowing asps:
  - *Local:* single fang puncture mark common, severe pain, some swelling, lymphadenopathy, occasional local necrosis

- *Systemic:* nausea, vomiting, diaphoresis, fever, respiratory distress, cardiac arrhythmias
- For colubrids:
  - *Local:* mild to moderate local swelling, pain, ecchymosis, bloody exudate from fang marks
  - *Systemic:* nausea, vomiting, coagulopathy, renal dysfunction, headache

Treatment

1. Initiate same field treatment as for North American pit viper envenomation. Use the pressure immobilization technique for bites of elapids, sea snakes, burrowing asps, colubrids, and any unknown snake when the bite does not produce significant local pain.
2. Avoid wasting time on potentially dangerous therapies with no proven benefit (see Box 37.1).
3. Treat pain (acetaminophen or opiates preferred, avoid nonsteroidal antiinflammatory drugs [NSAIDs] because of increased risk for bleeding).
4. Treat nausea with ondansetron 4 to 8 mg PO or IV or promethazine 12.5 to 25 mg IM.
5. Anaphylaxis should be treated with aqueous epinephrine 0.1% (1:1000) (0.3 to 0.5 mL in adults, 0.01 mL/kg in children) by intramuscular injection, followed by a histamine-1 blocker such as chlorpheniramine maleate (10 mg in adults, 0.2 mg/kg in children).
6. Treat respiratory distress by placing patient in the recovery position and providing supplemental oxygen if available. Patients with severe respiratory distress may require endotracheal intubation and mechanical ventilation.
7. If in a remote or wilderness setting, follow the algorithm in Fig. 37.3 and arrange to transport the patient as quickly as possible to the nearest appropriate medical facility where antivenom therapy can be initiated (see Appendix S).

VENOMOUS LIZARD BITES

The Gila monster (see Plate 12) and Mexican beaded lizard (see Plate 13) are found in North America. Both possess venom glands and grooved teeth. Human envenomation most often occurs when the lizard retains its grasp and chews on the patient.

Signs and Symptoms

- Usually simple puncture wounds, although teeth may break off or be shed during the bite and remain in the wound
- Pain, often severe and burning, at the wound site within 5 minutes
  - Pain radiating up the extremity
  - Intense pain lasting 3 to 5 hours and then subsiding after 8 hours

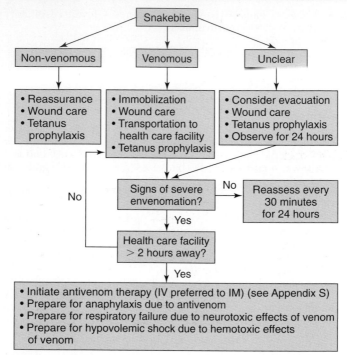

FIGURE 37.3 Algorithm indicating appropriate management for a suspected venomous snakebite in a patient while in a remote or wilderness location. Many health centers and district hospitals in non-US countries may be able to provide tetanus prophylaxis and wound care, but they may not have a supply of antivenom. If a suspected venomous snakebite has occurred or if the snake species is unclear, the 24-hour observation period is best done near a health care facility that has antivenom in the event symptoms develop. In remote settings, it may be appropriate to administer antivenom immediately in patients showing moderate or severe symptom. This should be performed only by a skilled health care provider who has the capacity to treat antivenom side effects (e.g., anaphylaxis, hypotension, respiratory arrest). If a provider has antivenom but not the capacity to treat severe side effects, it may be desirable to wait until the antivenom can be administered at a health care facility with more advanced capabilities. This decision should be guided by the severity of envenomation, type of antivenom (e.g., likelihood of anaphylaxis for the specific preparation), and time to evacuation to the health care facility. *IV*, Intravenous; *IM*, intramuscular.

- Edema at the wound site, usually within 15 minutes, that progresses slowly in variable degrees up the extremity
- Cyanosis or blue discoloration around the wound
- Weakness, fainting, diaphoresis, nausea, vomiting, difficulty breathing, paresthesias

- Tenderness at the wound site for 3 to 4 weeks after the bite but usually little tissue necrosis
- Hypotension rare; no coagulation defects noted

Treatment

A Gila monster may hang on tenaciously during a bite; mechanical means may be required to loosen the grip of the jaws.

1. Cleanse the wound thoroughly with a soap-and-water scrub or with a dilution of povidone-iodine.
2. Infiltrate the puncture wounds with 1% lidocaine using a 25-gauge needle and then probe the wounds to detect the presence of shed or broken teeth, thus helping to prevent future infection from a foreign body.
3. Administer an analgesic appropriate for the degree of pain.
4. A bandage to stop bleeding and provide immobilization may be beneficial.
5. As with snakebites, avoid use of suction devices, ligatures, pressure immobilization, incisions, electrotherapy, and ice compression (see Box 37.1).

Disorders involving the bites or stings of arthropods in this chapter include:
- Spiders
- Bees and wasps
- Ants
- Caterpillar spine irritations
- Sucking bugs
- Beetles
- Flies and other winged insects
- Lice, fleas, mites, chiggers
- Ticks
- Scorpions

DISORDERS
SPIDER BITES

Spiders use their venom to capture, immobilize, and/or predigest prey. Therefore the bites of many spiders cause local reactions in humans, which may include immediate pain, swelling, erythema, and blisters. The local skin reaction usually lasts from minutes to hours but occasionally may persist for days. Unless the venom is from a toxic species, there are few or no systemic symptoms and all treatment is symptomatic.

Brown ("Fiddleback" or "Recluse") Spiders

Necrotic arachnidism, or loxoscelism, is caused by spiders of the genus *Loxosceles* and other spiders that deposit a venom characterized by its local dermonecrotic activity. The fiddleback spider (see Plate 14) carries the characteristic violin-shaped marking on the dorsum of its cephalothorax. The clinical spectrum of loxoscelism ranges from mild and transient skin irritation to severe local necrosis accompanied by hematologic and renal pathologic conditions.

Signs and Symptoms

- The most common presentation is an isolated cutaneous lesion.
- Local symptoms begin at the moment of the bite, with a sharp stinging sensation, although some patients report no awareness of having been bitten.
- Stinging subsides over 6 to 8 hours and is then replaced by aching and pruritus.
- The site becomes edematous, with an erythematous halo surrounding an irregularly shaped violaceous center of incipient necrosis; a white ring of vasospasm and ischemia may be discernible between the central lesion and the halo.

- Often the erythematous margin spreads irregularly, in a gravitationally influenced pattern that leaves the original center near the top of the lesion.
- In more severe cases, serous or hemorrhagic bullae arise at the center within 24 to 72 hours, with an underlying eschar (see Plate 15).
- Systemic reactions: hemoglobinuria within 24 hours of envenomation; fever, chills, maculopapular rash, weakness, leukocytosis, arthralgias, nausea, and vomiting within 24 hours of the bite.

Treatment
1. Apply cold (ice) compresses intermittently for the first 4 days after the bite. Do not apply heat.
2. Elevation and loose immobilization of the extremity may help to limit swelling.
3. Pain control may require opiate therapy.
4. If the wound appears infected, apply a topical antiseptic (mupirocin, bacitracin) under a sterile dressing. Administer an oral antibiotic such as cephalexin, dicloxacillin, or erythromycin (see Appendix H).
3. Seek advanced medical care to consider adjunctive measures for the bite wound and to evaluate for hospitalization for coagulopathy or renal failure caused by hemolysis and hemoglobinuria.
4. Obtain appropriate tetanus prophylaxis (when available).
5. Reported therapies include dapsone, glucocorticoids, hyperbaric oxygen, electric shock, antivenom, metronidazole, diphenhydramine, phentolamine, and cyproheptadine, although there is scant evidence to support their efficacy.

Widow Spiders
Female spiders of the genus *Latrodectus* carry the characteristic hourglass marking on the ventral abdomen (see Plate 16).

Signs and Symptoms
- The initial bite is sometimes sharply painful but often nearly painless, with only a tiny papule or punctum visible; surrounding skin is slightly reddened and sometimes indurated; in many cases no further progression of symptoms occurs.
- Neuromuscular symptoms: these can become dramatic within 30 to 60 minutes as involuntary spasms and rigidity can affect the large muscle groups of the abdomen, limbs, and lower back; the worst pain usually occurs within the first 8 to 12 hours but may remain severe for several days.
- A predominantly abdominal presentation may resemble an acute abdomen.
- Priapism, fasciculations, weakness, ptosis, thready pulse, fever, salivation, diaphoresis, vomiting, bronchorrhea, pulmonary edema, rhabdomyolysis, and hypertension with or without seizures may occur.

- The characteristic pattern of facial swelling, known as *Latrodectus* facies, may develop hours after the bite.

Treatment

The natural course of an envenomation is to resolve completely after a few days, although pain may last for a week or more.

1. Cleanse the bite site. Apply a cold (ice) pack to the bite site. Provide tetanus prophylaxis if available.
2. For muscle spasm, administer a benzodiazepine (e.g., diazepam 5 to 10 mg IV/IM, or lorazepam 1 to 2 mg IV/IM) or opiates (e.g., morphine 4 to 8 mg IV/IM/SC).
3. Administer pain medication (IV opiates preferable).
4. Calcium gluconate infusion, advocated in the past, has proved only minimally useful and is **no longer** recommended.
5. Monitor the patient for hypertension.
   a. Administer a centrally acting or vasodilating antihypertensive if the patient develops urgent hypertension and such a drug is available (e.g., nifedipine 30 to 60 mg ER PO daily, nicardipine 20 to 40 mg PO q8hr, or nicardipine IV drip started at 5 mg/hr IV and increased 2.5 mg/hr q5–15 min prn to a maximum of 15 mg/hr).
   b. Be alert for a seizure associated with rapid elevation in blood pressure.
5. Antivenom is available in the United States from Merck and Co.; in Australia from Commonwealth Serum Laboratories; and in South Africa from the National Health Laboratory Service. In general antivenom is recommended for respiratory arrest, seizures, uncontrolled hypertension, or pregnancy. The usual dose is one to three vials or ampules intravenously.
6. Recent studies suggest that most patients require only one vial of antivenom, and anaphylactic complications are rare.
7. All symptomatic children, pregnant women, and patients with a history of hypertension with suspected or confirmed envenomations should be admitted to a hospital for treatment and observation.

Funnel-Web Spiders

Funnel-web spiders (see Plate 17) are large, aggressive spiders that deliver a potent neurotoxin.

Signs and Symptoms

- Intense pain at the bite site lasting for 30 minutes with or without a local wheal surrounded by erythema; localized sweating
- Phase I
  - Begins minutes after venom injection, with local piloerection and muscle fasciculation; becomes generalized over the next 10 to 20 minutes
  - Intense pain at the bite site; perioral tingling, nausea and vomiting, diaphoresis, salivation, lacrimation, diarrhea

- Severe hypertension, tachycardia, hyperthermia, and coma
- Sporadic apnea and intense muscle writhing
- Phase II
  - Begins 1 to 2 hours after envenomation, as phase I symptoms begin to subside
  - Return of consciousness (if lost) and the appearance of recovery
  - In severe cases, gradually worsening hypotension, with periods of apnea and the onset of pulmonary edema

Treatment

1. In the field, apply the pressure immobilization technique for venom sequestration at the bite site (see Chapter 37).
2. Give specific antivenom, which is developed in rabbits and is the mainstay of treatment. Adult and pediatric dose is two ampules (100 mg purified IgG per ampule) of antivenom administered intravenously every 15 minutes until symptoms improve.
3. Be aware that general management, in addition to antivenom administration, is supportive.
   a. Give oxygen and intravenous fluid support.
   b. Use atropine 0.5 to 1 mg IV in adults and 0.02 mg/kg in children to lessen salivation and bronchorrhea.
   c. Administer a β-adrenergic blocking agent as needed to control severe hypertension and tachycardia.

Banana (Brazilian Wandering or Armed) Spiders

The *Phoneutria* spiders of South America are large nocturnal creatures noted for their aggressive behavior and painful bites.

Signs and Symptoms

- Severe local pain that radiates up the extremity into the trunk, followed within 10 to 20 minutes by tachycardia, hypertension, hypothermia, profuse diaphoresis, salivation, vertigo, visual disturbances, nausea and vomiting, and priapism.
- If death occurs (usually in 2 to 6 hours), it is usually caused by respiratory paralysis.

Treatment

1. Treat mild envenomation symptomatically by infiltrating the bite site with a local anesthetic.
2. Be aware that narcotics may potentiate the venom's respiratory depressant effect and should not be used.
3. For severe envenomation, administer monovalent antivenom (Belo Horizonte) or polyvalent antivenom (Sero Antiaracidico Polivalente, Instituto Butantan, available in Brazil).

Wolf Spiders

Wolf spiders are diurnal predators that are usually a mottled dark gray or brown (Fig. 38.1).

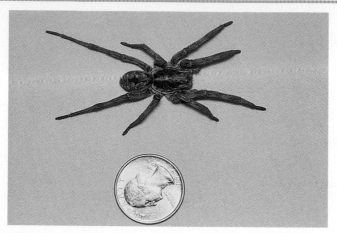

FIGURE 38.1 Wolf spider (*Lycosa* species). (Courtesy Arizona Poison & Drug Information Center, 1996.)

Signs and Symptoms
- Local pain, swelling, and erythema
- Rarely, necrosis

Treatment
1. Apply a cold (ice) pack to the bite site.
2. Administer oral pain medication or infiltrate the area with an anesthetic agent.

Tarantulas
Tarantulas are large, slow spiders (Fig. 38.2) capable of inflicting a painful bite when threatened. Several varieties possess urticating hairs, which they flick by the thousands through the air into an attacker's skin and eyes.

Signs and Symptoms
- Intense inflammation where hairs land, which may remain pruritic for weeks
- Aching or stinging pain at the bite site
- Keratoconjunctivitis

Treatment
1. Therapy is supportive and based on symptoms. To remove urticating hairs, apply and remove sticky tape from the skin in a few repeated applications.
2. Elevate the bitten extremity and immobilize it to reduce pain.
3. Administer analgesics as needed.
4. Topical or systemic corticosteroids and oral antihistamines may be used for urticating hair exposure.

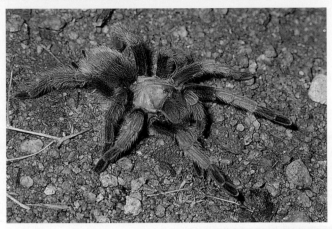

FIGURE 38.2   Mature female tarantula *Aphonopelma iodius*. (Courtesy Michael Cardwell & Associates, 1997.)

5. For eye exposure, irrigate the eyes and then consider ophthalmic antibiotic/corticosteroid ointment (e.g., combination bacitracin/ neomycin/polymyxin B/hydrocortisone ophthalmic ointment q3-4h for 5 to 7 days) for keratoconjunctivitis and follow up with an ophthalmologist as soon as possible.

Hobo Spiders
The bite of the hobo spider, also called the northwestern brown spider *(Tegenaria agrestis)*, can cause a necrotic reaction like that induced by the brown recluse spider.

Signs and Symptoms
- Local redness, vesiculation, and necrosis
- Systemic effects: headache, visual disturbances, hallucinations, weakness, and lethargy

Treatment
1. Apply cold (ice) compresses intermittently for the first 4 days after the bite. Do not apply heat.
2. If the wound appears infected, apply a topical antiseptic (mupirocin, bacitracin) under a sterile dressing. Administer an oral antibiotic such as cephalexin, dicloxacillin, or erythromycin (see Appendix H).

Running Spiders and Sac Spiders
Running and sac spiders are often nondescript spiders with yellow, brown, green, or olive coloration.

Signs and Symptoms
- Vary with species
- May include dyspnea, varying degrees of weakness, local redness, pain and edema, headache, fever, nausea, and necrosis

Treatment
1. Be aware that this lesion usually heals without problems provided that secondary infection does not develop.
2. Apply cool compresses, elevate the involved area, immobilize the patient, and give analgesics as needed.

HYMENOPTERA (BEES, WASPS, AND ANTS)
By far the most important venomous insects are members of the order Hymenoptera, including bees, wasps, and ants (Fig. 38.3). The abdomen and thorax are connected by a slender pedicle, which may be quite long in certain wasps and ants.

Signs and Symptoms
- Instantaneous pain, followed by a wheal-and-flare reaction, with variable edema. Most stings are on the head and neck, followed by the foot, leg, hand, and arm. Stings may occur in the mouth, pharynx, or esophagus if the insects are accidentally ingested.
- Fire ant stings may produce vesicles that subsequently become sterile pustules; this is caused by the ant grasping the skin with its mouthparts and inflicting multiple stings (Fig. 38.4).
- In the case of multiple bee, wasp, yellow jacket, or hornet stings, vomiting, diarrhea, generalized edema, dyspnea, hypotension, and collapse may develop. The lethal dose of honeybee venom has been estimated at 500 to 1500 stings.
- Large local reactions are relatively common, spreading more than 15 cm (5.9 inches) beyond the sting and persisting longer than 24 hours.
- Allergic sting reactions
  - Reactions occur in areas remote from the sting and typically include pruritus, hives, difficulty breathing, nausea, papular urticaria, and angioedema. Other symptoms include abdominal pain and vomiting.
  - When a reaction is life threatening, there is marked respiratory distress, hypotension, loss of consciousness, and arrhythmias.
  - Most fatalities occur from anaphylaxis, and most of these occur within 1 hour of the sting.

Treatment
1. The treatment of an anaphylactic reaction follows conventional guidelines, as follows:
   a. Maintain the airway and administer oxygen if available.
   b. Obtain intravenous or intraosseous access. Administer lactated Ringer's or normal saline solution to support the systolic blood pressure at a level of at least 90 mm Hg.
   c. Administer aqueous epinephrine 1:1000 intramuscularly in the prehospital setting at the first indication of serious

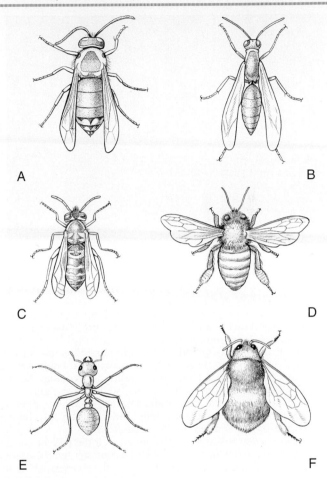

FIGURE 38.3 Representative venomous Hymenoptera. **A,** Hornet *(Vespula maculata)*; **B,** wasp *(Chlorion aerarium icheumerea)*; **C,** yellow jacket *(Vespula maculirons)*; **D,** honeybee *(Apis mellifera)*; **E,** fire ant *(Solenopsis invicta)*; **F,** bumblebee *(Bombus* species).

hypersensitivity. The dose for adults is 0.3 to 0.5 mL; for children younger than 12 years of age, it is 0.01 mL/kg, not to exceed 0.3 mL. An alternative is to inject the contents of an EpiPen or EpiPen Jr. intramuscularly into the lateral thigh region. An alternative is Adrenaclick or its authorized generic version. Repeat in 20 minutes for persistent symptoms. If the reaction is limited to pruritus and urticaria, there is no wheezing or facial swelling, and the patient is older than 45 years of age, administer an antihistamine and reserve epinephrine for a worsened condition.

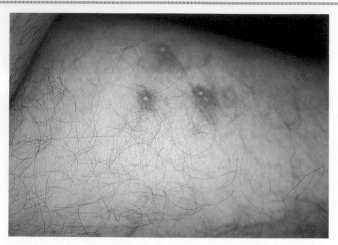

FIGURE 38.4   Fire ant lesions.

d. In the presence of profound hypotension, when the skin is not adequately perfused, 2 to 5 mL of a 1:10,000 epinephrine solution may be given by slow IV push, or an infusion may be initiated by mixing 1 mg in 250 mL and infusing at a rate of 0.25 to 1 mL/min.

e. Selective inhaled (nebulized) β_2-adrenergic agents, such as albuterol, can also be effective in relieving bronchospasm at doses of 2.5 mg/3 mL of a 0.08% solution. Local application of antihistamine lotions or creams, such as tripelennamine, may be helpful. An oral antihistamine, such as diphenhydramine, 25 to 50 mg for adults and 1 mg/kg for children every 6 hours is often an effective adjunct.

f. If the reaction is severe or prolonged or if the patient is regularly medicated with corticosteroids, administer hydrocortisone 200 mg, methylprednisolone 50 mg, or dexamethasone 15 mg IV with a 5-day oral course or 10-day oral taper to follow. The parenteral dose of hydrocortisone for children is 2.5 mg/kg. If the therapy is initiated orally, administer prednisone, 60 to 100 mg for adults and 1 mg/kg for children.

2. For mild hymenopteran stings, apply ice packs to provide relief.

3. Be aware that a honeybee or yellow jacket may leave an embedded stinger. Remove the stinger (and possibly, attached venom sac) as quickly as possible with a sharp edge or forceps. Do not be overly concerned about squeezing the sac—it is more important to remove the stinger and sac as quickly as possible.

4. Note that a home remedy such as a paste of unseasoned meat tenderizer or baking soda is of variable usefulness, although some report the former to be effective. Topical anesthetics in "sting sticks" have limited usefulness.

5. Because infection is common, apply antimicrobial ointment such as mupirocin to cover the wound. Debridement of fire ant blisters is not recommended.
6. Envenomation from multiple hymenopteran stings may require more aggressive therapy, including intravenous calcium gluconate (5 to 10 mL of 10% solution) in conjunction with a parenteral antihistamine and corticosteroid to relieve pain, swelling, and nausea and vomiting. A corticosteroid, such as methylprednisolone, 24 mg the first day then tapered over 5 days, often hastens resolution of a large local reaction to a bee or wasp sting.
7. Manage delayed serum sickness in response to multiple hymenopteran stings with a corticosteroid such as prednisone, 60 to 100 mg for adults and 1 mg/kg for children, tapered over 2 weeks.

LEPIDOPTERA (CATERPILLARS)

Injury usually follows contact with caterpillars and is less frequent with the cocoon or adult stage. The largest outbreaks have been associated with spines detached from live or dead caterpillars and cocoons.

Signs and Symptoms

- With caterpillars that have hollow spines and venom glands, instant nettling pain, followed by redness and swelling, after direct contact with the live insect
  - Ordinarily no systemic manifestations; symptoms subsiding within 24 hours
  - Possibly intense pain with central radiation, accompanied by nausea and vomiting, headache, fever, and lymphadenopathy
  - Rarely, coagulopathy
- With attached or detached spines from certain caterpillars or moths, itching and erythematous, papular, or urticarial rash within a few hours to 2 days after contact
  - Rash persisting for up to 1 week
  - Lesions rarely bullous
  - Conjunctivitis, upper respiratory tract irritation, rare asthma-like symptoms with or without dermatitis

Treatment

1. Apply adhesive tape, a commercial facial peel, or a thin layer of rubber cement to remove spines.
2. Administer an oral nonsteroidal anti-inflammatory drug.
3. If the dermatitis is severe and persistent, consider administering a corticosteroid such as prednisone, 60 to 100 mg for adults and 1 mg/kg for children, tapered over 10 days.
4. An oral antihistamine such as fexofenadine may be helpful.
5. Pain medication is added as needed to control discomfort.

HEMIPTERA (SUCKING BUGS)

"Sucking bugs" have sucking mouthparts, generally in the form of a beak. Included are the assassin bugs, kissing bugs (see

Fig. 38.6B), and flying bedbugs. Many of these bugs bite at night on exposed parts of the body. The bites themselves may be painless.

Signs and Symptoms
- On initial exposure, usually no reaction
- With repeated bites, erythematous pruritic papules that may persist for up to 1 week; bites are often grouped in a cluster or line and may be accompanied by giant urticarial wheals, lymphadenopathy, hemorrhagic bullae, and fever
- Systemic anaphylaxis possible
- Possible pain at the sting site
  - Local swelling that lasts several hours
  - With bedbugs, usually a pruritic wheal with central hemorrhagic punctum, followed by a reddish papule that persists for days

Treatment
Treatment is supportive.

BEETLES
Several families of beetles, such as blister and rove beetles, produce toxic secretions that may be deposited on the skin.

Signs and Symptoms
- With the blister beetle, contact is painless and seldom remembered by the patient; blisters induced by cantharidin toxin appear 2 to 5 hours after contact, generally as single or multiple areas, usually 5 to 50 mm (0.2 to 2 inches) in diameter and thin walled; unless broken or rubbed, they are not usually painful.
- The vesicant substance of the rove beetle is an alkaloid; if the beetle is crushed or rubbed on the skin, redness occurs after several hours, followed by a crop of small blisters that persist for 2 to 3 days; conjunctivitis occurs if the secretion is rubbed into the eyes.

Treatment
1. Treat beetle vesication as a superficial chemical burn.
2. Topical preparations containing corticosteroids and antihistamines are not particularly effective.

DIPTERA (TWO-WINGED FLIES, BITING MIDGES, AND MOSQUITOES)
Insects of this order have one pair of wings and are indiscriminate feeders on feces and human foodstuffs (Fig. 38.5). These habits make them by far the most important arthropod vectors of human disease. See Chapter 39 for information about protection against blood-feeding arthropods.

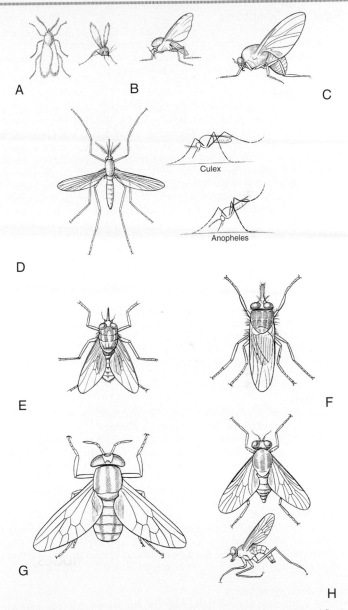

FIGURE 38.5   Blood-feeding biting flies (not drawn to scale). **A,** Sand fly; **B,** biting midge; **C,** blackfly; **D,** mosquito; **E,** stable fly; **F,** tsetse fly; **G,** tabanid fly; **H,** snipe fly.

Signs and Symptoms

- Immediate pruritic wheals followed in 12 to 24 hours by red, swollen, itchy lesions; can cause blistering or necrosis.
- Rarely, immune response leading to asthma, bullous eruptions, fever, lymphadenopathy, or hepatomegaly.

Mosquitoes

Mosquitoes are characterized by scaled wings, long legs, and a slender body. The size of these insects varies, but they rarely exceed 15 mm (0.6 inch) in length. They can fly at 1.4 to 2.6 km/hr (0.9 to 1.6 mph). Mosquitoes do not sting because there is no stinger; they pierce the skin and suck blood with their mouthparts. They identify their targets by scent as well as by the carbon dioxide of exhaled breath and some chemicals found in sweat. The female mosquito requires about 50 seconds to attach and approximately 2 minutes to finish feeding. Given their ability to transmit viruses, many of which are without immunizations or specific treatment, mosquitoes are of public health concern (Table 38.1). Mosquitos transmit many travel-acquired illnesses. (See Chapter 48 for further discussion on dengue fever, yellow fever, Zika virus, and Japanese encephalitis; see Chapter 47 for more discussion on malaria.)

Clinical Manifestations of Mosquito Bites

- Local irritation with soft pale wheal, with itching
- Papular urticaria with itching
- Occasional hive-like skin lesion, with itching
- Rare blisters, bullae, erythema multiforme, or purpura, with or without itching

Treatment

1. Immediately after the bite, apply a cold (ice) pack.
2. Apply a topical antipruritic lotion or cream.
3. If the reaction is severe or prolonged, consider the administration of a corticosteroid such as prednisone, 60 to 100 mg for adults and 1 mg/kg for children, for a 5-day course or tapered over 7 to 14 days.
4. A topical corticosteroid cream or ointment may be helpful.

West Nile Virus

West Nile virus is a single-stranded ribonucleic acid (RNA) virus. Mosquitoes are the vectors for this virus, and birds are the most common reservoir. Disease usually occurs in temperate zones either in late summer, early fall, or year-round in milder climates.

Signs and Symptoms

- The incubation period from bite to clinical infection is 3 to 14 days.
- Most infections are asymptomatic or associated with a mild influenza-like illness with fever, malaise, fatigue, difficulty

Table 38.1 Characteristics of Mosquito-Borne Viral Diseases						
VIRUS	FAMILY	GEOGRAPHIC DISTRIBUTION	MAIN AGE GROUP AFFECTED	MORTALITY (%)	SPECIFIC TREATMENT	HUMAN VACCINE AVAILABLE
Dengue fever virus	Flaviviridae	Central and South America, Africa, Asia, southeastern United States	Adults	Dengue: <1% Severe Dengue: >20	No	Limited*
Yellow fever virus	Flaviviridae	Africa and South America	Men ages 15–45	20	No	Yes
Japanese encephalitis	Flaviviridae	Japan, China, Southeast Asia, India	Children and adults	20–30	No	Yes
West Nile virus	Flaviviridae	Africa, West Asia, Middle East, Europe, United States	Adults	3–15	No	No
St Louis encephalitis	Flaviviridae	Central, western, southern United States	Adults	5–30	No	No
Eastern equine encephalitis	Togaviridae	East and Gulf Coasts of United States, southern United States, South America	Children and adults	33	No	No
Murray Valley encephalitis	Flaviviridae	Australia, Papua New Guinea	Children and adults	15–30	No	No

Continued

Table 38.1 Characteristics of Mosquito-Borne Viral Diseases—cont'd

VIRUS	FAMILY	GEOGRAPHIC DISTRIBUTION	MAIN AGE GROUP AFFECTED	MORTALITY (%)	SPECIFIC TREATMENT	HUMAN VACCINE AVAILABLE
La Crosse virus (California)	Bunyaviridae	Midatlantic and southeastern United States	Children	<1	No	No
Ross River virus	Togaviridae	Australia, Papua New Guinea, South Pacific	Children and adults	Rare	No	No
Jamestown Canyon virus	Bunyaviridae	United States (including Alaska) and Canada	Children and adults	Unknown	No	No
Chikungunya virus	Togaviridae	Africa, Asian Subcontinent, Southeast Asia, Americas	All	<1%	No	No
Zika virus	Flaviviridae	Central and South America, Africa, Southeast Asia, the Philippines	Children and adults	Unknown	No	No

*There is currently no dengue vaccine approved for use in the United States. A vaccine was approved for use in Mexico, but has yet to come to market as of publication. Various other dengue vaccines are currently under development.

concentrating, headache, nausea, vomiting, anorexia, lymph-adenopathy, and rash.
- Severe infections include encephalitis, meningitis, or menin-goencephalitis. Encephalitis may present with parkinsonian features or other movement disorders, such as myoclonus or intention tremor, or with acute flaccid paralysis or asymmetric weakness.

Treatment
No specific treatment is available. Therapy is symptomatic and supportive.

CUTANEOUS MYIASIS
Parasitism by fly larvae occurs when an insect such as the human botfly *(Dermatobia hominis)* deposits an egg on human skin. The egg hatches immediately, and the larva enters the skin through the bite of the carrier or through some other small break in the skin. The larvae grow to 15 to 20 mm (0.6 to 0.8 inch) under the skin.

Signs and Symptoms
- As the larvae grow under the skin, the initial pruritic papule becomes a furuncle with a characteristic central opening, from which serosanguineous fluid exudes (see Plate 18).
- Pain often accompanies movement of the older larvae, but lesions are not particularly tender to palpation.
- The tip of a larva may protrude from the central opening, or bubbles produced by its respiration may be seen.
- Lymphadenopathy, fever, and secondary infection are rare.

Treatment
1. Sometimes simple pressure will extrude the organism, particularly if it is small.
2. Occlusion of the breathing hole with heavy oil, nail polish, or animal fat (e.g., bacon) may cause the larva to emerge sufficiently for it to be grasped and withdrawn.
3. Alternatively, inject about 2 mL of local anesthetic into the base of the lesion, thus extruding the larva by fluid pressure.
4. If you attempt surgical excision under local anesthesia, take care not to break or rupture the larva, because this might result in an inflammatory reaction that predisposes to infection.

LICE (ORDER ANOPLURA)
Lice are very active, but nits (eggs) are easily identified as whitish ovals, about 0.5 mm (0.02 inch) long, attached firmly to one side of the hair. Machine washing and drying of sheets and clothing at hot settings will kill lice and nits.

Signs and Symptoms
- Small, red macule in response to secretions released by the louse during biting and feeding

- Characteristic body louse bite: a central hemorrhagic punctum in many of the macules
- Excoriations, crusts, eczematization in a parallel pattern from scratching, particularly on the shoulders, trunk, and buttocks (favorite sites for bites)
- Severe pruritus and inflammation caused by sensitization after repeated exposure to bites; patient possibly infested for weeks before pruritus becomes marked
- Occipital and posterior cervical adenopathy associated with head lice

Treatment

1. Treat head lice with one application of 1% permethrin cream rinse or 0.5% malathion lotion. Hair should be washed, rinsed, and dried and the treatment preparation applied for 10 to 20 minutes before being washed off. A fine-toothed comb may be used to remove nits after rinsing.
2. Combing should be repeated in 1 to 2 days to confirm treatment success. If head lice are resistant, use 0.3% pyrethrins and 3% piperonyl butoxide in combination. Use 1% hexachlorocyclohexane (lindane) shampoo for patients intolerant of permethrin. Note that lindane is contraindicated in children, infants, and pregnant women and should be used only as a last resort in elders. Apply it to the wet hair, lather, and leave it in place for 4 minutes before rinsing.
3. Repeat the treatment 7 to 10 days later as a precaution in case some nits were not killed by the first application.
4. Treat body lice with the same medications, but be aware that parasites and nits are not usually found on the skin. These must be eradicated from the clothing. Take a good bath and launder all clothing.
5. Treat pubic lice with the same medications. One method is to apply permethrin 1% cream rinse for 10 to 20 minutes and then rinse. Another method is to rub crotamiton lotion into the affected area daily for several weeks to destroy hatching ova and prevent a persistent infection.
6. Manage eyelash infection by careful application of physostigmine ophthalmic ointment using a cotton-tipped applicator.

FLEAS (ORDER SIPHONAPTERA) (Fig. 38.6A)

Signs and Symptoms

- Small, central, hemorrhagic puncta surrounded by erythema and urticaria; bullae or even ulceration after bite in highly sensitive individuals.
- Intensely pruritic, with scratching often resulting in crusting and the development of impetigo.
- Tungiasis caused by burrowing flea (jigger, chigo, sand flea), usually on the feet, buttocks, or perineum of a person who wears no shoes or frequently squats.

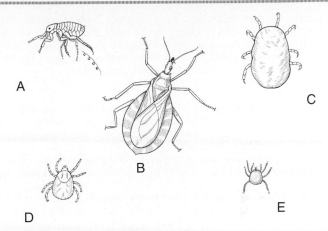

FIGURE 38.6   Various blood-feeding arthropods (not drawn to scale). **A,** Flea; **B,** kissing bug; **C,** soft tick; **D,** hard tick; **E,** chigger mite.

- Firm itchy nodule with posterior end of the flea visible as a dark plug or spot in the center of the nodule.
- Numerous papules aggregating into plaques with a honeycomb appearance.
- Secondary infection around each flea inevitable, resulting in ulceration and suppuration.

Treatment
1. Relieve pruritus by applying corticosteroid creams or calamine lotion with phenol.
2. Administer a systemic antihistamine to help control itching.
3. Clean excoriations and apply a topical antiseptic ointment such as mupirocin.
4. With a burrowing flea infestation (tungiasis), remove the burrowing flea or a pustule will rupture, leaving an ulcer.
5. Preparations containing 9.1% imidacloprid eliminate or reduce fleas on dogs when applied to the skin. An oral preparation used for dogs and cats contains lufenuron, an inhibitor of insect development.

MITES (CLASS ARACHNIDA, ORDER ACARINA)
The human scabies mite is *Sarcoptes scabiei* var. *hominis*. The adult female burrows into the epidermis.

Signs and Symptoms
- Hallmark of scabies: severe nocturnal pruritus
  - Itching also provoked by any warming of the body
  - Elapsed time of 4 to 6 weeks between infestation and onset of severe pruritus

- Cutaneous manifestations: an epidermal burrow (a linear or serpentine track, rarely longer than 5 to 10 mm [0.2 to 0.4 inch]) with a predilection for the interdigital spaces, palms, flexor surfaces of the wrists, elbows, feet, ankles, belt line, anterior axillary folds, lower buttocks, penis, and scrotum.

Treatment

1. A single overnight application of 5% permethrin cream is curative. Also apply the chemical beneath the fingernails. Symptoms may persist for more than a month until the mite and mite products are shed with the epidermis.
2. One percent hexachlorocyclohexane (lindane) cream or lotion is curative, although it is contraindicated in infants and pregnant women.
3. Sulfur in petrolatum 5% to 10% or another suitable vehicle applied for three consecutive nights is an alternative, as is crotamiton cream 10% or lotion applied for two consecutive nights.
4. Treat contacts simultaneously. Clothing and linens should be laundered the morning after treatment to kill mites that may have strayed from the skin.

TROMBICULID (CHIGGER) MITES (See Fig. 38.6E)

In the United States the most important mite species of the family Trombiculidae is *Eutrombicula alfreddugèsi,* known as the red bug, chigger, or harvest mite. Adult mites lay eggs in vegetation, and newly hatched larvae crawl up the vegetation, from which they attach themselves to human skin with hooked mouthparts.

Signs and Symptoms

- Maddeningly pruritic hemorrhagic puncta that usually become surrounded by intense erythema within 24 hours.
- Bites may number in the hundreds and can be associated with an allergic reaction.
- Blisters, purplish discoloration, swelling of feet and ankles, secondary infection in excoriated skin.

Treatment

1. Treatment is symptomatic and consists of topical antipruritic agents, corticosteroids, and systemic antihistamines.
2. Consider superpotent topical corticosteroid cream or ointment, such as 0.05% clobetasol, applied sparingly several times daily.
3. Phenol 1% in calamine may be effective for itching.

TICKS (See Fig. 38.6C and D)
Local Reaction to Tick Bites
Signs and Symptoms

- Vary from small pruritic nodule to extensive area of ulceration, erythema, and induration
- Possibly accompanied by fever, chills, and malaise

Treatment

1. If tick mouthparts or heads remain embedded in the wound, remove them surgically using a needle or the sharp tip of a knife or scalpel.
2. Manage wound infection with an antibiotic.

Tick Paralysis

Tick paralysis occurs most frequently during the spring and summer, when ticks are feeding. Girls are more often affected than boys because the ticks can hide more easily in girls' longer scalp hair. In the United States, the Pacific Northwest and Rocky Mountain areas account for the vast majority of cases. Neurotoxic venom from 43 different argasid (soft-shelled) and ixodid (hard-shelled) tick species is released from their salivary glands during feeding, resulting in sodium channel blockade and inhibition at the neuro-muscular junction.

Signs and Symptoms

- From 5 to 6 days after the adult female tick attaches: restlessness, irritability, paresthesias in the hands and feet
- Over the ensuing 24 to 48 hours: ascending, symmetric, and flaccid paralysis with loss of deep tendon reflexes; weakness usually greater in the lower extremities
- Within 1 to 2 days: severe generalized weakness possible, accompanied by bulbar and respiratory paralysis
  - Cerebellar dysfunction with incoordination and ataxia possible
  - Facial paralysis an isolated finding in persons with ticks embedded behind the ear

Treatment

1. Note that the diagnosis is established when paralysis resolves after tick removal. In North America, most patients show improvement within hours of tick removal, with return to normal in several days.
2. Aside from tick removal, treatment is supportive.

Lyme Disease

Lyme disease, caused by *Borrelia burgdorferi,* is transmitted most often by the deer tick *Ixodes scapularis* and the western black-legged tick *Ixodes pacificus.*

Signs and Symptoms

Stage I (early localized)

- Average 7 to 10 days (range: 3 to 32 days) after inoculation, patient develops an expanding, annular, and erythematous skin lesion (erythema migrans) (Fig. 38.7; see Plate 19).
- Initially, central red macule or papule; but as lesion expands, partial central clearing is usually seen while outer borders remain bright red.

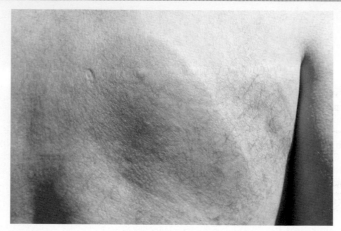

FIGURE 38.7 Rash of erythema migrans. (Photo courtesy of Paul Auerbach, MD.)

- Borders usually flat but may be raised.
- Centers of some early lesions intensely red and indurated, vesicular, or necrotic; sometimes affected area develops multiple red rings within the outside margin, or the central area turns blue before clearing.
- Lesion diameter 15 cm (5.9 inches) (range: 2 to 60 cm [0.8 to 23.6 inches]) and may be anywhere on the body, although the most common sites are thigh, groin, and axilla.
- Lesion is warm to the touch and usually described as burning, but occasionally as itching or painful.
- Rash fades after an average of 28 days (range: 1 to 14 weeks) without treatment; with antibiotics, lesion resolves after several days.
- Constitutional symptoms accompany erythema migrans, but are usually mild and consist of regional lymphadenopathy, fever, fatigue, neck stiffness, arthralgia, myalgia, and malaise.
- Annular erythematous lesions occur hours after being bitten, representative of a hypersensitivity reaction and not to be confused with erythema migrans.

Stage II (early disseminated)
- During hematogenous spread of microorganisms (a few days to weeks after the bite), multiple annular skin lesions appear in 20% to 50% of patients.
  - Generally they are smaller, migrate less, and lack indurated centers.
  - Located anywhere except palms and soles.
  - No blistering or mucosal involvement.
- Other skin manifestations: malar rash; rarely, urticaria.

- The most common constitutional symptoms: malaise and fatigue, which may be severe and are usually constant throughout the duration of the illness.
- Fever, typically low-grade and intermittent, is common.
- Tender regional lymphadenopathy along the distribution of erythema migrans or posterior cervical chains.
- Generalized lymphadenopathy and splenomegaly.
- Symptoms of meningeal irritation in some patients, including severe intermittent headaches, stiff neck with extreme forward flexion, and lack of Kernig or Brudzinski signs.
- Mild encephalopathy with somnolence, insomnia, memory disturbances, emotional lability, dizziness, poor balance, and clumsiness.
- Dysesthesias of the scalp.
- Musculoskeletal complaints, including arthralgias; migratory pain in tendons, bursae, and bones; and generalized stiffness or severe cramping pain, particularly in the calves, thighs, and back.
- Symptoms of hepatitis and generalized abdominal pain.
- Conjunctivitis in 10% to 15% of patients.
- Neurologic manifestations appear an average of 4 weeks after the onset of erythema migrans, including meningoencephalitis, with headache as a major symptom; facial nerve palsy (in 11% of Lyme disease patients and 50% of patients with Lyme disease meningitis, but this may be an isolated finding); radiculoneuritis (triad of meningitis, cranial neuritis, and radiculoneuritis suggests Lyme disease in the differential diagnosis).
- Cardiac abnormalities in 4% to 10% of patients, including atrioventricular block, which can progress to complete heart block.
- Arthritis in about 60% of untreated persons with erythema migrans.
  - Develops in a few weeks to 2 years (median 4 weeks) after onset of illness.
  - Typical pattern of brief recurrent episodes of asymmetric oligoarticular swelling and pain in large joints, separated by longer periods of complete remission.
- Knee most frequently involved, followed by the shoulder, elbow, temporomandibular joint, ankle, wrist, hip, and small joints of the hands and feet.

Stage III (late disease)

- The above symptoms begin a year or more after the onset of infection, although patients may present with stage III disease as the initial manifestation of Lyme disease.

Treatment

If the diagnosis of Lyme disease is made by clinical or serologic determination, initiate antibiotic therapy (Table 38.2).

Prophylaxis

Recent studies have been conflicting on the efficacy and cost-effectiveness of antibiotic prophylaxis for tick bites in the prevention

Table 38.2   Antimicrobial Recommendations for Lyme Disease

DRUG	DOSE*	DURATION (DAYS)
Early Localized Disease		
Adults		
Doxycycline	100 mg PO bid	14
Tetracycline	250–500 mg PO qid	14
Amoxicillin	500 mg PO tid	14
Cefuroxime	500 mg PO tid	14
Erythromycin	1–4 g/day divided PO qid	14 (max 4 g daily)
Children		
Amoxicillin	50 mg/kg/day PO divided tid	14
Doxycycline (>8 years)	100 mg PO bid or <45 kg at 5 mg/kg/day divided bid	14 (max 200 mg/day)
Erythromycin	30–50 mg/kg/day PO divided qid	14 (max 4 g daily)
Tetracycline (>8 years)	250 mg PO qid	14
Cefuroxime axetil	30–40 mg/kg/day PO divided bid	14
Early Disseminated and Late Diseases[†] and Late Disseminated Neurologic Disease[‡] (Treatment Duration Based on Severity of Disease;14 Days in Nonneurologic and Noncardiac Cases)		
Adults		
Ceftriaxone	2 g IV/IM daily	14–28
Cefotaxime	2 g IV q8h	14–28
Penicillin G	20 million IU/day IV divided q4h	14–28 (max 20 million IU/day)

Table 38.2 Antimicrobial Recommendations for Lyme Disease—cont'd

DRUG	DOSE*	DURATION (DAYS)
Children		
Ceftriaxone	80–100 mg/kg/day IV daily	14–28 (max 2 g/day)
Cefotaxime	90–180 mg/kg/day IV q8h	14–28
Penicillin G	300,000 IU/kg/day IV divided q4–6h	14–28 (max, 24 million IU/day)
Late Disseminated Arthritis		
Adults		
Amoxicillin	500 mg PO qid	14–28
Doxycycline	100 mg PO bid	14–28
Ceftriaxone	80–100 mg/kg/day IV daily	14 (max, 4 g/day)
Children		
Amoxicillin	50 mg/kg/day PO divided tid	14–28
Ceftriaxone	80–100 mg/kg/day IV/IM daily	14–28 (max 2 g/day)
Disseminated Disease and Cardiac Involvement		
Adults		
Doxycycline§	100 mg PO bid	14–28
Amoxicillin§	500 mg PO q8h	14–28
Ceftriaxone¶	2 g/day IV daily	14–28
Children		
Ceftriaxone	75–100 mg/kg/day IV/IM daily	14–21 (max, 2 g/day)
Penicillin G	300,000 IU/kg/day IV divided q4–6h	14–21 (max, 24 million IU/day)

Continued

DRUG	DOSE*	DURATION (DAYS)
Table 38.2 Antimicrobial Recommendations for Lyme Disease—cont'd		
Lyme Disease in Pregnancy		
Cutaneous involvement only, or tick bite in endemic area	50 mg/kg/day PO divided tid	21
Amoxicillin		
Severe acute disease or late/ disseminated disease	20 million IU/d IV divided q4h	21
Penicillin G		

*Total daily dose shown to be divided, if necessary, as indicated.
†For multiple lesions of erythema migrans, use treatment for early localized disease for at least 21 days. For isolated facial palsy, use treatment for early localized disease for 21 days.
‡Neurologic involvement limited to an isolated facial palsy should be treated as early disease.
§For mild cardiac involvement (i.e., first-degree atrioventricular block with PR interval less than 0.30 second).
¶For second- or third-degree heart block, although no evidence indicates that intravenous regimen is better than oral regimens; 28-day course recommended.
**In pregnancy, penicillin is preferred. If pregnant patient is allergic to penicillin, use erythromycin at 15 to 20 mg/kg/day IV divided qid.
bid, Twice a day; *IM*, intramuscularly; *IU*, international units; *IV*, intravenously; *PO*, orally; *qid*, four times a day; *tid*, three times a day.

of Lyme disease. The current guidelines of the Infectious Diseases Society of America are as follows. Patients must meet ALL the following criteria:
• Attached tick identified as an adult or nymphal *I. scapularis* tick (deer tick).
• Tick is estimated to have been attached for 36 hours or longer (by degree of engorgement or time of exposure).
• Prophylaxis is begun within 72 hours of tick removal.
• Local rate of infection of ticks with *B. burgdorferi* is 20% or higher (e.g., New England, parts of the mid-Atlantic states, and parts of Minnesota and Wisconsin).
• Doxycycline is not contraindicated (i.e., the patient is not younger than 8 years, pregnant, or lactating).
The recommended dose of doxycycline is 200 mg for adults and 4 mg/kg up to a maximum dose of 200 mg in children 8 years or older given as a single dose. Only patients meeting all the stated criteria should be given antibiotic prophylaxis.

Relapsing Fever

Relapsing fever is an acute disease caused by *Borrelia* and characterized by recurrent paroxysms of fever separated by afebrile periods.

Signs and Symptoms

- Abrupt onset of fever lasting about 3 days, afebrile period of variable duration (average 6 to 7 days), and relapse with return of fever and other clinical manifestations.
- Fever usually high, greater than 39°C (102.2°F)
- Initial febrile period averaging 3 days but possibly lasting 1 to 17 days
- Febrile period terminating with rapid defervescence (the crisis), accompanied by drenching sweats and intense thirst
- Pruritic eschar at the site of the tick bite possible but usually absent by the onset of clinical symptoms
- Incubation period of about 7 days, then fever, frequently accompanied by shaking chills, severe headache, myalgias, arthralgias, muscular weakness, lethargy, upper abdominal pain, nausea, and vomiting
- Splenomegaly, hepatomegaly, altered sensorium, peripheral neuropathy, pupillary abnormalities, pathologic deep tendon reflexes
- Rash, ranging from a macular eruption to petechiae and erythema multiforme, developing in about 25% of patients

Treatment

1. Tetracycline and erythromycin are both effective. A 7- to 10-day course (500 mg PO q6h) of either drug is recommended.
2. A Jarisch-Herxheimer reaction is common after the first dose of antibiotics. It is often severe and may be fatal.
   a. The reaction begins with a rise in body temperature and exacerbation of existing signs and symptoms. Vasodilation and declining blood pressure follow.
   b. Pretreat any patient with relapsing fever who will be receiving the initial dose of an antibiotic with an intravenous infusion of isotonic saline solution in anticipation of the Jarisch-Herxheimer reaction.
   c. A lower initial dose of antibiotic may reduce the frequency of this reaction.

Rocky Mountain Spotted Fever

Rocky Mountain spotted fever (RMSF) is caused by *Rickettsia rickettsii*. Most cases in the United States occur between the months of April and September, when the vector ticks are active.

Signs and Symptoms

- Ranges from mild, subclinical illness to fulminant disease with vascular collapse and death within 3 to 6 days of onset.
- Incubation period 2 to 14 days, with severe disease associated with the shorter incubation period.

- Typically there is a sudden onset of fever, chills, headache, and myalgias; fever is usually high, greater than 39°C (102.2°F).
- The most characteristic feature is rash, which develops 2 to 5 days after the onset of illness in 85% to 90% of patients.
  - Typically develops first on the wrists, hands, ankles, and feet, spreading rapidly in centripetal fashion to cover most of the body, including the palms, soles, and face.
  - Lesions are initially pink macules, 2 to 5 mm (0.1 to 0.2 inch) in diameter, and readily blanch with pressure.
  - After 2 to 3 days lesions are fixed, darker red, papular, and finally petechial.
  - Hemorrhagic lesions coalesce to form large areas of ecchymosis.
  - Unfortunately, rash is often absent on initial presentation, making the diagnosis more difficult; in 10% to 15% of patients, no rash is ever noted ("spotless fever").
- Other signs and symptoms include abdominal pain, vomiting, diarrhea, confusion, conjunctivitis, and peripheral edema.
- Seizures are possible during the acute phase of illness but they rarely persist.
- Lethargy and confusion common, possibly progressing to stupor or coma.
- Cough, chest pain, dyspnea, or coryza also noted.

Treatment
1. Initiate antibiotic therapy at the earliest suggestion of RMSF. Unfortunately the classic triad of rash, fever, and tick bite is rarely present.
2. Give either tetracycline or chloramphenicol, both of which are very effective, although neither drug is rickettsicidal. These antibiotics inhibit the rickettsiae until an adequate immune response by the patient eradicates the infection.
   a. Give tetracycline 500 mg PO q6h in adults and 25 to 50 mg/kg/day PO divided q6h in children.
   b. Alternatively, give doxycycline 100 mg twice daily intravenously in severely ill adult patients or orally in mildly or moderately ill patients.
   c. In rare clinical settings, give chloramphenicol 50 mg/kg/day PO for adults and 75 mg/kg/day for children.
3. Continue treatment until the patient is afebrile for 48 hours or for a minimum of 5 to 7 days. Be aware that relapses are common but may be treated with the same drug when they occur.

Ehrlichiosis
Ehrlichieae are tick-borne rickettsial organisms that cause disease in humans and animals throughout the world. Human ehrlichiosis has a broad clinical spectrum, ranging from a subclinical infection to a mild viral-like illness to a life-threatening disease.

Signs and Symptoms

- After an average incubation period of 7 days (range: 1 to 21 days): high fever, headache, chills or rigors, malaise, myalgia, anorexia.
- Rash, which may be maculopapular or petechial, in 20% to 40% of patients about 8 days after onset of illness.
- Severe complications: more likely in older persons and include cough, pneumonitis, dyspnea, respiratory failure, meningoencephalitis, and renal failure.

Treatment

- Give doxycycline 100 mg PO or IV q12h or tetracycline 500 mg PO q6h for 7 to 10 days.
- For children younger than 8 years of age or pregnant women, consider rifampin or chloramphenicol (see Appendix H).

Colorado Tick Fever

Colorado tick fever is caused by a small RNA virus that is transmitted to humans by ticks. The incubation period is 3 to 6 days (range: 0 to 14 days).

Signs and Symptoms

- Usually begins with an abrupt onset of fever.
  - The most characteristic feature of illness (seen in 50% of patients): biphasic, or "saddleback," fever pattern.
  - The first 2 to 3 days of fever are followed by 1 or 2 days of remission and then an additional 2 to 3 days of fever.
  - During fever, patients also have severe headache, myalgias, lethargy.
- Photophobia, ocular pain, anorexia, nausea, vomiting, abdominal pain.
- Macular or maculopapular rash in 5% to 12% of patients.
- Usually mild illness, but severe complications possible, especially in children younger than 10 years of age, including meningoencephalitis or hemorrhagic diathesis.
- Three weeks or longer required for full recovery, with the most common persistent symptoms being malaise and weakness.

Treatment

Treatment is symptomatic and supportive.

Babesiosis

Babesia organisms are intraerythrocytic protozoan parasites. The vector tick may be the same as which carries the infectious agent of Lyme disease. The presence of an intact spleen appears to play an important role in resistance to *Babesia* organisms.

Signs and Symptoms

- Acute babesiosis: gradual onset of malaise, anorexia, and fatigue followed within several days to a week by fever, sweats, and myalgias

- Less common symptoms: headache, nausea, vomiting, depression, shaking chills, splenomegaly, jaundice, hepatomegaly
- No rash associated with disease
- Hemolytic anemia more pronounced in splenectomized patients

Treatment

1. Currently treatment is recommended only for the seriously ill patient or the patient with asplenia, immunosuppression, or elder status.
2. For severe infections, give azithromycin 500 mg PO on day 1, followed by 250 mg PO on days 2 through 7, combined with atovaquone 750 mg PO q12h for 7 days.
3. Alternative therapy with similar efficacy but more side effects is a combination of clindamycin and quinine.

Prevention of Tick-Borne Diseases

Close and regular inspection of all parts of the body should be performed when traveling in tick-infested areas. Protective clothing (long pants cinched at the ankles or tucked into boots and socks) should be worn when in tick-infested areas. Spraying clothes with an insect repellent may provide an additional barrier against ticks (Box 38.1; see also Fig. 39.1). Adult ixodid ticks are generally on the body for 1 to 2 hours before attaching. See Chapter 39 for more information.

Tick Removal

See Fig. 39.2 and page 480.

BOX 38.1 Protection Against Insects

- Wear proper clothing to prevent the insect from obtaining access to the skin. Light-colored clothing makes it easier to spot ticks and is less attractive to biting flies.
- Use screens over windows, screened enclosures, or bed nets with fine mesh.
- Avoid unnecessary use of lights. Camp in a site that is high, dry, open, and uncluttered.
- Apply a repellent containing N,N-diethyl-3-methylbenzamide, commonly known as DEET (from its former chemical name). Bathing, excessive sweating, wiping, or other abrasive actions that deplete the supply of available repellent on skin may justify reapplication. Avoid prolonged use of high concentrations (more than 35%) of DEET, particularly in small children.
- Use permethrin-impregnated fabric (see Fig. 39.1). Note that the insecticidal action can noticeably reduce the density of the biting population in the immediate area. After contact, pests drop or fly away from the treated clothing, but they are not necessarily killed.

SCORPIONS

Centruroides exilicauda, the bark scorpion (see Plate 20) of Arizona, is usually less than 5 cm (2 inches) long, yellow to brown, and possibly striped. It carries the identifying subacular tooth beneath its stinger. Some scorpions fluoresce under a "black light," which can be used to inspect clothing, sleeping bags, etc. Other scorpions worldwide cause similar syndromes.

Signs and Symptoms

- Begin immediately after envenomation and progress to maximum severity in 5 hours
- Infants: extreme illness possible 15 to 30 minutes after a sting
- Improvement without administration of antivenom within 9 to 30 hours
- Paresthesias and pain persisting for days to 2 weeks
- *Grade I:* local pain and paresthesias at the site of envenomation, which can be elicited by tapping on the sting site
- *Grade II:* pain and paresthesias remote from the sting bite, along with local findings. The patient may complain of a "thick tongue" and "trouble swallowing." Children and adults frequently rub their noses, eyes, and ears, and infants may show unexplained crying.
- *Grade III:* either cranial nerve or somatic skeletal neuromuscular dysfunction.
  - Cranial nerve dysfunction: blurred vision, wandering eye movements (involuntary, conjugate, slow, roving); hypersalivation; difficulty swallowing; tongue fasciculation; upper airway obstruction; slurred speech.
  - Somatic skeletal neuromuscular dysfunction: jerking of the upper extremities, restlessness, arching of the back, and severe involuntary shaking and jerking that may be mistaken for a seizure (true seizures are caused by some scorpion species).
- *Grade IV:* both cranial nerve and somatic skeletal neuromuscular dysfunction.
- Hypertension, nausea, vomiting, hyperthermia, tachycardia, and respiratory distress also possible.

Treatment

1. Control local pain with ice packs, which may be applied for 30 minutes each hour. Give oral analgesics as needed. Infiltration with a local anesthetic or application of a digital or regional nerve block may be used. Although not studied, topical anesthetic patches (e.g., Lidoderm patch) can also be used.
2. Observe the patient with mild to moderate (grade I to II) envenomation for progression to more severe symptoms (grade III to IV).
3. Avoid the use of narcotics, barbiturates, benzodiazepines, or other potent analgesics to control symptoms of agitation or motor hyperactivity unless prepared to definitively manage the

airway because these agents may lead to apnea and loss of protective airway reflexes.

4. Manage hyperthermia from uncontrolled muscular activity with administration of acetaminophen or, if extremely severe, physical cooling methods.

5. Atropine may be used for severe bradycardia.

6. Sublingual (oral) nifedipine (5 to 10 mg by puncturing and swallowing the gelatin capsule) may be used to block excessive adrenergic tone. Alternatively, prazosin, a selective α-adrenergic blocker, may be given at an initial dose of 0.5 mg PO for adults and 0.25 mg PO for children, repeated at 4 hours and then q6h as needed for up to 24 hours.

7. Antivenom administration is controversial worldwide. Some recommend it for reversal of grade III envenomation with respiratory distress or grade IV envenomation. Administration carries the risk for anaphylaxis. Ideally it should be administered in a hospital critical care setting as soon as possible.

8. Prospective studies of anti-inflammatory corticosteroids have not shown a benefit.

Protection From Blood-Feeding Arthropods

Of all the hazards, large and small, that might befall the outdoor enthusiast, perhaps the most vexatious comes from the smallest perils—blood-feeding arthropods. Mosquitoes, flies, fleas, mites, midges, chiggers, and ticks all readily bite humans (Box 39.1).

Mosquitoes vector serious or sometimes fatal diseases to humans, so strategies to minimize exposure can not only prevent annoyance but also save lives.

PERSONAL PROTECTION

Personal protection against insect bites can be achieved in three ways:
- By avoiding infested habitats
- By using protective clothing and shelters
- By applying insect repellents

Habitat Avoidance

Avoiding infested habitats reduces the risk for being bitten.
- Mosquitoes and other nocturnal bloodsuckers are particularly active at dusk, making this a good time to be indoors.
- To avoid the usual resting places of biting arthropods, campgrounds should be situated in areas that are high, dry, open, and as free from vegetation as possible.
- Areas with standing or stagnant water should be avoided because these are ideal breeding grounds for mosquitoes.
- Attempts should be made to avoid the unnecessary use of lights, which attract many insects.

Physical Protection

- Physical barriers can be extremely effective in preventing insect bites, by blocking arthropods' access to the skin.
- Long-sleeved shirts, socks, long pants, and a hat will protect all but the face, neck, and hands.
- Tucking pants into the socks or boots makes it much more difficult for ticks or chigger mites to gain access to the skin.
- Light-colored clothing is preferable because it makes it easier to spot ticks, and it is less attractive to mosquitoes and biting flies.
- Ticks will find it more difficult to cling to smooth, tightly woven fabrics (e.g., nylon).
- Loose-fitting clothing, made of tightly woven fabric, with a tucked-in T-shirt undergarment is particularly effective at reducing bites on the upper body.

BOX 39.1   Mosquito Facts (Family Culicidae)

Mosquitoes are responsible for more arthropod bites than any other blood-sucking organism. They can be found all over the world except in Antarctica.

1. Mosquitoes rely on visual, thermal, and olfactory stimuli to help them locate a blood meal.
2. For mosquitoes that feed during the daytime, host movement and dark-colored clothing may initiate orientation toward an individual.
3. Visual stimuli appear to be important for in-flight orientation, particularly over long ranges.
4. Olfactory stimuli become more important as a mosquito nears its host.
5. Carbon dioxide serves as a long-range attractant, luring mosquitoes at distances of up to 36 m (118 ft).
6. At close range, skin warmth and moisture serve as attractants.
7. Volatile compounds—derived from sebum, eccrine and apocrine sweat, and/or the bacterial action of cutaneous microflora on these secretions—may also act as chemoattractants.
8. Floral fragrances found in perfumes, lotions, soaps, and hair-care products can also lure mosquitoes.
9. Alcohol ingestion may increase the likelihood of being bitten by mosquitoes.
10. Significant variability in the attractiveness of different individuals to the same or different species of mosquitoes can exist.
11. Men tend to be bitten more readily than women.
12. Adults are more likely to be bitten than children.
13. Heavy-set people are more likely to attract mosquitoes, perhaps because of their greater relative heat or carbon dioxide output.
14. During the day, mosquitoes tend to rest in cool, dark areas such as on dense vegetation or in hollow tree stumps, animal burrows, and caves. To complete their life cycle, mosquitoes also require standing water, which may be found in tree holes, woodland pools, marshes, or puddles. To minimize the chance of being bitten by mosquitoes, campsites should be situated as far away from such sites as possible.

- A light-colored full-brimmed hat will protect the head and neck.
  - Deerflies tend to land on the hat instead of the head.
  - Blackflies and biting midges are less likely to crawl to the shaded skin beneath the brim.
- Mesh garments or garments made of tightly woven material are available to protect against insect bites.
  - Head nets, hooded jackets, pants, and mittens are available from a number of manufacturers in a wide range of sizes and styles (Box 39.2).

BOX 39.2   Manufacturers of Protective Clothing, Protective Shelters, and Insect Nets

Protective Clothing (Includes Hooded Jackets, Pants, Head Nets, Ankle Guards, Gaiters, and Mittens)
Bug Baffler, Inc.
  P.O. Box 444
  Goffstown, NH 03045
  800-662-8411
  bugbaffler.com
The Original Bug Shirt Company
  P.O. Box 127
  Trout Creek, Ontario, Canada
  800-998-9096
  bugshirt.com
Outdoor Research
  2203 1st Avenue South
  Seattle, WA 98134-1424
  206-971-1496
  outdoorresearch.com
Shannon Outdoors Bug Tamer
  P.O. Box 444
  Louisville, GA 30434
  800-852-8058
  shannonoutdoors.com/bugtamer

Protective Shelters and Insect Nets
Long Road Travel Supplies
  111 Avenida Drive
  Berkeley, CA 94708
  800-359-6040
  longroad.com
Travel Medicine, Inc.
  369 Pleasant Street
  Northampton, MA 01060
  800-872-8633
  travmed.com
Wisconsin Pharmacal Company
  1 Repel Road
  Jackson, WI 53037
  800-558-6614
  atwater-carey.com

- With a mesh size of less than 0.3 mm (0.01 inch), many of these garments are woven tightly enough to exclude even biting midges and ticks.
- As with any clothing, bending or crouching may still pull the garments close enough to the skin surface to enable insects to bite through.

- Shannon Outdoors addresses this potential problem with a double-layered mesh that reportedly prevents mosquito penetration.
- Although mesh garments are effective barriers against insects, some people may find them uncomfortable during vigorous activity or in hot weather.
- Lightweight insect nets and mesh shelters are available to protect travelers sleeping indoors or in the wilderness (see Box 39.2).
  - Their effectiveness may be enhanced by treating them with a permethrin-based contact insecticide, which can provide weeks of efficacy after a soak or spray-on application that will endure through several wash cycles (Fig. 39.1).

REPELLENTS

For many people, applying an insect repellent may be the most effective and easiest way to prevent arthropod bites.

Chemical Repellents

See Table 39.1.

Table 39.1 Chemical Insect Repellents			
MANUFAC-TURER	**PRODUCT NAME**	**FORMS**	**CHEMICAL**
Sawyer Products Safety Harbor, FL 800-940-4664	Sawyer Controlled Release	Lotion	20% DEET
	Sawyer Ultra 30 Insect Repellent	Lotion	30% DEET
		Aerosol spray	30% DEET
	Sawyer Maxi-DEET	Pump spray	100% DEET
S.C. Johnson Racine, WI 800-558-5566	OFF! Family Care Insect Repellent (Tropical Fresh)	Pump spray	5% DEET
	OFF! Family Care Unscented	Pump spray	7% DEET
	OFF! Family Care	Aerosol spray	15% DEET
	OFF! Active	Aerosol spray	15% DEET
	OFF! Deep Woods	Aerosol spray, pump spray, towelettes	25% DEET

Table 39.1 Chemical Insect Repellents—cont'd			
MANUFAC- TURER	**PRODUCT NAME**	**FORMS**	**CHEMICAL**
S.C. Johnson Racine, WI 800-558-5566	OFF! Deep Woods Sportsmen	Pump spray	25% DEET
	OFF! Deep Woods Sportsmen	Aerosol spray	30% DEET
	OFF! Deep Woods Sportsmen	Pump spray	98% DEET
Tender Corporation Littleton, NH 800-258-4696	Ben's Tick and Insect Repellent	Aerosol spray, pump spray, wipes	30% DEET
	Ben's 100 Tick and Insect Repellent	Pump spray	100% DEET
Spectrum Brands Alpharetta, GA 800-336-1372	Cutter All Family Insect Repellent	Aerosol spray, pump spray	7% DEET
	Cutter Skinsations Insect Repellent	Aerosol spray, pump spray	7% DEET
	Cutter Dry	Aerosol spray	10% DEET
	Cutter Unscented	Aerosol spray	10% DEET
	Repel Family Dry	Aerosol spray, pump spray	10% DEET
	Cutter Sport	Aerosol spray	15% DEET
	Repel Sportsmen Formula	Aerosol spray, stick	25% DEET
	Repel Hunter's Formula with Earth Scent	Aerosol spray	25% DEET
	Cutter Backwoods	Aerosol, pump spray	25% DEET
	Repel Sportsmen Max	Pump spray, aerosol spray, lotion	40% DEET
	Repel 100 Insect Repellent	Pump spray	100% DEET

Continued

Table 39.1 Chemical Insect Repellents—cont'd			
MANUFAC-TURER	**PRODUCT NAME**	**FORMS**	**CHEMICAL**
Coleman Company Jackson, WI 800-558-6614	Coleman Insect Repellent	Aerosol spray	25% DEET
	Coleman Insect Repellent	Aerosol spray	40% DEET
	Coleman Insect Repellent	Pump spray	100% DEET
3M St Paul, MN 888-364-3577	Ultrathon	Pump spray	19% DEET
	Ultrathon	Aerosol spray	25% DEET
	Ultrathon	Lotion	35% DEET
S.C. Johnson Racine, WI 800-558-5566	OFF! Family Care Insect Repellent II Clean Feel	Pump spray	Picaridin 5%
Avon Products, Inc. New York, NY 800-367-2866	Skin So Soft Bug Guard Plus Picaridin	Aerosol spray, pump spray, towelettes	Picaridin 10%
Spectrum Brands Alpharetta, GA 800-336-1372	Repel Sportsman Gear Smart Insect Repellent	Pump spray, wipes	Picaridin 15%
	Repel Tick Defense	Aerosol spray	Picaridin 15%
Tender Corporation Littleton, NH 800-258-4696	Natrapel 12-Hour	Pump spray, aerosol spray, wipes	Picaridin 20%

DEET

- N,N-diethyl-3-methylbenzamide (previously called N,N-diethyl-m-toluamide), or DEET, remains the gold standard of presently available insect repellents.
- DEET has been registered for use by the general public since 1957. It is a broad-spectrum repellent that is effective against many species of crawling and flying insects, including mosquitoes, biting flies, midges, chiggers, fleas, and ticks.
- DEET may be applied directly to skin, clothing, mesh insect nets or shelters, window screens, tents, or sleeping bags.
- Care should be taken to avoid inadvertent contact with plastics (e.g., watch crystals, eyeglass frames), rayon, spandex, leather, or painted and varnished surfaces because DEET may damage these. DEET does not damage natural fibers like wool and cotton.

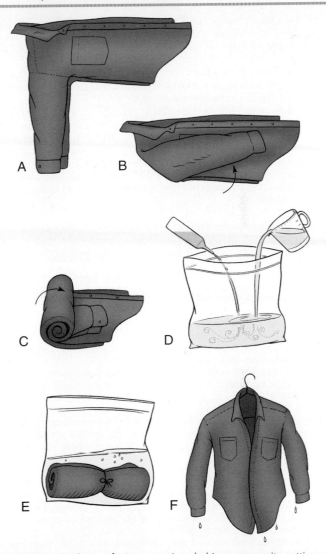

FIGURE 39.1 Technique for impregnating clothing or mosquito netting with permethrin solution. **A** to **C,** Lay jacket flat and fold it shoulder to shoulder. Fold sleeves to inside, roll tightly, and tie middle with string. For mosquito net, roll tightly and tie. **D,** Pour 60 mL (2 oz) of permethrin into plastic bag. Add 1 L (1 qt) water. Mix. Solution will turn milky white. **E,** Place garment or mosquito netting in bag. Shut or tie tightly. Let rest 10 minutes. **F,** Hang garment or netting for 2 to 3 hours to dry. Fabric can also be laid on a clean surface to dry. (Redrawn from Rose S: *International travel health guide,* Northampton, MA, 1993, Travel Medicine, with permission.)

- In the United States, DEET is sold in concentrations from 5% to 100% in multiple formulations, including lotions, solutions, gels, sprays, roll-ons, and impregnated towelettes (see Table 39.1).
- As a general rule, higher concentrations of DEET provide longer-lasting protection. For most uses, however, there is no need to use the highest concentrations of DEET.
- Products with 10% to 35% DEET provide adequate protection under most conditions. In fact, most manufacturers, responding to consumer demand, offer a greater variety of low-concentration DEET products, and the vast majority of products now contain DEET concentrations of 35% or less.
- Persons averse to applying DEET directly to the skin may get long-lasting repellency by applying it only to their clothing (Box 39.3).

BOX 39.3   Guidelines for Safe and Effective Use of DEET Insect Repellents

- When only short-term protection is needed, repellents with 10% DEET or less may provide adequate protection.
- Use just enough repellent to lightly cover exposed skin; do not saturate the skin.
- Repellents should be applied only to exposed skin and clothing. Do not use under clothing.
- To apply to the face, dispense into palms, rub hands together, and then apply thin layer to face.
- Young children should not apply repellents themselves.
- Avoid contact with the eyes and mouth. Do not apply to children's hands so as to prevent possible subsequent contact with mucous membranes.
- After applying, wipe repellent from the palmar surfaces to prevent inadvertent contact with eyes, mouth, and genitals.
- Never use repellents over cuts, wounds, or inflamed, irritated, or eczematous skin.
- Do not inhale aerosol formulations or get them in the eyes. Do not apply when near food.
- Frequent reapplication is rarely necessary unless the repellent seems to have lost its effectiveness. Reapplication may be necessary in very hot, wet environments because of rapid loss of repellent from the skin surface.
- Once inside, wash treated areas with soap and water. Washing the repellent from the skin surface is particularly important when a repellent is likely to be applied for several consecutive days.
- If you suspect that you are having a reaction to an insect repellent, discontinue its use, wash the treated skin, and consult a physician.

Modified from US Environmental Protection Agency, Office of Pesticide Programs, Prevention, Pesticides and Toxic Substances Division: *Reregistration Eligibility Decision (RED): DEET*, (EPA-738-F-95-010), 1998, Washington. DC.

- Stored in a plastic bag between wearings, DEET-treated garments maintain their repellency for several weeks.
- Products with a DEET concentration higher than 35% are probably best reserved for circumstances when the wearer will be in an environment with a high density of insects (e.g., a rain forest), when there is a high risk for disease transmission from insect bites, or when there may be rapid loss of repellent from the skin surface, as under conditions of high temperature and humidity or rain. Under these circumstances, reapplication of the repellent will most likely be necessary to maintain its effectiveness.
- Sequential application of a DEET-based repellent and a sunscreen can reduce the efficacy of the sunscreen.
- Some products contain a combination of sunscreen and DEET; they will deliver the sun protection factor (SPF) stated on the label.
- 3M and Sawyer Products manufacture extended-release formulations of DEET that make it possible to deliver long-lasting protection without relying on high concentrations:
  - The 3M product Ultrathon is an acrylate polymer formulation containing 35% DEET; it is as effective as 75% DEET, providing up to 12 hours of greater than 95% protection against mosquito bites.
  - Sawyer Products' controlled-release 20% DEET lotion traps the chemical in a protein particle that slowly releases it to the skin surface, providing repellency equivalent to a standard 50% DEET preparation and lasting about 5 hours.
- Case reports of potential DEET toxicity exist in the medical literature and have been extensively reviewed.
  - Fewer than 50 cases of significant toxicity from DEET exposure have been documented in the medical literature; more than three-quarters of these resolved without sequelae.
  - Studies find DEET use safe in pregnancy; formulations of up to 30% may be used in children older than 2 months.
  - The Environmental Protection Agency (EPA) has issued guidelines to ensure safe use of DEET-based repellents (see Box 39.3). Careful product choice and commonsense application greatly reduce the possibility of toxicity.
  - Questions about the safety of DEET may be addressed to the EPA-sponsored National Pesticide Information Center, available every day from 8:00 AM to 12:00 PM PST at 800-858-7378 or via their website at npic.orst.edu/.

IR3535 (Ethyl Butylacetylaminoproprionate)

- IR3535 is an analog of the amino acid β-alanine; it has been sold in Europe as an insect repellent for more than 20 years.
- In the United States this compound is classified by the EPA as a biopesticide, effective against mosquitoes, ticks, and flies.
- IR3535 was brought to the US market in 1999 and sold by Avon Products, Inc., and Sawyer Products in concentrations from 7.5% to 20%, with and without sunscreen.

- Depending on the species of mosquito and the testing method, this repellent has demonstrated widely variable effectiveness, with complete protection times ranging from 23 to 360 minutes.
- In general IR3535 provides longer-lasting repellency than the botanical citronella-based repellents, but it does not match the overall efficacy of DEET.

Picaridin
- The piperidine derivative picaridin (also known as KBR 3023) is the newest insect repellent to become available in the United States.
- Picaridin-based insect repellents have been sold in Europe since 1998 under the brand name Bayrepel.
- This nearly odorless, nongreasy repellent is effective against mosquitoes, biting flies, and ticks.
- Studies have shown that when used at higher concentrations of up to 20%, picaridin repellents can offer an efficacy comparable to that of DEET, giving up to 8 hours of protection.
- The chemical is aesthetically pleasant and, unlike DEET, shows no detrimental effects on contact with plastics.
- The EPA found picaridin to have a low toxicity risk.
- Picaridin is superior to DEET as a tick repellent.

Botanical Repellents
- Thousands of plants have been tested as sources of insect repellents.
- Although none of the currently available plant-derived chemicals tested to date demonstrates the broad effectiveness and duration of DEET, a few show repellent activity.
- Plants with essential oils that have been reported to possess repellent activity include citronella, neem, cedar, verbena, pennyroyal, geranium, catnip, lavender, pine, cajeput, cinnamon, vanilla, rosemary, basil, thyme, allspice, garlic, and peppermint. When tested, most of these essential oils tended to show short-lasting protection from minutes to 2 hours.
- A summary of readily available plant-derived insect repellents is shown in Table 39.2.

Citronella
- In general, studies show that citronella-based repellents are less effective than DEET repellents.
- Citronella provides a shorter protection time (in some studies, 40 minutes to 2 hours); this may be partially overcome by frequent reapplication of the repellent.
- The EPA concluded that citronella-based insect repellents must contain the following statement on their labels: "For maximum repellent effectiveness of this product, repeat applications at 1-hour intervals."

Table 39.2   Botanical Insect Repellents (Registration Exempt)

MANUFAC-TURER	PRODUCT NAME	FORM(S)	ACTIVE INGREDI-ENTS
TyraTech, Inc. Morrisville, NC 855-373-7210	Guardian	Pump spray	Geraniol 5%
HOMS, LLC Pittsboro, NC 800-270-5721	BiteBlocker Xtreme Sportsman	Lotion, pump spray	Soybean oil 3%, geranium oil 6%, castor oil 8%
	BiteBlocker Herbal	Pump spray	Soybean oil 2%, geranium oil 5%
All Terrain Company Newport, NH 800-246-7328	Herbal Armor	Pump spray and lotion	Soybean oil 11.5%, citronella oil 10%, peppermint oil 2%, cedar oil 1.5%, lemongrass oil 1%, geranium oil 0.05%, in a slow-release encapsulated formula
	Kids Herbal Armor	Pump spray	
Quantum, Inc. Eugene, OR 800-448-1448	Buzz Away Extreme	Pump spray, towelettes	Soybean oil 3%, geranium oil 6%, castor oil 8%, cedarwood oil 1.5%, citronella 1%, peppermint oil 0.5%, lemongrass oil 0.25%
Spectrum Brands Alpharetta, GA 800-336-1372	Cutter Natural	Pump spray	Geraniol 5%, soybean oil 2%
	Repel Natural	Pump spray	Geraniol 5%, soybean oil 2%

- Citronella candles have been promoted as an effective way to repel mosquitoes from one's local environment and may decrease bites by 42%.

Bite Blocker

- Bite Blocker is a "natural" repellent in a formulation that combines soybean oil, geranium oil, and coconut oil.
- Studies showed that this product can provide more than 97% protection against *Aedes* species mosquitoes under field conditions even 3.5 hours after application. Bite Blocker provides a mean of 200 ± 30 minutes of complete protection from mosquito bites.

- Laboratory studies using three different species of mosquitoes have shown that Bite Blocker provides an average protection time of about 7 hours and about 10 hours of protection against biting blackflies.

BioUD (2-Undecanone)

BioUD (2-undecanone) is a repellent derived from the wild tomato plant. It was registered by the EPA in 2007 as a biopesticide for use against mosquitoes and ticks. In field studies against mosquitoes, 7.75% BioUD provided repellency comparable with 25% DEET. BioUD repelled the American dog tick *Dermacentor variabilis* from human skin for more than 2.5 hours and was still effective 8 days after application to cotton fabric. Laboratory testing demonstrated that BioUD was two to four times more effective than 98% DEET at repelling *Amblyomma americanum, D. variabilis,* and *Ixodes scapularis.*

Lemon Eucalyptus

- A eucalyptus derivative (*p*-menthane-3,8-diol, or PMD) isolated from oil of the lemon eucalyptus plant has a strong lemony scent and has shown promise as an effective "natural" repellent.
- Field tests of this repellent have shown mean complete protection times ranging from 4 to 8 hours, depending on the mosquito species.
- PMD-based repellents can cause significant ocular irritation, so care must be taken to keep them away from the eyes. They should not be used in children younger than 3 years.

Ingested Repellents

There has always been great interest in finding an oral insect repellent. Oral repellents would be convenient and would eliminate the need to apply creams to the skin or put on protective clothing. Unfortunately no effective oral repellent has been discovered. Tests of over 100 ingested drugs, including vitamins and foods such as garlic, failed to reveal any that worked well against mosquitoes.

Table 39.2 lists botanical repellents currently on the market.

INSECTICIDES
Permethrin

- Pyrethrum is a powerful, rapidly acting insecticide originally derived from crushed dried flowers of the daisy *Chrysanthemum cinerariifolium.*
- It is effective against mosquitoes, flies, ticks, fleas, lice, and chiggers. It does not repel insects but works as a contact insecticide, causing nervous system toxicity, leading to death or "knockdown" of the insect.
- Permethrin has low mammalian toxicity, is poorly absorbed by the skin, and is rapidly metabolized by skin and blood esterases.

Table 39.3 Permethrin Insecticides			
MANUFAC-TURER	**PRODUCT NAME**	**FORM(S)**	**ACTIVE INGREDIENT**
Sawyer Products Safety Harbor, FL 800-940-4464	Permethrin Clothing Gear and Tents Insect Repellent	Aerosol and pump sprays	Permethrin 0.5%
Spectrum Brands, Alpharetta, GA 800-336-1372	Repel Permethrin Clothing and Gear Insect Repellent	Aerosol spray	Permethrin 0.5%
Coleman (Wisconsin Pharmacal), Jackson, WI 800-558-6614	Coleman Gear and Clothing	Aerosol spray	Permethrin 0.5%
3M, St Paul, MN 888-364-3577	Ultrathon Clothing and Gear Insect Repellent	Pump spray	Permethrin 0.5%

- Permethrin should be applied directly to clothing or to other fabrics (tent walls or mosquito nets), not to skin.
- Permethrin is nonstaining, nearly odorless, resistant to degradation by heat or sun, and maintains its effectiveness for at least 2 weeks and through several launderings.
- The combination of permethrin-treated clothing and skin application of a DEET-based repellent creates a formidable barrier against biting insects.
- Permethrin-based insecticides currently available in the United States are listed in Table 39.3.
- To apply to clothing do the following:
  - Spray each side of the fabric (outdoors) for 30 to 45 seconds, just enough to moisten the fabric.
  - Allow the clothing to dry for 2 to 4 hours before wearing.
- Permethrin solution is also available for soak-treating large items such as mesh bed nets or for treating multiple garments simultaneously (see Fig. 39.1).
- Permethrin-pretreated shirts, pants, socks, and hats can also be purchased.

REDUCING LOCAL MOSQUITO POPULATIONS

Consumers may still find advertisements for small ultrasonic electronic devices that are meant to be carried on the body and claim to repel mosquitoes by emitting "repellent" sounds such as that of a dragonfly (claimed to be the natural enemy of the mosquito), male mosquito, or bat.

- Multiple studies conducted in the field and in the laboratory show that these devices do not work.
- Mass-marketed backyard "bug zappers," which use ultraviolet light to lure and electrocute insects, are also ineffective: Mosquitoes continue to be more attracted to humans than to the devices.
- DEET-impregnated wristbands offer no protection against mosquito bites. But in one study, wearing impregnated anklets, wristbands, shoulder strips, and pocket strips provided up to 5 hours of complete protection.
- Using more specific bait such as a warm moist plume of carbon dioxide as well as other known chemical attractants (e.g., octenol) may prove to be a more successful way to lure and selectively kill biting insects.
- Pyrethrin-containing yard foggers set off before an outdoor event can temporarily reduce the number of biting arthropods in a local environment. These products should be applied before any food is brought outside and should be kept away from animals and fishponds.
- Burning coils that contain natural pyrethrins or synthetic pyrethroids (such as D-allethrin or D-trans-allethrin) can also temporarily reduce local populations of biting insects. Some concerns have been raised about the cumulative safety of long-term use of these coils in an indoor environment.
- Wood smoke from campfires can also reduce the likelihood of being bitten by mosquitoes. The smoke's ability to repel insects may vary depending on the type of wood or vegetation burned.

INTEGRATED APPROACH TO PERSONAL PROTECTION

An integrated approach to personal protection is the most effective way to prevent arthropod bites regardless of where one is in the world and which species of insects may be attacking.

- Maximal protection is best achieved by avoiding infested habitats and using protective clothing, topical insect repellents, and permethrin-treated garments.
- When appropriate, mesh bed nets or tents should be used to prevent nocturnal insect bites.
- DEET-containing insect repellents are the most effective products currently on the US market, providing broad-spectrum, long-lasting repellency against multiple arthropod species.
- The Centers for Disease Control (CDC) has approved picaridin, IR3535, and oil of lemon eucalyptus as alternative repellents that can be used to reduce the likelihood of contracting insect-borne disease.

- Insect repellents alone, however, should not be relied on to provide complete protection.
  - Mosquitoes, for example, can find and bite any untreated skin and may even bite through thin clothing.
  - Deerflies, biting midges, and some blackflies prefer to bite around the head and readily crawl into the hair to bite where there is no protection.
- Wearing protective clothing, including a hat, reduces the chances of being bitten.
- Treating clothes, including the hat, with permethrin maximizes their effectiveness by causing knockdown of any insect that crawls or lands on the treated clothing.
- To prevent chiggers or ticks from crawling up the legs, pants should be tucked into boots or stockings.
- Persons traveling to parts of the world where insect-borne disease is a potential threat can protect themselves best if they learn about indigenous insects and the diseases they might transmit. This information may be found at cdc.gov/travel or by telephoning 800-CDC-INFO.

TICKS

Awareness of ticks and the diseases they transmit is a necessary first step in prevention. Other steps include the following:

- Proper clothing should be light-colored, because this makes ticks easier to spot.
- The avoidance of heavily infested areas reduces exposure, as does reducing contact with leaf litter.
- Boots provide better protection than do tennis shoes and socks. Tucking pant legs into the tops of the socks reduces the ticks' ability to climb up the legs of potential hosts. A ring of masking tape or duct tape at the tops of the socks further reduces exposure.
- Topical DEET and permethrin-impregnated gear and clothing round out an effective protection strategy against ticks.

Frequent inspection of the body should be performed when one is in a tick-infested area. Although some diseases require as much as 24 to 48 hours of tick attachment to allow transmission, others are transmitted within an hour.

Removal of attached ticks should never be done by bare or even gloved hands. The procedure for removing an embedded tick is as follows:

1. Use fine-tipped forceps.
2. Gently grasp the tick as close to the skin as possible and gradually retract it outward in a straight line (Fig. 39.2).
3. The area should then be cleaned with a local antiseptic.
4. Other methods for tick removal—such as applying petroleum jelly to the tick or using a lighted match or cigarette, isopropyl alcohol, or fingernail polish—do not ease removal of the tick. These and other "remedies" most likely increase the expression of tick saliva and foregut contents, thus increasing the chance of disease transmission.

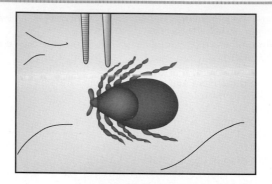

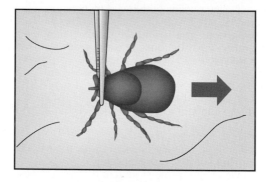

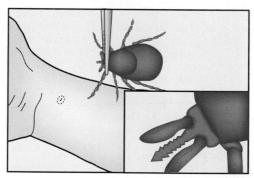

FIGURE 39.2   Ideal tick removal method. Grasp the tick near the surface of the skin and withdraw it from the skin in a steady, constant motion. Do not turn, jerk, or twist as you do this. (From US Army Center for Health Promotion and Preventive Medicine. Focus on Lyme Disease, Issue 9, Fall 1996.)

5. Removal of larval ticks is easier because their size and mouthparts are extremely tiny. A piece of tape, such as duct tape, applied to the skin and then removed easily removes free-crawling or attached larval ticks. Alternatively, the thin edge of a plastic object such as a credit card or driver's license scraped along the skin easily removes attached larvae. This method is appropriate only for larval ticks, not for nymphs or adults.

40 | Toxic Plants

TOXIC PLANT INGESTIONS
General Considerations
- For most toxic plant ingestions, the treatment is supportive and symptomatic care, as specific therapies often do not exist.
- Supportive care takes priority over plant identification.
- Airway, breathing, and circulation are assessed, including hydration status, end-organ perfusion, and urine output.
- Oral administration of activated charcoal (1 g/kg), up to 50 g, may aid gastrointestinal (GI) decontamination.
- History should include the following:
  - Time of ingestion
  - Amount and part of plants ingested
  - Initial symptoms
  - Time between ingestion and onset of symptoms
  - Method of preparation (e.g., drying, cooking, boiling)
  - Number of persons who ate the same plant and their symptoms

ORGAN SYSTEM PRINCIPLES
Toxic effects of certain plants can be grouped into categories designated by major effects on the central nervous, cardiovascular, GI, renal, endocrine-metabolic, hematopoietic, and reproductive systems.

Central Nervous System
Anticholinergic Plants (Tropane Alkaloids)
Plants causing human toxicity include *Atropa belladonna* (deadly nightshade), *Mandragora* spp. (mandrake), *Hyoscyamus niger* (black henbane), *Datura* spp. (jimsonweed), and *Brugmansia* spp. (angel's trumpet).

Anticholinergic Syndrome
Central
- Central nervous system (CNS) excitation
- Agitation
- Hallucinations
- Lethargy
- Coma
- Respiratory depression
- Mumbling speech
- Muteness
- Undressing behavior
- Repetitive picking behavior

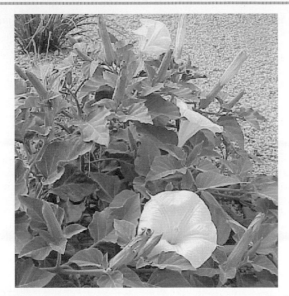

FIGURE 40.1   Jimsonweed (*Datura* spp.) is a bush with trumpet-like flowers.

Peripheral
- Tachycardia
- Mydriasis
- Blurred vision
- Inability to accommodate (visually)
- Flushed skin
- Hyperthermia
- Absent bowel sounds
- Urinary retention
- Dry mucous membranes

Jimsonweed (Fig. 40.1)

Young, thin, tender stems of jimsonweed contain the highest concentration of tropane alkaloids. However, the seeds also contain high concentrations of the alkaloids, and as little as one-half teaspoon of seeds can cause death from cardiopulmonary arrest.

Symptoms may appear within minutes and may last for days. These include the following:
- Tachycardia
- Dry mouth
- Agitation
- Nausea and vomiting
- Incoherence
- Disorientation
- Auditory and visual hallucinations

- Mydriasis (blurred vision and photophobia are sequelae); anisocoria if one eye has topical contact
- Decreased bowel sounds
- Slurred speech
- Hyperthermia
- Flushed skin
- Urinary retention
- Hypertension
- Seizures, flaccid paralysis, and coma

Deadly Nightshade

All parts of deadly nightshade contain tropane alkaloids, but the highest concentrations are in the ripe fruit and green leaves; each berry may contain up to 2 mg of atropine. The berries may be mistaken for bilberries (hurtleberries). The most severely poisoned patients have anticholinergic symptoms, with hypertonia, hyperthermia, respiratory failure, and coma. Other common symptoms include meaningless speech, lethargy, tachycardia, mydriasis, and flushing.

Treatment

1. Provide decontamination and supportive care, including oral administration of activated charcoal, airway protection, intravenous (IV) fluids, and vasopressors for hypotension resistant to IV fluids.
2. Treat hyperthermia.
3. Agitation can be treated with administration of a benzodiazepine. Haloperidol and phenothiazines should not be used because these agents may enhance toxicity.
4. Foley catheterization and nasogastric tube placement may be necessary if bladder distention and decreased gut motility develop.

Nicotinic Plants (Pyridine-Piperidine Alkaloids)

Nicotine alkaloids are found mainly in the Solanaceae family of plants. Other families containing nicotine alkaloids include Hippocastanaceae (horse chestnut) and Asclepiadaceae (milkweed).

Tobacco Plants

Nicotiana tabacum is the major source of commercial tobacco. One to two cigarettes, ingested and absorbed, can be lethal to a child.

Nicotinic Syndrome

Early Stage
- Hypertension
- Tachycardia
- Vomiting
- Diarrhea
- Muscle fasciculations
- Convulsions

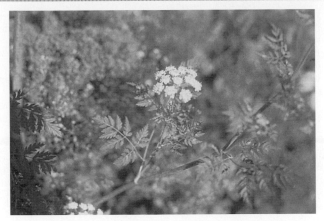

FIGURE 40.2   Poison hemlock *(Conium maculatum)*.

Late Stage
- Hypotension
- Bradyarrhythmias
- Paralysis
- Coma

Conium maculatum (poison hemlock) (Fig. 40.2) is also known as spotted hemlock, California or Nebraska fern, stinkweed, fool's parsley, and carrot weed. It has a mousy odor and an unpleasant bitter taste; it burns the mouth and throat. All plant parts are poisonous; the roots are especially toxic. Poisoning may also occur after eating birds that have consumed poison hemlock.

Initially, stimulation causes the following:
- Sialorrhea
- Nausea and vomiting
- Diarrhea
- Abdominal cramping
- Tremor
- Tachycardia
  followed by
- Dry mucosae
- GI hypotonia
- Diminished cardiac contraction
- Bradycardia
- Muscle swelling and stiffness

Betel Nut
Areca catechu (areca palm) produces betel nut.

Clinical effects resemble nicotinic syndrome and cholinergic toxicity; they include the following:
- CNS effects (dizziness, euphoria, subjective arousal, altered mental status, hallucinations, psychosis, convulsions)

- Cardiac effects (tachycardia, hypertension, palpitations, arrhythmias, bradycardia, hypotension, chest discomfort, and acute myocardial infarction in susceptible individuals)
- Pulmonary effects (bronchospasm, tachypnea, dyspnea), GI effects (salivation, vomiting, diarrhea)
- Urogenic effects (urinary incontinence) and musculoskeletal effects (weakness and paralysis)
- Other: flushing, diaphoresis, warm sensations, red- or orange-stained oral mucosa and saliva, and dark brown– or black-stained teeth

Quinolizidine Alkaloids
Common toxic plants in this group include the golden chain tree *(Laburnum anagyroides)*, Kentucky coffee tree *(Gymnocladus dioica)*, necklace pod sophora *(Sophora tomentosa)*, and mescal bean bush *(Sophora secundiflora)*.

Treatment
1. Supportive care with attention to airway protection and ventilation is necessary.
2. Seizures should be treated with benzodiazepines and barbiturates.
3. Treat with IV fluids to ensure adequate urine output (1 mL/kg per hour).
4. Urine may be alkalinized with IV sodium bicarbonate to achieve a urine pH of 7.5.
5. Treating initial excessive adrenergic stimulation with excessive adrenergic antagonists is not advised because this complicates the nicotinic blockade that follows.
6. Symptomatic bradycardia can be treated with atropine and hypotension with IV fluids and inotropic agents if needed.

Hallucinogenic Plants
Chemical relationships exist between serotonin, psilocybin *(Psilocybe* spp.), and D-lysergic acid diethylamide (LSD).

Morning Glory (Ipomoea violacea)
About 300 seeds, or enough to fill a cupped hand, are equivalent to 200 to 300 mg of LSD, with similar systemic and hallucinatory effects. Ingestion of Hawaiian baby woodrose seeds *(Argyreia nervosa)* presents similarly.

Nutmeg (Myristica fragrans)
Nutmeg contains myristicin, which is metabolized to amphetamine-like compounds.

Cannabis (Cannabis sativa)
The primary psychoactive component is most concentrated in the flowering tops.

Effects include mild mood-altering qualities, euphoria, altered perceptions, time distortion, intensification of ordinary sensory experiences, impairment of short-term memory and attention, impairment of motor skills and reaction times, anxiety, psychotic symptoms, and tachycardia.

Peyote Cactus (Lophophora williamsii)

Effects include a slight rise in blood pressure and heart rate, tachypnea, hyperreflexia, mydriasis, ataxia, perspiration, flushing, salivation, and urination.

Mescal Bean Bush or Texas Mountain Laurel (S. secundiflora)

The beans contain the toxic alkaloid cytisine, which causes nausea, numbing sensations, hallucinations, unconsciousness, convulsions, and death due to respiratory failure.

Khat or Evergreen Khat Tree (Catha edulis)

Khat is also known as chat, qat, eschat, miraa, qaad, and jaad. Khat leaves and bark are chewed, with the juice of the masticated plant being swallowed for stimulatory effects. Khat contains cathinone, cathine (norpseudoephedrine), and norephedrine. Structurally cathinone is like amphetamines. Synthetic cathinones (known as "bath salts") have been manufactured and used illicitly.

Effects include increased energy and alertness, feelings of increased endurance and self-esteem, enhanced imaginative ability, higher capacity to associate ideas, euphoria, tachycardia, increased blood pressure, tachypnea, mydriasis, anorexia, hypomania, insomnia, delusions, paranoid psychosis, aggression, depression, anxiety, hyperthermia, and endocrine disturbances.

Anticholinergic Plants

Henbane *(H. niger)*, jimsonweed *(Datura stramonium)*, and mandrake *(Mandragora officinarum)* contain tropane alkaloids and can produce hallucinations.

Treatment

Treatment of patients exposed to hallucinogenic plants is supportive. Benzodiazepines are first-line treatment for agitation.

Sedating Plants (Isoquinoline Alkaloids)
Poppy
Papaver somniferum flowers yield opium.

Neuromuscular-Blocking Plants (Indole Alkaloids)
Yellow or Carolina Jasmine (Gelsemium sempervirens)

Convulsant Plants (Indoles, Resins)
Strychnine
Strychnine, found in seeds of the tree *Strychnos nux-vomica*, is a powerful CNS stimulant.

Symptoms include hyperreflexia, hypersensitivity to stimuli, migratory rippling movements of the muscles, twitching, severe muscle spasm, rigidity, and spinal convulsions (generally, flexor spasm of the upper limbs, extensor spasm of the lower limbs, opisthotonic posturing, and spasms of the jaw muscles, all without loss of consciousness or postictal states). In between the spasms, which last from 30 seconds to 2 minutes, the muscles become completely relaxed. Respiratory and secondary cardiac failure may ensue during severe convulsions.

Treatment
1. Provide decontamination and supportive treatment, including activated charcoal, benzodiazepines, and barbiturates.
2. Chemical paralysis with a nondepolarizing agent, endotracheal intubation, and mechanical ventilation may be required for severely poisoned patients.

Water Hemlock
Water hemlock *(Cicuta maculata)* and chinaberry *(Melia azedarach)* are two of the most toxic resin-containing plants. Chinaberry produces primarily GI symptoms (see later). The resin of *C. maculata*, an unsaturated aliphatic alcohol called cicutoxin, possesses convulsion-inducing properties.

Symptoms
- Early symptoms are primarily GI, including abdominal pain, vomiting, and diarrhea.
- Profuse perspiration, salivation, and respiratory distress.
- Tachycardia and hypertension or bradycardia and hypotension.
- Epileptiform seizure activity or spastic and tonic movements, including opisthotonus without seizure activity.
- Pupils may be any size.
- Rhabdomyolysis and renal failure.
- Death associated with persistent seizures, cerebral edema, ventricular fibrillation, pulmonary edema, cardiopulmonary arrest, and disseminated intravascular coagulation.

Treatment
1. Symptomatic and supportive with attention to the airway.
2. Activated charcoal.
3. Benzodiazepine and barbiturate administration for seizure control.
4. Phenytoin is contraindicated because it is ineffective for seizure control.
5. Anticholinergic agents are not recommended because they do not reduce seizure activity.
6. Maintenance of adequate urine output and alkalization of urine to treat rhabdomyolysis.

Cardiovascular System
Purine Alkaloids
Cardiotoxins That Inhibit Na⁺, K⁺-ATPase (Cardiac Glycosides)

Cardiac glycosides are found in *Digitalis purpurea* (foxglove; Fig. 40.3), *Digitalis lanata, Nerium oleander* (common oleander; Fig. 40.4), *Thevetia peruviana* (yellow oleander), *Convallaria majalis* (lily of the valley), *Urginea maritima* (squill or sea onion), *Urginea indica, Strophanthus gratus* (ouabain), *Asclepias* spp. (balloon cotton, red-headed cotton bush, milkweeds), *Calotropis procera* (king's crown), *Carissa spectabilis* (wintersweet), *Carissa acokanthera* (bushman's poison), *Cerbera manghas* (sea mango), *Plumeria rubra* (frangipani), *Cryptostegia grandiflora* (rubber vine), *Euonymus europaeus* (spindle tree), *Cheiranthus, Erysimum* (wallflower), and *Helleborus niger* (hellebore).

Clinical Presentation
- Nausea and vomiting
- Visual changes (yellow and green colors, "halos," geometric shapes, scintillations, photophobia)
- Mental status changes (disorientation, psychosis, lethargy, stupor, dysarthria, weakness, dizziness, seizures)
- Cardiac disturbances (palpitations, bradycardia, atrioventricular block, sinus node block, extrasystoles, ventricular arrhythmias, syncope)
- Hyperkalemia
- When death occurs, it is generally caused by cardiotoxicity

Treatment
Cardiac glycoside toxicity from plant ingestions has been successfully treated with the following:
1. Activated charcoal
2. Cardiac pacing
3. Antiarrhythmic agents
4. Digoxin-specific Fab fragments (e.g., Digibind)
5. Maintenance of fluid and electrolyte balance
6. Avoid calcium administration (theoretically harmful)

Steroid Alkaloids Cardiotoxins That Block Sodium Channels
Steroid alkaloids form principal toxic components of several common cardiotoxic plants: *Aconitum* spp. (monkshood; Fig. 40.5), *Veratrum viride* (American hellebore), and *Zigadenus* spp. (death camas).

Symptoms
- Begin within 3 minutes to 6 hours of ingestion and may persist for several days
- Nausea and vomiting
- Salivation

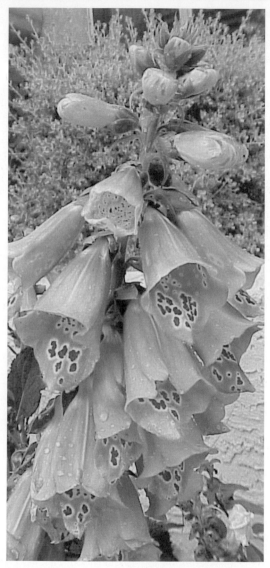

FIGURE 40.3 *Digitalis purpurea* (foxglove). (Photo courtesy Kimberlie Graeme, MD.)

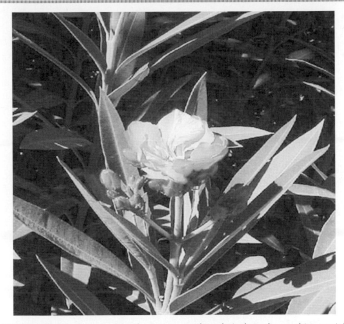

FIGURE 40.4 *Nerium oleander* (common oleander) plants have white or pink flowers. (Photo courtesy Kimberlie Graeme, MD.)

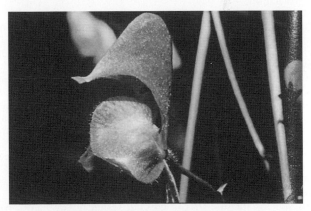

FIGURE 40.5 Monkshood (*Aconitum* spp.).

- Diaphoresis
- Dyspnea
- Restlessness
- Cardiac effects are clinically like cardiac glycoside toxicity, with enhanced vagal tone, bradycardia, heart block, ectopic beats, supraventricular tachycardia, bundle branch block, junctional escape rhythms, ventricular tachycardia, bifascicular ventricular tachycardia, polymorphic ventricular tachycardia, torsades de pointes, ventricular fibrillation, asystole, and hypotension.
- Occasionally death ensues, generally from ventricular arrhythmias such as refractory ventricular fibrillation.

Veratrum Alkaloids
Veratrum and *Zigadenus* species belong to the lily family.

Symptoms
- Generally occur within 30 minutes to 3 hours and resolve within 24 to 48 hours
- Diaphoresis, nausea, vomiting, diarrhea, abdominal pain, hypotension, bradycardia, arrhythmias, and shock
- Syncope, respiratory depression, scotomata, paresthesias, fasciculations, muscle spasticity, hyperreflexia, vertigo, ataxia, dizziness, coma, seizures, and sometimes death

Treatment
1. Treatment of cardiotoxic steroid alkaloid poisoning is supportive and includes atropine, crystalloid fluids, and vasopressors.
2. Patients may require mechanical ventilation and cardiopulmonary resuscitation.
3. Magnesium may suppress ventricular tachycardia.
4. Lidocaine, amiodarone, and hemoperfusion have also been used to treat ventricular arrhythmias.

Grayanotoxins
Resins called grayanotoxins are found in rhododendrons, mountain laurels, and azaleas. Grayanotoxins produce toxicity similar to that of the steroid alkaloids, veratrum, and aconite by binding to myocardial sodium channels and increasing their permeability. Symptoms include salivation, emesis, hypotension, bradycardia, arrhythmias, hypotension, chest pain, dizziness, circumoral and extremity paresthesias, incoordination, and muscular weakness.

Other Cardiotoxins
Taxine Alkaloids
Taxus species include *Taxus baccata* (English yew) and *Taxus brevifolia* (western yew).

Although GI toxicity is most common, dizziness, pupillary dilation, muscle weakness, and convulsions have also been reported. Severe toxicity is characterized by bradycardia, heart block, ventricular tachycardia, ventricular fibrillation, widened QRS complexes, and cardiac arrest.

Lidocaine administration and cardiac pacing have also been reportedly beneficial in the treatment of humans poisoned with yew.

Oral and Gastrointestinal System
Gastrointestinal Irritants
Chinaberry Trees

M. azedarach plants contain toxins that induce gastroenteritis. Immature berries are green but turn yellow and wrinkle with age. After ingestion of as little as one berry, severe gastroenteritis and often bloody diarrhea ensue. Symptoms may be rapid or delayed for several hours after ingestion.

Treatment is supportive, with replacement of fluids and electrolytes and administration of activated charcoal. Hypotension generally resolves with administration of IV fluids.

Solanum

The *Solanum* species include *Solanum tuberosum* (potato), *Solanum gracile* (wild tomato), *Solanum carolinense* (horse nettle), *Solanum pseudocapsicum* (Jerusalem cherry), *Solanum dulcamara* (woody nightshade), *Solanum nigrum* L. var. *americanum* (black nightshade), and other nightshade plants.

Solanine generally produces gastroenteritis, but bradycardia, weakness, and CNS and respiratory depression may also be seen. Treatment is supportive, with replacement of fluids and electrolytes and administration of activated charcoal. Hypotension generally resolves with administration of IV fluids. Atropine may be beneficial if bradycardia develops.

Saponin Glycosides (Pokeweed)

Phytolacca americana, or *Phytolacca decandra*, is most commonly known as pokeweed but is also known as Virginia poke, inkberry, pocan, pigeonberry, American cancer root, garget, red ink, American nightshade, scoke, jalap, and redwood. The root is the most toxic part of the plant.

Symptoms

- Fulminant gastroenteritis with vomiting and diarrhea 2 to 4 hours after ingestion.
- Diarrhea may appear foamy from the sudsing effect of saponin glycosides.
- Hypotension may follow significant GI fluid losses.
- Severe ingestions may result in weakness, loss of consciousness, seizures, and respiratory depression.

Treatment

1. Administration of activated charcoal.
2. Fluid replacement for dehydration secondary to GI fluid losses.
3. Airway support.

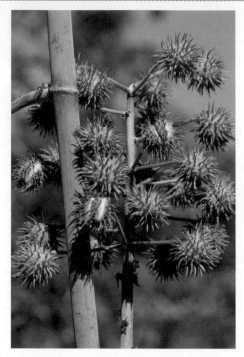

FIGURE 40.6 Guatemalan castor bean plant. (Photo courtesy Paul Auerbach, MD.)

4. Seizures should be treated with benzodiazepines. Hematologic changes generally resolve within weeks.

Anthraquinone Glycosides

Herbal teas that contain leaves, flowers, or bark of senna *(Cassia senna)*, leaves of aloe *(Aloe barbadensis)*, and bark of buckthorn *(Rhamnus frangula)* can cause severe diarrhea. Treatment is supportive, emphasizing adequate volume and electrolyte replacement.

Toxins That Inhibit Protein Synthesis (Phytotoxins)
Phytotoxins (Ricin, Abrin)

Phytotoxins are found in the families Fabaceae—including *Abrus precatorius* (jequirity bean, rosary pea, prayer bead), which contains abrin—and Euphorbiaceae, including the *Ricinus communis* (castor bean), which contains ricin (Fig. 40.6).

Symptoms

- The oral lethal dose is estimated to be 1 mg/kg, theoretically as little as one castor bean in a child and 8 to 10 in an adult.

- There is a latent period of 1 to 6 hours, followed by nausea, vomiting, diarrhea, hemorrhagic gastritis, abdominal pain, thirst, dehydration, hypotension, and shock.
- Death may occur from dehydration and electrolyte imbalances; convulsions may precede death. Death usually occurs after 72 hours because of multiorgan failure.

Treatment
Treatment is supportive, including fluid and electrolyte replacement and activated charcoal administration. Ricin antibody administered intravenously shortly after exposure could be beneficial.

Toxins That Inhibit Cell Division
Colchicine
Colchicine toxicity can occur after ingestion of *Sandersonia aurantiaca* (Christmas bells, Chinese lantern lily); *Gloriosa superba* (glory lily); and, more commonly, *Colchicum autumnale*, all in the lily family.

Symptoms
- Acute poisoning may occur after a latent period of several hours.
- Initial GI effects are severe abdominal pain, nausea, vomiting, diarrhea, and hemorrhagic gastroenteritis.
- Electrolyte abnormalities, volume depletion, acidosis, shock, arrhythmias, and multiorgan failure may occur.
- Muscular weakness and ascending paralysis may cause respiratory arrest, which may occur with a clear sensorium.

Treatment
1. Symptomatic and supportive.
2. Assisted ventilation as needed.
3. Parenteral analgesics to relieve severe abdominal pain should be used cautiously because colchicine sensitizes patients to CNS depressants.
4. Fluid and electrolyte replacement.

Podophyllum
Podophyllum peltatum is most commonly known as the mayapple but has also been called American mandrake. Treatment is similar to that for colchicine.

Hepatotoxic Agents
Pyrrolizidine Alkaloids
Plants containing pyrrolizidine alkaloids include *Senecio vulgaris* (groundsel), *Senecio longilobus* (gordolobo), *Senecio jacobaea* (tansy ragwort), *Senecio latifolius* (Dan's cabbage or "muti"), *Symphytum officinale* (comfrey), *Gynura segetum*, *Ilex paraguariensis* (mate), *Heliotropium* spp., *Crotalaria* spp. (rattlebox), *Amsinckia intermedia* (fiddleneck or tar weed), *Baccharis pteronoides*, *Astragalus lentiginosus*, *Gnaphalium*, *Cynoglossum*, *Echium*, *Tussilago farfara*,

and *Adenostyles alliariae* (alpendost). These plants are consumed in herbal preparations, in breads made with grains that are contaminated with pyrrolizidine-containing weeds ("bread poisoning"), and in teas. Toxicity is associated with hepatic venoocclusive disease; hepatomegaly; cirrhosis; and Budd-Chiari syndrome, which are characterized by obstruction of the trunk or large branches of the hepatic vein. Treatment is supportive.

Oral Irritants (Glycosides, Oxalates)
Daphne
Daphne *(Daphne mezereum),* with its fragrant succulent berries, represents a significant risk to curious children, in whom only a few ingested berries may be lethal. The fruits contain a coumarin glycoside and a diterpene that irritate mucous membranes, with swelling of the tongue and lips. Blisters form if berries are rubbed on the skin. Severe gastroenteritis with GI bleeding may occur after ingestion. In addition, progressive weakness, paralysis, seizures, and coma may develop. Treatment is supportive.

Insoluble Oxalates
Philodendron, Dieffenbachia (dumb cane), *Spathiphyllum* spp. (peace lily), and *Colocasia* spp. (elephant's ear, common cala) contain insoluble oxalates arranged in numerous needles of calcium oxalate (raphides).

Symptoms
- Painful edematous swelling, including angioedema
- Dysphagia
- Vesicles, bullae, or ulcer formation of the oral mucous membranes
- Esophageal erosions
- Respiratory obstruction caused by edema

Treatment is supportive, with special attention to maintaining a patent airway.

Plants That Induce Hypoglycemia
Ackee Fruit
Unripe ackee fruit, *Blighia sapida,* contains hypoglycemic compounds.

Symptoms
- Vomiting, abdominal pain, hypotonia, convulsions, and coma
- Severe hypoglycemia

Treatment is largely supportive and consists of securing an airway and administering activated charcoal, glucose, and IV fluids.

Plants That Inhibit Cellular Respiration
Cyanogenic Plants
Amygdalin is the cyanogenic glycoside found in the seeds of apples and pits of cherries, peaches, plums, and apricots. Black or wild

cherries *(Prunus serotina)* are considered the most dangerous. Linseeds *(Linum usitatissimum)* and cycad seeds *(Cycas* spp.) are also cyanogenic.

Symptoms
- GI distress, bitter almond breath
- CNS (agitation, anxiety, excitement, weakness, numbness, hypotonia, spasticity, coma, seizures)
- Respiratory (hyperpnea, dyspnea, apnea, cyanosis)
- Cardiovascular (tachycardia and hypertension followed by bradycardia and hypotension, heart block, ventricular arrhythmias, asystole)
- Metabolic acidosis
- Pink or cyanotic skin color

Treatment
1. 100% oxygen.
2. Treat cyanide poisoning with hydroxocobalamin at a dose of 5 g IV for adults (70 mg/kg for children); may be repeated for a total dose of 10 g in adults.
3. Alternative cyanide antidote therapy includes amyl nitrite pearls, sodium nitrite, and sodium thiosulfate (cyanide antidote kit), but these are being phased out and may be unavailable in some locations.
4. Supportive care, including mechanical ventilation, IV fluids, and vasopressors as needed.

Plant-Induced Dermatitis
Cutaneous exposure to plants may cause a wide array of skin problems. Plant-induced dermatitis can manifest in multiple fashions, including weeping eczematous patches and plaques, vesicles and bullae, fine scaly patches, or any combination of these. The most common injury to skin caused by plants is a simple scratch, laceration, or puncture wound. This can lead to either bacterial or fungal infection. Plant-induced dermatitis reactions can be further subclassified into irritant contact dermatitis, allergic contact dermatitis, contact urticaria, and less common phototoxic dermatitis and photoallergic dermatitis. Plants can also cause contact urticaria and foreign-body reactions.

Irritant Contact Dermatitis
Plants with sharp leaves, thorns, or spines are the most common cause of irritant contact dermatitis. Examples include the cactus and rose thorns. Chemical irritation can also occur with plants such as the white mustard.

Signs and Symptoms
- Caused by direct contact with the offending plant.
- Most of these rashes are mild and self-limited, typically involving 1% to 2% of body surface area.

- Irritant contact dermatitis causes transient redness and pruritus of the contacted skin.
- The spectrum of reactions ranges from linear scratch marks to weeping ulcerated red scaly plaques.

Treatment
1. Remove patient from exposure to the irritant chemicals or ensure barrier protection with clothing.
2. Gently cleanse the wound with antibacterial soap, apply cool compresses, and watch for infection.
3. Antihistamines, such as hydroxyzine 10 to 25 mg PO four times daily or diphenhydramine 25 mg PO two to four times daily can help with itching.
4. A topical medium-strength steroid, such as triamcinolone 0.1% cream, may be applied twice a day to the affected areas for up to 2 weeks.
5. Clobetasol 0.05% cream or ointment (an ultrapotent topical steroid) can also be used in severe cases.
6. In the case of topical medium-strength and ultrapotent topical steroids, care should be taken to avoid application to the groin, axillae, and face.
7. Typical steroid application regimens are twice daily for 1 to 2 weeks.
8. Cool compresses with aluminum acetate solution (Domeboro, Burow solution) diluted 1:40 in water are very helpful in soothing pruritus and exudative skin irritation.
9. Dermatitis generally heals in less than 7 days if no complications develop and tissue damage is minimal.

Allergic Contact Dermatitis
Allergic contact dermatitis is a type IV delayed hypersensitivity reaction. The most common cause of acute allergic contact dermatitis in the United States is from exposure to poison ivy, oak, and sumac plants (see Plate 21).

Signs and Symptoms
- The most common acute presentation is linearly arranged eczematous edematous patches and plaques with varying amounts of vesiculation and the eruption of bullae.
- Occasionally the eruption is widespread.
- If the face is involved, there can be severe eyelid swelling and patients may be quite distressed by their appearance.
- In severe cases, patients can have systemic symptoms of fever, chills, fatigue, and lethargy.
- In its more chronic form, allergic contact dermatitis presents with lichenified eczematous plaques in exposed areas.

Treatment
1. Systemic corticosteroids are the first line of treatment for moderate to severe disease.

2. In mild cases, use an ultrapotent topical steroid alone, such as clobetasol 0.05% ointment applied to the affected areas twice daily for 2 weeks.

3. If the reaction is of less than 2 hours' duration, IV hydrocortisone (adult dose 100 to 200 mg) or methylprednisolone (adult dose 500 mg to 1 g) can be curative.

4. After a patient has suffered 4 to 6 hours with massive edema, erythema, and pruritus, IV therapy is highly effective, but it must be followed by more prolonged oral or intramuscular administration of corticosteroids for 2 to 3 weeks.

5. If the patient presents after 8 to 16 hours, administer prednisone, 1 mg/kg per day up to 60 mg/d for 3 to 4 days followed by a slow taper over 2 to 3 weeks.

6. A bath with one cup of Aveeno oatmeal per tub of water, in addition to therapy with an antihistamine such as hydroxyzine or diphenhydramine, is helpful for the itching.

7. Together, pimecrolimus (Elidel) 1% cream and tacrolimus (Protopic) 0.03% and 0.1% creams represent new topical immunomodulators that offer a noncorticosteroid treatment alternative.

Contact Urticaria

Contact urticaria can be classified as immunologically or nonimmunologically induced. The immunologic subtype is due to an immediate hypersensitivity reaction requiring antibody formation to a substance.

- Common causes include fruits (e.g., apple and tomato), grains, tulips, spices (e.g., cinnamon, mustard, and rapeseed), trees (e.g., birch and cedar), and vegetables (e.g., carrot, celery, chive, garlic, lettuce, onion, parsley, and potato).

- Type I hypersensitivity reactions show a broad clinical spectrum, from mild skin hives to anaphylaxis. Patients typically present with urticarial wheals in the areas of exposure within 1 to 2 hours of handling a plant.

- Occasionally there is oral involvement with tongue and lip swelling. When there is prominent oral involvement, one must also consider consumed food as a cause. Nonimmunologic plant contact dermatitis is caused by the direct release of urticating substances onto or into the skin.

- The most common plant causing contact urticaria is the stinging nettle, *Urtica dioica* (see Plate 22).

- Urticarial reactions are typically acute and resolve spontaneously, so the advice of a physician is rarely sought. Persistent paresthesia lasting hours has been reported.

Treatment

1. All patients with a risk for severe urticaria should always carry a self-administered epinephrine injection with them.

2. Other supportive treatments for anaphylactic shock—such as histamine$_1$ (H$_1$) and histamine$_2$ antagonists, IV steroids, albuterol,

---

BOX 40.1   Topical Phototoxic Plants

Angelica
Carrot
Celery
Cow parsley
Dill
Fennel
Fig
Gas plant
Giant hogweed
Lemon
Lime
Meadow grass
Parsnip
Stinking mayweed
Yarrow

and oxygen—may be required. Diphenhydramine (Benadryl), in an adult dose of 25 to 50 mg IV/IM usually stops the progression of wheal formation and can be followed by oral hydroxyzine (10–25 mg three times daily) or cyproheptadine (4 mg three times daily) for 2 to 5 days.
3. Pure H_1 blockers, such as fexofenadine (60 mg bid), are also effective and do not depress the CNS.

Phytophotodermatitis
Many plants can produce phototoxic reactions in exposed skin (Box 40.1), resulting in *phytophotodermatitis*. The two types of phytophotodermatitis are phototoxic and photoallergic.
- *Phototoxic* reactions, which appear clinically as an exaggerated sunburn, are analogous to irritant contact dermatitis.
- *Photoallergic* reactions, which appear as eczematous reactions, are analogous to allergic contact dermatitis. Phototoxic reactions are encountered more frequently and are often recognized by a clinician's knowledge of offending agents and the morphology of the exanthem.
- The reactions most frequently appear as linear red patches and plaques with or without edema, but they can also be bullous in nature.
- Common chemical precipitants are furocoumarins, especially psoralens, which are found in limes, lemons, and certain other plants.
- Phytophotodermatitis is common among farm workers, bartenders, cannery packers, and vacationers to sunny climates.
- Meadow-grass dermatitis among hikers is caused by contact with various common weeds (e.g., meadow parsnip) containing furocoumarins. This leads to whip-like erythematous streaks

and postinflammatory hyperpigmentation after exposure to sunlight.

Treatment
1. Sun-protective clothing and emollients
2. Avoidance of causative agents
3. High-potency topical corticosteroids
4. Alternatively, topical tacrolimus
5. Consider systemic immunosuppressants or psoralen plus ultraviolet A (PUVA) with oral glucocorticosteroids for refractory cases

41 | Mushroom Toxicity

There are four major types of mushroom toxins:
1. Gastrointestinal irritants
2. Disulfiram-like toxins
3. Neurotoxins
   a. Muscarinic
   b. Isoxazole derivatives
   c. Psilocybin—hallucinogenic
4. Protoplasmic
   a. Gyromitrin—hepatotoxic
   b. Amatoxin—hepatotoxic
   c. Orellanine—nephrotoxic

If a toxic mushroom ingestion is suspected, follow this guide to mushroom identification:
1. Collect any specimens left at home—preferably uncooked.
2. Collect fresh specimens from gathering sites.
3. Transport and store mushrooms in paper bags.
4. Spores can be recovered from gastrointestinal fluid.
5. Note initial toxicity and time since ingestion. Note symptoms or lack of symptoms among others ingesting mushrooms.
6. Contact a regional poison control center for assistance in locating an expert in identification.
7. When symptoms are not consistent with the identified species, consider that the person might have ingested another type of mushroom.

DISORDERS CAUSED BY GASTROINTESTINAL TOXINS (Table 41.1)
Signs and Symptoms
- Nausea, vomiting, intestinal cramping, and diarrhea within 1 to 2 hours of ingestion
- Stools usually watery and occasionally bloody with fecal leukocytes
- Chills, headaches, and myalgias
- Spontaneous remission of symptoms in 6 to 12 hours

Treatment
1. Initiate supportive treatment, including intravenous or oral fluid and electrolyte replacement.
2. Note time since ingestion. If more than 2 hours have passed between ingestion and symptoms, ingestion of a more serious protoplasmic toxin may have occurred. Monitor liver transaminases.

Table 41.1 Gastrointestinal Disorders: Causative Mushrooms and Identification

NAME	DESCRIPTION
Chlorophyllum molybdites (green-spored parasol) (see Plate 23)	This summer mushroom has a large whitish cap (often 10–40 cm [3.9–15.7 inches] in diameter) that is initially smooth and becomes convex with maturity. Tan or brown warts may be present. The gills are free from the stalk, initially white to yellow and becoming green with maturity. The stalk is 5–25 cm (2–9.8 in) long, smooth, and white. The ring is generally brown on the underside.
Omphalotus olearius (jack-o'-lantern) (see Plate 24)	This bright orange to yellow mushroom has sharp-edged gills. It often grows in clusters at the base of stumps or on buried roots of deciduous trees. The cap is 4–16 cm (1.6–6.3 inches) in diameter on a stalk that is 4–20 cm (1.6–7.9 inches) long. The gills are olive to orange, with white to yellow spores.
Amanita flavorubescens and *Amanita brunnescens*	Both have broad caps (3–15 cm [1.2–5.9 inches] in diameter) with loosely attached warts. The caps are yellowish to brown. The stalks are 3–18 cm (1.2–7.1 inches) long, enlarging toward the base with a superior ring.

3. For a severe case, administer an antiemetic, such as prochlorperazine (Compazine) 2.5 to 10 mg IV, a 25-mg suppository, or ondansetron 4 to 8 mg IV or oral disintegrating tablet.
4. Treat diarrhea with loperamide 4 mg initially, followed by 2 mg after each loose stool up to 16 mg/day.

DISORDERS CAUSED BY DISULFIRAM-LIKE TOXINS (Table 41.2)
Signs and Symptoms
If a person ingests these mushrooms and subsequently ingests alcohol, symptoms like those of an alcohol-disulfiram (Antabuse) reaction can begin within 2 to 6 hours and can last up to 72 hours.
- Severe headache, flushing, and tachycardia within 15 to 30 minutes of alcohol ingestion

Table 41.2 Disulfiram-Like Disorders: Causative Mushroom and Identification	
NAME	**DESCRIPTION**
Coprinus atramentarius (inky cap) (see Plate 25)	This mushroom has a 2–8 cm (0.8–3.1 in) cylindric cap on a 4–5 cm (1.6–2 in) thin stalk. The cap is white, occasionally orange or yellow at the top, with a surface that is characteristically shaggy. The mature cap often develops cracks at its margins, which turn up. The cap blackens as it matures and then liquefies.

- Hyperventilation, shortness of breath, palpitations
- Chest pain and orthostatic hypotension in severe cases; may be confused with an allergic reaction or acute myocardial infarction

Treatment
1. Generally requires only supportive care.
2. Hypotension responds to fluid or, if necessary, norepinephrine (2 to 4 mcg/min IV or 0.05 to 0.1 mcg/kg/min in children, increasing as needed every 5 to 10 minutes).
3. Severe symptomatic supraventricular tachycardia can be controlled with propranolol (0.5 to 3 mg IV in adults; 0.01 to 0.02 mg/kg in children up to a maximum of 1 mg/dose, repeated after 5 to 10 minutes as needed).
4. Symptoms may resolve spontaneously within 3 to 6 hours.
5. Activated charcoal is not beneficial.

DISORDERS CAUSED BY NEUROLOGIC TOXINS (MUSCARINE) (Table 41.3)
Signs and Symptoms
- Symptoms develop within 15 to 30 minutes of ingesting muscarine-containing mushrooms.
- Symptoms include salivation, lacrimation, urination, diarrhea, diaphoresis, gastrointestinal upset, and emesis (SLUDGE).
- Bradycardia and bronchospasm.
- Constricted pupils.
- Copious bronchial secretions that may cause respiratory failure, requiring mechanical ventilation.

Treatment
1. Supportive care with oxygen, suctioning, and endotracheal intubation as needed.
2. Fluid and electrolyte replacement.
3. Atropine (if symptoms are life threatening) 0.01 mg/kg IV every 5 to 10 minutes until secretions are controlled. There is no

Table 41.3 Muscarine Disorders: Causative Mushrooms and Identification	
NAME	**DESCRIPTION**
Amanita muscaria (see Plate 26)	This mushroom has a cap 5–30 cm (2–11.9 inches) in diameter that is scarlet red with white warts. The stalk is white, often hollow, and grows 15–20 cm (5.9–7.9 inches) long, tapering upward. It has a prominent cup and volva and numerous rings. The gills are free and white.
Inocybe cookei (see Plate 27)	The Inocybaceae family contains small brown mushrooms with conical caps up to 6 cm (2.4 inches) in diameter. Stalks are 2–10 cm (0.8–3.9 inches) long and covered with fine brown to white hairs. The gills are brown and notched.
Clitocybe dealbata	*Clitocybe* mushrooms are whitish tan to gray, with 15–33 mm (0.6–1.3 inches) caps on hairless stalks 1–5 cm (0.4–2 inches) long. The gills run down the stalk.

Table 41.4 Isoxazole Reactions: Causative Mushrooms and Identification	
NAME	**DESCRIPTION**
Amanita muscaria	See Table 41.3.
Amanita pantherina (see Plate 28)	This mushroom is 5–15 cm (2–5.9 inches) long with a cap 5–15 cm in diameter. The cap is white to pink early and becomes reddish-brown or brown with maturity. The stalk has a distinct ring with a volva or cup at the bottom. When the flesh is cut or injured, it develops a pinkish tinge. The gills are free and produce white spores.

upper limit to the dose if secretions are excessive. Atropine may worsen the central nervous system (CNS) effects of some mushrooms, such as *Amanita muscaria.*

ISOXAZOLE REACTIONS (Table 41.4)
Signs and Symptoms
Symptoms usually begin within 30 minutes of ingestion and last up to 2 hours.

With ingestion of <15 mg, the following may appear:
- Dizziness
- Ataxia

Table 41.5　Hallucinogenic Disorders: Causative Mushrooms and Identification	
NAME	**DESCRIPTION**
Species of *Psilocybe* (see Plate 29)	These are little brown mushrooms with 0.5–4 cm (0.2–1.6 in) broad caps that are smooth and become sticky or slippery when wet. The stalks are slender and 4–15 cm (1.6–5.9 in) long. The gills are gray to purple-gray. The flesh of these mushrooms turns blue or greenish when bruised or cut.
Species of *Panaeolus*	These little brown mushrooms are about the same size as *Psilocybe*. The gills are dark gray or black with black spores. Unlike *Psilocybe*, the caps are not sticky or slippery when wet.

With ingestion of ≥15 mg, the following may appear:
- Pronounced ataxia, visual disturbances
- Delirium or manic behavior
- Visual hallucinations, seizures, muscle twitching, hyperactivity

Treatment
1. Supportive care
2. Sedation as needed with a benzodiazepine (e.g., diazepam 2 to 5 mg IV q10min as needed) or phenobarbital (30 mg IV hourly).
3. If hyperpyrexia occurs (primarily seen in children), consider external cooling.

DISORDERS CAUSED BY HALLUCINOGENIC MUSHROOMS (Table 41.5)
Signs and Symptoms
With ingestion of 10 mg of the mushroom, the following may appear:
- Moderate euphoria
  With ingestion of 20 mg of the mushroom, the following may appear:
- Hallucinations and a loss of time sensation
- Heightened imagination developing within 15 to 30 minutes of ingestion
- Hallucinations lasting 4 to 6 hours
- Fever and seizures in children

Treatment
1. Supportive care
2. Sedation as needed with a benzodiazepine (e.g., diazepam 2 to 5 mg IV q10min as needed) or phenobarbital (30 mg IV hourly).

Table 41.6 Protoplasmic Disorders: Causative Mushrooms and Identification	
NAME	**DESCRIPTION**
Gyromitra Toxin	
Gyromitra esculenta (false morel) (see Plate 30)	This mushroom grows in the spring near pines and in sandy soil. It is 5–16 cm (2–6.3 inches) in height with a reddish-brown to dark-brown irregularly shaped cap. The cap's surface is curved and folded, resembling a human brain. The stalk is often as thick as the cap. The inside of the cap and the stalk are hollow.
Amatoxin	
Amanita phalloides (death cap) (see Plate 31)	This mushroom grows under deciduous trees in the fall and has a white to greenish cap 4–16 cm (1.6–6.3 inches) in diameter, often with remnants of the veil (warts). The stalk is thick, 5–18 cm (2–7 inches) long, with a large bulb at the base, often with a volva or cup. A thin ring is usually present on the stalk. The gills are generally free and white to green.
Amanita virosa (see Plate 32)	This mushroom resembles *Amanita phalloides*, but the cap is more yellowish or white.

3. If hyperpyrexia occurs (primarily seen in children), consider external cooling.

DISORDERS CAUSED BY PROTOPLASMIC POISONS (Table 41.6)
Gyromitra Toxin
Signs and Symptoms
- Onset of nausea, vomiting, and diarrhea within 4 to 50 (average 5 to 12) hours
- Neurologic symptoms of dizziness, weakness, and loss of muscle coordination
- Severe neurologic symptoms including coma, delirium, and seizures
- Hepatic failure beginning 2 to 4 days after ingestion
- Hepatic failure often associated with hypoglycemia

Treatment
1. Activated charcoal if the patient presents within 1 hour of ingestion. Note that most of these patients will be asymptomatic.

2. Fluid and electrolyte replacement as needed.
3. Glucose replacement. Treat hypoglycemia with glucose infusion.
4. Pyridoxine 25 mg/kg up to 20 g/day IV to control seizures or coma
5. If significant hepatic failure occurs, transfer the patient to a transplant facility.

Amatoxin (See Table 41.6)
Signs and Symptoms
- Onset of nausea, vomiting, and diarrhea 4 to 16 hours after ingestion
- Resolution of gastrointestinal symptoms 12 to 24 hours later
- Onset of hepatic and occasionally renal failure 48 to 72 hours after ingestion
- Possibly coagulopathy and pancreatitis associated with the hepatotoxicity

Treatment
Established
1. Activated charcoal (1 g/kg orally or via gastric tube) if the ingestion has occurred within 5 hours.
2. Silymarin (silibinin) 20 to 40 mg/kg per day IV, 1.4 to 4.2 g/day orally.

Experimental
3. Hyperbaric oxygen if available.
4. Cimetidine 4 to 10 g IV divided over 48 hours.
5. If significant hepatic failure develops, transfer the patient to a transplant facility.

Animal Attacks

Recommended oral antibiotics for prophylaxis of animal and human bite wounds are listed in Appendix J.

WOUND CARE

Evaluate for potential blunt trauma and injury to deep and vital structures by penetrating teeth, claws, or horns. When the patient reaches definitive care, make sure that he or she receives appropriate immunizations to enable tetanus immunity.

1. Irrigate the wound, using boiled or otherwise treated and potable water (see Chapter 20 for a further discussion of irrigation).
2. If possible, add a germicidal agent to the irrigating solution. In order of preference, use 1% povidone-iodine solution (not "scrub"), 1% benzalkonium chloride, or ordinary hand (camping) soap.
3. Complete the irrigation with a germicide-free solution (e.g., potable water) to rinse all irritating chemicals from the wound. Use 2% benzalkonium chloride or potable water with dish soap to cleanse wounds inflicted by animals suspected of being rabid (see Chapter 43).
4. Clean the wound, if necessary, by swabbing with a soft, clean cloth or sterile gauze. Follow with a repeat irrigation.
5. Determine whether the injury is high or low risk for infection to make decisions about closure, need for antibiotics, and evacuation (Box 42.1).
6. If the wound edges are macerated, crushed, or extremely contaminated, perform sharp debridement.
7. If the wound must be closed to control bleeding, allow dressing, or facilitate evacuation, do so in a manner that allows drainage. Use tape, surgical adhesive strips, or loose approximating sutures or staples in preference to a tight closure.
   a. High-risk wounds should be irrigated, debrided, and if possible left open for closure later. Do not primarily close bite wounds older than 6 to 12 hours (limbs) or 12 to 24 hours (face).
   b. Immobilize high-risk wounds of the hand with a bulky mitten dressing in an elevated position and start the patient promptly on an antibiotic (see Appendix J).
8. Cover the wound with a sterile dressing or clean dry cloth.

BOX 42.1 Risk Factors for Infection From Animal Bites

High Risk
Location
Hand, wrist, or foot
Scalp or face in patients with high risk for cranial perforation; computed tomography or skull radiograph examination is mandatory
Over a joint (possibility of perforation)
Through-and-through bite of cheek or chin

Type of Wound
Punctures that are difficult or impossible to irrigate adequately
Tissue crushing that cannot be debrided (typical of herbivores)
Carnivore bite over vital structure (e.g., artery, nerve, joint)

Patient
Older than 50 years
Asplenic
Chronic alcoholic
Altered immune status (e.g., chemotherapy, acquired immunodeficiency syndrome, immune defect)
Diabetic
Peripheral vascular insufficiency
Chronic corticosteroid therapy
Prosthetic or diseased cardiac valve (consider systemic prophylaxis)
Prosthetic or seriously diseased joint (consider systemic prophylaxis)

Species
Large cat (canine teeth produce deep punctures that can penetrate joints and the cranium)
Primates
Pigs (anecdotal evidence only)
Alligators and crocodiles

Low Risk
Location
Face, scalp, ears, and mouth (all facial wounds should be sutured)
Self-bite of buccal mucosa that does not go through to skin (i.e., is not through and through)

Type of Wound
Large clean lacerations that can be thoroughly cleansed (the larger the laceration, the lower the infection rate)
Partial-thickness lacerations and abrasions

Species
Rodents
Quokkas
Bats (although there is a high risk for rabies)

9. Apply a splint if appropriate to restrict motion.
10. If the wound is of the high-risk type (see following features) or treatment is hours away, administer a prophylactic antibiotic as listed in Appendix J. High-risk wounds have the following features:
    - Location: hand, scalp or face in infants, over a major joint (possible perforation), through-and-through wound of cheek
    - Type of wound: puncture, tissue crush, carnivore bite over a vital structure (artery, nerve, or joint)
    - Patient risk factor: elderly, asplenic, chronic alcoholic, immunosuppressed, diabetic, peripheral vascular insufficiency, receiving chronic corticosteroid therapy, prosthetic or diseased cardiac valve, prosthetic or seriously diseased joint
    - Animal species: feline, human, primate, pig

WOUND INFECTION

The causative organisms in a wound infection after an animal bite are most often *Staphylococcus* or *Streptococcus,* but anaerobic infection may occur. Less common pathogens, such as *Pasteurella* or *Eikenella,* are usually sensitive to and effectively treated with the antibiotics discussed in Appendix J.

SPECIFIC ANIMAL CONSIDERATIONS
Dog
- If a dog's large teeth cause facial or scalp wounds in a small child, particularly an infant, be alert for the possibility of an underlying skull or facial bone fracture.
- For a bite made by a large dog or any other animal with large teeth and when the bite is close to a major vessel, examine the wound for absent or diminished pulse, sensory or motor deficit, large or expanding hematoma, or extremely active bleeding. Any of these may indicate an arterial injury that will require immediate evacuation to a center equipped with vascular imaging and surgeons.

Cat
- Do not primarily repair a cat bite puncture because of the high likelihood of infection.
- *Pasteurella multocida* causes an infection that may follow a cat or ungulate bite.
- With bites from large cats, suspect deep penetration, even with a seemingly trivial surface wound.

Porcupine
- Be aware that porcupine quills not only penetrate human skin but also can migrate up to 25 cm (9.8 inches). The quills are barbed, with spongy cores, allowing them to absorb body fluid and expand, which makes removal even more difficult.

- Pull the quill straight out. If the quill is deeply penetrated, make a small nick in the skin to allow egress of the entrapped barb.

Skunk

- The skunk sprays its victim with musk from anal sacs. The musk causes skin irritation, keratoconjunctivitis, temporary blindness, nausea, and occasionally seizures and loss of consciousness. The chief component of the musk is butyl mercaptan.
- Neutralize the butyl mercaptan with a strong oxidizing agent such as sodium hypochlorite in a 5.25% solution (household bleach) further diluted 1:5 or 1:10 in water. Then cleanse the area with tincture of green soap, followed by a dilute bleach rinse. Tomato juice as a shampoo has been advocated for deodorizing hair, which should then be washed and can be mildly bleached or cropped short.

Herbivores

High-risk bites from horses, donkeys, cattle, sheep, camels, deer, and most other herbivores are treated with the same antibiotics as bites from dogs, cats, and humans.

Pigs

Bites from domestic pigs may pose a risk for infections from bacteria that are resistant to routinely recommended prophylactic antibiotics. Add ciprofloxacin 500 mg q12h to the regimen (see Appendix J).

Alligators and Crocodiles

Victims of alligator or crocodile attack typically sustain wounds contaminated with freshwater or seawater, depending on the location; antibiotic choice should be directed against *Aeromonas hydrophila* and *Vibrio* species.

AVOIDING AND MITIGATING ANIMAL ATTACKS

To avoid animal attacks and bites,

- Do not leave young children alone with wild or potentially biting animals.
- Never pet an unfamiliar dog, especially if it is tied up or confined.
- Avoid sudden movements around animals.
- Never try to separate fighting animals unless you are well protected; instead, use a bucket of water or a hose.
- Do not invade the territory of nursing animals or animals with young offspring.
- Do not corner or threaten animals unless in a purposeful defensive gesture (as when under attack by a cougar).
- Know which animals you might encounter and their likely behaviors when frightened, hungry, irritated, and threatened, and know how they will respond to your behaviors for the purposes of pacification, intimidation, and defense.

BEAR ATTACK PREVENTION AND RISK REDUCTION
Prevent Predatory Behavior
- Avoid camping along bear travel corridors or at feeding sites.
- Use proper food storage to render human food unavailable to bears.
- Avoid campsites littered with human refuse.
- Reduce food odors by cooking and eating at a site away from the sleeping area. Do not sleep in clothes worn while cooking or eating.
- Do not leave garbage or food buried or poured into the ground at the campsite.
- Keep sleeping bags at least partially unzipped to facilitate a quick exit.
- Sleep in a tent. Equip each tent with a flashlight. Consider equipping yourself with pepper spray.

Avoiding an Encounter
- Make noise so that the bear knows a person is present. Bear bells may not be sufficiently loud.
- Remain alert to the terrain and environment in bear country. An "upwind bear" is more likely to be surprised by you, as is one in heavy forestation, near loud rushing water, in the rain, or in fog.
- Avoid ripened berry patches, streams with spawning fish, and elk calving grounds. A collection of ravens may indicate carrion and the presence of feeding bears.
- If you see bear signs (e.g., tracks, scratching, droppings, or a prey carcass), suspect that a bear is in the vicinity.
- Do not approach bears or any wild animals too closely for a better view or photograph.

Avoiding an Attack
- Allow the bear to know that you are human and not a prey species. Once the bear sees you, step out away from any visual obstruction and make it clear that you are a human. If you attempt to hide, you may confuse the bear. Speak in a calm voice to allow the bear to identify you.
- Do not make sudden movements or yell out.
- Do not stare directly at the bear. Look to the side or stand sideways to the bear. Never turn your back on any wild carnivore.
- Do not climb a tree or run away.

If a Grizzly Bear Attacks
- Do not run, try to climb a tree, fight, or scream.
- Drop to the ground and protect your head and neck by interlocking your hands behind your head (ear level) and flexing your head forward, either in the fetal position or flat on the ground face-down (Fig. 42.1). If a curious bear turns you supine, continue rolling to the face-down position.

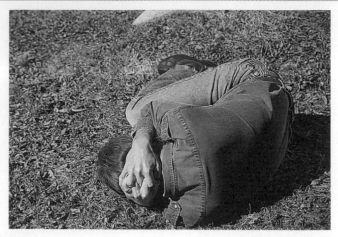

FIGURE 42.1   Curling into the fetal position to defend against a grizzly bear attack. (Courtesy Marilynn G. French.)

- Do not hold out an arm to ward off the attack.
- Never try to look at the bear during an attack.
- After the attack, minimize any perceived threat and stay down until you are sure the bear has left the area.
- When you believe the bear has left the area, peek around while moving as little as possible, try to determine which way the bear went, and then pick the best option for leaving the area.

If a Black Bear Attacks

If the attack is by a black bear, a different set of guidelines (from grizzly bear defense) should be followed. Black bear aggression should be countered with aggression, such as shouting, yelling, throwing rocks or sticks, or whatever means are available. The person should never lie down in a protective, submissive position because black bears are more likely to prey on humans they encounter at close range than are grizzly bears.

43 | Zoonoses

DEFINITION
Zoonoses are diseases of animals that may be transmitted to humans under natural conditions.

DISORDERS
Rabies
Globally, rabies is the tenth most frequent cause of death from infectious disease. The World Health Organization (WHO) currently estimates the number of annual rabies deaths globally at 40,000 to 70,000, although the median number of 55,000 deaths is widely accepted. That is an average of approximately one death every 10 minutes.

In the United States, rabies viruses in dogs and from wildlife spillover are rare. Rabies surveillance data have identified the four major animal reservoirs to be bats, raccoons, skunks, and foxes. Bat exposures may go unrecognized, because of the minimal injury or pain from a bite, and are the most common cause of human rabies. Small rodents, such as chipmunks, squirrels, gerbils, rabbits, rats, and mice, are not a risk for viral transmission to humans. Rabies is not rare in other domestic animals, including cattle, horses, mules, sheep, and goats.

Rabies virus is transmitted in saliva or by aerosols of saliva, secretions, and excretions (bats). Because the virus is sensitive to desiccation and ultraviolet light, once contaminated materials are dry or exposed to sunlight, they rapidly become noninfectious.

Physical contact with wild animals should be avoided. If wild animals are observed, certain symptoms (which if lacking by no means excludes rabies) are indicative of rabies (Box 43.1). If rabies is suspected, a complete set of samples should be collected for testing by all currently available diagnostic procedures. Consultation is available from the Centers for Disease Control and Prevention (CDC) 24 hours a day, 7 days a week, and should be obtained (877-554-4625; http://www.cdc.gov/rabies/).

Signs and Symptoms
- Incubation period: 9 days to more than 1 year, usually (in humans) 2 to 12 weeks
- Initial symptoms are nonspecific
  - Malaise, fatigue, anxiety, agitation, irritability, insomnia, depression, fever, headache, nausea, vomiting, sore throat, abdominal pain, anorexia

---

BOX 43.1   Symptoms Possibly Indicative of Rabies

- Unprovoked aggression ("furious" rabies). Some animals may attack anything that moves, or even inanimate objects.
- Unusual friendliness ("dumb" rabies).
- The animal may stumble, fall, appear disoriented or uncoordinated, or wander aimlessly.
- Paralysis, often beginning in the hind legs or throat. Paralysis of the throat muscles can cause the animal to bark, whine, drool, choke, or froth ("foam") at the mouth.
- Atypical vocalizations ranging from chattering to shrill screams.
- Nocturnal animals may become unusually active during the day.
- Raccoons walk as if on very hot pavement.
- Skunks, raccoons, foxes, and dogs usually display furious rabies. Bats often display dumb rabies and may be found on the ground, unable to fly. This can be very risky for children, who are more likely than adults to handle wild animals.

- Early pain, pruritus, or paresthesias at the site of the bite in approximately half of patients
- Neurologic symptoms after prodromal period, which lasts 2 to 10 days; may be in the form of furious or paralytic (dumb) rabies
- Furious rabies: increasing agitation, hyperactivity, seizures, and episodes in which the patient may thrash about, bite, and become aggressive, alternating with periods of relative calm
  - Hallucinations possible
  - Severe laryngeal spasm or spasm of respiratory muscles possible when the patient attempts to drink, or even looks at, water (hydrophobia)
  - Pharyngeal spasm possible when air is blown on the patient's face (aerophobia)
- Paralytic (dumb) rabies: progressive lethargy, incoordination, ascending paralysis, coma

Postexposure Treatment

1. Observe the offending animal (Fig. 43.1).
2. Wash the area thoroughly with soap and water to reduce contamination. Cleanse the wound with either povidone-iodine solution or benzalkonium chloride (Zephiran). If neither of these agents is available, use 70% alcohol (ethanol) solution.
3. Infiltrate the wound edges with local anesthetic (e.g., procaine hydrochloride 1%).
4. Administer rabies immune globulin.
   a. The drug of choice is human rabies immune globulin (HRIG, 150 international units of neutralizing antibody per milliliter), administered as a single dose of 20 international units/kg. Theoretically, HRIG may be effective at any time before development of symptoms and should be given regardless

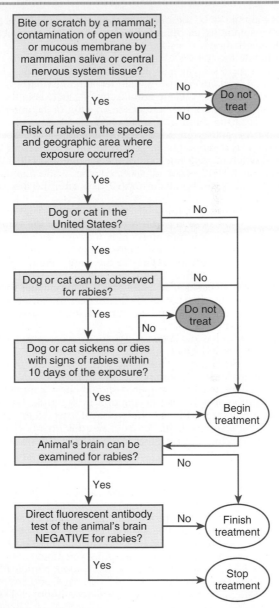

FIGURE 43.1 Postexposure Prophylaxis. Decision tree for human rabies postexposure prophylaxis. (From Bennett JE, Dolin R, Blaser MJ, editors: *Mandell, Douglas, and Bennett's principles and practices of infectious diseases*, ed 8, Philadelphia, 2015, Elsevier.)

of the time since the biting accident. An alternative is equine rabies immune globulin (ERIG), which is given at a dose of 40 international units/kg.

b. Infiltrate the full dose around the bite wound. If the wound is in a small site, such as the finger, inject as much as feasible in that area. Inject the remainder intramuscularly at a site distant from the vaccine administration, such as in the upper outer quadrant of the buttocks in an adult or the anterolateral aspect of the thigh in a small child.

c. Give the antiserum while active immunization (vaccine) is started, as described next. Be certain to use a different syringe and different anatomic site for the vaccine and HRIG administration. If HRIG is not administered when active immunization is started, it can be given up to 7 days after the first vaccine dose.

5. Administer human diploid cell vaccine (HDCV). The vaccine is given as a 1-mL dose regardless of the patient's age on days 0, 3, 7, and 14. Inject it intramuscularly into the deltoid muscle in an adult and into an anterior thigh muscle in an infant or small child. Do not give the vaccine in the same syringe or site as HRIG, and do not give it into the buttock (to avoid a poorly immunogenic deposition into fat). The WHO continues to recommend a fifth dose on day 28 for immunocompromised patients. Pregnancy is not considered a contraindication to postexposure prophylaxis (PEP).

6. A person who has undergone preexposure immunization with HDCV or purified chick embryo cell vaccine (PCEC) should receive booster doses of the same vaccine on days 0 and 3.

7. After immunization, antirabies titers 2 to 4 weeks after the immunization series is completed should show complete virus neutralization at a 1:5 serum dilution in the rapid fluorescent focus inhibition test (RFFIT) or a titer of at least 0.5 international units. If the response is inadequate, an additional booster dose of rabies vaccine can be given each week until a satisfactory response is obtained.

Prevention

The CDC and other institutions now advocate the following measures:

1. Dwellings should be "bat-proofed" by tightly covering all possible entrances, particularly roof ventilation openings, with wire screens. Protection from bats in unscreened dwellings or when sleeping outdoors can be achieved with mosquito netting.

2. Contact with bats must be assiduously avoided, particularly bats that are behaving unusually. Bats are nocturnal, and any activity during daylight hours should be considered abnormal. Diseased bats often are unable to fly.

3. Any person who has contact with a bat, regardless of whether a bite is thought to have been inflicted, should receive PEP unless the bat has been caught and examined for rabies.

4. Any person, particularly a child, who awakens from sleep and finds a bat in the room should receive PEP unless the bat has been caught and examined. Several recent bat rabies victims have been children who experienced this type of exposure.

Preexposure Prophylaxis

1. Obtain preexposure immunization in humans by administering either HDVC or PCEC in three 1-mL intramuscular (deltoid muscle in adults and anterior thigh muscle in children) injections on days 0, 7, and 21 or 28.
2. Check the antirabies titer, and give a booster dose of vaccine if the titer drops below complete virus neutralization at a 1:5 serum dilution in the RFFIT or a titer of at least 0.5 international units.

Cat-Scratch Disease

Cat-scratch disease has been linked to the organism *Bartonella* (formerly *Rochalimaea*) *henselae*. Most cases are caused by scratches from cats, but dog and monkey bites, as well as thorns and splinters, have been implicated. Most cases occur in children, with an average incubation period of 3 to 10 days.

Signs and Symptoms

- Characteristic feature: regional lymphadenitis, usually involving lymph nodes of the arm or leg
  - May affect only one lymph node
  - Nodes often painful and tender, and about 25% suppurate
- Raised, red, slightly tender, and nonpruritic papule with a small central vesicle or eschar that resembles an insect bite at the site of primary inoculation
- Mild systemic symptoms including fever (usually <39° C [102.2° F]), chills, malaise, anorexia, and nausea
- Evanescent morbilliform and pleomorphic rashes lasting up to 48 hours
- Parinaud's oculoglandular syndrome: conjunctivitis and ipsilateral, enlarged, tender preauricular lymph node
- Rarely, encephalopathy, seizures, transverse myelitis, arthritis, splenic abscess, optic neuritis, or thrombocytopenic purpura

Treatment

1. Cat-scratch disease usually resolves spontaneously in weeks to months. In approximately 2% of patients (usually adults), the course is prolonged and involves systemic complications.
2. Antibiotics that may help shorten the course of illness include trimethoprim/sulfamethoxazole, rifampin, gentamicin, and ciprofloxacin (see Appendix H).
3. For isolated lymph node involvement, treat with azithromycin (10 mg/kg on day 1 [500 mg maximum], followed by 5 mg/kg/day for 4 days [up to 250 mg/day]) for a 5-day course.
4. The following antibiotics have been studied and found to be

ineffective: amoxicillin/clavulanate, erythromycin, dicloxacillin, cephalexin, ceftriaxone, cefaclor, and tetracycline.

Leptospirosis

Leptospirosis is caused by *Leptospira interrogans,* which infects many wild and domestic animals. Dogs are the most common vectors. The organism is shed in the urine. Humans contract the disease when they encounter contaminated water or soil.

Signs and Symptoms

- After incubation period (average 7 to 12 days, range 1 to 26 days), initial phase (4 to 7 days) of abrupt high fever, chills, headache, malaise, prostration, myalgias, lymph node enlargement, nonproductive cough, and prominent conjunctival suffusion without exudate; nausea, vomiting, and abdominal pain possible
- Apparent recovery for a few days, followed by return of less dramatic fever associated with relentless headache with meningeal signs; severe cases initially interpreted as aseptic meningitis, infectious hepatitis, or fever of unknown origin (FUO)
- Maculopapular, petechial, or purpuric rash; uveitis (iridocyclitis); arrhythmias; splenic enlargement
- Weil's syndrome (icteric form): jaundice, petechial hemorrhages, renal insufficiency

Treatment and Prevention

1. The treatment of choice is doxycycline, 100 mg orally (PO) twice daily for 7 days, or for children 8 years or older, 2 mg/kg/day in two equally divided doses, not to exceed 200 mg daily.
2. Azithromycin, 10 mg/kg PO on day 1 (maximum 500 mg/day), followed by 5 mg/kg/day PO once daily on subsequent days (maximum 250 mg/day), or amoxicillin, 25 to 50 mg/kg in three equally divided doses (maximum 500 mg/dose), can also be used, especially for children less than 8 years old and pregnant women.
3. Alternative regimens for hospitalized patients include penicillin, 250,000 to 400,000 units/kg/day IV in four to six divided doses (maximum 6 to 12 million units daily); ceftriaxone, 80 to 100 mg/kg IV once daily (maximum 2 g daily); cefotaxime, 100 to 150 mg/kg/day IV in three to four equally divided doses; or doxycycline, 4 mg/kg/day IV in two equally divided doses (maximum 200 mg/day, not in children or pregnant women).
4. Several studies have demonstrated comparable efficacy for doxycycline, penicillin, ceftriaxone, cefotaxime, and azithromycin. A Jarisch-Herxheimer reaction may be seen within a few hours of initial treatment.
5. Doxycycline 200 mg PO once weekly may be used to prevent illness when traveling in endemic countries and participating in high-risk activities such as rafting, kayaking, or swimming in fresh water.

Rat-Bite Fever

Rat-bite fever is an acute illness caused by *Streptobacillus monili-formis* or *Spirillum minus,* which are part of the oral flora of rodents, including squirrels. It may also result from bites by weasels, dogs, cats, and pigs.

Signs and Symptoms

- Streptobacillary rat-bite (Haverhill) fever:
  - Incubation period of 1 week to several weeks; disease transmitted by contaminated food, milk, or water or by simply playing with pet rats, without a history of bite or injury
  - Initial symptoms: fever, chills, cough, malaise, headache
  - Less frequently lymphadenitis, followed by a nonpruritic morbilliform or petechial rash that frequently involves the palms and soles
  - Migratory polyarthritis in 50% of patients that may last several years
  - Centralized lymphadenitis, absence of meningeal signs
- Spirillary rat-bite fever:
  - Incubation period of 7 to 21 days, during which the bite lesion heals
  - Onset heralded by chills, fever, lymphadenitis, and dark-red macular rash
  - Myalgias common, but arthritis absent, which helps in the differentiation from streptobacillary rat-bite fever
  - Disease episodic and relapsing, with a 24- to 72-hour cycle

Treatment

1. The treatment of choice is IV penicillin G, 200 000 units every 4 hours for 7 to 10 days, followed by an oral course (penicillin V, 500 mg PO four times daily, ampicillin, 500 mg four times daily), or amoxicillin (500 mg three times daily) to complete a 14-day course of therapy.
2. Alternatives for penicillin-allergic patients:
   - Doxycycline, 100 mg IV or PO twice daily
   - Tetracycline, 30 mg/kg/day PO in four divided doses
   - Streptomycin, 15 mg/kg/day IM in two divided doses
3. Erythromycin is not effective.
4. Complications such as endocarditis should be treated with high-dose IV potassium penicillin G, 10 to 20 million units/day, or alternatively IV ceftriaxone 2 g daily.
   - Doxycycline can be used at dosing noted above as an alternative for penicillin allergic patients with severe complications.

Tularemia

Tularemia represents a variety of syndromes caused by *Francisella tularensis*. This bacterium is a common parasite of rabbits, rodents, hares, moles, beavers, muskrats, squirrels, rats, and mice. The primary mode of transmission to humans is via a blood-sucking arthropod such as a tick or by skin or eye inoculation resulting from skinning, dressing, or handling a diseased animal.

Signs and Symptoms

* Abrupt onset of fever, often with chills and temperature up to 41.5° C (106.7° F)
* Headache, which may mimic meningitis in severity
* Hepatomegaly, splenomegaly
* Six clinical presentations
  * Ulceroglandular form (most common)
    * Typical skin lesion beginning as red papule or nodule that indurates and ulcerates
    * Frequently painful and tender
    * Ulcers associated with handling infected animals usually located on the hand, with associated lymphadenopathy in the epitrochlear or axillary area
    * Infection transmitted by tick bite, usually initiated on the lower extremity and associated with inguinal or femoral lymphadenopathy
    * Possible exudative pharyngitis
  * Oculoglandular form
    * Unilateral conjunctivitis in and around a nodular lesion on the conjunctiva, extreme ocular pain, photophobia, itching, lacrimation, mucopurulent eye discharge
    * Enlargement of the ipsilateral preauricular lymph node
  * Glandular form: enlarged, tender lymph nodes without an associated skin lesion
  * Typhoidal form: fever, chills, debility, possible exudative pharyngitis
  * Oropharyngeal form
    * Exudative pharyngitis associated with cervical lymphadenitis
    * Also, may be seen with typhoidal or oculoglandular form
  * Pneumonic form: pneumonia, with cough, chest pain, shortness of breath, sputum production, and hemoptysis

Treatment

1. Streptomycin is the drug of choice; administer in a dose of 30 to 40 mg/kg/day IM divided q12h for 3 days, followed by half the dose for another 4 to 7 days.
2. Alternative antibiotics include intravenous gentamicin or oral tetracycline or chloramphenicol. The latter two drugs are given as 50 to 60 mg/kg/day divided q6h for 14 days. Relapse may occur with the oral drugs.
3. For mild infections, doxycycline, 100 mg twice daily for 14 days in adults, and for children over 8 years old, 2 to 4 mg/kg/day PO in two divided doses for 14 days (daily dose not to exceed 200 mg), or ciprofloxacin, 500 to 750 mg twice daily for 14 days, is appropriate.
4. Ceftriaxone is not effective.

Brucellosis

Brucella organisms are carried chiefly by swine, cattle, goats, and sheep. They are usually transmitted to humans by direct skin contact or from the ingestion of contaminated milk products. The incubation period in humans is 1 to 15 weeks.

Signs and Symptoms

- No specific symptoms or signs; thus the nickname "mimic" disease
- Most characteristic clinical manifestation: undulating fever
- Acute form: headache, weakness, diaphoresis, myalgias, arthralgias, anorexia, constipation, weight loss, hepatomegaly, and splenomegaly
- Subacute or "undulant" form: like acute, but milder symptoms, with addition of arthritis and orchitis
- Chronic form: symptoms persist for more than 1 year; arthralgias and extra-articular rheumatism, mimics chronic fatigue syndrome
- Rare but serious complications include endocarditis, neurobrucellosis with meningitis, and hepatic abscess.

Treatment

1. Administer doxycycline 100 mg PO twice daily for 6 weeks plus either streptomycin 1 g IM daily for the first 14 to 21 days, gentamicin 5 mg/kg/day IM for 7 days, or rifampin 600 to 900 mg PO once daily for 6 weeks.
2. In pregnancy treat with rifampin 900 mg PO once daily for 6 weeks, with the addition of trimethoprim/sulfamethoxazole in the second trimester.
3. For children younger than 8 years also give oral trimethoprim/sulfamethoxazole and rifampin for 4 to 6 weeks, with gentamicin added for the first 14 days if osteoarticular, neural, or endocarditis manifestations are present. For children older than 8 years, antibiotic choices are the same as for adults.

Trichinellosis

Trichinellosis, also known as trichinosis, is an infection caused by nematodes of the genus *Trichinella*. The infection is acquired by ingesting larvae encysted in skeletal muscle, usually raw or undercooked pork. It can also be acquired from wild game such as bear, raccoon, horse, walrus, cougar, and wild swine.

Signs and Symptoms

- Nausea, vomiting, and abdominal pain approximately 5 days after ingestion of infective meat; diarrhea or fever possible; gastrointestinal symptoms persisting for 4 to 6 weeks
- Larvae invade skeletal muscle as early 7 days after ingestion.
  - Capillary damage during larval migration, which appears as facial (especially periorbital) edema, photophobia, blurred vision, diplopia, and complaints of pain associated with eye movements

- Splinter hemorrhages in the nail beds, along with cutaneous petechiae and hemorrhagic lesions in the conjunctivae
- Fever up to 41° C (105.8° F)
- After 2 weeks: cough, dyspnea, pleuritic chest pain, hemoptysis, meningitis symptoms, headache
- After 3 weeks: myalgias, muscle stiffness

Treatment

1. Management of symptomatic *Trichinella* infection consists of anthelmintic therapy and corticosteroids.
2. Albendazole and mebendazole are the primary anthelmintic drugs used. Albendazole is slightly preferred because it does not require as much monitoring as mebendazole. The recommended dose for albendazole is 400 mg twice daily for 8 to 14 days. The recommended dose for mebendazole is 200 to 400 mg three times daily for 3 days, followed by 400 to 500 mg three times daily for 10 days.
3. Steroids (e.g., prednisone, 30 to 60 mg/day PO for 10 to 30 days) can be given for relief of severe illness, such as myocarditis caused by migrating larvae or nervous system involvement.
4. Dosage and duration of treatment are individually determined by clinical response.
5. Steroids reduce the inflammatory response to larvae, but can also interfere with rejection of adult females in the intestine, thus prolonging the period of larva deposition.
6. Early treatment before larvae have established themselves in the muscle is most effective.
7. There is no satisfactory, safe, and effective drug for elimination of harbored larvae.

Prevention

1. Cook meat to an internal temperature of 65.6° C to 77° C (150° F to 170.6° F).
2. Most *Trichinella* larvae are killed by freezing. Holding the meat at −15° C (5° F) for 20 days, −23.3° C (−9.9° F) for 10 days, or −28.9° C (−20° F) for 6 days is recommended.
3. Salting, drying, and smoking are not always effective. *Trichinella nativa* found in Arctic mammals is resistant to freezing.

Hantavirus Pulmonary Syndrome

Hantavirus pulmonary syndrome (HPS; also known as hantavirus cardiopulmonary syndrome, HCPS) is a severe viral respiratory illness predominantly transmitted through a rodent vector such as the deer mouse. Other small mammals such as brush mice and western chipmunks may be infected. The animals shed virus in saliva, urine, and feces for weeks.

Signs and Symptoms

- Incubation period ranging from 10 days to 6 weeks and consists of five stages that may overlap: febrile, hypotensive, oliguric, diuretic, and convalescent.

- Prodrome of fever, myalgia, and variable respiratory symptoms, which may include cough and shortness of breath with minimal broncho-spasm, followed by rapid onset of acute respiratory distress
- Headache, chills, abdominal pain, nausea, vomiting; possible hemorrhage related to thrombocytopenia
- Rapid deterioration, including respiratory failure and hypotension
- The mortality from hemorrhagic fever with renal syndrome (HFRS) is 1% to 40% (depending on the strain), and recovery may take months.
- CDC screening criteria include febrile illness with temperature higher than 38.3° C (101° F) in a previously healthy person characterized by unexplained acute respiratory distress syndrome (ARDS) or bilateral interstitial pulmonary infiltrates developing within 72 hours of hospitalization, with respiratory compromise requiring supplemental oxygen.

Treatment
1. Therapy is supportive and based on symptoms.
2. Ribavirin was studied, but the CDC has stated that the drug is of no use with hantavirus pulmonary syndrome and is not available for use under any current research protocol as of 2004.
3. Intensive care unit management of symptoms is recommended with pressors, avoidance of fluid overload, and possible use of extracorporeal membrane oxygenation in the most severe cases.
4. Glucocorticoids are not recommended for treatment of patients with HPS.

Prevention
1. Eliminate rodents, and reduce the availability of food sources and nesting sites used by rodents inside the home. Maintain snap traps and use rodenticides.
2. Keep food and water covered and stored in rodent-proof metal or thick plastic containers. Keep cooking areas clean.
3. Dispose of clutter. Contain and elevate garbage.
4. Remove food sources that might attract rodents. Avoid feeding or handling rodents.
5. Spray dead rodents, nests, and droppings with a general-purpose household disinfectant or 10% bleach solution before handling. Dispose of all excreta and nesting materials in sealed bags. Always wear rubber or plastic gloves.
6. Avoid contact with rodents and rodent burrows. Do not disturb dens.
7. Do not use cabins or other enclosed shelters that are rodent infested until they have been appropriately cleaned and dis-infected. Seal holes and cracks in dwellings to prevent entrance by rodents. Avoid sweeping, vacuuming, or stirring dust until the area is thoroughly wet with disinfectant.
8. Do not pitch tents or place sleeping bags in areas close to rodent feces or burrows or near possible rodent shelters (garbage dumps, woodpiles).

9. If possible, do not sleep on bare ground.
10. Burn or bury all garbage promptly. Clear brush and trash from around homes and outbuildings.
11. Use only bottled water or water that has been disinfected for oral consumption, cooking, washing dishes, and brushing teeth.

Plague

Plague is a bacterial illness caused by *Yersinia pestis*. Plague is carried by various rodent reservoirs and transmitted by fleas. Carnivorous mammals can acquire plague by ingesting infected rodents or by being bitten by their fleas. Plague in cats is a serious problem.

Signs and Symptoms
Bubonic Plague
- Incubation period of 2 to 6 days, then appearance of enlarged, tender lymph nodes (buboes) proximal to the point of percutaneous entry
- Inguinal nodes most often involved because fleas usually bite humans on the legs; axillary buboes from skinning an animal as the mode of transmission
- High fever, chills, malaise, headache, myalgias
- Cardiovascular collapse with shock and hemorrhagic phenomena possible, with blackened, hemorrhagic skin lesions

Septicemic Plague
- Fever, chills, malaise, headache, abdominal pain, nausea, vomiting, diarrhea
- Eventual cardiovascular collapse with disseminated intravascular coagulation

Pneumonic Plague
- Incubation period of 2 to 3 days, then acute, fulminant disease
- Characterized by symptoms of pneumonia, including fever, cough, shaking chills, headache, tachypnea, and bloody sputum

Treatment for All Types of Plague
1. Streptomycin was the original agent used in treatment, but because of availability, the generally preferred drug is gentamicin, 5 mg/kg IV or IM once or 2-mg/kg loading dose, followed by 1.7 mg/kg IV or IM three times daily for 10 days.
2. Aminoglycosides penetrate poorly into the CSF and therefore are not recommended for treatment of meningeal plague.
3. An acceptable alternative is doxycycline in a loading dose of 200 mg IV, followed by 100 mg IV twice daily for 10 days.
4. Although limited clinical trials have been done on humans, animal studies suggest that fluoroquinolones are effective agents against plague. As such, levofloxacin is also an acceptable alternative, but it should only be used in patients who cannot tolerate aminoglycosides or tetracyclines.

5. Chloramphenicol or TMP-SMX may also be used. Chloramphenicol is administered in a loading dose of 25 mg/kg PO up to 3 g total, followed by 50 to 75 mg/kg/day PO in four divided doses for 10 to 14 days. If the patient does not tolerate oral therapy, chloramphenicol can be given IV, 25 mg/kg as a loading dose followed by 60 mg/kg in four divided doses every 6 hours until PO therapy is tolerated.

6. It is preferable to use chloramphenicol in the event of meningitis or endophthalmitis because of good penetration into affected tissues.

7. TMP-SMX (320/1600 mg) twice daily for 10 to 17 days was found effective in treating plague.

8. Recent literature shows that sulfonamides should be used in the treatment of bubonic plague only.

9. Infants born to plague-infected mothers may have congenital infection. They can be treated with kanamycin, 15 mg/kg/day IV or IM in four divided doses every 6 hours, or streptomycin, 10 to 20 mg/kg/day in four divided doses every 6 hours.

10. Some experts recommend treatment of children with TMP-SMX, 4 mg/kg of trimethoprim twice daily for 7 to 10 days.

Prevention

1. The greatest risk for contagion is by aerosol transmission from patients with pneumonic plague.

2. Keep infected patients in strict quarantine for a minimum of 48 hours after antibiotic therapy is begun (suspected case) or 4 days after beginning antibiotic therapy (confirmed case).

3. Contact personnel should wear gloves, gowns, masks, and eye protection.

4. Treat individuals directly exposed to pneumonic plague prophylactically with tetracycline, 500 mg PO q6h for 6 days, for adults, or cotrimoxazole (otitis media dose) for children.

5. In areas where plague occurs, control fleas with insecticides.

Anthrax

Anthrax is a bacterial illness caused by *Bacillus anthracis*. Naturally occurring anthrax is acquired from contact with infected animals (usually herbivores) or contaminated animal products but has become an agent of bioterrorism. It can be transmitted by inhalation, inoculation, or ingestion. The spore form of anthrax is highly resistant to physical and chemical agents and can persist in the environment for years. Anthrax is not transmitted from person to person.

Signs and Symptoms

The incubation period is 1 to 5 (range up to 60) days. Cutaneous anthrax is the most common form.

Inhalation Anthrax
- First stage is a few hours to a few days of a flu-like illness: nonspecific symptoms of fever, dyspnea, cough, headache, vomiting, chills, weakness, abdominal pain
- Second stage is abrupt onset of acute hemorrhagic mediastinitis, characterized by fever, dyspnea, diaphoresis, and hypotension
- Mortality rate approaches 90%, even with treatment; hemorrhagic meningitis with meningismus, delirium, and obtundation; shock and death within 24 to 36 hours

Cutaneous Anthrax
- Variable local edema, followed by pruritic macule or papule by second day, with or without tiny vesicles
- Blackened, painless, and depressed eschar, often with extensive local edema; eschar dries and falls off in 7 to 14 days
- Lymphangitis, painful lymphadenopathy

Gastrointestinal (Ingestion) Anthrax
- Germination of spores in the upper gastrointestinal tract leads to oral or esophageal ulcer(s), with regional lymphadenopathy, edema, and sepsis.
- Germination of spores in terminal ilium or cecum leads to local lesions, nausea, vomiting, and malaise progressing to bloody diarrhea, peritonitis, and sepsis.
  - Ascites, acute abdomen

Treatment of Anthrax
1. Treatment for cutaneous anthrax without systemic involvement is oral ciprofloxacin or doxycycline, twice daily for 60 days. In children, the dose of ciprofloxacin is 20 to 30 mg/kg/day divided every 12 hours (not to exceed the adult dose of 500 mg every 12 hours), or doxycycline, 4.4 mg/kg/day divided every 12 hours (not to exceed the adult dose of 100 mg every 12 hours).
2. If patients are clinically improved, therapy may be changed to amoxicillin, 500 mg three times daily for adults, or 80 mg/kg/day divided three times daily for children.
3. For systemic anthrax (GI, inhalation, meningitis, injection), treatment should begin with a three-drug regimen, to include two bacteriocidal agents with good central nervous system (CNS) penetration and one protein synthesis inhibitor; preferred agents are ciprofloxacin and meropenem plus linezolid or clindamycin.
4. If meningitis is ruled out, CDC recommendations include 2 weeks of IV ciprofloxacin as well as one additional agent (e.g., clindamycin, linezolid, or doxycycline).
5. If symptoms improve, treatment switches to an oral regimen of ciprofloxacin or doxycycline for a total course of 60 days.
6. Treatment is the same during pregnancy; the risk of doxycycline or ciprofloxacin during pregnancy is outweighed by the potential mortality resulting from undertreated anthrax infection.

Prevention

1. In the event of potential exposure to inhaled anthrax spores, the CDC recommends 60 days of ciprofloxacin or doxycycline in combination with a three-dose regimen (0, 2, 4 weeks) of anthrax vaccine (BioThrax, formerly known as AVA) as an emergency public health intervention.
2. PEP is not recommended for exposure to cutaneous anthrax alone.

Glanders

Glanders occurs in a few Asian and African countries such as India, China, Mongolia, and Egypt and is primarily a disease of horses. Occasionally infections occur in dogs, cats, sheep, and goats. Humans are infected by exposure to sick horses. Infection can occur by inhalation of respiratory droplets or by contact with infected discharges.

Signs and Symptoms

- Incubation period of 1 to 5 days
- Pustular cutaneous eruptions
- Thick indurated lymphatics that may ulcerate
- Mucopurulent discharge from the eyes or nose
- Pneumonia
- Depending on the severity, the patient may have anorexia, fever, weight loss, headache, nausea, diarrhea, or septicemic shock.

Treatment

1. Administer sulfadiazine, 100 mg/kg/day divided q8h for 3 weeks.
2. Treatment with tetracyclines and streptomycin is also recommended.

Prevention

Glanders can be transmitted from one person to another, so strict infection control should be exercised with suspected patients.

Avian/Swine Influenza

The highly pathogenic H5N1 avian influenza virus has been reported mainly in Vietnam, Indonesia, Hong Kong, Thailand, China, Egypt, and Eastern Europe. Most infections in humans result from contact with infected birds or their contaminated feces. In 2009, H1N1 swine flu pandemic began in Mexico and spread to over 200 countries, including the United States and Canada, likely spread by air travel.

Signs and Symptoms

- Sudden onset of high fever, headache, malaise, cough, sore throat, and myalgias
- Gastrointestinal manifestations such as diarrhea may also occur.

Table 43.1　Pediatric Dose of Oseltamivir for Treatment of Influenza
>1 year: 　<15 kg: 30 mg PO bid for 5 days 　15–23 kg: 45 mg PO bid 　24–40 kg: 60 mg PO bid 　>40 kg: Administer as in adults

Table 43.2　Pediatric Dose of Oseltamivir for Prophylaxis of Influenza
>1 year: 　<15 kg: 30 mg PO daily for 10 days 　15–23 kg: 45 mg PO daily for 10 days 　24–40 kg: 60 mg PO daily for 10 days 　>40 kg: Administer as in adults

Treatment

1. Treatment is recommended for patients with confirmed or suspected influenza who require hospitalization; have progressive, severe, complicated illness; and those at risk for severe disease (children <2 years, adults >65 years, pregnant women or those less than 2 weeks postpartum, and persons with severe medical conditions). More information can be found at http://www.cdc.gov/flu.
2. Administer oseltamivir (Tamiflu) 75 mg PO q12h (adult dose and adolescents 13 years and older) for 5 days. Treatment should begin within 48 hours of symptom onset. The recommended dose of oseltamivir for pediatric patients older than 1 year is shown in Table 43.1.
3. Oseltamivir capsules may be opened and mixed with sweetened liquids.

Prevention

1. The recommended dose of oseltamivir for prophylaxis of influenza in adults and adolescents 13 years and older following close contact with an infected individual is 75 mg once daily for 10 days. The recommended dose for pediatric patients older than 1 year and older is shown in Table 43.2.

44

Diarrhea and Constipation

TRAVELER'S DIARRHEA

Traveler's diarrhea (TD) is the most important travel-related illness in terms of frequency and economic impact. Episodes of TD are nearly always self-limited, but the dehydration associated with an episode may be severe and poses a great health hazard. Rates of diarrhea for persons traveling from industrialized countries to developing regions are in the order of 40% to 60% over a 2- to 3-week period. The risk for TD is high among travelers to the developing tropical regions of Latin America, southern Asia, and Africa. Medications that reduce gastric acid (e.g., histamine blockers or proton pump inhibitors) or alter upper gastrointestinal motility may increase the risk for development of TD.

Definition

TD refers to a diarrheal illness contracted while traveling, although in about 15% of patients, symptoms begin after return home. Most clinical studies define TD as the passage of three or more unformed stools in a 24-hour period in association with one or more enteric symptoms, including the following: abdominal cramps; fever; fecal urgency; tenesmus; passage of bloody, mucoid stools; nausea; and vomiting.

Etiology

Diarrheal disease in travelers may be caused by a variety of bacterial, viral, and parasitic organisms that are most often transmitted by food and water. Bacteria account for 50% to 80% of TD in developing countries; the most common organism is enterotoxigenic *Escherichia coli*, followed by *Salmonella* species, *Campylobacter jejuni*, and *Shigella* species (Table 44.1).

Signs and Symptoms

- Acute diarrhea can be accompanied by nausea, loss of appetite, abdominal cramps, low-grade fever, and malaise (Table 44.2).
- Symptoms begin as early as 8 to 12 hours after contaminated food or water has been ingested.
- Dysentery (i.e., invasive disease) is present in 10% to 15% of cases, particularly associated with *Shigella*, *C. jejuni*, or *Salmonella*.
  - Passage of bloody stools
  - Fever up to 40° C (104° F)
  - Often associated with abdominal cramps, tenderness, and tenesmus

Table 44.1 Major Pathogens in Traveler's Diarrhea (Travel to Developing Tropical Regions)	
AGENT	**FREQUENCY (%)**
Bacteria	50–80
Enterotoxigenic *Escherichia coli*	5–50
Enteroaggregative *E. coli*	5–30
Salmonella species	1–15
Shigella species	1–15
Campylobacter jejuni	1–30
Aeromonas species	0–10
Plesiomonas shigelloides	0–5
Other	0–5
Viruses	0–20
Rotavirus	0–20
Norovirus	1–20
Protozoa	1–5
Giardia lamblia	0–5
Entamoeba histolytica	0–5
Cryptosporidium parvum	0–5
Unknown	10–40

- Dehydration (manifestations include tachycardia, orthostatic vital signs, dry mucous membranes, dark yellow urine and decreased urine output, lethargy, poor skin turgor) may be present and is most common in pediatric and geriatric populations.
- Vomiting as the predominant symptom suggests food intoxication secondary to enterotoxin produced by *Staphylococcus aureus*, *Bacillus cereus*, or *Clostridium perfringens*, or gastroenteritis secondary to viruses, such as rotavirus in infants or norovirus in any age group.
- An abdominal examination of persons with TD often shows mild tenderness, but there should not be signs of peritonitis.
- With persistent diarrhea (longer than 14 days' duration), consider possible infection with intestinal parasites such as *Giardia lamblia*, *Entamoeba histolytica*, *Cryptosporidium*, *Isospora*, *Cyclospora*, or less common entities that include the following:
  - Pseudomembranous enterocolitis *(Clostridium difficile)* after recent antibiotic use or spontaneously
  - Lactase deficiency induced by small-bowel pathogens

Table 44.2 Pathophysiologic Syndromes in Diarrheal Disease	
SYNDROME	**AGENT**
Acute watery diarrhea	Any agent, especially with toxin-mediated diseases (e.g., enterotoxigenic *Escherichia coli*, *Vibrio cholerae*)
Febrile dysentery	*Shigella*, *Campylobacter jejuni*, *Salmonella*, enteroinvasive *E. coli*, *Aeromonas* species, *Vibrio* species, *Yersinia enterocolitica*, *Entamoeba histolytica*, inflammatory bowel disease
Vomiting (as predominant symptom)	Viral agents, preformed toxins of *Staphylococcus aureus* or *Bacillus cereus*
Persistent diarrhea (>14 days)	Protozoa, small bowel bacterial overgrowth, inflammatory or invasive enteropathogens (*Shigella*, enteroaggregative *E. coli*)
Chronic diarrhea (>30 days)	Small-bowel injury, inflammatory bowel disease, irritable bowel syndrome (postinfectious), Brainerd diarrhea

- Viral enteropathogens such as rotavirus or Norwalk virus
- Small-bowel bacterial overgrowth syndrome
- *Strongyloides stercoralis* or *Trichuris trichiura*
- Postinfective malabsorption syndrome
- Tropical sprue
- Brainerd diarrhea
- Inflammatory bowel disease

Treatment (Tables 44.3 and 44.4)

1. TD typically runs a self-limited course of less than 1 week. Although recovery without antimicrobial treatment normally occurs in healthy adults, most travelers choose to mitigate the inconvenience and discomfort of diarrhea by seeking medical treatment.
2. Severe, watery TD can cause life-threatening fluid loss. Treating dehydration is an urgent priority, especially in older persons, young children, and infants. Fluid replacement is the cornerstone of therapy.
   a. Treating dehydration often significantly decreases malaise.
   b. Urine volume (decreased urine output for an adult is less than 500 mL in a 24-hour period) and color (one field indicator of dehydration is dark-yellow urine) can serve as markers of adequate hydration and should be monitored.
   c. If patients are otherwise healthy and not dehydrated, adequate oral intake can be achieved with soft drinks, fruit juice, broth, and soup, along with salted crackers. In those with excessive

Table 44.3 Nonspecific Drugs for Symptomatic Therapy in Adults	
AGENT	**THERAPEUTIC DOSE**
Attapulgite	3 g initially, then 3 g after each loose stool or every 2 hr (not to exceed 9 g/day); should be safe during pregnancy and childhood. (available in 600-mg tablets or liquid 600 mg/tsp)
Loperamide	4 mg initially; this is usually sufficient. If nonresponsive, can give 2 mg (one capsule) after each loose stool not to exceed 8 mg (four capsules)/day; do not use in dysenteric or febrile diarrhea
Bismuth subsalicylate	30 mL or two 262-mg tablets every 30 min for eight doses; may repeat on day 2
Probiotics	Dose according to package, because products and formulations vary. Daily dose may make diarrhea less severe and shorten its duration; consider in postinfectious or postantibiotic diarrhea

fluid losses and dehydration, oral rehydration therapy with electrolyte solutions containing glucose should be instituted. Reduced osmolarity (245 mOsm/L compared with the previous 311 mOsm/L) oral rehydration solutions (ORSs) are now recommended by the World Health Organization (WHO) for treating acute diarrhea (Table 44.5). The lower osmolarity reduces stool output (volume), vomiting, and need for intravenous (IV) therapy. Rehydration Project is a nonprofit international development group that maintains an up-to-date website on rehydration options (http://rehydrate.org/ors/low-osmolarity-ors.htm).

- Add one packet of ORS to 1 L (1 qt) of clean drinking or boiled water (after it is cooled). Many pharmacies or clinics may still stock the "old" WHO 1975 formula. It can be used to make a lower osmolarity solution that still meets new WHO parameters by mixing it in 1.2 L (1.2 qt) of water rather than in 1 L.
- Sports drinks, such as Gatorade, also provide adequate fluid replacement if diluted to about to about one-half their strength (add 0.5 L [0.5 qt] of water to 1 L [1 qt] of Gatorade). Full-strength sports drinks are often more hypertonic than 245 mOsm/L (the osmolality of Gatorade is approximately 360 mOsm/L) and may delay gastric absorption.
- A number of other ORSs are also available for children, including Pedialyte, Rehydralyte, Ricelyte, Infalyte, and Resol.
- Elete is a concentrated electrolyte solution that may be added to water to create a dehydration-sparing beverage.

Table 44.4 Oral Agents for Self-Treatment of Traveler's Diarrhea in Adults

AGENT	DOSE	DURATION	COMMENT
Azithromycin	1000 mg once	Single dose*	Preferred for dysentery or febrile diarrhea, travelers from Southeast Asia, and pregnant women
	500 mg once daily	3-day course	The 1000 mg dose may be associated with nausea
Levofloxacin	500 mg once daily	Single dose* or 3-day course	Fluoroquinolones are associated with multiple adverse events
Ciprofloxacin	750 mg once	Single dose*	
	500 mg twice daily	3-day course	
Ofloxacin	400 mg once daily	Single dose* or 3-day course	
Rifaximin	200 mg three times daily	3-day course	Not for use with dysentery or febrile diarrhea

If symptoms have not resolved after 24 hours, the regimen can be extended to complete a 3-day course (using the dosing listed for the 3-day course).
(From Riddle MS, Connor BA, Beeching NJ, et al. Guidelines for the prevention and treatment of travelers' diarrhea: a graded expert panel report. J Travel Med 2017; 24:S57.)

Table 44.5 Reduced Osmolarity Oral Rehydration Solution

REDUCED OSMOLARITY ORS	MMOL/L
Sodium	75
Chloride	65
Glucose, anhydrous	75
Potassium	20
Citrate	10
Total Osmolarity	245

ORS, Oral rehydration solution.

3. To make an improvised ORS, one of the following methods can be used:
   a. Add 30 mL (6 tsp) of sugar and 2.5 mL (½ tsp) of salt to 1 L (1 qt) of clean drinking water (or boiled water that has cooled).
   b. Add 2.5 mL (½ tsp) salt, 5 mL (1 tsp) baking soda, 40 mL (8 tsp) sugar, and 236 mL (8 oz) orange juice, diluted to 1 L (1 qt) with water.
4. Fluids should be given at rates of 50 to 200 mL/kg/24 hr, depending on the patient's hydration status.
5. Treatment with IV fluids is indicated for patients with severe dehydration and for those who cannot tolerate oral fluids.
6. Total food abstinence is unnecessary and not recommended. Patients should be encouraged to eat easily digested foods such as bananas, applesauce, rice, potatoes, noodles, crackers, toast, and soups. Dairy products should be avoided, because transient lactase deficiency can be caused by enteric infections. Caffeinated beverages and alcohol, which can enhance intestinal motility and secretions, should be avoided.

Symptomatic Therapy

Symptomatic medications are useful for treatment of diarrhea because they decrease symptoms and fluid loss and allow patients to return more quickly to normal activities (see Table 44.3).
1. Antimotility drugs
   a. Narcotic analogs related to opiates are the major antimotility drugs. In addition to slowing intestinal motility, these drugs alter water and electrolyte transport, probably affecting both secretion and absorption. Use over-the-counter agent loperamide (Imodium) or prescription agent diphenoxylate plus atropine (Lomotil) to offer relief to patients with watery diarrhea and cramps. Of the two drugs, loperamide is better tolerated and has fewer central opiate effects.
   b. The adult dose for loperamide is 4 mg for the initial dose and 2 mg after every loose stool, up to a total dose of 8 mg/day.
   c. These drugs can be valuable for long bus rides or summit bids where social constraints make frequent rest stops impractical.
   d. Antimotility drugs can be important for controlling fluid balance in a patient with profuse diarrhea who is unable to tolerate sufficient oral fluids to maintain a positive fluid balance.
   e. Avoid antimotility drugs alone (i.e., without antibiotics) if blood or mucus is present in the stool or if patient has signs of serious illness (high fever, recurrent vomiting, severe abdominal pain) because the inhibition of gut motility may facilitate intestinal infection by invasive bacterial enteropathogens. This theoretically deleterious effect does not appear to be an issue when loperamide is used concurrently with an effective antimicrobial agent.
   f. Antimotility drugs should be used only up to a maximum of 48 hours in acute diarrhea.

2. Bismuth subsalicylate (BSS; Pepto-Bismol) reduces the number of stools passed in TD by approximately 16% to 18%. Although BSS is recommended for mild diarrhea, for moderate to severe disease, loperamide works better and with a faster onset of action.
   a. Administer 30 mL (6 tsp) BSS liquid or 2 BSS tablets PO q30min, maximum eight doses in 24 hours.
3. Probiotics appear to reduce stool frequency and shorten the duration of acute infectious diarrhea by 1 day. The most extensively studied probiotics for diarrhea are *Lactobacillus*, *Bifidobacterium*, and *Saccharomyces*; however, optimal species and dosing have not been established. Potential mechanisms for their therapeutic action include protection of intestinal epithelial cells and barrier function, prevention of enterotoxin binding to intestinal epithelial cells, and regulation of intestinal microbial environment. Probiotics lose activity quickly, so should not be stored for long periods of time.

Antimicrobial Therapy

1. TD can be relieved in a little over 1 day after empiric antimicrobial therapy is instituted. With the concurrent use of loperamide, relief is realized in a matter of hours. Table 44.6 lists antimicrobial therapy for organism-specific diarrhea in adults.
2. With reports of increasing resistance among enteric enteropathogens worldwide, trimethoprim/sulfamethoxazole can no longer be recommended. Until recently, one of the fluoroquinolones had been the drug of choice for empiric treatment of TD. With recognition that *C. jejuni* is a common cause of traveler's diarrhea in Southeast Asia and that there is emerging resistance (up to 90%) to fluoroquinolones for *Campylobacter* in this region, the preferred agent for the empiric treatment of TD has become azithromycin for countries such as Thailand and India. Rifaximin, a nonabsorbed agent with broad activity against enteric pathogens, is effective in the treatment of TD in regions of the world where enterotoxigenic *E. coli* is the predominant pathogen. It is not recommended for treatment of bloody diarrhea or when an invasive pathogen is suspected, limiting its usefulness as a therapeutic agent in regions like Southeast Asia. However, because rifaximin can prevent diarrhea, including that caused by invasive pathogens, the most appropriate use of rifaximin might be as a chemoprophylactic agent. Recommended dosages of antimicrobial agents are shown in Tables 44.4 and 44.6. Often a single dose suffices. Travelers who do not respond to empiric antibiotic treatment or who have persistent diarrhea of more than 1 week's duration should seek medical attention. In the wilderness, *Giardia* can be an important cause of ongoing diarrhea unresponsive to antibiotics (see later).
3. Travelers with severe and incapacitating symptoms, or with dysentery, should be treated with empiric antimicrobial therapy immediately after the first passage of unformed stool.
4. Additional considerations follow:
   a. Azithromycin is an effective antibiotic for the treatment of many forms of TD and is the preferred agent for children.

Table 44.6 Antimicrobial Therapy for Organism-Specific Diarrhea in Adults

DIAGNOSIS	RECOMMENDATION
Enterotoxigenic and enteroaggregative *Escherichia coli* diarrhea	Rifaximin, 200 mg tid for 3 days *or* Ciprofloxacin, 500 mg bid for 1–3 days *or* Other fluoroquinolone for 3 days *or* Azithromycin, 1000-mg single dose
Cholera	Doxycycline, 300-mg single dose
Systemic salmonellosis (typhoid fever or bacteremic infection)	Ciprofloxacin, 500 mg bid for 5–7 days *or* Levofloxacin, 500 mg qd for 7–10 days
Salmonellosis (intestinal nontyphoid salmonellosis without systemic infection)	Antimicrobial therapy controversial if systemically ill (high fever and toxicity) or in a high-risk group: sickle cell anemia, age <3 mo or >64 yr, taking corticosteroids, undergoing dialysis, those with inflammatory bowel disease (if decision to treat, use regimen as for systemic salmonellosis)
Shigellosis	Ciprofloxacin, 500 mg bid for 3 days *or* Levofloxacin, 500 mg bid for 3 days
Campylobacteriosis	Erythromycin, 500 mg qid for 5 days *or* Azithromycin, 500 mg qd for 3 days, or 1000 mg in single dose

bid, Twice daily; *qd,* daily; *qid,* four times daily; *tid,* three times daily.

Azithromycin administered as a single 1-g oral dose has as high a cure rate as does 500 mg/day for 3 days.
b. Loperamide 4 mg should be administered concomitant with an antibiotic.
c. If the patient has begun initial treatment of diarrhea with BSS therapy, at least 8 hours must elapse before optimum antibiotic therapy can occur because BSS impairs absorption of oral antimicrobial agents.
d. Advise any patient who does not respond to empiric antibiotic treatment or who has diarrhea for more than 1 week to obtain clinical follow-up that includes a complete workup for bacterial and parasitic pathogens.

Prevention

1. Take dietary precautions. The risk for illness is lowest when a traveler's meals are self-prepared in a private home, highest when food is obtained from street vendors, and intermediate when food is consumed at public restaurants. Unfortunately, many studies evaluating risk have found little correlation between routine precautions and illness. Dietary recommendations to decrease the potential for transmission of fecal pathogens through food and water are as follows:

   a. Avoid tap water and ice made from untreated water (most enteric organisms can survive freezing).

   b. Bottled noncarbonated water may be contaminated with fecal coliforms.

   c. Bottled and carbonated drinks, beer, and wine are probably safe.

   d. Boiled or chemically disinfected water is safe.

   e. Alcohol in mixed drinks does not disinfect.

   f. Homemade beverages may not be safe.

   g. Ice in block form is often handled with unsanitary methods.

   h. Avoid unpasteurized cheese and dairy products.

   i. Avoid raw vegetables and salads, which may be contaminated by fertilization with human waste, or washing with contaminated water.

   j. Anything that can be peeled or have the surface removed is generally safe.

   k. Fruits and hearty vegetables can be disinfected by immersion and washing in iodinated water or by exposure to boiling water for 30 seconds.

   l. Avoid raw seafood and fish.

   m. Avoid raw meat because adequate cooking kills all microorganisms and parasites. If the meat is left at room temperature and recontaminated, cooked food can incubate pathogenic bacteria. Casseroles are notorious for reheating and contamination.

   n. Avoid eating foods upon which you have observed many flies to be resting.

2. Use of prophylactic medications to prevent TD

   a. Of the nonantibiotic drugs, only BSS has been shown by controlled studies to offer reasonable protection and safety. The current recommended dose of BSS (for prevention) is 2 tablets 4 times per day. Mild side effects include constipation, nausea, and blackened tongue or stools. BSS taken concurrently with antibiotics should be avoided because of the potential binding of BSS to the antibiotic, which prevents absorption.

   b. Do not give BSS to someone with a history of aspirin allergy.

   c. Give BSS with caution to small children; people with gout or renal insufficiency; and those taking probenecid, methotrexate, anticoagulants, or products containing aspirin.

3. Antimicrobial prophylaxis for TD
    a. A broad-spectrum antibiotic taken during travel can effectively prevent illness, but resolution of TD within a few hours can usually be obtained after oral antibiotic therapy with an appropriate antibiotic. It is probably unnecessary for the average traveler to ingest an antibiotic for the full duration of a trip.
    b. Antimicrobial prophylaxis of TD might be a reasonable strategy for residents of a low-risk country going to a high-risk area for fewer than 5 weeks with one or more of the following:
        • Underlying illness such as acquired immunodeficiency syndrome (AIDS); inflammatory bowel disease; or a cardiac, renal, or central nervous system disorder
        • An itinerary that is so rigid and critical that a person cannot tolerate any inconvenience caused by TD; such travelers include competitive athletes, politicians, sales representatives, and people going to special events
    c. For specific antibiotic therapy recommended to prevent TD, see Table 44.6.
    d. Despite its protection against diarrhea, the routine use of antimicrobial prophylaxis by travelers is not recommended because of the following:
        • Potential for adverse side effects
        • Alteration of normal bacterial flora
        • Tendency to "lower one's guard." Travelers taking prophylactic antibiotics may relax their vigilance, which can increase their risk for acquiring other nonbacterial infections

CHOLERA

Cholera has become a scourge of refugees afflicted by natural disasters or humanitarian crises. It is a severe form of diarrheal illness caused by *Vibrio cholerae* serogroups 01 and 0139, and characterized by profound fluid losses leading to dehydration, classic watery diarrhea sometimes with "rice water stools," vomiting, and debility. It is easily spread among groups of people and can rapidly cause hypotension and collapse. In addition to aggressive rehydration, effective antibiotics include doxycycline (300 mg PO), azithromycin (1 g PO; first choice in children in pediatric dose), and ciprofloxacin (500 mg PO bid for 5 to 7 days).

FOOD POISONING

Food poisoning results when toxins produced by bacteria are found in foods in concentrations sufficient to produce symptoms. This is not an infection, but a true poisoning. Most food poisoning is caused by *S. aureus* or *B. cereus*.

Signs and Symptoms

• Diarrhea that develops within 6 to 12 hours after a suspicious meal, most likely caused by ingesting a preformed toxin

- A common source is often found to have affected multiple persons
- Usually preceded by severe nausea and vomiting
- Symptoms usually limited to 24 hours
- Physical examination nonspecific

Treatment
- Treatment is directed toward fluid and electrolyte replacement (see earlier) and control of nausea.
- No specific antibiotic therapy exists.

INFECTION CAUSED BY INTESTINAL PROTOZOA
All intestinal protozoa are transmitted by the fecal-oral route. Protozoa typically cause subacute or chronic gastrointestinal symptoms but may also invade the bowel wall and cause severe dysentery with an acute presentation.

Giardia lamblia
G. lamblia (also known as *intestinalis* or *duodenalis*) is a flagellate protozoan with a life cycle that involves two forms. Trophozoites are responsible for symptomatic illness. They are rarely infective because they die quickly outside of the body. Some trophozoites encyst and are passed in the stools of infected hosts. Cysts are typically the form passed through fecal-oral contact and cause infection. Cysts are hardy in the external environment and retain viability in cold water for as long as 2 or 3 months. The infective dose of *Giardia* for humans is 10 to 25 cysts.

Giardiasis is a zoonosis with cross-infectivity from animals to humans. Animals that have been implicated as carriers include beavers, cattle, dogs, cats, rodents, sheep, and deer. In North America, *Giardia* is transmitted primarily through drinking water. Worldwide, person-to-person transmission may be more common.

Signs and Symptoms
- The severity of clinical manifestations is variable. In general, about half of exposed individuals clear the infection without clinical symptoms, and approximately 5% to 15% of individuals shed cysts asymptomatically.
- Average incubation period of 7 to 14 days (range 1 to 45 days)
- Sometimes abrupt onset of explosive, watery diarrhea accompanied by abdominal cramps, foul flatus, vomiting, fever, and malaise; typically lasts 3 to 4 days before transition to subacute syndrome
- Onset usually insidious, with symptoms that wax and wane
- Stools becoming mushy and malodorous
- Watery diarrhea alternating with soft stools and even constipation
- Middle and upper abdominal cramping, substantial burning acid indigestion, sulfurous belching, nausea, bowel distention, early satiety, foul flatus

- Dysenteric symptoms (blood and pus in the stool) are not features of giardiasis; fever and vomiting are infrequent except during initial onset.
- May develop into a chronic process associated with malabsorption and weight loss

Treatment

1. Treatment in the wilderness is usually initiated empirically based on the typical manifestations listed earlier.
2. Note that a cure can be achieved with one of several drugs. However, no drug is effective in all cases. In resistant cases, longer courses of two drugs taken concurrently may be effective.
3. Relapse may occur up to several weeks after treatment, which requires a second course of the same medication or an alternative drug.
4. Three antimicrobial drugs are currently recommended: tinidazole, metronidazole, and nitazoxanide.
5. Tinidazole (2000 mg adult dose; 50 mg/kg for children in a single dose) is highly effective and approved by the Food and Drug Administration (FDA) for treatment of giardiasis in persons older than 3 years. It should be taken with food. Tinidazole has a longer half-life than metronidazole and offers the advantage of a single-dose treatment. For those unable to swallow tablets, Tinidazole tablets may be compounded into an oral suspension.
   a. Procedure for compounding of the oral suspension of tinidazole (66.7 mg/mL):
      - Crush 4 tinidazole 500-mg tablets into a fine powder with a mortar and pestle.
      - Add approximately 10 mL of cherry syrup to the powder, and mix until smooth.
      - Transfer the suspension to a container using additional cherry syrup (30 mL total).
      - The suspension of crushed tablets in cherry syrup is stable for 7 days at room temperature.
6. Metronidazole can be used in children and adults (although giardiasis is not an FDA-approved indication for metronidazole). Adult dose is 250 mg tid for 5 to 7 days, and for children the dose is 15 mg/kg/day. Side effects are common and include nausea, gastrointestinal discomfort, and a metallic taste. Metronidazole may have a disulfiram-like effect, so alcohol consumption should be avoided.
7. Nitazoxanide, a nitrothiazolyl-salicylamide derivative, has been approved by the FDA for the treatment of giardiasis in children older than 1 year. In clinical trials it has been shown to be more effective than metronidazole in relieving symptoms in individuals with giardiasis. In addition, nitazoxanide is effective in treating multiple other infections caused by intestinal parasites (e.g., cryptosporidiosis and amebiasis). Nitazoxanide is available in liquid and tablet form but is expensive, and many pharmacies

do not stock it. The recommended oral doses are as follows:

a. *Adults:* 500 mg q12h for 3 days
b. *Children 1 to 3 years:* 100 mg q12h for 3 days
c. *Children 4 to 11 years:* 200 mg q12h for 3 days
d. *Children 12 years and older:* 500 mg q12 h for 3 days

8. The nonabsorbable drug paromomycin (Humatin, 25 to 30 mg/kg in three divided doses for 5 to 10 days) has been effective and may be used during pregnancy. When considering treatment during pregnancy, when possible, withhold treatment until after discussing with an obstetrician because none of the treatment options is considered completely safe.

Entamoeba histolytica

E. histolytica is found worldwide. Approximately 10% of the world's population carries the parasite. The prevalence in tropical countries is 30% to 50%. Despite its high prevalence, amebiasis accounts for less than 1% of cases of TD. As with *Giardia*, the life cycle of *E. histolytica* involves two forms. When a cyst is ingested through fecal contamination of food or water or via person-to-person contact, it divides and produces trophozoites. The trophozoites are the reproductive form, residing in the host and causing illness. Extraintestinal disease sometimes occurs by hematogenous spread. Abscesses develop primarily in the liver but may also involve the brain and lungs.

NONDYSENTERIC DISEASE
Signs and Symptoms

Eighty percent to 99% of infections result in an asymptomatic carrier state. In individuals who develop illness, the following may be noted:

- Most often, colonic inflammation without dysentery, causing lower abdominal cramping and altered stools
- Weight loss, anorexia, nausea
- Subacute infection developing into a nondysenteric bowel syndrome with symptoms of intermittent diarrhea, abdominal pain, weight loss, and flatulence

DYSENTERIC (INVASIVE) DISEASE
Signs and Symptoms

- Dysentery developing suddenly or after a period of mild symptoms
- Symptoms developing in as few as 8 to 10 days, but more often after weeks to months
- Ill appearance, with frequent bloody stools, tenesmus, moderate to severe abdominal pain and tenderness, and fever (considerable variation in severity)
- Rarely, significant fever

- Complications in 1% to 4% of patients: bowel perforation, toxic megacolon, strictures, or an ameboma (inflammatory lesion containing trophozoites that develops in the colon)
- Amoebic liver abscess acutely or years after infection
- In the wilderness, diagnosis considered in any patient with dysentery who is not responding to an appropriate antibiotic
- Asymptomatic cyst shedding and active gastrointestinal illness that persist for years if amebiasis is not treated

Treatment

1. Invasive colitis is treated with metronidazole (alternative therapies include tinidazole or nitazoxanide), followed by a luminal agent (such as paromomycin, diiodohydroxyquin, or diloxanide furoate) to eliminate intraluminal cysts.
   a. Dosing for metronidazole is 500 to 750 mg PO q8h for 7 to 10 days in adults and 35 to 50 mg/kg/day in three divided doses for 7 to 10 days in children.
   b. Dosing for tinidazole is 2 g PO daily for 3 days in adults. The dose for children older than 3 years is 50 mg/kg/day for 3 days (maximum dose: 2 g/day).
   c. Dosing for nitazoxanide is the same as for giardiasis (see earlier).
   d. Dosing for paromomycin is 25 to 30 mg/kg/day PO in three divided doses for 7 days.
   e. Dosing for diiodohydroxyquin is 650 mg PO q8h for 20 days for adults and 30 to 40 mg/kg/day in three divided doses for 20 days for children. This drug causes frequent systemic side effects, including cardiac arrhythmias requiring hospitalization for cardiac monitoring. Because this drug is related to ipecac, it may also cause vomiting.
2. In general, treatment is effective for invasive infections but disappointing for luminal infections (no regimen is completely effective in eradicating intestinal infection).

CRYPTOSPORIDIUM

Cryptosporidium is a protozoan parasite that is associated with self-limited diarrhea in immunocompetent hosts and severe debilitating diarrhea with weight loss and malabsorption in HIV-infected patients. A major source of infection is contaminated drinking or swimming water, which causes community outbreaks and TD. *Cryptosporidium* oocysts are present in 65% to 97% of surface waters and are difficult to eradicate because they are resistant to chlorine and iodine. Foodborne outbreaks are less common than are waterborne outbreaks. Person-to-person transmission is common, particularly among household members, health care workers, and children in day care centers.

Signs and Symptoms

- Incubation period usually 7 to 10 days (range 3 to 28 days)
- Syndrome generally mild and self-limited (typical duration of 5 to 6 days, range 2 to 26 days)

- Asymptomatic infection may occur
- Watery diarrhea (without blood or pus); abdominal cramps; nausea; flatulence; and, at times, vomiting and low-grade fever
- Immunocompromised hosts experience more frequent and prolonged infections, with profuse chronic watery diarrhea, malabsorption, and weight loss lasting months to years.
- Definitive diagnosis by stool examination or serologic techniques

Treatment
1. Recovery from infection depends upon the immune status of the patient. Immunocompetent patients usually recover without treatment within 1 to 2 weeks while receiving supportive therapy for vomiting and dehydration.
2. When therapy is required, nitazoxanide is the preferred drug. The adult dose is 500 mg q12h for 3 days. Dosing for children is as follows:
   a. *Children 1 to 3 years:* 100 mg q12h for 3 days; may consider increasing duration up to 14 days in HIV-exposed or HIV-infected patients
   b. *Children 4 to 11 years:* 200 mg q12h for 3 days; may consider increasing duration up to 14 days in HIV-exposed or HIV-infected patients
   c. *Children 12 years or older:* adult dosing

CYCLOSPORA CAYETANENSIS
C. cayetanensis is a protozoan parasite found in groundwater of developing countries. The organism has been shown to be an important cause of acute and protracted diarrhea. *Cyclospora* is endemic in many developing countries on all continents, with the highest rates occurring in Nepal, Haiti, and Peru. In the United States, most of the native outbreaks have been from areas east of the Rocky Mountains, usually associated with ingestion of contaminated imported raspberries.

Signs and Symptoms
- The onset of diarrhea is usually abrupt.
- *Cyclospora* causes a protracted watery diarrhea that can persist for weeks. Anorexia, nausea, and fatigue are common.
- Definitive diagnosis is made by finding the microorganism in a stool sample treated with a modified acid-fast stain.

Treatment
1. *Cyclospora* resists halogen-based (e.g., iodine and chlorine) water disinfection methods.
2. It is best killed by bringing drinking water to a boil.
3. The treatment of choice is trimethoprim/sulfamethoxazole; adult dose is one double-strength 160 mg/800 mg tablet PO q12h for 7 to 10 days. Ciprofloxacin 500 mg PO q12h for 7 days may be used as an alternative therapy for patients with a sulfa allergy.

CONSTIPATION

Constipation is a common malady during many wilderness sojourns. The most common cause for constipation during backcountry trips is dehydration. In addition, lack of roughage from eating foods that are often devoid of natural fiber may contribute. On certain trips, apprehension about using primitive toilet facilities and simple inconvenience may be factors.

Treatment

1. Increase fluid intake (approximately 2 L of fluid daily in adults).
2. Patients should try to drink an extra glass of water for every glass of diuretic beverage (i.e., coffee, tea, or alcohol).
3. Increase dietary fiber.
   a. It is helpful to bring along bran or psyllium seed (e.g., Metamucil) or methylcellulose (Citrucel) for this purpose.
   b. Patients should drink plenty of water; otherwise, ingesting fiber can be counterproductive.
   c. Fiber is not a laxative and will not typically induce an immediate bowel movement.
   d. Fiber-containing products, such as psyllium or methylcellulose, may cause gas or bloating.
   e. Fruits and vegetables may help prevent constipation.
4. Stool softeners such as docusate sodium (Colace) 50 to 500 mg/day PO in one to four divided doses enhance absorption of water and fat into stool, causing stool to soften. These drugs can be helpful, but they often lose their effectiveness over time.
5. At times a stronger stimulant medication may be indicated.
6. Bisacodyl (Dulcolax) is generally safe and effective.
   a. Bisacodyl should be taken with a full glass of water.
   b. The patient should swallow the tablets or capsules whole (i.e., do not chew or crush them).
7. Bisacodyl is also available as a rectal suppository. To use a rectal suppository, follow these steps:
   a. If the suppository is soft (such as in warm weather), insert it (in its wrapping) into cold water for 1 or 2 minutes before use.
   b. After removing the wrapper, moisten the suppository with water or petroleum jelly.
   c. The patient should lie on his or her side.
   d. With the pointed end forward, push the suppository into the rectum.
   e. The suppository should be retained for 15 to 20 minutes.
8. Polyethylene glycol 3350 is available as MiraLax. The dose is one heaping teaspoon of this osmotic laxative in at least 236 mL (8 oz) of beverage once a day. It may require 2 to 4 days for the first bowel movement to occur. Because it can be habit forming, it should not be used consecutively for more than 2 weeks.

45

Field Water Disinfection

RISK AND ETIOLOGY

Infectious agents in contaminated drinking water most commonly associated with the potential for causing illness in a wilderness setting include bacteria, viruses, and protozoa. The main reason for treating drinking water is to prevent gastrointestinal illness from fecal pollution with enteric pathogens. Appearance, odor, and taste do not reliably estimate water safety. Risk for waterborne illness depends on the number of organisms consumed, which is determined by the volume of water, concentration of organisms, and treatment system efficiency (Boxes 45.1 and 45.2).

Specific Etiologic Agents

Viruses

- The infectious dose of enteric viruses is only a few infectious units in the most susceptible people.
- Many other viruses are capable and suspected of waterborne transmission, and more than 100 different virus types are known to be excreted in human feces.

Protozoa

- Protozoa that cause enteric disease most often in wilderness travelers and that may be passed via waterborne transmission are *Giardia lamblia* and *Cryptosporidium parvum*.
- *Giardia* cysts have been found as frequently in pristine water and protected sources as in unprotected waters.
- Many of the species seemingly capable of passing *Giardia* cysts to humans, including dogs, cattle, ungulates (deer), and beavers, are present in wilderness areas.

Chemical Hazards

Chemical hazards are also an alarming source of pollution in surface water. Wilderness users must consider the possible presence of chemical, as well as microbiologic, contaminants.

DEFINITIONS

- Disinfection, the desired result of field water treatment, means the removal or destruction of harmful microorganisms.
- Pasteurization is similar to disinfection, but specifically refers to the use of heat, usually at temperatures below 100° C (212° F), to kill most pathogenic organisms.
- Sterilization is the destruction or removal of all life forms.

BOX 45.1 Waterborne Enteric Pathogens

Bacteria
Escherichia coli
Shigella
Campylobacter
Vibrio cholerae
Salmonella
Yersinia enterocolitica
Aeromonas

Viruses
Hepatitis A
Hepatitis E
Norovirus
Poliovirus
Miscellaneous viruses (more than 100 types: e.g., adenovirus, enterovirus, calicivirus, echovirus, astrovirus, coronavirus)

Protozoa
Giardia lamblia
Entamoeba histolytica
Cryptosporidium
Blastocystis hominis
Isospora belli
Balantidium coli
Acanthamoeba
Cyclospora

Parasites
Ascaris lumbricoides
Ancylostoma duodenale (hookworm)
Taenia spp. (tapeworm)
Fasciola hepatica (sheep liver fluke)
Dracunculus medinensis
Strongyloides stercoralis (pinworm)
Trichuris trichiura (whipworm)
Clonorchis sinensis (Oriental liver fluke)
Paragonimus westermani (lung fluke)
Diphyllobothrium latum (fish tapeworm)
Echinococcus granulosus (hydatid disease)

- Purification is the removal of organic or inorganic chemicals and particulate matter to remove offensive color, taste, and odor. Note that purification may not remove or kill enough microorganisms to ensure microbiologic safety.

HEAT
- Easy to use except when fuel is limited.
- Enteric pathogens, including cysts, bacteria, viruses, and parasites, can be killed at a temperature well below boiling (Table 45.1).

BOX 45.2   Water Quality: Key Points

- In general, cloudiness indicates higher risk for contamination; however, in remote wilderness water, most sediment is inorganic and clarity is not an indication of microbiologic purity.
- The major factor determining amount of microbe pollution in surface water is human and animal activity in the watershed.
- Streams do not purify themselves but may dilute a limited source of contamination.
- Settling effect of lakes may make them safer than streams, but care should be taken not to disturb bottom sediments when obtaining water.
- Groundwater (springs and protected wells) are generally cleaner than surface water because of the filtration action of overlying sediments.

Table 45.1   Heat

ADVANTAGES	DISADVANTAGES
Does not impart additional taste or color to water	Does not improve the taste, smell, or appearance of poor-quality water
Single-step process that inactivates all enteric pathogens	Fuel sources may be scarce, expensive, or unavailable
Efficacy is not compromised by contaminants or particles in the water, as happens with halogenation and filtration	Does not prevent recontamination during storage
Can pasteurize water without sustained boiling	

Relative susceptibility of microorganisms to heat: protozoa > bacteria > viruses.

Table 45.2   Boiling Temperatures at Various Altitudes

ALTITUDE (FT)	ALTITUDE (M)	BOILING POINT
5,000	1,524	95°C (203°F)
10,000	3,048	90°C (194°F)
14,000	4,267	86°C (186.8°F)
19,000	5,791	81°C (177.8°F)

- Thermal death is a function of both time and temperature; therefore, lower temperatures are effective with longer contact times.
- The boiling point decreases with the lower atmospheric pressure present at high elevations (Table 45.2).
- The majority of the time required to raise the temperature of water to its boiling point works toward disinfection, so water

is safe to drink by the time it has reached a full rolling boil. For an extra margin of safety, keep the water covered and hot for several minutes after boiling.

- Pasteurization (at subboiling temperatures with extended contact times) has been successfully achieved using solar heating. A solar cooker constructed from a foil-lined cardboard box with a glass window in the lid can be used for disinfecting large amounts of water by pasteurization. This could be a low-cost method for improving water quality, especially in refugee camps and disaster areas.

- When no other means are available, using hot tap water as drinking water may prevent traveler's diarrhea in developing countries. As a rule of thumb, water too hot to touch is within the pasteurization range. However, lukewarm tap water can contain pathogenic microorganisms.

FILTRATION, ADSORPTION, AND CLARIFICATION (Fig. 45.1)
Filtration
- Field filters that rely solely on the mechanical removal of microorganisms may be adequate for cysts and bacteria but may not reliably remove viruses unless tested for this function.

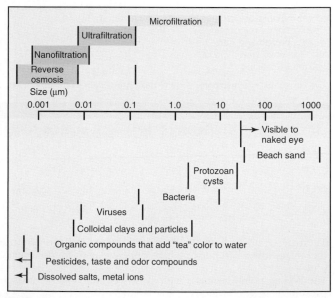

FIGURE 45.1 Relative size of microorganisms determines susceptibility to mechanical filtration. Mechanical filters span a wide range of pore sizes.

- They have the advantages of being simple and requiring no holding time.
- Most viruses adhere to larger particles or clump together into larger aggregates that may be removed by a filter. Filters are often expensive and can add considerable weight and bulk to a backpack.
- Some devices are designed as purely mechanical filters, whereas others combine filtration with granular activated carbon (GAC).
- The size of a microorganism is the primary determinant of its susceptibility to filtration.
- All filters eventually clog from suspended particulate matter, present even in clear streams, requiring cleaning or replacement of the filter. Flow can be partially restored to a clogged filter by back flushing or surface cleaning, which removes the larger particles trapped near the surface.

Microfiltration, Ultrafiltration, and Nanofiltration
- In general, portable filters for water treatment can be divided into microfiltration with pores down to 0.1 μm, ultrafiltration that can remove particles as small as 0.01 μm, and nanofiltration with pore sizes as small as 0.001 μm or less.
- Microfilters are effective for removing protozoa and bacteria, algae, most particles, and sediment, but allow dissolved material, small colloids, and some viruses to pass through.
- Ultrafiltration membranes are required for complete removal of viruses, colloids, and some dissolved solids.
- Nanofilters can remove other dissolved substances, including sodium chloride, from water. All filters require pressure to drive the water through the filter element. The smaller the pore size, the more pressure required.
- Some ceramic filters now remove 99% to 99.9% of viruses.

Adsorption Using Granular Activated Carbon
Granular carbon (i.e., charcoal) is widely used for water treatment and is the best means for removing toxic organic and inorganic chemicals from water (including disinfection by-products) and for improving odor and taste. GAC also removes radioactive contamination.
- Some, but not all, viral particles, bacteria, and protozoan cysts are removed by GAC filters.
- GAC does not kill microorganisms.
- No reliable means are available for determining precisely when GAC saturation is reached. Presence of unpleasant taste or color in the water can be the first sign that the charcoal is ineffective. To test the activity of the charcoal, one may filter iodinated water or water tinted with food coloring. With regular use, the lifetime of GAC is probably measured in months; it is substantially longer with infrequent use.
- With increasing industrial and agricultural contamination of distant groundwater, final treatment of drinking water with GAC may be important for some wilderness users.

Reverse Osmosis

- A reverse osmosis filter uses high pressure (100 to 800 psi) to force water through a semipermeable membrane that filters out dissolved ions, molecules, and solids.
- Reverse osmosis is generally used for desalinating water
- It may also be used to remove biologic contaminants.
- Small hand-pumped reverse osmosis units have been developed. High price and slow output currently limit their use by land-based wilderness travelers.
- It is an essential survival item for ocean travelers.

Forward Osmosis

Osmotic pressure also can be used to draw water through a membrane to create highly purified drinking water from low-quality source water, including brackish water. These products use a double-chamber bag or container with the membrane in between.

Clarification of cloudy water can be achieved by sedimentation, coagulation-flocculation (C-F), or adsorption (Table 45.3).

- Large particles settle by gravity over 1 to 2 hours in sedimentation. Although filters remove particulate debris, thus improving the appearance and taste of "dirty" water, they clog quickly if the water contains large particles.
- Smaller suspended particles can be removed by C-F. This is accomplished in the field by adding alum (aluminum potassium sulfate). Alum is used in the food industry as a pickling powder

Table 45.3 Summary of Clarification Techniques		
TECHNIQUE	**PROCESS USES**	**ADVANTAGES**
Sedimentation	Settling by gravity of large particulates	Greatly improves water aesthetics; however, requires a long time
Coagulation-flocculation	Removes suspended particles, most microorganisms, some dissolved substances	Simple process, easily applied in field Greatly improves water quality Improves efficacy of filtration and chemical disinfection
Activated charcoal	Removes organic and some inorganic chemicals	Removes toxins, such as pesticides, and removes chemical disinfectants Improves taste of water
Filtration	Physical and chemical process	Removes microorganisms If charcoal stage, may improve taste and remove chemicals

and is nontoxic. C-F will remove contaminants that cause an unpleasant color and taste, some dissolved metals, and some microorganisms.

CHEMICAL DISINFECTION (Tables 45.4 and 45.5)
Halogens (Chlorine and Iodine)

Worldwide, chemical disinfection is the most widely used method for improving and maintaining microbiologic quality of drinking water. Halogens, chiefly chlorine and iodine, are the most common chemical

Table 45.4 Water Disinfection Techniques and Halogen Doses		
Added to 1 L or Quart of Water		
IODINATION TECHNIQUES	**AMOUNT FOR 4 PPM**	**AMOUNT FOR 8 PPM**
Iodine tabs	½ tab	1 tab
Tetraglycine hydroperiodide		
EDWGT		
Potable Aqua		
Globaline		
2% Iodine solution (tincture)*	0.2 mL or 4 gtt	0.4 mL or 8 gtt
10% Povidone-iodine solution*†	0.35 mL or 7 gtt	0.70 mL or 14 gtt
Saturated solution: iodine crystals in water	13 mL	26 mL
Saturated solution: iodine crystals in alcohol	0.1 mL or 2 gtt	0.2 mL or 4 gtt
CHLORINATION TECHNIQUES	**AMOUNT FOR 5 PPM**	**AMOUNT FOR 10 PPM**
Sodium hypochlorite (household bleach 5%)†	0.1 mL or 2 gtt	0.2 mL or 4 gtt
Calcium hypochlorite (Redi-Chlor [$\frac{1}{10}$ g tab])		¼ tab/2 qt
Sodium dichloroisocyanurate (AquaClear)		1 tab (8.5 mg NaDCC)
Chlorine plus flocculating agent (Chlor-Floc)		1 tab

*Measure with dropper (1 drop = 0.05 mL) or tuberculin syringe.
†Povidone-iodine solutions release free iodine in levels adequate for disinfection, but scant data are available.
EDWGT, Emergency drinking water germicidal tablet; *gtt*, drops; *ppm*, parts per million.

disinfectants used in the field; however, chlorine dioxide is available in small-use applications. These agents are active against bacteria, viruses, *Giardia*, and cysts of amebae, excluding *Cryptosporidium*.

Factors Affecting Halogen Disinfection (Table 45.6)

Concentration and Demand

Disinfection with halogens depends on the following:

- The concentration of halogen
- The amount of time the halogen is in contact with the water (contact time)
- The water temperature (cold slows reaction time)
- The presence of organic contaminants in the water, which react with halogen and decrease its disinfectant action
- Water pH

Cold and Concentration (See Table 45.5)

Use four parts per million (ppm) as a target concentration for surface water, and allow extra contact time, especially if the water is cold. In cold water, the contact time or dose should be increased; in polluted water, the dose must be increased.

If there is no urgency, time can be increased instead of dose. Data for killing *Giardia* in very cold water (5° C [41° F]) with both chlorine and iodine indicate that contact time must be prolonged three to four times, not merely doubled, to achieve high levels of inactivation. If feasible, raising the temperature by 10°C to 20° C (18°F to 36° F) allows a lower dose of halogen and more reliable disinfection at a given dose.

Contaminants

- In cloudy water that will not settle out by sedimentation, the halogen dose should be at least 8 ppm. Ideally, use C-F to clarify the water before halogenation, and then use a smaller amount of halogen.

Table 45.5 Recommendations for Contact Time With Halogens in the Field			
	Contact Time in Minutes at Various Water Temperatures		
CONCENTRATION OF HALOGEN	**5°C (41°F)**	**15°C (59°F)**	**30°C (86°F)**
2 ppm	240	180	60
4 ppm	180	60	45
8 ppm	60	30	15

NOTE: Data indicate that very cold water requires prolonged contact time with iodine or chlorine to kill *Giardia* cysts. These contact times have been extended from the usual recommendations in cold water to account for this and for the uncertainty of residual concentration.

Table 45.6   Factors Affecting Halogen Disinfection

	EFFECT	COMPENSATION
Primary Factors		
Concentration	Measured in milligrams per liter (mg/L) or the equivalent, parts per million (ppm); higher concentration increases rate and proportion of microorganisms killed.	Higher concentration allows shorter contact time for equivalent results. Lower concentration requires increased contact time for equivalent levels of kill.
Contact time	Usually measured in minutes; longer contact time ensures higher proportion of organisms killed.	Contact time is inversely related to concentration; longer time allows lower concentration.
Secondary Factors		
Temperature	Cold slows reaction time.	Some treatment protocols recommend doubling the dose (concentration) of halogen in cold water, but if time allows, exposure time can be increased instead, or the temperature of the water can be increased.
Water contaminants, cloudy water (turbidity)	Halogens react with organic nitrogen compounds from decomposition of organisms and their wastes to form compounds with little or no disinfecting ability, effectively decreasing the concentration of available halogen. In general, turbidity increases halogen demand.	Doubling the dose of halogen for cloudy water is a crude means of compensation that often results in a strong disinfectant taste on top of the taste of the contaminants. A more rational approach is to first clarify water to reduce halogen demand.
pH	The optimal pH for disinfection is 6.5–7.5. As water becomes more alkaline, approaching pH 8.0, much higher doses of halogens are required.	Compensating for pH is not necessary for most surface water.

- Several simple color strip tests are available for field use, like those used for swimming pools and spas to measure the amount of free (residual) halogen in water. Testing in the wilderness for halogen residual may be reasonable for large groups but is not practical for most. Smell of chlorine usually indicates some free residual. Color and taste of iodine can be used as indicators. Above 0.6 ppm, a yellow to brown tint is noted.

pH
The optimal pH for halogen disinfection is 6.5 to 7.5. As water becomes more alkaline, approaching pH 8.0, much higher doses of halogens are required.

Pathogen Sensitivity
- Bacteria are extremely sensitive to halogens.
- Viruses and *Giardia* require higher concentrations or longer contact times.
- *Cryptosporidium* cysts are extremely resistant to halogens.
- The resistance of *Cryptosporidium* will require an alternative to halogens or a combination of methods to ensure removal and inactivation of all pathogens.
- Relative resistance between organisms is similar for iodine and chlorine.
- The physical state of the microbes also determines their susceptibility. Microbes that are aggregated in clumps or embedded in other matter or organisms may be shielded from disinfectants.

Chlorine
Chlorine has been used as a disinfectant for 200 years. The CDC-WHO Safe Water System for household disinfection in developing countries provides a dosage of 3.75 mg/L of sodium hypochlorite with a contact time of 30 minutes, sufficient to inactivate most bacteria, viruses, and some protozoa that cause waterborne diseases.

Iodine
Iodine is effective in low concentrations for killing bacteria, viruses, and cysts and in higher concentrations against fungi and even bacterial spores, but it is a poor algicide.

Recommendations
- Available data suggest the following:
  - High levels of iodine, such as those produced by recommended doses of iodine tablets, should be limited to periods of 1 month or less.
  - Iodine treatment that produces a low residual (1 mg/L or less) appears safe, even for long periods in people with normal thyroid function. This would require very low doses of iodine added to the water or an activated charcoal stage to remove residual iodine.

- Persons planning to use iodine for a prolonged period should have the thyroid gland examined and thyroid function measured to ensure that a state of euthyroidism exists.
- The following groups should not use iodine for water treatment because of their increased susceptibility to thyroid problems:
  - Pregnant women
  - Persons with known hypersensitivity to iodine
  - Persons with a history of thyroid disease, even if controlled by medication
  - Persons with a strong family history of thyroid disease (thyroiditis)
  - Persons from areas with chronic dietary iodine deficiency

Improving the Taste of Water Disinfected With Halogens

- Add flavoring to the water only *after* adequate contact time. Iodine will react with sugar additives, thereby reducing the free iodine available for disinfection.
- Use charcoal (GAC) to remove halogen *after* adequate contact time.
- Reduce the concentration and increase the contact time in clean water. For a small group of people, use a collapsible plastic container to disinfect water with low doses of iodine during the day or overnight.
- Iodine and chlorine taste and iodine color can be removed by chemical reduction. In addition, a much higher halogen dose (shorter contact time) can be used if followed by chemical reduction. To remove iodine and chlorine taste and iodine color by chemical reduction:
  - Add a few granules per liter of ascorbic acid (vitamin C, available in powder or crystal form) or sodium thiosulfate (nontoxic) after the required contact time (reduces iodine or chlorine to iodide or chloride, which has no taste or color).

Superchlorination-Dechlorination

- High doses of chlorine are added to the water in the form of calcium hypochlorite crystals to achieve concentrations of 30 to 200 ppm of free chlorine.
- These extremely high levels are above the margin of safety for field conditions and rapidly kill all bacteria, viruses, and protozoa and could kill *Cryptosporidium* with overnight contact times.
- After at least 10 to 15 minutes, several drops of 30% hydrogen peroxide solution are added. This reduces hypochlorite to chloride, forming calcium chloride and oxygen.
- The minor disadvantage of a two-step process is offset by excellent taste.
- This is a good technique for highly polluted or cloudy water and for disinfecting large quantities. It is the best technique for

storing water on boats or for emergency use. Water is then dechlorinated in needed quantities when ready to use.
- The ingredients can be easily obtained and packaged in small Nalgene bottles.

MISCELLANEOUS DISINFECTANTS
Chlorine Dioxide (Table 45.7)
- Chlorine dioxide is capable of inactivating most waterborne pathogens, including *Cryptosporidium parvum* oocysts, at practical doses and contact times.
- It is at least as effective a bactericide as chlorine and in many cases is superior.
- It is far superior as a virucide.
- It does not form chlorinated compounds in the presence of organics and is efficacious over a wide pH range.
- Cost-effective and portable chlorine dioxide treatment products include Micropur MP1, Aquamira, and Miox.

Mixed Species Disinfection (Miox Purifier)
- Passing a current through a simple brine salt solution generates free available chlorine, as well as other "mixed species" disinfectants that have been demonstrated effective against bacteria, viruses, and bacterial spores.
- The resulting solution has greater disinfectant ability than a simple solution of sodium hypochlorite.
- It has even been demonstrated to inactivate *Cryptosporidium*.
- Potential for malfunction and battery depletion exists.

Silver
Silver ion has bactericidal effects in low doses. The literature on antimicrobial effects of silver is confusing and contradictory.

Table 45.7 Chlorine Dioxide	
ADVANTAGES	**DISADVANTAGES**
Effective against all microorganisms, including *Cryptosporidium*	Volatile, so do not expose tablets to air and use generated solutions rapidly
Low doses have no taste or color	No persistent residual, so does not prevent recontamination during storage
Portable device now available for individual and small-group field use and simple to use	Sensitive to sunlight, so keep bottle shaded or in pack during treatment
More potent than equivalent doses of chlorine	
Less affected by nitrogenous wastes	

Relative susceptibility of microorganisms to chlorine dioxide: bacteria > viruses > protozoa.

- The use of silver as a drinking water disinfectant has been much more popular in Europe, where silver tablets (Micropur) are sold widely for field water disinfection.
- Silver ion has not been approved by the Environmental Protection Agency (EPA) for this purpose in the United States, but was approved as a water preservative to prevent bacterial growth in previously treated and stored water.
- Micropur Forte tablets release free chlorine for disinfection and silver for prolonged persistence of antimicrobial activity.
- Silver impregnation of filters may inactivate pathogens that pass through the filter pores or limit bacterial growth in the filter itself (bacteriostatic). Ceramic filters coated with silver have higher removal rates of bacteria than non-coated filters.

Potassium Permanganate

Potassium permanganate is a strong oxidizing agent with some disinfectant properties.

- It is used in municipal disinfection to control taste and odor.
- It has been used in a 1% to 5% solution as a drinking water disinfectant and is still used for this purpose in some countries, as well as for washing fruits and vegetables.
- Although potassium permanganate clearly has disinfectant action and is frequently used in some parts of the world, it cannot be recommended for point-of-use water disinfection unless no other means are available, because quantitative data are not available for viruses and no data are available for protozoan cysts.
- Packets of 1 g to be added to 1 L of water are sold in some countries.

Hydrogen Peroxide

Hydrogen peroxide is a strong oxidizing agent but a weak disinfectant. Although hydrogen peroxide can sterilize water, lack of data for protozoal cysts and quantitative data for dilute solutions prevents it from being useful as a field water disinfectant.

Ultraviolet Light and Sunlight

- Using sufficient doses, all waterborne enteric pathogens are inactivated by ultraviolet (UV) radiation (Table 45.8).
- UV treatment does not require chemicals and does not affect the taste of the water.
- UV works rapidly, and an overdose to the water presents no danger.
- UV light has no residual disinfection power; water may become recontaminated, or regrowth of bacteria may occur.
- Particulate matter can shield microorganisms from UV radiation.
- Portable field units, such as SteriPEN and AquaStar UV Portable Water Purifier, require a power source (battery, human powered, and solar-charged units are available). Users must prefilter or clarify cloudy water.

Table 45.8 Ultraviolet Irradiation	
ADVANTAGES	**DISADVANTAGES**
Effective against all microorganisms	Requires clear water
Imparts no taste	Does not improve water aesthetics
Portable device now available for individual and small-group field use; simple to use	Does not prevent recontamination during storage
Available from sunlight	Expensive
	Requires power source
	Requires direct sunlight, prolonged exposure; dose low and uncontrolled

- A new technology is the SolarBag.
  - The SolarBag disinfects 3 L at a time and can be used several times per day, on sunny or cloudy days.
  - It uses sunlight to activate a mesh insert coated with titanium dioxide.
  - For disinfection, the bag is placed flat or hanging in direct sunlight.
  - Disinfection requires 1 to 2 hours on a sunny day and 2 to 4 hours on a cloudy day.
  - For unknown water sources, a food-safe dye can be used as a tracer and timer. When the color has cleared, the water has been disinfected.
  - No chemicals or pumps are required, and it can be reused.
- A unique, low-tech approach uses a simple solar disinfection ("SODIS") technique (see http://www.sodis.ch/).
  - Transparent bottles (e.g., clear plastic beverage bottles), preferably lying on a dark surface, are exposed to sunlight for a minimum of 4 hours. Because ultraviolet radiation is reduced at increasing water depth, the containers used for SODIS should not exceed a water depth of 10 cm (4 inches).
  - Oxygenation induces greater reductions of bacteria, so agitation is recommended before solar treatment in bottles.
  - Where strong sunshine is available, solar disinfection of drinking water is an effective, low-cost method for improving water quality and may be of particular use in refugee camps and disaster areas.
  - With a water temperature of 30° C (86° F), 6 hours of midlatitude midday summer sunshine are required to achieve a 3-log reduction of fecal coliforms.
  - Treatment efficiency can be improved if bottles are exposed on sunlight-reflecting surfaces such as aluminum or corrugated iron sheets. Use of a simple reflector or solar cooker can achieve pasteurization temperatures of 65° C (149° F).

Table 45.9 Summary of Field Water Disinfection Techniques					
	BACTERIA	VIRUSES	GIARDIA/AMEBAE	CRYPTOSPORIDIUM	NEMATODES/CERCARIAE
Heat	+	+	+	+	+
Filtration	+	+/−*	+	+	+
Halogens	+	+	+	−	+/−†
Chlorine dioxide	+	+	+	+	+/−†

*Most filters make no claims for viruses. Reverse osmosis is effective. The General Ecology filtration system claims virus removal.
†Eggs are not very susceptible to halogens but have very low risk of waterborne transmission.

- Effects can also be enhanced by adding small amounts of hydrogen peroxide, lemon juice, or lime juice.

CHOOSING THE PREFERRED TECHNIQUE (Table 45.9)

- The best technique for disinfection for either an individual or a group depends on the number of persons, space and weight available, quality of source water, personal taste preferences, and availability of fuel.
- Optimal protection for all situations may require a two-step process of filtration or C-F and halogenation because halogens do not kill *Cryptosporidium* and filtration misses some viruses.
- Heat works as a one-step process, but it will not improve the taste and appearance of water.

HYDRATION AND DEHYDRATION ASSESSMENT AND TREATMENT

Water accounts for 50% to 70% of the body's weight. Because sweating involves loss of body mass, measuring changes in body weight is the simplest way to rapidly assess hydration status. However, wilderness first aid kits will almost never include an accurate scale with which to weigh a patient, so estimation of hydration status must rely on other observations (Table 46.1). Prevention of dehydration is key (Table 46.2).

URINE MARKERS

Urinary markers for dehydration include urine volume, urine specific gravity, urine osmolality, and urine color and are most accurately employed using the first morning void.

Urine Color

In the backcountry, the color of urine can be used as a rough guide to monitor hydration status. Under ideal circumstances the urine (first morning) should be in a clean, clear vial or cup and the color assessed against a white background. Urine color can be compared against a urine color chart or assessed relative to the degree of darkness.

- Strongly yellow-colored urine (similar to apple juice) is indicative of dehydration.
- Pale urine (similar to lemonade color or less color intense) indicates adequate hydration.

Dark yellow or orange urine can also be caused by recent use of laxatives or consumption of B complex vitamins or carotene. Orange urine may be caused by phenazopyridine (used in the treatment of urinary tract infections), rifampin, and warfarin. Red urine may be caused by ingestion of beets.

Urine Specific Gravity and Osmolality

Urine dipsticks that measure specific gravity are light and easily carried on backcountry trips and can be used as a marker of hydration. A urine specific gravity of more than 1.02 indicates a state of dehydration. Urine osmolality <700 mOsmol is consistent with euhydration.

Treatment

- Administer oral rehydration fluids to patients who are conscious and coherent.

Table 46.1	Signs and Symptoms of Dehydration		
SIGNS/ SYMPTOMS	**MILD DEHYDRATION**	**MODERATE DEHYDRATION**	**SEVERE DEHYDRATION**
Level of consciousness	Alert	Lethargic	Obtunded
Capillary refill	2 sec	2–4 sec	>4 sec, cool limbs
Mucous membranes	Normal	Dry	Parched, cracked
Tears	Normal	Decreased	Absent
Heart rate	Slight increase	Increased	Very increased
Respiratory rate	Normal	Increased	Increased and hyperpnea
Blood pressure	Normal	Normal, but orthostasis	Decreased
Pulse	Normal	Thready	Faint or impalpable
Skin turgor	Normal	Slow	Tenting
Eyes	Normal	Sunken	Very sunken
Urine output	Decreased	Oliguria	Oliguria/anuria

- Administer intravenous fluids (2 L normal saline over 4 hours for adults and 20 mL/kg for children) to patients who are severely dehydrated or unable to ingest oral fluids.

HYDRATION STRATEGIES

After significant body water deficits, such as those associated with physical work or heat stress, many hours of rehydration and electrolyte consumption may be needed to reestablish body water balance. For example, if hypohydrated by more than about 4% of total body mass, it may take more than 24 hours to fully rehydrate through water and electrolyte replacement.

- Drink 500 mL (2 cups) of fluid about 4 hours before endurance or strenuous activity to promote adequate hydration and allow time for excretion of excess water. If no urine, or concentrated urine, follows, drink another 300 mL (1¼ cups) 2 hours before activity.
- Replace water losses caused by sweating at a rate equal to the sweat rate (see Table 46.2).
  - Sweat losses range from 0.3 to 1.2 L/hr for an individual doing mild work while wearing cotton clothes.
  - Sweat losses range from 1 to 2 L/hr for an individual doing mild work and wearing nonpermeable clothing.

Table 46.2 Fluid Replacement Guidelines for Warm-Weather Training (Applies to Average Acclimated Soldier Wearing Battle Dress Uniform in Hot Weather)*

HEAT CATEGORY	WBGT INDEX (°F)	Easy Work		Moderate Work		Hard Work	
		WORK/REST CYCLE	WATER INTAKE (Q/HR)	WORK/REST CYCLE	WATER INTAKE (Q/HR)	WORK/REST CYCLE	WATER INTAKE (Q/HR)
1	78–81.9 (26°C–28°C)	NL	½	NL	¾	40/20 min	¾
2 (green)	82–84.9 (28°C–29.4°C)	NL	½	50/10 min	¾	30/30 min	1
3 (yellow)	85–87.9 (29.4°C–31°C)	NL	¾	40/20 min	¾	30/30 min	1
4 (red)	88–89.9 (31°C–32.2°C)	NL	¾	30/30 min	¾	20/40 min	1
5 (black)	>90	50/10 min	1	20/40 min	1	10/50 min	1

NL, No limit to work time per hour; WBGT, wet bulb global temperature.

Rest means minimal physical activity (sitting or standing), accomplished in shade if possible.

CAUTION: Hourly fluid intake should not exceed 1½ quarts. Daily fluid intake should not exceed 12 quarts.

Wearing body armor: Add 5°F to WBGT index. Wearing mission-oriented protective posture (MOPP, chemical protection) overgarment, add 10°F to WBGT index.

EASY WORK: Weapon maintenance; walking hard surface at 2.5 mph, ≤30-lb load; manual handling of arms; marksmanship training; drill and ceremony.

MODERATE WORK: Walking in loose sand at 2.5 mph, no load; walking hard surface at 3.5 mph, ≤40-lb load; calisthenics; patrolling; individual movement techniques (e.g., low crawl, high crawl); defensive position construction; field assaults.

HARD WORK: Walking on hard surface at 3.5 mph, ≥40-lb load; walking in loose sand at 2.5 mph with load.

1 quart = 946 mL.

*The work/rest times and fluid replacement volumes will sustain performance and hydration for at least 4 hr of work in the specified heat category. Individual water needs will vary ±¼ quart per hour.

From Montain SJ, Latzka WA, Sawka MN: Fluid replacement recommendations for training in hot weather, *Mil Med* 164:502, 1999.

- Sweat losses range from 1 to 2.5 L/hr for an individual doing strenuous work or during high exercise intensity in a hot climate.
- The perception of thirst is a poor indicator of hydration. Individuals can be 2% to 8% dehydrated before feeling thirsty.
- Unless an activity is prolonged and in hot weather with large volumes of sweat loss, beverages containing electrolytes and carbohydrates offer little advantage over water in maintaining hydration or electrolyte concentration or in improving intestinal absorption. The Institute of Medicine recommends that in the instance of prolonged activity in hot weather, fluid replacement should contain 20 to 30 mEq/L sodium (chloride as the anion), approximately 2 to 5 mEq/L potassium, and approximately 5% to 10% carbohydrate.
- Fluid-replacement beverages that are sweetened (with carbohydrates or artificial sweeteners) and cooled (to between 15°C and 21°C [59°F and 69.8°F]) stimulate ingestion of more fluid.
- Meals should be consumed regularly to return normal electrolyte losses.
- During prolonged exercise, frequent (every 15 to 20 minutes) consumption of moderate (150 mL [½ cup]) to large (350 mL [1½ cups]) volumes of low-osmolarity fluid may improve the gastric emptying rate.
- Optimal performance is attainable only with sufficient drinking during exercise to minimize dehydration. Even low levels of dehydration (1% loss of body mass) impair cardiovascular and thermoregulatory responses and reduce capacity for exercise.
- To restore hydration status after exercise, a person should consume 1 L (4¼ cups) of fluid for every kilogram of weight lost during the activity. Consumption of normal meals and snacks with sufficient volume of plain water will restore euhydration.

Malaria is a mosquito-transmitted, blood-borne, parasitic infection present throughout tropical and developing areas of the world. Parasites are transmitted by 30 to 40 (out of 430) species of the female *Anopheles* mosquito, which tends to bite between dusk and dawn. The World Health Organization (WHO) estimated 212 million cases of malaria worldwide in 2015, with an overall 21% decrease in incidence and 29% decrease in global mortality between 2010 and 2015.

Malaria infection causes a severe febrile illness that is potentially fatal, with most deaths occurring from *Plasmodium falciparum* infection in children in sub-Saharan Africa. *Plasmodium* sporozoites enter the bloodstream following inoculation from the mosquito and pass to the liver, where they develop into schizonts. Hepatic cells containing schizonts then rupture, releasing merozoites that then invade erythrocytes. These further develop into trophozoites or gametocytes within the erythrocyte. Free gametocytes invade the intestinal wall of feeding mosquitoes and develop into sporozoites, thus perpetuating the cycle of inoculation (Fig. 47.1).

Pathologic presentations of malaria, such as fever and anemia, occur during the asexual phase of the parasitic infection, in which the malaria parasite invades the healthy erythrocytes (erythrocytic phase). Parasitic replication over the subsequent 2 to 3 days following initial infection of healthy erythrocytes is followed by cell rupture and subsequent exponential parasite reproduction.

Five species of malaria typically cause disease in humans:
1. *Plasmodium vivax* (worldwide distribution, but uncommon in sub-Saharan Africa)
2. *P. falciparum* (worldwide distribution, predominant in sub-Saharan Africa, Amazon basin, Haiti, limited in Asia and Oceania)
3. *Plasmodium ovale* (West Africa, Amazon basin)
4. *Plasmodium malariae* (worldwide distribution)
5. *Plasmodium knowlesi* (limited to Southeast Asia)

Clinical Manifestations and Complications (Table 47.1)
- Clinical manifestations first evident 1 to 2 weeks after entry into endemic area (sooner if infected blood obtained through transfusion or shared needles)
- No pathognomonic signs, but common symptoms
  - Fever
  - Chills
  - Diaphoresis
  - Headaches
  - Nausea and vomiting

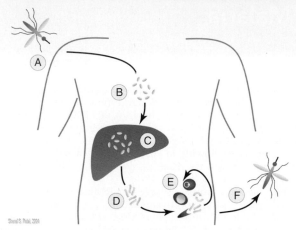

FIGURE 47.1   Malarial Parasite Life Cycle. During the malarial parasite life cycle, sporozoites are transmitted through the bite of a nocturnal feeding female *Anopheles* mosquito **(A)**. Sporozoites then migrate to the liver **(B)** and mature to merozoites **(C)**. A subset of *P. vivax* and *P. ovale* parasites remains dormant as hypnozoites, emerging months to years after the initial infection to cause disease. Eight to 25 days after the initial infection, 10,000 to 30,000 merozoites are released to invade erythrocytes **(D)**. Asexual parasites mature in 48 to 72 hours, each releasing 6 to 24 merozoites to invade more erythrocytes **(E)**. Some parasites develop into gametocytes (sexual stages), which are taken up during a mosquito blood meal. Diploid zygotes form ookinetes and develop into haploid sporozoites **(F)**. The sporozoites migrate to the mosquito salivary gland and continue the life cycle in humans with the next blood meal. (Courtesy Sheral S. Patel, with permission.)

- Abdominal pain, diarrhea
- Myalgias
- Paroxysms of chills followed by high fever and sweating
  - May last several hours and occur every 2 to 3 days
  - Classic periodic attacks often not observed in severe *P. falciparum* malaria; fever possibly constant
- Cerebral malaria (associated with high levels of *P. falciparum* parasitemia), characterized by high fevers, confusion, seizures, and eventually coma and death
- Acute renal failure, pulmonary edema
- Definitive diagnosis only by the presence of parasite-containing red blood cells (detected on thick and thin blood smears [see Plate 33])
- Clinical attacks during the first 4 to 8 weeks after return from the area of exposure
- Prolonged latent incubation times (up to 3 years) reported
- Severe manifestations and complications are more common with *P. falciparum* infection than with other species of malaria (Table 47.2).

Table 47.1   Key Clinical Manifestations and Complications of Human *Plasmodium* Infection

PLASMODIUM SPECIES	MANIFESTATIONS AND COMPLICATIONS
All species	Fever, chills, rigors, sweats, and headaches
	Weakness
	Myalgias
	Vomiting
	Diarrhea
	Hepatomegaly
	Splenomegaly
	Jaundice
	Anemia
	Thrombocytopenia
Plasmodium falciparum	Hyperparasitemia
	Cerebral malaria: seizures, obtundation, and coma
	Severe anemia
	Hypoglycemia
	Acidosis
	Renal failure
	Pulmonary edema (noncardiogenic)
	Vascular collapse
Plasmodium vivax and *Plasmodium ovale*	Splenic rupture
	Relapse months to years after primary infection because of latent hepatic stages
Plasmodium malariae	Low-grade fever and fatigue
	Chronic asymptomatic parasitemia
	Immune complex glomerulonephritis
Plasmodium knowlesi	Like *P. falciparum*, exception without cerebral malaria

Table 47.2 Severe Manifestations of *Plasmodium falciparum* Malaria in Children and Adults

CLINICAL MANIFESTATIONS	Prognostic Value (+ to +++)		Frequency (+ to +++)	
	CHILDREN	ADULTS	CHILDREN	ADULTS
Impaired consciousness	+++	+++	+++	++
Respiratory distress (acidotic breathing)	+++	+++	+++	++
Multiple convulsions	+	++	+++	+
Prostration	+	+	+++	+++
Shock	+++	+++	+	+
Pulmonary edema (radiologic)	+++	+++	+/−*	+
Abnormal bleeding	+++	++	+/−*	+
Jaundice	++	+	+	+++
Laboratory indices				
Severe anemia	+	+	+++	+
Hypoglycemia	+++	+++	+++	++
Acidosis	+++	+++	+++	++
Hyperlactatemia	+++	+++	+++	++
Renal impairment†	++	++	+	+++
Hyperparasitemia	+/−	++	++	+

*Infrequent.
†Acute kidney injury.
From World Health Organization: Severe malaria. *Trop Med Int Health* 19(Suppl 1):7–131, 2014.

- Epidemiologic and research definitions of severe *P. falciparum*, which are indicators of a poor prognosis (Table 47.3).

Diagnosis
History
Early and prompt diagnosis of malaria, particularly in nonendemic areas, requires the health care provider to take an appropriate travel history in the febrile patient and include malaria in the differential diagnosis. Most malaria cases in the United States occur among travelers who have visited malaria-endemic areas. A thorough travel history must be obtained, including travel dates, destinations, and any chemoprophylaxis taken. Because of drug resistance and potential medication noncompliance, chemoprophylaxis in a returned traveler does not exclude a diagnosis of malaria.

Patients may not have typical malarial paroxysms of fever and chills. Nonspecific symptoms (e.g., fatigue, diarrhea, headache, myalgias, and sore throat) may lead the clinician to another diagnosis, such as a viral syndrome. In semi-immune individuals, fever and persistent malaise may be present. Clinicians in endemic areas must add severe malaria to the differential diagnosis of an ill-appearing child.

Blood Smears
Thin and thick blood smears are the gold standard for the clinical diagnosis of malaria (see Plate 33). Blood smears should be interpreted by skilled microscopists trained in malaria diagnosis. The diagnosis of malaria and assessment of the severity of infection depend on parasite morphologic characteristics and the density of parasitemia. The Centers for Disease Control and Prevention (CDC) resource page on PDPx with instructions on collection and preparation of both thick and thin smears can be found at https://www.cdc.gov/dpdx/diagnosticprocedures/blood/specimenproc.html.

Antibody-Based Rapid Diagnostic Tests
Rapid diagnostic tests (RDTs) and microscopy should be primary diagnostic tools for confirmation and management of suspected malaria in all epidemiologic situations. Antibody-based RDTs are relatively simple to perform and interpret, and do not require specialized equipment or electricity. RDTs allow a provider to exclude malaria infection in settings where reliable, experienced microscopy is unavailable.

- Test results typically appear in 5 to 20 minutes as a colored test line.
- Antibody-based RDTs detect *Pf*HRP2, malaria-specific lactate dehydrogenase, or aldolase antigens in fingerprick blood samples.
- WHO's testing program and interactive guide of various products can be found online at http://finddiagnostics.org/programs/malaria-afs/malaria/current-projects/rdt_quality_control/interactiveguide-intro/interactive-guide/index.jsp.
- All malaria RDTs should be followed by malaria microscopy.

Table 47.3   Epidemiologic and Research Definitions of Severe *Falciparum* Malaria*

CHARACTERISTIC	LABORATORY MEASUREMENT OR SCORE
Impaired consciousness	Glasgow Coma Scale score <11 in adults or Blantyre Coma Scale score <3 in children
Acidosis	Base deficit of >8 mEq/L or, if unavailable, a plasma bicarbonate of <15 mmol/L or venous plasma lactate >5 mmol/L. Severe acidosis manifests clinically as respiratory distress (rapid, deep, labored breathing).
Hypoglycemia	Blood or plasma glucose <2.2 mmol/L (<40 mg/dL)
Severe malarial anemia	Hemoglobin concentration <5 g/dL or a hematocrit of <15% in children <12 years of age (<7 g/dL and <20%, respectively, in adults) together with a parasite count >10,000/µL
Renal impairment (acute kidney injury)	Plasma or serum creatinine >265 µmol/L (3 mg/dL) or blood urea >20 mmol/L
Jaundice	Plasma or serum bilirubin >50 µmol/L (3 mg/dL) together with a parasite count >100,000/µL
Pulmonary edema	Radiologically confirmed, or oxygen saturation <92% on room air with a respiratory rate >30/min, often with chest indrawing and crepitations on auscultation
Significant bleeding	Including recurrent or prolonged bleeding from nose gums or venipuncture sites; hematemesis or melena
Shock	Compensated shock is defined as capillary refill ≥3 s or temperature gradient on leg (mid to proximal limb), but no hypotension. Decompensated shock is defined as systolic blood pressure <70 mm Hg in children or <80 mm Hg in adults with evidence of impaired perfusion (cool peripheries or prolonged capillary refill)
Hyperparasitemia	*Plasmodium falciparum* parasitemia >10%

*For epidemiologic and research purposes, severe malaria is defined as one or more of the characteristics in the table, occurring in the absence of an identified alternative cause, and in the presence of *P. falciparum* asexual parasitemia.
From World Health Organization: Severe malaria. *Trop Med Int Health* 19(Suppl 1):7–131, 2014.

- A positive malaria RDT can inform the health care worker to urgently initiate malaria treatment.
- A negative RDT does not exclude the diagnosis of malaria.
- RDT result is qualitative, so microscopy must be used to quantify infection and the response to therapy.

Prevention

- Counseling
  - Importance of chemoprophylaxis
  - Potential adverse reactions or side effects from chemoprophylaxis
  - Clinical manifestations of malaria (see Table 47.1)
  - Plan for urgent medical care
- Personal protective measures
  - Minimize outdoor activity at dusk and night
  - Wear long sleeves, long pants, and hats at dusk and night
  - Use insect repellent
    - 10% to 35% *N,N*-diethyl-3-methylbenzamide (DEET) for exposed skin
    - Permethrin for clothes, shoes, mosquito nets, tents, and other gear
    - Insecticide-treated bed nets
    - Mosquito coils and candles
- Chemoprophylaxis
  - Assess considerations when choosing a drug for malaria prophylaxis (Table 47.4).
  - For a complete list of drugs used for the prevention of malaria, see Table 47.5.
  - Assess malaria risk based on geographic location.
    - Use map to identify malaria-endemic countries (Fig. 47.2).
    - Use CDC Malaria Information and Prophylaxis, by Country site https://www.cdc.gov/malaria/travelers/country_table/a.html for specific recommendations and prophylaxis.
  - Determine malaria resistance patterns (using the above CDC web URL).
  - Consider the following:
    - Age
    - Underlying medical conditions
    - Allergies
    - Tolerability
    - Length of stay
    - Advise when to start medication and how long to continue after return.
    - Determine whether medication should be prescribed for presumptive self-treatment.

Treatment of Uncomplicated Malaria
Presumptive Self-Treatment
1. If treatment is required, it implies failure of malaria chemoprophylaxis. Taking prophylactic medications does not exclude the

Text continued on p. 580

Table 47.4	Considerations When Choosing a Drug for Malaria Prophylaxis	
DRUG	**REASONS TO CONSIDER USE OF THIS DRUG**	**REASONS TO CONSIDER AVOIDING USE OF THIS DRUG**
Atovaquone-proguanil	Good for last-minute travelers because the drug is started 1–2 days before travel Some people prefer to take a daily medicine Good choice for shorter trips because you have to take the medicine for only 7 days after traveling, rather than for 4 weeks Well tolerated; side effects uncommon Pediatric tablets are available and may be more convenient	Cannot be used by women who are pregnant or breastfeeding a child that weighs <5 kg (11.02 b) Cannot be taken by people with severe renal impairment Tends to be more expensive than some of the other options (especially for long trips) Some people (including children) would rather not take a medicine every day
Chloroquine	Some people would rather take medicine weekly Good choice for long trips because it is taken only weekly Some people are already taking hydroxychloroquine chronically for rheumatologic conditions; such persons may not have to take an additional medicine Can be used in all trimesters of pregnancy	Cannot be used in areas with chloroquine or mefloquine resistance May exacerbate psoriasis Some people would rather not take a weekly medication For short trips, some people would rather not take medication for 4 weeks after travel Not a good choice for last-minute travelers, because drug needs to be started 1–2 weeks before travel
Doxycycline	Some people prefer to take a daily medicine Good for last-minute travelers because the drug is started 1–2 days before travel Tends to be the least expensive antimalarial People who are already taking doxycycline chronically to prevent acne do not have to take an additional medicine Doxycycline also can prevent some additional infections (such as rickettsial infections and leptospirosis), so it may be preferred by people planning to hike, camp, and swim in freshwater	Cannot be used by pregnant women and children <8 years of age Some people would rather not take a medicine every day For short trips, some people would rather not take medication for 4 weeks after travel Women prone to getting vaginal yeast infections when taking antibiotics may prefer taking a different medicine People may want to avoid the increased risk of sun sensitivity Some people are concerned about the potential of developing gastric distress from doxycycline

| Mefloquine | Some people would rather take medicine weekly
Good choice for long trips because it is taken only weekly
Can be used in all trimesters of pregnancy | Cannot be used in areas with mefloquine resistance
Cannot be used in patients with certain psychiatric conditions
Cannot be used in patients with a seizure disorder
Not recommended for people with cardiac conduction abnormalities
Not a good choice for last-minute travelers because the drug needs to be started ≥2 weeks before travel
Some people would rather not take a weekly medication
For short trips, some people would rather not take medication for 4 weeks after travel |
| Primaquine | It is the most effective medicine for preventing *Plasmodium vivax* infection, so it is a good choice for travel to places with more than 90% *P. vivax* as the cause of malaria
Good choice for shorter trips because you only have to take the medicine for 7 days after traveling, rather than for 4 weeks
Good for last-minute travelers because the drug is started 1–2 days before travel
Some people prefer to take a daily medicine | Cannot be used in patients with G6PD deficiency
Cannot be used in patients who have not been tested for G6PD deficiency
There are costs and delays associated with getting a G6PD test; however, it only has to be done once; once a normal G6PD level is verified and documented, the test does not have to be repeated the next time primaquine is considered
Cannot be used by pregnant women
Cannot be used by women who are breastfeeding, unless the infant has also been tested for G6PD deficiency
Some people (including children) would rather not take a medicine every day
Some people are concerned about the potential of having gastric distress from primaquine |

G6PD, Glucose-6-phosphate dehydrogenase.

From Centers for Disease Control and Prevention: CDC Health Information for International Travel, 2018, Atlanta, Georgia, 2018, US Department of Health and Human Services, Public Health Service, Centers for Disease Control and Prevention, National Center for infectious Diseases, Division of Global Migration and Quarantine; https://wwwnc.cdc.gov/travel/yellowbook/2018/infectious-diseases-related-to-travel/malaria#5216.

Table 47.5 Drugs Used for the Prevention of Malaria (in Alphabetical Order)*

DRUG	TRADE NAMES	ADULT DOSE	PEDIATRIC DOSE[†]	WHEN TO START BEFORE TRAVEL TO MALARIOUS AREA
Atovaquone-proguanil	Malarone	1 adult tablet[‡] orally, daily	5–8 kg (11.02–17.6 lb): ½ pediatric tablet[§] daily >8–10 kg (22 lb): ¾ pediatric tablet[§] daily >10–20 kg (44.1 lb): 1 pediatric tablet[§] daily >20–30 kg (66.14 lb): 2 pediatric tablets[§] daily >30–40 kg (66.14–88.2 lb): 3 pediatric tablets[§] daily ≥40 kg (88.2 lb): 1 adult tablet[§] daily	1–2 days
Chloroquine phosphate	Aralen, generic	300-mg base (500-mg salt) orally, once/week	5-mg/kg base (8.3-mg/kg salt) orally, once/week, up to maximum adult dose of 300-mg base	1–2 weeks
Doxycycline	Vibramycin, Vibra-Tabs, Doryx, Periostat, and others; generic	100 mg orally, daily	≥8 years: 2.2 mg/kg up to adult dose of 100 mg/day	1–2 days
Hydroxychloroquine sulfate	Plaquenil, generic	310-mg base (400-mg salt) orally, once/week	5-mg/kg base (6.5-mg/kg salt) orally, once/week, up to maximum adult dose of 310-mg base	1–2 weeks

HOW LONG TO CONTINUE AFTER RETURN	ADVERSE EFFECTS	COMMENTS
7 days	Headache, nausea, vomiting, abdominal pain, diarrhea, increased transaminase levels, and seizures	Take with food or milk. Contraindicated in persons with severe renal impairment (i.e., creatine clearance of <30 mL/min). Not recommended for children <5 kg (11.02 lb), pregnant women, and women breastfeeding infants <5 kg (11.02 lb). Partial-tablet doses should be prepared and dispensed by a pharmacist. For children weighing 5–<11 kg (24.25 lb), off-label use is recommended by the CDC.
4 weeks	Pruritus, nausea, headache, skin eruptions, dizziness, blurred vision, and insomnia	Has been used extensively and safely during pregnancy. May exacerbate psoriasis.
4 weeks	Gastrointestinal upset, vaginal candidiasis, photosensitivity, allergic reactions, blood dyscrasias, azotemia in renal diseases, and hepatitis	Take with food. Contraindicated in children <8 years of age and pregnant women.
4 weeks	Pruritus, nausea, headache, skin eruptions, dizziness, blurred vision, and insomnia	Has been used extensively and safely during pregnancy. May exacerbate psoriasis.

Continued

Table 47.5   Drugs Used for the Prevention of Malaria (in Alphabetical Order)*—cont'd

DRUG	TRADE NAMES	ADULT DOSE	PEDIATRIC DOSE†	WHEN TO START BEFORE TRAVEL TO MALARIOU AREA
Mefloquine	Lariam, Mephaquin, generic	228-mg base (250-mg salt) orally, once/ week	≤9 kg: 4.6-mg/kg base (5-mg/kg salt) orally, once/week >9–19 kg: ¼ tablet once/ week >19–30 kg: ½ tablet once/ week >30–45 kg: ¾ tablet once/ week ≥45 kg: 1 tablet, once/week	≥2 weeks
Primaquine primary prophylaxis	—	30-mg base (52.6-mg salt) orally, daily	0.5-mg/kg base (0.8-mg/kg salt) up to adult dose, orally, daily	1–2 days

HOW LONG TO CONTINUE AFTER RETURN	ADVERSE EFFECTS	COMMENTS
4 weeks	Gastrointestinal disturbances, headache, insomnia, vivid dreams, visual disturbances, depression, anxiety disorder, and dizziness	Contraindicated in persons with active depression or a recent history of depression, generalized anxiety disorder, psychosis, schizophrenia, other major psychiatric disorders, or seizures. Rare serious adverse reactions reported with treatment doses include psychoses and seizures. These reactions are seen more frequently at the higher doses used for treatment. Contraindicated in people allergic to mefloquine or related compounds (quinine, quinidine). Not recommended for persons with cardiac conduction abnormalities. Use with caution in travelers with psychiatric disturbances or a history of depression. In the United States, 250-mg tablet of mefloquine contains 228-mg mefloquine base. Outside the United States, 275-mg mefloquine tablet contains 250-mg mefloquine base. For children weighing <5 kg, off-label use is recommended by the CDC.
7 days	Nausea, abdominal pain, and hemolytic anemia (especially in patients with G6PD deficiency)	An option for primary prophylaxis in special circumstances such as short-duration travel to areas with principally *Plasmodium vivax*. Take with food. All persons taking primaquine should have a documented normal G6PD level before beginning the medication. Contraindicated in persons with G6PD deficiency, during pregnancy, and during breastfeeding, unless the infant being breastfed has a documented normal G6PD level.

Continued

Table 47.5   Drugs Used for the Prevention of Malaria (in Alphabetical Order)*—cont'd

DRUG	TRADE NAMES	ADULT DOSE	PEDIATRIC DOSE[†]	WHEN TO START BEFORE TRAVEL TO MALARIOUS AREA
Primaquine presumptive antirelapse therapy (terminal prophylaxis)	—	30-mg base (52.6-mg salt) orally, daily	0.5-mg/kg base (0.8-mg/kg salt) up to adult dose, orally, daily	Not applicable

*Caused by *Plasmodium falciparum*, *P. ovale*, *P. vivax*, and *P. malariae*.
[†]Should never exceed adult dose.
[‡]Adult tablets contain 250 mg atovaquone and 100 mg proguanil hydrochloride.
[§]Pediatric tablets contain 62.5 mg atovaquone and 25 mg proguanil hydrochloride.
CDC, Centers for Disease Control and Prevention.
Modified from Centers for Disease Control and Prevention: CDC Health Information for International Travel, 2018, Atlanta, Georgia, 2018, U.S. Department of Health and Human Services, Public Health Service, Centers for Disease Control and Prevention, National Center for infectious Diseases, Division of Global Migration and Quarantine; https://wwwnc.cdc.gov/travel/yellowbook/2018/infectious-diseases-related-to-travel/malaria#5216.
Refer to the U.S. Centers for Disease Control and Prevention for most recent destination specific risks and chemoprophylaxis and treatment guidelines.

possibility of becoming infected because no current drug or drug regimen provides 100% protection against malaria.
2. Presumptive self-treatment should be used only as an interim measure, and travelers should be advised to seek medical evaluation as soon as possible so that thick and thin blood smears can be obtained for precise diagnosis.
3. A reliable supply of self-treatment medication is a complete course of an approved malaria treatment regimen obtained preferably from a reliable pharmacy before travel. A reliable supply:
   a. is not counterfeit or substandard
   b. will not interact adversely with the patient's other medications, including chemoprophylaxis
   c. will not deplete local resources in the destination country
4. Presumptive self-treatment should be taken immediately if the traveler develops an influenza-like illness with fevers and chills,

HOW LONG TO CONTINUE AFTER RETURN	ADVERSE EFFECTS	COMMENTS
14 days	Nausea, abdominal pain, and hemolytic anemia (especially in patients with G6PD deficiency)	Indicated for people who have had prolonged exposure to *P. vivax*, *Plasmodium ovale*, or both. Take with food. All persons taking primaquine should have a documented normal G6PD level before beginning the medication. Contraindicated in persons with G6PD deficiency, during pregnancy, and during breastfeeding, unless the infant being breastfed has a documented normal G6PD level.

and professional medical care is not available within 24 hours.

Note the drugs used for the reliable supply treatment of presumed malaria infection (Table 47.6). Have the patient take a treatment dose of one of the antimalarial agents when signs and symptoms suggest an acute attack and prompt medical attention is not available.

General Approach

1. In addition to supportive care, treatment consists of rapid and appropriate antimalarial therapy for uncomplicated (Table 47.7) and severe malaria (Table 47.8).
2. Therapeutic agents should be chosen based on prophylaxis used (if any), age of the patient, pregnancy and lactation status, species of malaria and their reported resistance patterns endemic to the region of likely inoculation, drug availability, cost, and side effects.
3. Care should be taken to assess for signs or symptoms of severe malaria (see Table 47.3).

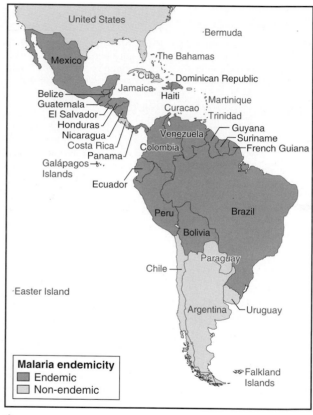

A

FIGURE 47.2 A, Malaria-endemic countries in the Western Hemisphere. **B,** Malaria-endemic countries in the Eastern Hemisphere. (From Centers for Disease Control and Prevention: *CDC health information for international travel 2018: The yellow book,* New York, 2018, Oxford University Press.)

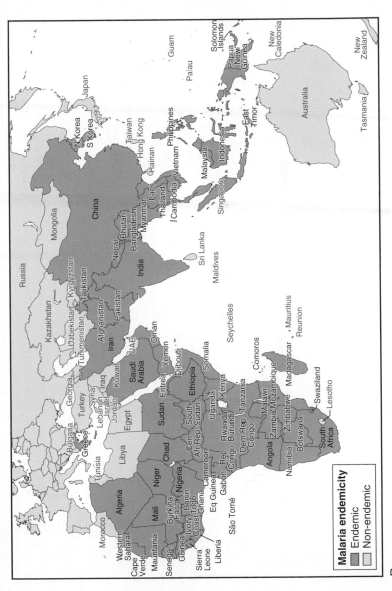

Malaria endemicity
- Endemic
- Non-endemic

B

Table 47.6	Reliable Supply Regimens for the Treatment of Malaria*†		
DRUG	ADULT DOSE	PEDIATRIC DOSE	COMMENTS
Atovaquone-Proguanil Adult tablet contains 250 mg atovaquone and 100 mg proguanil. Pediatric tablet contains 62.5 mg atovaquone and 25 mg proguanil.	4 adult tablets, orally as a single daily dose for 3 consecutive days	Daily dose to be taken for 3 consecutive days: 5–8 kg (11.02–17.6 lb): 2 pediatric tablets 9–10 kg (19.8–22.04 lb): 3 pediatric tablets 11–20 kg (24.25–44.09 lb): 1 adult tablet 21–30 kg (46.3–66.14 lb): 2 adult tablets 31–40 kg (68.34–88.14 lb): 3 adult tablets >41 kg (90.39 lb): 4 adult tablets	Contraindicated in people with severe renal impairment (creatinine clearance <30 mL/min) Not recommended for people taking atovaquone-proguanil prophylaxis Not recommended for children weighing <5 kg (11.02 lb), pregnant women, and women breastfeeding infants weighing <5 kg (11.02 lb)
Artemether-Lumefantrine One tablet contains 20 mg artemether and 120 mg lumefantrine.	A 3-day treatment schedule with a total of 6 oral doses is recommended for both adult and pediatric patients based on weight. Patient should receive initial dose, followed by second dose 8 hours later, then 1 dose twice per day for the following 2 days. 5 to <15 kg (11.02 to <33.07 lb): 1 tablet per dose 15 to <25 kg (33.07 to <55.12 lb): 2 tablets per dose 25 to <35 kg (55.12 to <77.16 lb): 3 tablets per dose ≥ 35 kg (≥77.16 lb): 4 tablets per dose		Not for people taking mefloquine prophylaxis Not recommended for children weighing <5 kg (<11.02 lb), pregnant women, and women breastfeeding infants weighing <5 kg (<11.02 lb)

*If used for presumptive self-treatment, medical care should be sought as soon as possible.
†Refer to the U.S. Centers for Disease Control and Prevention for most recent destination-specific risks and malaria chemoprophylaxis and treatment guidelines.

From Centers for Disease Control and Prevention: CDC Health Information for International Travel, 2018, Atlanta, Georgia, 2018, U.S. Department of Health and Human Services, Public Health Service, Centers for Disease Control and Prevention, National Center for Infectious Diseases, Division of Global Migration and Quarantine 2018.
https://wwwnc.cdc.gov/travel/yellowbook/2018/infectious-diseases-related-to-travel/malaria#5216

4. Patient can be given acetaminophen (paracetamol) 1 g PO q6h to q8h or 15 mg/kg/dose q6h to q8h in children.
5. Nonsteroidal antiinflammatory drugs should be avoided because of the possible renal complications of malaria.
6. Oral hydration should be continued because patients often have insensible losses through fever, nausea, and vomiting.

Treatment of Uncomplicated Malaria
Plasmodium falciparum, or a Species Not Identified, Acquired in Areas With Chloroquine-Sensitive Malaria

1. Chloroquine and hydroxychloroquine are the drugs of choice for infections with chloroquine-susceptible malarial parasites (see Table 47.7).
2. In addition, any regimen recommended for treatment of chloroquine-resistant malaria can be used for treatment of chloroquine-sensitive malaria.

Plasmodium falciparum, or Species Not Identified, Acquired in Areas With Chloroquine-Resistant Malaria

1. Four treatment regimens are options for treatment of chloroquine-resistant *P. falciparum* infection (see Table 47.7).
   a. Two fixed-dose combination products (atovaquone-proguanil and artemether-lumefantrine)
   b. Quinine or quinidine, in conjunction with doxycycline, tetracycline, or clindamycin
   c. Mefloquine should only be used when there is no other alternative, due to rare but potentially serious severe neuropsychiatric reactions at treatment doses.
2. Treatment options for children are the same as for adults. Weight-based dosing should not exceed recommended adult doses.
3. If no other treatment options are available, doxycycline or tetracycline can be used in children 8 years of age or less. Quinine can be given for a full 7 days, regardless of where the infection was acquired.
4. Do not treat malaria with the same medication used for malaria prophylaxis.
5. Mefloquine should not be used to treat malaria infection acquired in areas of reported mefloquine resistance.
6. Outside the United States, artemisinin-based combination therapy (artemether plus lumefantrine, artesunate plus amodiaquine, artesunate plus mefloquine, or artesunate plus sulfadoxine-pyrimethamine) is recommended for treatment of uncomplicated malaria.
7. For persons living in a low malaria-transmission area, the WHO recommends that a single gametocytocidal dose of primaquine (0.25 mg base per kg) be added to all artemisinin combination treatments for falciparum malaria (except in infants and pregnant

Text continued on p. 596

Table 47.7   Medications Used for the Treatment of Uncomplicated Malaria
(Based on Drug Available in the United States)*

DRUG	TRADE NAMES	ADULT DOSE
Plasmodium falciparum, or species not identified, acquired in areas with chloroquine-sensitive malaria **Two recommended options (A or B). If species subsequently identified as Plasmodium vivax or Plasmodium ovale, treatment with primaquine also needed.**		
A. Chloroquine phosphate[‡]	Aralen, generic	600-mg base (=1000-mg salt) orally immediately, followed by 300-mg base (=500-mg salt) orally at 6, 24, and 48 hr Total dose: 1500-mg base (=2500-mg salt)
B. Hydroxychloroquine sulfate	Plaquenil, generic	620–mg base (=800-mg salt) orally immediately, followed by 310-mg base (=400-mg salt) orally at 6, 24, and 48 hr Total dose: 1550-mg base (=2000-mg salt)
P. falciparum, or species not identified, acquired in areas with chloroquine-resistant malaria or unknown resistance **Four recommended options (A through D). If species subsequently identified as P. vivax or P. ovale, treatment with primaquine also needed.**		
A. Atovaquone-proguanil	Malarone	4 adult tablets[§] (1 g atovaquone/400 mg proguanil) orally qd × 3 days

PEDIATRIC DOSE[†]	ADVERSE EFFECTS	COMMENTS
10-mg base/kg (max. 600-mg base) orally immediately, followed by 5-mg base/kg orally at 6, 24, and 48 hr Total dose: 25-mg base/kg	Pruritus, nausea, headache, skin eruptions, dizziness, blurred vision, and insomnia.	Has been used extensively and safely during pregnancy. May exacerbate psoriasis.
10-mg base/kg orally immediately, followed by 5-mg base/kg orally at 6, 24, and 48 hr Total dose: 25-mg base/kg	Pruritus, nausea, headache, skin eruptions, dizziness, blurred vision, and insomnia.	Has been used extensively and safely during pregnancy. May exacerbate psoriasis.
<5 kg (<11.02 lb): not indicated 5–8 kg (11.02–17.64 lb): 2 pediatric tablets[‡] orally/day × 3 days 9–10 kg (19.8–22.05 lb): 3 pediatric tablets[‡] orally/day × 3 days 11–20 kg (24.25–44.1 lb): 1 adult tablet orally/day × 3 days 21–30 kg (46.3–66.14 lb): 2 adult tablets orally/day × 3 days 31–40 kg (68.34–88.18 lb): 3 adult tablets[¶] orally/day × 3 days >40 kg (88.18 lb): 4 adult tablets[¶] orally q day × 3 days	Headache, nausea, vomiting, abdominal pain, diarrhea, increased transaminase levels, and seizures.	Take with food or milk. Contraindicated for persons with severe renal impairment (i.e., creatine clearance of <30 mL/min). Not recommended for children <5 kg (11.02 lb), pregnant women, women breastfeeding infants <5 kg (11.02 lb), and persons who received atovaquone-proguanil prophylaxis.

Continued

Table 47.7   Medications Used for the Treatment of Uncomplicated Malaria (Based on Drug Available in the United States)—cont'd

	DRUG	TRADE NAMES	ADULT DOSE
B.	Artemether-lumefantrine	Coartem, Riamet	1 tablet (20 mg artemether and 120 mg lumefantrine); six oral doses over 3 days (0, 8, 24, 36, 48, and 60 hr) 4 tablets/dose if ≥35 kg; if <35 kg, refer to pediatric dosing
C.	Quinine sulfate	—	542-mg base (=650-mg salt) orally TID × 3 or 7 days
PLUS	Doxycycline	Vibramycin, Vibra-Tablets, Doryx, Periostat, and others; generic	100 mg orally BID × 7 days

PEDIATRIC DOSE[†]	ADVERSE EFFECTS	COMMENTS
1 tablet (20 mg artemether and 120 mg lumefantrine). Six oral doses over 3 days (0, 8, 24, 36, 48, and 60 hr) 5 to <15 kg (11.02 to <33.07 lb): 1 tablet/dose 15 to <25 kg (33.07 to <55.12 lb): 2 tablets/dose 25 to <35 kg (55.12 to <77.16 lb): 3 tablets/dose ≥35 kg (≥77.16 lb): 4 tablets/dose	Headache, anorexia, dizziness, asthenia, arthralgias, and myalgia.	Take with food. Contraindicated during first trimester of pregnancy. Safety during second and third trimesters of pregnancy is unknown. Contraindicated for persons taking strong CYP3A4 inducers. Warnings and precautions on the package insert include prolongation of the QT interval, concomitant use of QT-prolonging drugs and other antimalarials, drug interactions with CYP3A4, and drug interactions with CYP2D6. Should not be used in patients with cardiac arrhythmias, bradycardia, severe cardiac disease, or a prolonged QT interval. Has not been studied for efficacy and safety in patients with severe hepatic and/or renal impairment.
8.3-mg base/kg (=10-mg salt/kg) orally TID × 3 or 7 days	Cinchonism, hypoglycemia, sinus arrhythmias, atrioventricular block, prolonged QT interval, ventricular tachycardia, and ventricular fibrillation.	In Southeast Asia, continue treatment for 7 days because of increased relative resistance to quinine. Continue treatment for 3 days for infections acquired in Africa or South America. Contraindicated in patients with a history of blackwater fever, thrombocytopenic purpura, cardiac conduction defects and arrhythmias, myasthenia gravis or optic neuritis.
>8 years: 2.2 mg/kg orally q 12 hr × 7 days	Gastrointestinal upset, vaginal candidiasis, photosensitivity, allergic reactions, blood dyscrasias, azotemia in renal diseases, and hepatitis.	Take with food. Contraindicated in children <8 years and pregnant women.

Continued

Table 47.7 Medications Used for the Treatment of Uncomplicated Malaria (Based on Drug Available in the United States)—cont'd

	DRUG	TRADE NAMES	ADULT DOSE
OR PLUS	Tetracycline	Achromycin, Sumycin, Panmycin, and others; generic	250 mg orally QID × 7 days
OR PLUS	Clindamycin	Cleocin and others; generic	20 mg base/kg/day orally divided TID × 7 days
D.	Mefloquine	Lariam, Mephaquin, generic	684-mg base (=750-mg salt) orally as initial dose, followed by 456-mg base (=500-mg salt) orally 6–12 hr after initial dose. Total dose: =1250-mg salt.

PEDIATRIC DOSE†	ADVERSE EFFECTS	COMMENTS
>8 years: 25 mg/kg/day orally divided QID × 7 days	Gastrointestinal upset, vaginal candidiasis, photosensitivity, allergic reactions, blood dyscrasias, azotemia in renal diseases, and hepatitis.	Take with food. Contraindicated in children <8 years and pregnant women.
20 mg base/kg/ day orally divided TID × 7 days	Diarrhea, nausea, vomiting, abdominal pain, rash, pruritus, jaundice, and urticaria.	Take with food. Contraindicated in individuals with a history of antibiotic-associated colitis or ulcerative colitis. Use with caution in individuals with hepatic or renal impairment.
13.7-mg base/kg (=15-mg salt/kg) orally as initial dose, followed by 9.1-mg base/kg (=10-mg salt/kg) 6–12 hr after initial dose. Total dose: =25-mg salt/kg.	Gastrointestinal disturbances, headaches, insomnia, vivid dreams, visual disturbances, depression, anxiety disorders, and dizziness.	Contraindicated in persons with active depression or a recent history of depression, generalized anxiety disorder, psychosis, schizophrenia, other major psychiatric disorders, or seizures. Rare serious adverse reactions reported with treatment doses include psychoses and seizures. These reactions are seen more frequently at the higher doses used for treatment. Contraindicated in people allergic to mefloquine or related compounds (quinine, quinidine). Not recommended for persons with cardiac conduction abnormalities. Use with caution in travelers with psychiatric disturbances or a previous history of depression. In the United States, 250-mg tablet of mefloquine contains 228-mg mefloquine base. Outside the United States, 275-mg mefloquine tablet contains 250-mg mefloquine base. For children weighing <5 kg (11.02 lb), off-label use is recommended by the Centers for Disease Control and Prevention.

Continued

Table 47.7 Medications Used for the Treatment of Uncomplicated Malaria (Based on Drug Available in the United States)—cont'd

	DRUG	TRADE NAMES	ADULT DOSE
Plasmodium malariae and Plasmodium knowlesi acquired in all regions Two recommended options (A or B).			
A.	Chloroquine phosphate	As above	As above
B.	Hydroxychloroquine sulfate	As above	As above
P. vivax and P. ovale acquired in areas with chloroquine-sensitive P. vivax malaria Two recommended options (A or B).			
A.	Chloroquine phosphate	As above	As above
PLUS	Primaquine phosphate	—	30-mg base (52.6-mg salt) orally, daily for 14 days after departure from the malarious area
OR			
B.	Hydroxychloroquine sulfate	As above	As above
PLUS	Primaquine phosphate	As above	As above

PEDIATRIC DOSE†	ADVERSE EFFECTS	COMMENTS
As above	As above	As above
As above	As above	As above
As above	As above	As above
0.5-mg/kg base (0.8-mg/kg salt) up to adult dose, orally, daily for 14 days after departure from the malarious area	Nausea, abdominal pain, and hemolytic anemia, especially in patients with G6PD deficiency.	Use with any of the above drug regimens to prevent relapse of *P. vivax*. Take with food. All persons taking primaquine should have a documented normal G6PD level before beginning the medication. Contraindicated in persons with G6PD deficiency and during pregnancy and breastfeeding unless the infant being breastfed has a documented normal G6PD level.
As above	As above	As above
As above	As above	As above

Continued

	DRUG	TRADE NAMES	ADULT DOSE
Table 47.7 Medications Used for the Treatment of Uncomplicated Malaria (Based on Drug Available in the United States)—cont'd			

P. vivax and _P. ovale_ acquired in areas with chloroquine-resistant _P. vivax_ malaria
Three recommended options (A–C).

	DRUG	TRADE NAMES	ADULT DOSE
A.	Quinine sulfate	As above	As above
PLUS	Doxycycline or tetracycline	As above	As above
PLUS	Primaquine phosphate	As above	As above
_OR_			
B.	Atovaquone-proguanil	As above	As above
PLUS	Primaquine phosphate	As above	As above
_OR_			
C.	Mefloquine	As above	As above
PLUS	Primaquine phosphate	As above	As above

Pregnant women
P. falciparum, or species not identified, acquired in areas with chloroquine-sensitive malaria
Two recommended options (A or B).
If species subsequently identified as _P. vivax_ or _P. ovale,_ patient should be maintained on chloroquine prophylaxis for the duration of the pregnancy. After delivery, pregnant patients who do not have G6PD deficiency should receive terminal prophylaxis with primaquine.

	DRUG	TRADE NAMES	ADULT DOSE
A.	Chloroquine phosphate[‡]	As above	As above
B.	Hydroxychloroquine sulfate	As above	As above

PEDIATRIC DOSE[†]	ADVERSE EFFECTS	COMMENTS
As above	As above	As above
As above	As above	As above
As above	As above	As above
As above	As above	As above
As above	As above	As above
As above	As above	As above
As above	As above	As above
Not applicable	As above	As above
Not applicable	As above	As above

Continued

Table 47.7 Medications Used for the Treatment of Uncomplicated Malaria (Based on Drug Available in the United States)—cont'd		
DRUG	**TRADE NAMES**	**ADULT DOSE**
Pregnant women *P. falciparum,* **or species not identified, acquired in areas with chloroquine-resistant malaria** *Two recommended options (A or B).* **If species subsequently identified as** *P. vivax* **or** *P. ovale,* **patient should be maintained on chloroquine prophylaxis for the duration of the pregnancy. After delivery, pregnant patients who do not have G6PD deficiency should receive terminal prophylaxis with primaquine.**		
A.	Quinine sulfate plus clindamycin	As above	As above
B.	Mefloquine	As above	As above

*Caused by *Plasmodium falciparum, P. ovale, P. vivax, P. malariae,* and *P. knowlesi.*
†Should never exceed the adult dose.
‡Pediatric tablets contain 62.5 mg atovaquone and 25 mg proguanil hydrochloride.
§Adult tablets contain 250 mg atovaquone and 100 mg proguanil hydrochloride.
¶Refer to the U.S. Centers for Disease Control and Prevention for most recent destination-specific risks and malaria chemoprophylaxis and treatment guidelines.
Health care professionals requiring assistance with diagnosis and treatment of suspected or confirmed cases of malaria should refer to the CDC website https://www.cdc.gov/malaria/diagnosis_treatment/treatment.html or call the CDC Malaria Hotline (770-488-7788, or toll-free 855-856-4713, from 9:00 AM to 5:00 PM Eastern Standard Time, Monday through Friday) or the Emergency Operations Center during evenings, weekends, and holidays (770-488-7100); ask to page the person on-call for the Malaria Branch).
G6PD, Glucose-6-phosphate dehydrogenase.
Modified from 1. Centers for Disease Control and Prevention: CDC Health Information for International Travel, 2014, Atlanta, Georgia, 2014, U.S. Department of Health and Human Services, Public Health Service, Centers for Disease Control and Prevention, National Center for infectious Diseases, Division of Global Migration and Quarantine; and 2. Centers for Disease Control and Prevention: Malaria Treatment (United States). 11-9-2012. 12-24-0014.

women) to sterilize infection and reduce transmission of artemisinin-exposed, and potentially resistant, *P. falciparum* strains.

Plasmodium malariae and Plasmodium knowlesi
Chloroquine and hydroxychloroquine can be used for both *P. malariae* and *P. knowlesi* infections (see Table 47.7). In addition, any regimen recommended for treatment of chloroquine-resistant malaria can be used for treatment of *P. malariae* and *P. knowlesi.*

Plasmodium vivax and Plasmodium ovale
1. Chloroquine and hydroxychloroquine can be used for most *P. vivax* and *P. ovale* infections (see Table 47.7).

PEDIATRIC DOSE[†]	ADVERSE EFFECTS	COMMENTS
Not applicable	As above	As above
Not applicable	As above	As above

2. Regimens for treatment of *P. falciparum* acquired from areas of chloroquine resistance can also be used.
3. Treatment of *P. vivax* and *P. ovale* should be followed by a 14-day course of primaquine to eradicate hypnozoites that remain dormant in the liver.
4. Screen patients for G6PD deficiency prior to initiating primaquine therapy to avoid the complication of hemolytic anemia and methemoglobinemia.
5. Treatment options for children are the same as for adults. Weight-based dosing should not exceed recommended adult doses.

Text continued on p. 604

Table 47.8   Medications Used for the Treatment of Severe Malaria (Based on Drugs Available in the United States)*

DRUG	TRADE NAMES	ADULT DOSE

Severe malaria treatment: All *Plasmodium* species, all regions
Two recommended options (A or B). Initiate therapy immediately. If species subsequently identified as *Plasmodium vivax* or *Plasmodium ovale* treatment with primaquine also needed (see uncomplicated malaria treatment).

A. Quinidine gluconate plus one of the following: doxycycline, tetracycline, or clindamycin

	DRUG	TRADE NAMES	ADULT DOSE
A.	Quinidine gluconate (IV)	—	6.25-mg base/kg (=10-mg salt/kg) loading dose IV (maximum of 600-mg salt) in normal saline slowly over 1–2 hr, followed by continuous infusion of 0.0125-mg base/kg/min (=0.02-mg salt/kg/min) for at least 24 hr. Alternative regimen: 15-mg base/kg (=24-mg salt/kg) loading dose IV infused over 4 hr, followed by 7.5-mg base/kg (=12-mg salt/kg) infused over 4 hr every 8 hr, starting 8 hr after the loading dose (see package insert). Once parasite density <1% and able to take oral medication, complete course with oral quinine (dose as per uncomplicated malaria).

PEDIATRIC DOSE[†]	ADVERSE EFFECTS	COMMENTS
Same as adult dose	Cinchonism, tachycardia, prolonged QRS and QTc intervals, flattened T wave, ventricular arrhythmias, hypotension, and hypoglycemia.	For infections acquired in Southeast Asia, continue treatment for 7 days because of increased relative resistance to quinine. Continue treatment for 3 days for infections acquired in Africa or South America. Continuous electrocardiography, blood pressure, and glucose monitoring are recommended, especially for pregnant women and children. The loading dose should be decreased or omitted for patients who have received quinine or mefloquine. For problems with quinidine availability, call the manufacturer (Eli Lilly, 800-821-0538) or the Malaria Hotline at the Centers for Disease Control and Prevention. If >48 hr of parenteral therapy is required, the quinine or quinidine dose should be decreased by $\frac{1}{3}$ to $\frac{1}{2}$. Contraindicated in people with a history of blackwater fever, thrombocytopenic purpura, cardiac conduction defects and arrhythmias, myasthenia gravis, and optic neuritis.

Continued

Table 47.8 Medications Used for the Treatment of Severe Malaria (Based on Drugs Available in the United States)*—cont'd

	DRUG	TRADE NAMES	ADULT DOSE
PLUS	Doxycycline	Vibramycin, Vibra-Tablets, Doryx, Periostat and others; generic	100 mg BID orally × 7 days. If unable to take oral medication, give 100 mg IV every 12 hr. Switch to oral doxycycline when patient can take oral medication. Total treatment course = 7 days.
OR PLUS	Tetracycline	Achromycin, Sumycin, Panmycin, and others, generic	Dose as per uncomplicated malaria.
OR PLUS	Clindamycin	Cleocin and others, generic	20-mg base/kg/day orally divided TID × 7 days. If unable to take oral medication, give 10-mg base/kg loading dose IV followed by 5-mg base/kg IV every 8 hr. Switch to oral clindamycin as soon as patient can take oral medication. Total treatment course = 7 days.

PEDIATRIC DOSE†	ADVERSE EFFECTS	COMMENTS
>8 years: 2.2 mg/kg orally q 12 hr × 7 days. If unable to take oral medication, give IV. For children <45 kg, give 2.2 mg/kg IV every 12 hr. For children ≥45 kg, use same dosing as for adults. Switch to oral doxycycline as soon as patient can take oral medication. Total treatment course = 7 days.	Gastrointestinal upset, vaginal candidiasis, photosensitivity, allergic reactions, blood dyscrasias, azotemia in renal diseases, and hepatitis.	Take with food. Contraindicated in children <8 years and pregnant women.
Dose as per uncomplicated malaria.	See uncomplicated malaria treatment.	See uncomplicated malaria treatment.
20-mg base/kg/day orally divided TID × 7 days. If unable to take oral medication, give 10-mg base/kg loading dose IV followed by 5-mg base/kg IV every 8 hr. Switch to oral clindamycin as soon as patient can take oral medication. Total treatment course = 7 days.	Diarrhea, nausea, vomiting, abdominal pain, rash, pruritus, jaundice, and urticaria.	Take with food. Contraindicated in individuals with a history of antibiotic-associated colitis or ulcerative colitis. Use with caution in individuals with hepatic or renal impairment.

Continued

Table 47.8   Medications Used for the Treatment of Severe Malaria (Based on Drugs Available in the United States)*—cont'd

	DRUG	TRADE NAMES	ADULT DOSE
B. Artesunate followed by one of the following: atovaquone-proguanil, doxycycline (clindamycin in pregnant women), or mefloquine			
B.	Artesunate	—	2.4 mg/kg/dose IV × 3 days at 0, 12, 24, 48, and 72 hr
Followed by	Atovaquone–proguanil	Malarone	Dose as per uncomplicated malaria.
OR	Doxycycline	Vibramycin, Vibra-Tablets, Doryx, Periostat and others; generic	Dose as per uncomplicated malaria.
OR	Clindamycin	Cleocin and others, generic	Dose as per uncomplicated malaria.
OR	Mefloquine	Lariam, Mephaquin; generic	Dose as per uncomplicated malaria.

PEDIATRIC DOSE†	ADVERSE EFFECTS	COMMENTS
2.4 mg/kg/dose IV × 3 days at 0, 12, 24, 48, and 72 hr	Gastrointestinal upset, bradycardia, rash, and fever	Available in the United States through an investigational new drug protocol from the Centers for Disease Control and Prevention. For use in patients with severe disease who do not have timely access or who cannot tolerate or fail to respond to IV quinidine. Information regarding use in pregnant women is limited. Use with caution for individuals with renal or hepatic impairment.
Dose as per uncomplicated malaria.	See uncomplicated malaria treatment.	See uncomplicated malaria treatment.
Dose as per uncomplicated malaria.	See uncomplicated malaria treatment.	See uncomplicated malaria treatment.
Dose as per uncomplicated malaria.	See uncomplicated malaria treatment.	See uncomplicated malaria treatment.
Dose as per uncomplicated malaria.	See uncomplicated malaria treatment.	See uncomplicated malaria treatment.

Continued

Table 47.8   Medications Used for the Treatment of Severe Malaria (Based on Drugs Available in the United States)*—cont'd

DRUG	TRADE NAMES	ADULT DOSE
Prevention of relapses: *P. vivax* and *P. ovale* only		
Primaquine phosphate	—	Dose as per uncomplicated malaria.

*Caused by *Plasmodium falciparum*, *P. ovale*, *P. vivax*, and *P. malariae* in the United States.
†Should never exceed the adult dose.
‡Pediatric tablets contain 62.5 mg atovaquone and 25 mg proguanil hydrochloride.
§Adult tablets contain 250 mg atovaquone and 100 mg proguanil hydrochloride.
¶Refer to the U.S. Centers for Disease Control and Prevention for most recent destination-specific risks and malaria chemoprophylaxis and treatment guidelines.
Health care professionals requiring assistance with diagnosis and treatment of suspected or confirmed cases of malaria should refer to the CDC website at http://www.cdc.gov/malaria/diagnosis_treatment/treatment.html or call the CDC Malaria Hotline (770-488-7788, or toll-free 855-856-4713, from 9:00 AM to 5:00 PM Eastern Standard Time, Monday through Friday) or the Emergency Operations Center during evenings, weekends, and holidays (770-488-7100); ask to page the person on-call for the Malaria Branch.
G6PD, Glucose-6-phosphate dehydrogenase; *IV*, intravenous.
Modified from 1. Centers for Disease Control and Prevention: CDC Health Information for International Travel, 2014, Atlanta, Georgia, 2014, U.S. Department of Health and Human Services, Public Health Service, Centers for Disease Control and Prevention, National Center for infectious Diseases, Division of Global Migration and Quarantine; and 2. Centers for Disease Control and Prevention: Malaria Treatment (United States). 11-9-2012. 12-24-0014.

6. Because doxycycline and tetracycline are not indicated for use in children 8 years of age or less, quinine-based regimens that include either of these drugs should be avoided in this age group.
7. Mefloquine is the recommended treatment option for children less than 8 years old with chloroquine-resistant *P. vivax*. Atovaquone-proguanil or artemether-lumefantrine should be used if the benefits outweigh the risks of treatment, and mefloquine is not available.

Pregnant Women

Pregnant women are at high risk for developing severe malaria. Malaria infection during pregnancy is associated with perinatal morbidity (i.e., miscarriage, prematurity, low birth weight, congenital infections), as well as death.

1. For pregnant women with uncomplicated malaria caused by chloroquine-sensitive *P. falciparum*, *P. malariae*, *P. vivax*, and *P. ovale*, use the same treatment regimens as those recommended for nonpregnant adult patients (see Table 47.7).
2. In pregnant patients diagnosed with chloroquine-resistant *P. falciparum* infection, use mefloquine or a combination of quinine and clindamycin for treatment.

PEDIATRIC DOSE†	ADVERSE EFFECTS	COMMENTS
Dose as per uncomplicated malaria.	See uncomplicated malaria treatment.	See uncomplicated malaria treatment.

3. Doxycycline, tetracycline, atovaquone-proguanil, and artemether-lumefantrine should not be used in pregnant patients unless no other treatment options are available and benefits outweigh the risks.
4. Atovaquone-proguanil and artemether-lumefantrine are pregnancy class category C drugs and are generally not indicated for use in pregnant women.
5. In cases of *P. vivax* and *P. ovale*, terminal prophylaxis with primaquine should be given to pregnant patients with normal G6PD levels after delivery. Treat with chloroquine prophylaxis during pregnancy.
6. Primaquine can be given after delivery.

Treatment of Severe Malaria

Parenteral antimalarial therapy is recommended for patients with severe disease, regardless of the infecting malarial species.

1. Parenteral quinidine gluconate (or quinine dihydrochloride) combined with doxycycline, tetracycline, or clindamycin is recommended for treatment in the United States (see Table 47.8).
2. Blood pressure, cardiac rhythms, and blood glucose levels should be monitored closely in an intensive care setting during IV administration of quinidine or quinine.

3. At least 24 hours of continuous infusion or three intermittent doses of parenteral quinidine therapy is recommended.
4. Parenteral therapy should be continued until the parasite density is less than 1%, and the patient can take oral treatment.
5. Complete the treatment course with an oral regimen of quinine, atovaquone-proguanil, or artemether-lumefantrine.
6. Another option for parenteral therapy is artesunate in combination with a second oral drug (atovaquone-proguanil, doxycycline, clindamycin, or mefloquine).
7. In the United States, contact the CDC for artesunate, available under an Investigational New Drug protocol.

Supportive Care for Severe Malaria

1. Correct dehydration, hypoglycemia, and acidosis.
2. Admission to the intensive care unit is often required to manage complications (e.g., seizures, severe anemia, hypoglycemia, acidosis, renal failure, pulmonary edema, hypoxemia, and hypovolemia).
3. Place patients receiving intravenous quinine derivatives on a cardiac monitor in the intensive care unit and perform frequent blood pressure measurements.
4. Quinine or quinidine derivatives are typically given with a continuous infusion of 5% to 10% dextrose. Measure blood glucose levels every 4 to 6 hours.
5. Adjust drug dosages for patients with evidence of renal failure. Patients with renal insufficiency receiving quinine derivatives should be given a standard loading dose, but if more than 48 hours of parenteral treatment is required, the maintenance doses should be decreased by 30% to 50% to prevent drug accumulation.
6. Total plasma concentrations of 8 to 15 mg/mL for quinine and 3 to 8 mg/mL for quinidine are effective for treatment of severe malaria without causing toxicity.
7. Use anticonvulsants (e.g., benzodiazepines) for treatment of seizures.
8. Empirically treat with antibiotics for bacterial meningitis until a lumbar puncture can be performed to exclude this diagnosis.
9. Exchange transfusions have no proven benefit, as no survival advantage has been demonstrated in adequately powered randomized clinical trials.
10. Other adjunctive therapies that have no proven benefit, or are harmful, include dexamethasone for cerebral malaria, heparin for thrombocytopenia, iron chelators to reduce parasite clearance time, pentoxifylline for tumor necrosis factor synthesis inhibition, and dichloroacetate for metabolic acidosis.
11. In children, careful attention should be paid to airway compromise, altered breathing patterns, dehydration, compensated shock, and/or impaired consciousness.
12. All children with severe malaria should be treated with broad-spectrum antibiotics in addition to antimalarial therapy.

Management of severe malaria should preferably be carried out in consultation with a tropical medicine or infectious diseases specialist, or with the assistance of the CDC 770-488-7788 or toll free 855-856-4713. The WHO has created a practical handbook for health professionals who manage patients with severe malaria: apps.who.int/iris/bitstream/10665/79317/1/9789241548526_eng.pdf?ua–1.

48 Travel-Acquired Illnesses

SOURCES OF INFORMATION

The Centers for Disease Control and Prevention (CDC) publishes several authoritative sources of information on travel medicine. *Health Information for International Travel* (the "yellow book") is updated annually. Two other periodicals, the weekly *Morbidity and Mortality Weekly Report (MMWR)* and *Summary of Health Information for International Travel* (the "blue sheet," published biweekly), provide updated information on the status of immunization recommendations, worldwide disease outbreaks, and changes in health conditions. A reliable way to obtain current travel health information, including vaccine requirements, malaria chemoprophylaxis, and disease outbreaks for various regions of the world, is to consult the CDC Travelers' Health website at http://wwwnc.cdc.gov/travel/. See Chapter 49 for more information on immunizations for travel. For nonmedical information of interest to the traveler, the U.S. State Department can be accessed at http://travel.state.gov/. Additional resources for travel medicine information are listed at the end of the chapter.

Aside from traveler's diarrhea (see Chapter 44), traffic-related accidents, and purified protein derivative conversion, the major travel-acquired illnesses in descending order from most to least common are as follows:

- Malaria (see Chapter 47)
- Influenza A or B (see Chapter 49)
- Dengue fever
- Yellow fever
- Animal bite with rabies risk (see Chapter 43)
- Hepatitis
- Typhoid and paratyphoid fevers
- Human immunodeficiency virus infection (not discussed in this chapter)
- Cholera
- *Legionella* infection (not discussed in this chapter)
- Japanese B encephalitis
- Meningococcal disease
- Zika virus infection
- Poliomyelitis (see Chapter 49)

These disorders are often preventable if the traveler takes specific precautions or prophylactic agents. Influenza, acute HIV infection, *Legionella*, and poliomyelitis are not discussed in this chapter because they are generally preventable with standard immunizations, or their medical management is like that in developed countries. Travelers at risk for HIV exposure should consider bringing 72 hours of postexposure prophylaxis medication, because many developing countries do not have access to HIV drugs.

MALARIA

See Chapter 47.

DENGUE FEVER

(See Table 48.1 for comparison of clinical illness in malaria and Dengue fever.)

- Dengue viruses belong to the family Flaviviridae, genus *Flavivirus,* and have four distinct but closely related serotypes (DEN-1, DEN-2, DEN-3, and DEN-4), all of which cause infection.
- The incidence of dengue has increased by 30-fold over the past 5 decades, with the World Health Organization (WHO) identifying it as the most important mosquito-borne viral disease in the world.
- Several species of *Aedes* can transmit dengue, but the most important is *Aedes aegypti,* which is found in tropical and subtropical regions under 1000 meters and between 35 degrees north and 35 degrees south latitude globally.
- All four serotypes can cause DHF, and the four serotypes do not provide cross-protective immunity, so it is possible for one individual to sustain four separate dengue infections over a lifetime.

Table 48.1 Clinical Illness in Malaria and Dengue Fever		
SIGNS AND SYMPTOMS	**MALARIA**	**DENGUE FEVER**
Fever	+++	+++
Chills	+++	++
Headache	+++	+++
Malaise		++
Anorexia		++
Nausea, vomiting	++	++
Abdominal pain	++	
Myalgia	++	++
Arthralgia		++
Backache	+	
Dark urine	+	

+++, >90% of patients; ++, >50% of patients; +, <10% of patients.

- Although previous infection provides homologous immunity to one serotype, individuals who experience secondary infection by another serotype are at higher risk for more severe forms of disease.
- Immunofluorescence assay of serum or CSF with serotype specific monoclonal antibodies (IgM enzyme-linked immunosorbent assay [ELISA]) is the test of choice to confirm the diagnosis.

Signs and Symptoms
- From bite to clinical infection, 4- to 7-day incubation period
- High fever (≥38.5°C [101.3°F]), myalgias, headache, arthralgias, and rash
- Positive tourniquet test for capillary fragility: the appearance of 20 or more petechiae over a square-inch patch on the forearm after deflation of the blood pressure cuff (held for 5 minutes between systolic and diastolic pressures)
- Irritability, depression, encephalitis, seizures
- Differentiation between dengue fever and dengue hemorrhagic fever (DHF) is development of plasma leakage in DHF. Following 2 to 7 days of higher fever come bleeding (ranging from petechiae, ecchymoses, epistaxis, and mucosal bleeding to gastrointestinal bleeding and hematuria), thrombocytopenia (<100,000/mm³), hemoconcentration, and hepatomegaly.
- Other symptoms include abdominal pain, nausea and vomiting, and restlessness or lethargy.
- WHO defines severe dengue as having one of three criteria: (1) severe plasma leakage leading to shock or fluid accumulation with respiratory distress, (2) severe bleeding, or (3) severe organ involvement.
- WHO defines high-risk "warning signs" to designate increased risk for severe disease:
  - Abdominal pain or tenderness
  - Persistent vomiting
  - Clinical fluid accumulation
  - Mucosal bleed
  - Lethargy, restlessness
  - Liver enlargement >2 cm
  - Increase in HCT concurrent with rapid decrease in platelet count

Treatment
1. There are currently no effective antiviral agents, but substantial research is ongoing.
2. Current treatment recommendations developed by the WHO focus on supportive care and are divided across three groups (A, B, and C) stratified by risk for deterioration based on "warning signs."
3. Patients in group A (without warning signs) are likely to have mild disease and can be treated at home with supportive care.

   a. Electrolyte oral rehydration solution
   b. Acetaminophen for fevers at 6-hour intervals
   c. Close observation that includes daily ambulatory clinic visits
4. Group B includes patients with warning signs or coexisting factors (e.g., pregnant women, infants, or elderly persons; persons who are obese or have diabetes, renal failure, or chronic hemolytic diseases) that place them at higher risk, as well as social circumstances that would make outpatient management difficult.
   a. Admit and administer intravenous (IV) hydration with isotonic fluids.
   b. Recommended fluids include 0.9% saline, Ringer's lactate, and Hartmann's solution beginning at 5 to 7 mL/kg/hr for 1 to 2 hours, followed by 3 to 5 mL/kg/hr for 2 to 4 hours, and finally ongoing at 2 to 3 mL/kg/hr based on clinical response.
   c. A urine output of 0.5 mL/kg/hr should be maintained through the critical phase, through IV fluids switched to oral rehydration once that is possible.
   d. Any signs of decompensation, including an early rise in hematocrit and accompanying thrombocytopenia, indicate the need for more aggressive therapy.
5. Patients in group C have severe dengue or have failed to improve despite the treatments.
   a. For compensated shock, aggressive fluid resuscitation is indicated at 5 to 10 mL/kg/hr repeated in doses of 10 to 20 mL/kg/hr as needed.
   b. Frequent hematocrit checks are needed, and if decreasing, blood transfusion should be considered.
   c. Hypotensive patients require isotonic fluid boluses at 20 mL/kg over 15 minutes as needed.
   d. Transitioning to colloid fluids is recommended for a patient in shock with a rising hematocrit, because this suggests rapid plasma leakage.

YELLOW FEVER
Yellow fever is one of the viral hemorrhagic fevers. It is caused by a single-stranded RNA flavivirus that is transmitted by mosquitoes. The liver is the principal target organ. All recent cases of American yellow fever were acquired in the jungle environment; however, urban transmission continues to occur in Africa.

Signs and Symptoms
- May appear as an undifferentiated viral syndrome
- Specific diagnosis in the wilderness is extremely difficult; clinical suspicion is based on immune status, geographic distribution of the disease, travel history, and characteristic triphasic fever, as follows:
  - *Infection phase:* After 3 to 6 days of incubation period, onset of headache, photophobia, fever, malaise, back pain, epigastric pain, anorexia, and vomiting. May also have "Faget sign"

(bradycardia occurring at the height of the fever), conjunctival injection, and a coated tongue with pink edges.

- *Remission phase:* The 3 to 4 days of infection phase is followed by up to 48 hours of brief remission.
- *Intoxication phase (up to 15% of individuals infected with yellow fever virus):* Onset of jaundice, fever, encephalopathy, and in severe cases, hypotension, shock, oliguria, coma, and multiorgan failure. Hemorrhage usually manifested as hematemesis, but bleeding from multiple sites possible.
- Signs of a poor prognosis include early onset of the intoxication phase, hypotension, severe hemorrhage with disseminated intravascular coagulation, renal failure, shock, and coma.

Treatment

1. Perform a careful physical examination. Be aware that the laboratory evaluation includes thick and thin blood smears to rule out malaria and blood cultures for bacterial pathogens; both necessitate evacuation to a qualified medical facility. If the patient's condition progresses to the intoxication phase, arrange for immediate evacuation to an intensive care unit (ICU).
2. Note that no effective antiviral treatment is available for yellow fever.
3. Supportive care in the field includes the following:
   a. Control fever with acetaminophen (do not use salicylates).
   b. Give intravenous (IV) fluids and oral rehydration fluids.
   c. Transfer the patient to a hospital as quickly as possible.

Prevention

1. Give yellow fever vaccine (>95% of those vaccinated achieve significant antibody levels). Be aware that booster doses of vaccine are recommended every 10 years.
2. Current recommendations for yellow fever vaccine can be obtained online at http://wwwnc.cdc.gov/travel/ (see Chapter 49).
3. Avoid the causative organism through mosquito protection measures in endemic areas, including repellent and proper netting.

RABIES EXPOSURE

Rabies exists almost everywhere in the world except for Antarctica and a few island nations. Most cases of human disease in the developing world result from multiple, deep bites to the face, scalp, or upper extremities from an unimmunized canine. In more developed countries, however, most rabies transmission occurs from wild animal carriers (see Chapter 42). Travelers who plan on spending more than 1 month in regions at high risk for rabies should consider preexposure rabies immunization. CDC recommendations for rabies prophylaxis can be found at https://www.cdc.gov/rabies/index.html. Rabies is almost universally fatal within a few weeks of symptom onset. If a potential rabies exposure occurs, immunized patients will require only two subsequent rabies immunization boosters on days 0 and 3 post exposure with close follow-up. Patients without preexposure immunizations should receive rabies immune globulin and rabies immunization, as outlined in Chapter 43.

HEPATITIS VIRUSES

The causes of hepatitis may be divided into two groups. First, the *lettered* viruses now include hepatitis A to G. These are associated with defined clinical syndromes and elevated liver function test results. Second, other organisms that cause hepatitis as part of a more systemic infection include Epstein-Barr virus, cytomegalovirus, toxoplasmosis, and leptospirosis.

Hepatitis A

Hepatitis A virus (HAV) is transmitted mainly through the fecal-oral route, either by person-to-person contact or by ingestion of contaminated food or water. Occasional cases are associated with exposure to nonhuman primates. HAV is endemic worldwide, but developing regions have a significantly higher prevalence. In most instances, resolution of the acute disease is permanent, but rare cases of relapse have been noted. Death from HAV is rare. After natural infection, HAV antibodies confer immunity. HAV patients are infectious for approximately 2 weeks before the onset of symptoms. Viral shedding declines with the onset of jaundice. The patient is typically not infectious 1 to 2 weeks after the onset of clinical disease.

Signs and Symptoms

- Incubation period ranging from 2 to 7 weeks
- Infection is often asymptomatic or mild, especially in children.
- Classic syndrome: early onset of anorexia, followed by nausea, vomiting, fever, and abdominal pain
- Symptoms possibly accompanied by hepatosplenomegaly
- Jaundice after gastrointestinal syndrome by several days to a few weeks; resolution of jaundice lasting another 3 to 4 weeks
- Although rare, HAV sometimes follows a fulminant course (0.5% to 1% of patients), resulting in hepatic necrosis, hepatic encephalopathy, and death. The incidence of fulminant hepatitis increases with age.
- Clinical presentation is often milder than with other types of viral hepatitis, but not distinctive enough to allow clinical differentiation.
- Several laboratory tests are available to confirm the diagnosis, but diagnosis in the field is clinical.

Treatment

1. No specific therapy exists for HAV infection.
2. Instruct affected persons to adhere to enteric precautions to avoid transmission to others (compulsive hand washing).

3. Although infectivity drops sharply soon after the onset of jaundice, to be safe, continue enteric and blood-drawing precautions for 2 weeks.

Prevention
1. See discussion of HAV vaccine in Chapter 49.
2. Previously nonimmunized persons exposed to HAV should receive the vaccine within 2 weeks of exposure.
3. See discussion of water safety and dietary precautions in Chapter 45.

Hepatitis B
With the widespread use of serologic markers for hepatitis B disease, it became apparent that spread occurs through exchange of blood, semen, or, rarely, saliva of infected people. Although spread is possible from persons with acute disease, the primary sources of viral particles are chronic carriers. The carrier state follows acute infection in up to 90% of infected infants and 10% of adults. In many areas of the developing world, most infections occur in infancy or childhood, and chronic carriers may constitute as much as 10% to 20% of the total population; thus travelers are more likely to be exposed to carriers than is the nontraveling population. The risk is higher in persons regularly exposed to body fluids, including medical personnel and persons with many sexual partners.

Signs and Symptoms
- Range of incubation period is 7 to 22 weeks
- Manifestations are like those of HAV: fever, anorexia, nausea, vomiting, abdominal pain.
- Additional prodrome of rash, arthralgias, or arthritis and fever occurs in up to 20% of hepatitis B patients (rare in HAV).
- Jaundice developing a short time after gastrointestinal symptoms
- With self-limited disease, recovery is complete by 6 months.
- With fulminant course (1% to 3% of patients), hepatic necrosis, hepatic encephalopathy, and death can occur.
- Other possibilities:
  - Asymptomatic chronic carrier state
  - Chronic active hepatitis
  - Chronic progressive hepatitis
- Definitive diagnosis requires antigen and antibody tests.

Treatment
1. No specific field therapy exists for HBV.
2. Note that prolonged and sometimes persistent viremia makes blood and body fluid precautions necessary until antigen and antibody testing show noninfectivity.
3. The decision to start acute HBV therapy depends on the presence of cirrhosis, LFT levels, and HBV DNA levels. The use of antiviral therapy for HBV is beyond the scope of this book.

Prevention

Universal immunization of US infants beginning at birth and catch-up immunization of children and adolescents are the current recommendations. Vaccination for at-risk adults is also advised. Travelers to highly endemic areas who stay for 6 or more months or have close contact with inhabitants should be vaccinated (see Chapter 49).

Hepatitis C

This syndrome was previously termed *non-A, non-B (NANB) hepatitis* and was thought to be caused by a heterogeneous group of causes. It is now clear that most such cases were due to hepatitis C. Risk factors for hepatitis C include IV drug use and, before routine testing, transfusion of blood products. Nonparenteral routes of infection are less important for hepatitis C than for hepatitis B. Hepatitis C is a global problem. Approximately 80% of exposed individuals have historically developed chronic infection, which may lead to cirrhosis in 20% of subjects and hepatocellular carcinoma in up to 5% of this subset of infected persons. Rates of infection vary from 1% to 5% in most Western countries to 20% in parts of the Middle East, such as Egypt.

Signs and Symptoms

- Acute disease is indistinguishable from hepatitis A or hepatitis B virus infections.
- Most infections are asymptomatic with jaundice occurring in fewer than 20% of infected individuals.
- Transition to chronic hepatitis after an insidious asymptomatic infection is the usual pattern.
- Chronic hepatitis may be asymptomatic or associated with nonspecific symptoms, such as lethargy, nausea, and abdominal discomfort.
- Extrahepatic syndromes associated with hepatitis C infection include porphyria cutanea tarda, membranous glomerulonephritis, and mixed cryoglobulinemia.
- Definitive diagnosis requires antigen and antibody tests.

Treatment

1. Treatment of acute hepatitis C is supportive.
2. Avoid alcohol and drug use.
3. All patients with evidence of chronic hepatitis C virus infection should be considered for antiviral therapy.
4. Regimen selection is based on the HCV genotype, with specific considerations for patients with cirrhosis, HIV coinfection, post–liver transplant infection, and severe renal impairment.
5. Regimens based on oral direct-acting antiviral agents are highly efficacious, with cure rates greater than 90% in treatment-naive patients infected with HCV genotypes 1, 2, 3, and 4. Limited data are available regarding patients infected with the less common HCV genotypes 5 and 6.

6. The Infectious Diseases Society of America and American Association for the Study of Liver Diseases provide frequently updated recommendations on the management of chronic hepatitis C infection at http://www.hcvguidelines.org.

Prevention
1. Prevention of hepatitis C largely depends on risk reduction, especially with respect to IV drug use.
2. Pooled immunoglobulin has been used after exposure, but this should be procured from donors screened for hepatitis C. It is, however, not generally recommended.
3. Unlike hepatitis B, protective antibody responses have not been demonstrated.

Hepatitis D
- Hepatitis D infection is found only in patients concomitantly or previously infected with hepatitis B.
- Transmission follows a pattern like hepatitis B.
- In the United States, affected populations are IV drug abusers and multiply transfused hemophiliacs.
- Serologic evidence of hepatitis D disease has been documented in the Mediterranean basin, West Africa, and parts of South America.
- The diagnosis should be suspected in previously well patients infected with hepatitis B who are now having recurrent symptoms.
- The diagnosis is made based on serologic examination.
- Management is supportive, and only interferon-α has proved antiviral activity against hepatitis D virus. There are no specific vaccines for hepatitis D virus.

Hepatitis E, F, and G
- Hepatitis E is an RNA virus and is the second most common cause of viral hepatitis transmitted via the enteric route.
- The epidemiologic characteristics are like hepatitis A. However, hepatitis E has animals (pigs and deer) as its reservoir.
- This group of infections is especially important in the Indian subcontinent, the Middle East, and Africa.
- The incubation period is 2 to 6 weeks.
- The disease is usually self-limited but may be associated with severe illness in pregnant women.
- Diagnosis in travelers from endemic areas can be made based on IgM antibody to hepatitis E in serum or testing of stool for viral antigen.
- Vaccines are not available. Prophylaxis is appropriate advice for travelers and involves counseling with respect to precautions regarding ingestion of food and water in endemic areas.
- Hepatitis F is a putative hepatitis virus of uncertain significance, first described in France.
- Hepatitis G is a member of the flavivirus family with limited

homology to hepatitis C. Its significance as a cause of hepatitis is unclear.

TYPHOID AND PARATYPHOID FEVER

Typhoid fever occurs worldwide, but its prevalence and attack rates are much higher in developing countries. It is estimated to cause 26 million cases and 200,000 deaths annually. Humans arc the only host for *Salmonella typhi*, the most common cause of the typhoid fever syndrome. Nearly all cases are contracted through ingestion of contaminated food and water. The risk for transmission is relatively high in Mexico, Peru, India, Pakistan, Chile, sub-Saharan Africa, and Southeast Asia.

Salmonella species are gram-negative enteric bacilli. *S. typhi* is the prime cause of typhoid fever, but other species may cause a typhoid fever–like syndrome. The term *enteric fever* is used to describe a severe systemic infection with *Salmonella paratyphi* (paratyphoid fever). The clinical appearance of *S. paratyphi* infection is like that seen with typhoid (see Signs and Symptoms), but typically *S. paratyphi* infection runs a shorter course.

Signs and Symptoms

- Onset of illness is usually 10 to 14 days after exposure to the pathogen.
- Gastroenteritis is possible early during the disease with associated abdominal pain and constipation. Diarrhea is more common in younger children.
- Fever
  - Usually the first sign of disease
  - May be accompanied by bradycardia
  - Increases slowly over several days and remains constant for 2 to 3 weeks, after which defervescence begins
- Headaches, malaise, anorexia
- "Rose spots" (2- to 4-mm maculopapular blanching lesions) classically described on the trunk, although not seen in most patients
- Hepatomegaly, splenomegaly in many patients
- Uncomplicated, untreated typhoid fever usually resolves spontaneously in 3 to 4 weeks.
- Life-threatening complications:
  - Intestinal perforation leading to peritonitis
  - Gastrointestinal hemorrhage
  - Pneumonia
  - Multisystem failure with myocardial involvement
- Definitive diagnosis possible by bacterial culture
- Possible for patients to remain asymptomatic carriers and continue to shed organisms for years

Treatment

1. Give antibiotics:
   a. Ciprofloxacin 500 mg q12h for 2 weeks (or another quinolone)

b. In cases of quinolone resistance (either laboratory or clinical unresponsiveness), ceftriaxone or other third-generation cephalosporins are indicated.
c. Azithromycin is another useful alternative for treatment of uncomplicated enteric fever.
d. In the absence of the previously mentioned antibiotics, use one of the following, but remember that resistance has been noted:
- Ampicillin, 100 mg/kg per day in four divided doses for at least 2 weeks
- Co-trimoxazole: 80 mg trimethoprim plus 400 mg sulfamethoxazole per day in two divided doses for at least 2 weeks
- Chloramphenicol, 50 mg/kg per day in four divided doses for 2 weeks

2. Make certain that the patient has adequate nutrition and food support.
3. High-dose steroids are not recommended for those with mild to moderate disease but may be used cautiously in those with severe disease. The current recommendation in severe disease is dexamethasone 3 mg/kg for the first dose, followed by 1 mg/kg every 6 hours for eight more doses.
4. Be aware that relapse can occur after 2 weeks of therapy and necessitates retreatment with the same regimen.

Prevention
1. Because typhoid vaccine does not ensure protection, educate vaccinated travelers to avoid potentially contaminated food and drink (see Chapter 45).
2. See discussion of typhoid fever vaccine in Chapter 49.

CHOLERA
Cholera is a potentially lethal diarrhea disease in adults and children caused by *Vibrio cholerae* O1. Occasionally causing pandemic outbreaks, cholera is spread by contaminated water and food supplies in areas of poor sanitation. Cholera can be transmitted in crustaceans or survive in a dormant state in brackish water. Death usually occurs following voluminous diarrhea, dehydration, hypovolemia, and shock.

Signs and Symptoms
- Initial abdominal pain, cramping, nausea, and vomiting
- Subsequent "rice water" diarrhea with "fishy" smell
- Severe dehydration, dry mucous membranes, fast pulse rate, hypotension, sunken eyes, decreased skin turgor, decreased urine output
- Decreased level of consciousness, lethargy, stupor
- Muscle and abdominal cramping with electrolyte deficiency

Treatment
1. Aggressive oral, IV, or intraosseous (IO) fluid replacement in two phases: (1) rapid rehydration of existing fluid deficits over

2 to 4 hours, and (2) maintenance hydration for duration of illness.

2. Severe dehydration is typically 10% to 15% of patient's body weight; 30% of the estimated fluid losses should be replaced in the first 30 minutes in adults, and first hour in children, following fluid initiation.

3. After rehydration has been achieved, measure fluid losses over a 4-hour period and replace on top of maintenance fluids over the next 4 hours. Oral hydration should be attempted first, with IV or IO hydration reserved for significant ongoing fluid losses and inadequate oral hydration alone.

4. Oral hydration can be achieved with homemade or commercially available oral rehydration solution (ORS; see Chapter 44) or parenterally with lactated Ringer's solution with 20 mEq of KCl added to every 1 L of solution. Alternatively, normal saline with 20 mEq of KCl added to every 1 L of solution can be used if lactated Ringer's solution is not available.

5. If IV or IO access is unobtainable and the patient is not taking adequate volume of ORS, a nasogastric tube can be placed with administration of ORS at the same rate. Be sure to elevate the head of the bed 30 degrees to prevent aspiration.

6. Initiate antibiotic therapy with tetracycline 500 mg PO q6h in adults and 50 mg/kg per day PO divided q6h in children older than 8 years for 3 to 5 days. Alternatively, use doxycycline 300 mg PO once as a single dose in adults and 4 to 6 mg/kg PO once as a single dose in children older than 8 years. In pregnant women, children younger than 8 years, or in tetracycline/doxycycline-resistant areas, use azithromycin 1 g once as a single dose in adults or 20 mg/kg as a single dose in children, or ciprofloxacin 1 g PO once as a single dose in adults or 20 mg/kg PO once as a single dose in children.

7. Transport or evacuate the patient as soon as possible to definitive medical care while continuing rehydration and antibiotic therapy.

JAPANESE B ENCEPHALITIS

- Japanese encephalitis is a viral infection transmitted by *Culex* mosquitoes. Transmission takes place year-round in tropical and subtropical areas and during the late spring, summer, and early fall in temperate climates. This disease occurs primarily in rural areas, often associated with pig farming.
- Encephalitis is caused by a neurotropic flavivirus.
- After initial replication near the mosquito bite, viremia occurs and may seed infection to the brain.
- The virus causes central nervous system nerve cell destruction and necrosis.
- Most infections in endemic areas involve children, but this disease may occur in any age-group.
- Japanese encephalitis virus is the leading cause of viral encephalitis in Asia, with recent expansion into northern Australia.
- There have been rare reported outbreaks in US territories and in the western Pacific.

Signs and Symptoms
- No clinical illness in most infections
- Encephalitis (about 1 in 300 infections)
- Mild, undifferentiated febrile illness (encephalitis patients often with a similar prodrome)
- Headache, lethargy, fever, confusion, abdominal pain, nausea, and vomiting; possible tremors or seizures
- Approximately 30% reported mortality rate with clinical encephalitis; 50% of survivors have severe neurologic sequelae
- Encephalitis syndrome not easily distinguished from other arboviral encephalitis
- Definitive diagnosis is serologic testing (ELISA).

Treatment
1. No specific therapy exists for this disease.
2. Provide supportive care and hydration.
3. Transport severe cases to a medical facility with an ICU.
4. Practice blood and body fluid precautions.
5. Therapies such as corticosteroids, interferon-α, and ribavirin have all been studied in randomized, double-blind, placebo-controlled trials and do not seem to benefit patients with JE.

Prevention
1. The main interventions are prophylactic: vaccination and reduced arthropod exposure.
2. Vaccination is recommended for persons older than 9 months of age traveling to endemic areas during the transmission season who will be staying for longer than 1 month, and if travel includes rural areas.
3. See discussion of Japanese encephalitis vaccine in Chapter 49.

MENINGOCOCCAL DISEASE
Meningococcal disease is caused by *Neisseria meningitidis,* a gram-negative diplococcus. Meningococcal meningitis classically attacks children and young adults and is often seen in epidemic form. Despite effective antibiotic therapy and immunization, this disease remains problematic in many parts of the world. Epidemic situations pose the greatest health problem to both travelers and resident populations. Since 1970, large outbreaks have occurred in Brazil; China; sub-Saharan Africa; New Delhi, India; and Nepal.

Transmission of the organism occurs through respiratory secretions, so close contact is believed to be important in the spread of the disease.

Signs and Symptoms
- Variety of forms, including but not limited to the following:
  - Bacteremia with septic shock
  - Meningitis, often with bacteremia
  - Pneumonia

- Sustained meningococcemia may lead to severe toxemia with hypotension, fever, and disseminated intravascular coagulation.
- Meningitis caused by *N. meningitidis* is marked by the classic triad of fever, headache, and stiff neck and possibly accompanied by bacteremia and any of several skin manifestations including petechiae, pustules, or maculopapular rash.
- Severe meningitis may progress to mental status deterioration, hypotension, congestive heart failure, disseminated intravascular coagulation, and death.
- During an epidemic, a presumptive diagnosis can be made based on clinical presentation.
- Definitive diagnosis requires culture of the organism from cerebrospinal fluid or blood.
- Several commercial kits for measuring meningococcal antigen are now available for use on cerebral spinal fluid or blood samples.

Treatment

1. Be aware that meningococcal meningitis, or sepsis, is a medical emergency, with suspected patients requiring immediate evacuation to an appropriate medical facility.
2. Note that, fortunately, the organism remains sensitive to many antibiotics, such as the following:
   a. Penicillin G, 300,000 units/kg/ day (up to 24 million units/day) IV in divided doses q2h for 7 to 10 days for serious disease
   b. Ceftriaxone, 2 g q12h IV
   c. Chloramphenicol, 100 mg/kg/day divided q6h IV (note that there has been emergence of chloramphenicol-resistant strains of *N. meningitidis*)
3. Give supportive care, including close monitoring for hypotension and cardiac failure (will necessitate ICU-level care) and IV fluid support.
4. Dexamethasone may be of value for patients in a coma or with evidence of increased intracranial pressure.
5. Make sure that close contacts receive prophylaxis to eradicate the organism (ciprofloxacin 500 mg PO as a single dose, or rifampin 600 mg PO q12h for four doses).

Prevention

- Because the infectious agent has been found in household contacts and in persons exposed to oral secretions, contacts should receive prophylaxis to eradicate the organism.
- Rifampin, 600 mg orally every 12 hours for four doses, is standard adult prophylaxis.
- Children should receive 10 mg/kg of rifampin every 12 hours for four doses if older than 1 month and 5 mg/kg every 12 hours for four doses if younger than 1 month.
- More recently, alternate regimens using ceftriaxone and ciprofloxacin have also been proved to be efficacious, although rifampin remains the standard.

- Ceftriaxone is given intramuscularly as a single dose (125 mg for children <15 years and 250 mg for people >15 years). Ciprofloxacin is given at 20 mg/kg (maximum 500 mg) orally as a single dose.

See discussion of meningococcal vaccine in Chapter 49.

ZIKA VIRUS

- Zika virus is a single-stranded RNA flavivirus, like yellow fever, dengue, West Nile, and Japanese encephalitis viruses.
- Zika virus is transmitted primarily by *Aedes* species of mosquitoes, particularly *Aedes africanus*, *A. aegypti*, and *A. albopictus*.
- These are the same vectors responsible for transmission of dengue and chikungunya viruses. Co-transmission with these viruses has been reported.
- Transmission from human mother to newborn during pregnancy has been confirmed, as has sexual transmission from male travelers returning from Zika-prevalent regions.
- Sexual transmission has occurred both while the male was symptomatic and prior to symptom development, and the virus has been detected in sperm.
- Zika virus infection is a nationally notifiable condition.
- Diagnostic tests for Zika virus are not commercially available. Nucleic acid testing (NAT), RT-PCR and IgM antibody assays are performed at the CDC Division of Vector-Borne Diseases Arbovirus Diagnostic Laboratory.

Signs and Symptoms

- Approximately 20% of patients infected with Zika virus become symptomatic.
- Most patients with Zika virus infection have a mild, nonspecific, and self-limited acute illness.
  - Fever
  - Maculopapular rash
  - Arthralgias
  - Conjunctivitis
  - Myalgias
  - Uveitis
  - Retroorbital pain
- Most patients experience resolution of symptoms by 1 week.
- Very few require hospitalization, and death is rare.
- Guillain-Barré syndrome has become more prevalent in countries experiencing Zika outbreaks; an association is suspected though causality has not been established as of the time of this publication.
- Congenital Zika syndrome (among fetuses infected during pregnancy)
  - Severe microcephaly with partial skull collapse
  - Decreased brain tissue with pattern of brain damage
  - Damage to back of eye and pigment changes
  - Joint abnormalities (e.g., clubfoot)

- Increased overall muscle tone and restricted body movements

Treatment
1. No vaccine exists for Zika virus infection.
2. There is no specific treatment for Zika virus disease.
3. Treatment is supportive and includes hydration and antipyretics.
4. Administration of nonsteroidal antiinflammatory drugs should be avoided until dengue can be excluded, to avoid risk of hemorrhage.

Prevention
1. No vaccine exists to prevent Zika.
2. Condom use can reduce risk of transmission via sexual contact.
3. Prevention centers on avoiding exposure.
4. Travel to endemic areas should be avoided if possible, especially for pregnant women.
5. It is highly recommended to avoid mosquito bites by wearing long sleeves and tucked pant legs, sleeping under a mosquito net, and using effective insect repellents.

RESOURCES FOR TRAVEL MEDICINE INFORMATION
Telephone Information
Centers for Disease Control and Prevention (CDC) Traveler's Health Hotline: +1-800 CDC-INFO (+1-800-232-4636).

U.S. Department of State Overseas Citizens' Services: U.S.-based telephone number, 888-407-4747, and from overseas, +1-202-501-4444.

Official References
Centers for Disease Control and Prevention (CDC): *Health information for international travel,* New York, 2015, Oxford University Press (revised annually).

Morbidity and Mortality Weekly Report, Centers for Disease Control and Prevention, 1600 Clifton Rd, MS E-90. Atlanta, GA 30333. Telephone: +1-404-498-1150. Subscriptions are available at the website: http://www.cdc.gov.

World Health Organization (WHO): *International travel and health, vaccination requirements and health advice,* 2012, World Health Organization Publications Center USA, 49 Sheridan Avenue, Albany, NY 12215 (revised frequently).

Pretravel Clinic Directories
American Society of Tropical Medicine and Hygiene: http://www.astmh.org.

International Society of Travel Medicine: http://www.istm.org.

Travelers' Clinic Directory

English-Speaking Physicians: International Association for Medical Assistance to Travelers (IAMAT): https://www.iamat.org.

Locations: 1623 Military Rd #279, Niagara Falls, NY, USA, 14304-1745. Telephone; 716-754-4883.

67 Mowat Ave, Suite 036, Toronto, Ontario, M3K 3E3 Canada Telephone: 416-652 0137.

Immunizations may be divided into three categories: required, recommended, and routine. Table 49.1 details vaccine schedules and booster intervals for adult travelers who are assumed to have received the primary series of routine vaccines as children. The international traveler should have all current immunizations recorded in a World Health Organization (WHO) International Certificate of Vaccination. This yellow document is recognized worldwide and has a dedicated page for documentation of the yellow fever vaccine. If given, cholera vaccination can be recorded in the space provided for "Other Vaccinations" in the newer booklets.

Contraindications to vaccinations are often overstated. In general, live-virus vaccines and attenuated bacterial vaccines are contraindicated during pregnancy and in persons with impaired immune systems due to medical conditions (e.g., HIV, asplenia, congenital immune deficiencies) or medical therapy (e.g., corticosteroids, cancer chemotherapy, radiation therapy, or immune suppression therapy in the organ transplant patient). Box 49.1 outlines vaccination practices for the patient with HIV, which is a reasonable approach to vaccination in most immunocompromised hosts, in whom live-virus and live-attenuated bacterial vaccines should generally be avoided.

REQUIRED TRAVEL VACCINES

"Required" immunizations are not only those regulated by WHO, but also those required by some countries. For example, yellow fever vaccine may be required for entry into some WHO member countries, whereas smallpox and cholera vaccinations are no longer required for international travel according to WHO regulations. However, some countries continue to "require" cholera vaccination in practice. Meningococcal vaccine is not required by WHO but is by certain countries; for example, Saudi Arabia requires meningococcal vaccination for persons arriving for the Hajj or Umrah pilgrimages.

Yellow Fever Vaccine

Yellow fever (YF) is a viral infection transmitted by mosquitoes in equatorial South America and Africa (Table 49.2). Several countries require proof of YF vaccination from all arriving travelers (Table 49.3). YF vaccine is a live-attenuated viral vaccine that is highly protective and is given as a single dose for primary immunization. The booster interval is 10 years. Because of age-related risk of encephalitis after immunization, most authorities agree that the YF vaccine is contraindicated in infants less than 6 months of age,

Text continued on p. 633

Table 49.1 Vaccines and Immunoglobulin for Adult Travelers Who Completed Childhood Immunizations

VACCINE	ROUTE (DOSE)	SCHEDULE
Hepatitis A (Havrix and Vaqta)	IM (1.0 mL)	Primary: 2 doses Additional booster doses: not recommended
Hepatitis B (Recombivax HB and Engerix-B)	IM (adult and pediatric formulations)	Primary: 1 dose at 0, 1, and 6 months Booster: not routinely recommended Accelerated schedules (see text)
Hepatitis A and B antigens combined (Twinrix)	IM (1.0 mL)	Primary: 1 dose at 0, 1, and 6 months Booster: not routinely recommended Accelerated schedules (see text)
Influenza	IM (0.5 mL)	One dose of current vaccine annually
Influenza (FluMist)	Intranasal (0.5 mL)	Primary: 1 dose per season
Japanese B encephalitis (Ixiaro)	IM (0.5 mL) 2 months to 3 years: 0.25 mL >3 years: 0.5 mL	Primary: 1 dose at 0 and 28 days Booster: >1 year following primary series, booster if continued risk
Measles (monovalent or combined with rubella and mumps, MMR)	SC (0.5 mL)	Primary: 2 doses separated by at least 1 year Booster: none (Unless born prior to 1956; then see CDC recommendation.)

SIDE EFFECTS, PRECAUTIONS, AND CONTRAINDICATIONS*	COMMENTS
Local reactions: <56% Fever: <5% Headache: 16%	Prevaccine hepatitis A serology may be cost-effective for some travelers (see text).
Local reaction: 3%–29% Fever: 1%–6%	
Local reactions: approximately 56% Systemic reactions: similar to single-antigen products	Give at least 2 doses of vaccine before departure to provide protection against hepatitis A.
Local reactions: <33% Systemic reactions: occasional Allergic reaction: rare Avoid in those with history of anaphylaxis to eggs.	
Mild upper respiratory tract symptoms: occasional Avoid in those with history of anaphylaxis to eggs, Guillain-Barré syndrome, or immunosuppression.	Approved for persons 5 to 49 years old
	Ixiaro is a Vero cell culture–derived formulation. A single booster >1 year after completion of primary series if ongoing risk
Fever, 5–21 days after vaccination: 5%–15% Transient rash: 5% Local reaction among those who received killed vaccine (1963–67): 4%–55% Severe allergic reactions, CNS complications, thrombocytopenia (MMR): rare Avoid in pregnancy, immunocompromised hosts, and those with history of anaphylaxis to eggs or neomycin.	Do not give immune globulin within 3 months of vaccine dose. If MMR and yellow fever vaccine are not given simultaneously, separate by 28 days or longer.

Continued

Table 49.1   Vaccines and Immunoglobulin for Adult Travelers Who Completed Childhood Immunizations—cont'd

VACCINE	ROUTE (DOSE)	SCHEDULE
Meningococcal polysaccharide-protein conjugate quadrivalent vaccine (Menactra)	IM (0.5 mL)	Primary: single dose Booster: not recommended for routine use; every 5 years recommended for ongoing risk
Mumps	SC (0.5 mL)	Primary: 1 dose (usually as MMR) Booster: none
Pneumococcal polysaccharide Conjugate vaccine (PCV 13)	SC or IM (0.5 mL)	Primary: single dose at age 65 or age 60 if high risk Booster: high-risk patients after 5 years from initial dose
Poliomyelitis	SC or IM (0.5 mL)	Booster: one adult dose
Rabies Human diploid cell vaccine (HDCV); purified chick embryo cell (PCEC); rabies vaccine adsorbed (RVA)	IM (1.0 mL)	Preexposure: 1 dose at 0, 7, and 21 or 28 days Booster doses depend on ongoing risk and results of serology (see text)
Rubella	SC (0.5 mL)	Primary: 1 dose (usually as MMR) Booster: none

SIDE EFFECTS, PRECAUTIONS, AND CONTRAINDICATIONS*	COMMENTS
Local reactions: 10%–60% Systemic reactions: occasional fever, headache, and malaise	Replaces quadrivalent polysaccharide vaccine (Menomune)
Mild allergic reactions: uncommon Parotitis: rare Avoid in pregnancy, immunocompromised hosts, and those with history of anaphylaxis to eggs or neomycin.	Do not give immune globulin within 3 months of vaccine dose. If MMR and yellow fever vaccine are not given simultaneously, separate by 28 days or longer.
Mild local reactions: approximately 50% Systemic symptoms: <1% Arthus-like reaction with booster doses occurs. Avoid in those with moderate to severe acute illness.	Opportunity to update routine vaccination in older travelers
Local reactions: occasional	Additional boosters not recommended. Access CDC or WHO databases for current regions with polio transmission.
Mild local or systemic reactions: occasional Immune complex–like reactions after booster dose of HDCV (2–21 days after vaccination): 6%	Target children in endemic areas who might not tell parents about bites.
Transient arthralgias in adult women beginning 3–25 days after vaccination: up to 25% Arthritis: <2% Avoid in pregnancy, immunocompromised hosts, and those with history of anaphylaxis to neomycin.	Do not give immune globulin within 3 months of vaccine dose. If MMR and yellow fever vaccine are not given simultaneously, separate by 28 days or longer.

Continued

Table 49.1   Vaccines and Immunoglobulin for Adult Travelers Who Completed Childhood Immunizations—cont'd

VACCINE	ROUTE (DOSE)	SCHEDULE
Tetanus-diphtheria (Td)	IM (0.5 mL)	Booster dose every 10 years
Tetanus-diphtheria with acellular pertussis (Tdap)	IM (0.5 mL)	One-time dose (wait at least 2 years since last Td), then resume Td every 10 years.
Typhoid Ty21a	Oral capsules	Primary: 1 capsule every other day for 4 doses Booster: every 5 years if ongoing risk
Typhoid Vi polysaccharide	IM (0.5 mL)	Primary: single dose Booster: every 2 years if ongoing risk
Varicella	SC (0.5 mL)	Primary: 2 doses at 4-week interval or longer. No booster
Varicella-zoster virus (VZV) vaccine	SC (0.5 mL)	One dose

SIDE EFFECTS, PRECAUTIONS, AND CONTRAINDICATIONS*	COMMENTS
Local reactions: common Systemic symptoms: occasional Anaphylaxis: rare Arthus-like reactions possible after multiple previous boosters Avoid if Guillain-Barré syndrome occurs 6 weeks or earlier after previous dose.	Consider booster at 5 years for travelers to remote areas or regions without adequate health care facilities when sustaining punctures or other significant wounds is possible.
Like Td	Do not confuse Tdap with the pediatric formulation (TDaP), which can cause adverse reactions in adults.
Gastrointestinal upset or rash: infrequent Avoid in pregnancy and in persons with febrile illness, taking antibiotics, or in immunocompromised state.	Refrigerate capsules. If already taking mefloquine, separate doses by 24 hours.
Local reaction: 7% Headache: 16% Fever: <1%	
Local reactions: 20% Fever: 15% Localized or mild systemic varicella rash: 6% Avoid in immunocompromised hosts, if severe allergic reactions to gelatin or neomycin, or if serum immune globulin within 5 months.	Rare transmission of vaccine strain to susceptible hosts; therefore, avoid if close contacts are immunosuppressed.
	Recommended for all adults over 60 years old, including those with previous history of zoster Decreases the incidence of postherpetic neuralgia

Continued

VACCINE	ROUTE (DOSE)	SCHEDULE
Table 49.1 Vaccines and Immunoglobulin for Adult Travelers Who Completed Childhood Immunizations—cont'd		
Yellow fever	SC (0.5 mL)	Primary: single dose Booster: every 10 years

*Moderate or severe acute illness with or without fever or a serious reaction to a previous dose is a contraindication to all vaccines.
IM, Intramuscularly; *SC*, subcutaneously.
Modified from information in Centers for Disease Control and Prevention (CDC): *Health information for international travel,* 2018 https://wwwnc.cdc.gov/travel/page/yellowbook-home; and Hill DR, Ericsson CD, Pearson RD et al: Guidelines for the practice of travel medicine, *Clin Infect Dis* 43:1499, 2006.

BOX 49.1   Vaccination in HIV-Positive Adults

Generally Avoid
- Varicella-zoster virus vaccine
- Bacille Calmette-Guérin vaccine
- Oral polio vaccine
- Oral typhoid vaccine

Avoid if CD4+ Cells <200
- Yellow fever vaccine
- Measles vaccine

Give Routinely
- Tetanus/diphtheria (or Tdap) vaccine
- Hepatitis B vaccine
- *Streptococcus pneumoniae* vaccine
- *Haemophilus influenzae* type b vaccine
- Influenza vaccine, yearly
- Hepatitis A vaccine

Give if Indicated for Travel
- Typhoid Vi vaccine
- Meningococcal vaccine
- Polio, inactivated poliomyelitis vaccine
- Rabies vaccine
- Japanese encephalitis (JE)
- Tick-borne encephalitis (JE) vaccine

SIDE EFFECTS, PRECAUTIONS, AND CONTRAINDICATIONS*	COMMENTS
Mild headache, myalgia, fever (5–10 days after vaccination): 25% Immediate hypersensitivity: rare Viscerotropic syndrome or neurotropic disease: rare (see text) Avoid if allergic to eggs. Contraindicated in immunocompromised hosts	If person can eat eggs without a reaction, person can take vaccine.

and immunization should usually be delayed until the infant is 9 months or older. The vaccine is generally not recommended for persons older than 60 years, immunocompromised, or pregnant.

There are several potential complications to YF vaccine, including hypersensitivity reaction, vaccine-associated neurologic disease, and vaccine-associated viscerotropic disease (YEL-AVD). The latter of these is a severe reaction that mimics fulminant YF infection resulting in multisystem organ failure and death. The incidence of YEL-AVD in persons older than 60 is estimated at 1.4 to 1.8 cases per 100,000 doses, which is significantly higher than the estimated 0.3 to 0.4 cases per 100,000 doses in the general population. Despite these purported risks, the small number of cases makes accurate risk factor assessment difficult.

Cholera Vaccine

Cholera is an intestinal infection caused by *Vibrio cholerae* that involves profuse secretory diarrhea. The injectable cholera vaccine is not very efficacious, even when the primary series of two doses given 1 week or more apart is received. WHO no longer endorses a requirement for this vaccine before entry into any country. For countries that still require cholera vaccination for travelers arriving from cholera-endemic areas, recording a single cholera dose in the traveler's International Certificate of Vaccination should suffice to meet this regulation.

Two oral, whole-cell killed vaccines are available. Dukoral (Crucell, The Netherlands), licensed in many European countries

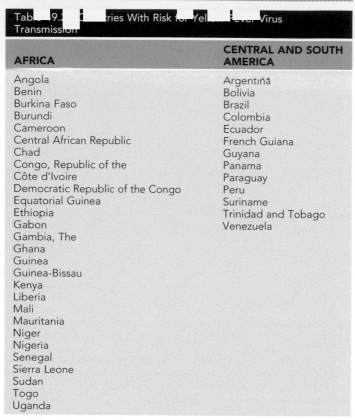

Table 19.2 Countries With Risk for Yellow Fever Virus Transmission	
AFRICA	**CENTRAL AND SOUTH AMERICA**
Angola	Argentina
Benin	Bolivia
Burkina Faso	Brazil
Burundi	Colombia
Cameroon	Ecuador
Central African Republic	French Guiana
Chad	Guyana
Congo, Republic of the	Panama
Côte d'Ivoire	Paraguay
Democratic Republic of the Congo	Peru
Equatorial Guinea	Suriname
Ethiopia	Trinidad and Tobago
Gabon	Venezuela
Gambia, The	
Ghana	
Guinea	
Guinea-Bissau	
Kenya	
Liberia	
Mali	
Mauritania	
Niger	
Nigeria	
Senegal	
Sierra Leone	
Sudan	
Togo	
Uganda	

From Centers for Disease Control and Prevention: https://wwwnc.cdc.gov/travel/yellowbook/2018/infectious-diseases-related-to-travel/yellow-fever Courtesy Centers for Disease Control and Prevention.

and Canada, is administered in two doses 1 to 6 weeks apart (three doses in children 2 to 6 years old). Shanchol (Shantha Biotechnics, India) is administered in two doses 2 weeks apart to persons older than 1 year old.

Smallpox Vaccine

The requirement for smallpox vaccine for international travel was removed from WHO regulations in 1982. The CDC has embarked on an initiative to immunize health care providers, first responders, and others involved in bioterrorism preparedness, but the vaccine is not otherwise available, and travel is not considered a sufficient reason for vaccination.

Table 49.3 Countries That Require Proof of Yellow Fever Vaccination From All Arriving Travelers*	
Angola	Ghana
Burundi	Guinea-Bissau
Central African Republic	Liberia
Congo, Republic of the	Mali
Côte d'Ivoire	Niger
Democratic Republic of Congo	Sierra Leone
French Guiana	Suriname
Gabon	Togo

*Country requirements for yellow fever vaccination are subject to change at any time; therefore CDC encourages travelers to check with the destination country's embassy or consulate before departure.

From Centers for Disease Control and Prevention: https://wwwnc.cdc.gov/travel/yellowbook/2018/infectious-diseases-related-to-travel/yellow-fever Courtesy Centers for Disease Control and Prevention.

RECOMMENDED TRAVEL VACCINES

"Recommended" vaccines are those that are not routinely given during childhood in the United States but are advised for travelers based on the travel health risk assessment. Vaccines in this category include those for hepatitis A and B, typhoid fever, meningococcal meningitis, Japanese encephalitis virus, rabies, tick-borne encephalitis, varicella-zoster virus (VZV), influenza, and bacille Calmette-Guérin (BCG). The VZV vaccine is supposed to be used routinely in the United States, but for many adult US travelers, it remains a vaccine that must be added. The influenza vaccine is often but not routinely used in children; it is recommended for many travelers. Although BCG vaccination is used in children in the developing world, it is not used in US children. Some vaccines are now routinely recommended for children. These include hepatitis B (since 1991), hepatitis A (more recently in United States), and meningococcal vaccine, which is recommended for all 11- to 12-year-olds and young adults before starting higher education. Because of these practices, in the future, more travelers will likely have been vaccinated with recommended vaccines.

Hepatitis A Vaccine

Hepatitis A is the second most common vaccine-preventable travel-associated infectious disease, after influenza, and hepatitis A virus (HAV) is the most common cause of viral hepatitis. In the absence of vaccination, HAV infection occurs in 6 to 30 persons per 100,000 travelers per month who visit high- and medium-endemic destinations. Risk is high even among those residing in "first-class" accommodations. Adventure travelers who venture off usual tourist routes may be at increased risk compared with other groups of travelers. Vaccination against HAV should be considered for all travelers to regions with moderate to high endemicity.

A single dose of monovalent hepatitis A vaccine leads to sero-conversion of 80% by 2 weeks and 99% after 1 month following vaccination. For most healthy people, one dose of the monovalent HAV vaccine administered at any time before departure should provide adequate protection. The HAV vaccine products are thought to be interchangeable. After two full doses separated by 6 to 12 months, protection is likely lifelong, so booster doses are not recommended in immunocompetent travelers. Travelers who fail to receive their second dose of HAV vaccine within 6 to 12 months should attempt to complete the series; however, protective antibody levels have been produced even when the second dose was given 8 years after the initial dose.

Hepatitis B Vaccine

Hepatitis B vaccine was added to the list of vaccines recommended for routine immunization of U.S. children in 1991, and consideration should be given to vaccinating all U.S. adults regardless of travel. Risk to short-term travelers is low; however, travelers should be vaccinated when contact with body fluids or blood is possible (e.g., through sex or medical work), when it is anticipated that medical care might be received in a developing country, or if the person is a frequent short-term traveler. Long-term travelers and expatriates should be vaccinated.

Two recombinant vaccines (Engerix-B and Recombivax HB) are thought to be interchangeable. The standard regimen for both vaccines is one dose at each of 0, 1, and 6 months. After any of the hepatitis B vaccination regimens, additional boosters are not recommended for normal hosts. Engerix-B is approved by the US Food and Drug Administration (FDA) for an accelerated dosage schedule of 0, 1, and 2 months, with a booster dose at 12 months for long-lasting protection. Although a highly accelerated 3-week schedule is not FDA approved, literature supports dosing at 0, 7, and 21 days, with a 12-month booster with either licensed vaccine. This regimen affords 65% protection at the end of 1 month and 100% seroconversion at 13 months. This is an attractive option for at-risk travelers who plan to depart in the next 3 to 4 weeks. An interrupted series can be completed without being restarted if the series cannot be completed before travel.

A combined hepatitis A and hepatitis B vaccine is dosed at 0, 1, and 6 months. Because a smaller dose of HAV antigen is used in this preparation, travelers must receive their second dose before travel for reliable protection. Literature supports a highly accelerated 3-week dosing regimen, with a 12-month booster using the combination vaccine.

Typhoid Fever Vaccine

Typhoid is an insidious febrile illness caused by *Salmonella enterica* serotype Typhi. The incidence of typhoid fever among American travelers is estimated at 1 to 10 cases per 100,000 travelers. Among reported cases in the United States, the majority were acquired during international travel. The risk to travelers is highest among visitors to the Indian subcontinent, where the incidence is estimated at more than 100 cases per 100,000 native persons. Travelers most at risk are those visiting friends and relatives (VFR). Visitors to Central and South America, Africa, and Asia should be considered for typhoid vaccination when they might be exposed to conditions of poor sanitation and hygiene, even for short periods.

The two vaccines currently available offer a similar degree of protection. The parenteral purified Vi polysaccharide typhoid vaccine is administered as a single injection, with a booster recommended every 2 years. The oral Ty21a typhoid vaccine uses a live-attenuated strain of *S. enterica* serotype Typhi. One capsule is taken every other day for four doses (a three-dose regimen is recommended in Europe). A booster regimen is recommended every 5 years.

Meningococcal Vaccine

Vaccine protection against meningococcal meningitis is recommended for long-term travelers to the sub-Saharan "meningitis belt." Short-term travelers to this region should receive vaccine if they will travel during the dry season (December to June) or have extensive contact with local people. The quadrivalent meningococcal vaccine is required for travel to Saudi Arabia for Umrah or the annual Hajj religious pilgrimages. Regardless of travel, the classic recommendation has been that young adults who will live in school dormitories and persons with complement deficiencies who will have prolonged contact with a local population, such as in a refugee camp, or with surgical or functional asplenia should be vaccinated. Travelers to regions where outbreaks are occurring should be vaccinated. Practitioners who do not subscribe to commercial information services that are routinely updated should check the CDC website (http://www.cdc.gov/travel) periodically to determine where epidemic disease of any causation is occurring.

Quadrivalent meningococcal polysaccharide vaccine induces immunity against serogroups A, C, Y, and W-135. A single dose appears to provide immunity for 5 years. However, a single-dose quadrivalent meningococcal polysaccharide-protein conjugate vaccine is the preferred vaccine for those older than 2 years, with a booster recommended every 5 years for ongoing risk. Travelers who had previously been vaccinated with polysaccharide vaccine and need revaccination should receive a conjugate vaccine. However, neither the polysaccharide nor the conjugate vaccine provides immunity against serogroup B. The FDA recently approved a vaccine (Trumenba) active against four *Neisseria meningitidis* serogroup B strains prevalent in the United States, for use in adolescents and young adults age 10 to 25 years. It has not been recommended for travelers because *N. meningitides* serogroup B infections are rare in sub-Saharan Africa.

Japanese Encephalitis Virus Vaccine

Japanese encephalitis (JE) is an arboviral infection transmitted by mosquitoes in Asia and Southeast Asia. Transmission is year-round in tropical and subtropical areas and during the late spring, summer, and early fall in temperate climates. JE virus is not considered a risk for short-term travelers visiting usual tourist destinations in urban and developed resort areas.

Personal protective measures to prevent mosquito bites can greatly reduce risk of infection. The overall incidence of JE among people from nonendemic countries traveling to Asia is estimated at less than 1 case per 1 million travelers. However, travelers who stay for prolonged periods (including expatriates) in rural areas with active JE virus transmission are likely to be at a risk like that of the susceptible resident population (~5 to 50 cases per 100,000 children per year). Persons on short trips may be at risk if they are staying in rural areas or have high mosquito exposure. Thus vaccination should be offered to both long- and short-term visitors to rural areas when travel will occur during transmission season, particularly when mosquito exposure might be high and significant time will be spent outdoors.

Two vaccines (JE-Vax, Ixiaro) are FDA approved, but only Ixiaro, a Vero cell culture–derived formulation, is available. Previously recommended only for use in persons 17 years or older, Ixiaro is now approved by the FDA for use in children 2 months or older. A single dose of Ixiaro has been shown to effectively boost antibody levels in persons previously vaccinated with JE-Vax, but the duration of protection is unknown. The primary immunization schedule for Ixiaro is two doses, on days 0 and 28, with therapy completed 1 week or longer before travel. In patients receiving JE-Vax, fewer than 1% of patients reported redness, swelling, tenderness, and pain after injection. Systemic adverse events reported included headache (26%), myalgias (21%), influenza-like illness (13%), and fatigue (13%).

The single-dose, live-attenuated SA 14-14-2 JE vaccine manufactured in Chengdu, China (available in destination countries such as Nepal), has been effectively used extensively in South and Southeast Asia for decades with an acceptable safety profile.

Rabies Vaccine
See Chapter 43.

Tick-Borne Encephalitis Vaccine
Tick-borne encephalitis (TBE) is a viral illness transmitted predominantly by bites of *Ixodes* ticks during spring and summer months in rural forested areas of central and eastern Europe, Scandinavia, Siberia, and northern Japan. Infection can lead to central nervous system (CNS) effects of meningitis, encephalitis, or meningoencephalitis in about 20% to 30% of infected persons. Infection can occur after ingestion of unpasteurized dairy products from infected cows, goats, or sheep.

There are no licensed vaccines for TBE in the United States. The standard dosing regimen is three doses given over 1 year. Accelerated schedules exist, but doses would likely need to be administered in the destination country. Whereas expatriates can consider obtaining vaccine at their new location, it is much more practical for most travelers to at-risk areas to use stringent tick bite precautions (e.g., repellents and insecticides, protective clothing, frequent tick surveillance) and to avoid unpasteurized dairy products.

Bacille Calmette-Guérin Vaccine for Tuberculosis

The BCG vaccine is intended to prevent tuberculosis (TB). The vaccine is currently not recommended for most US travelers, including expatriates. This is because it is believed to be of varying efficacy in preventing adult forms of TB. Persons taking short trips for tourism or business to developing countries where TB is common among the indigenous population are not at great risk for contracting TB. However, expatriates or travelers who will live among foreign residents or work in foreign orphanages, schools, hospitals, or similar facilities are at significant risk of exposure to TB infection. Such travelers should be tested with a purified protein derivative (PPD) skin test before the trip, and if the test is negative, they should be retested 3 months after their return to a developed country and yearly thereafter. In the setting of travel and exposure, persons who convert from a negative to a positive PPD skin test should be treated with isoniazid for 9 months, regardless of age. Interferon-γ release assays (IGRAs) are blood tests that measure host cell–mediated immune response to *Mycobacterium tuberculosis* antigen. IGRAs appear to have high specificity but variable sensitivity compared with the TB skin test. IGRAs may be most useful in BCG-vaccinated patients and in persons unlikely to return for reading of a skin test.

Varicella-Zoster Virus (Chickenpox) Vaccine

VZV infections are common throughout the world. Primary infection with VZV is known as chickenpox. After primary infection with VZV, the virus often stays dormant. It can reemerge as shingles later in life. A traveler with a history of chickenpox can be considered immune. Many adults have had exposure to VZV, so if time permits, serum immunity should be documented before considering vaccination. If a person is not immune, two doses of single-antigen varicella vaccine should be given 4 to 8 weeks apart.

Influenza Vaccine

Each year, the influenza vaccine antigen composition is based on projections of winter influenza activity in North America (or South America). The vaccine differs, depending on the hemisphere in which one lives, and therefore may not protect against the precise influenza strains circulating elsewhere in the world. Because of when the projections are made, the vaccination may not be available for at-risk travelers from the United States during late spring through early autumn.

Travelers from the United States may be exposed to influenza when traveling during winter months in the northern hemisphere, between April and September in the southern hemisphere, and year-round in the tropics. Travelers from diverse locations may be brought together during cruises, resulting in an outbreak of influenza during periods when influenza transmission might otherwise not frequently occur. Risk for acquiring influenza during long-haul flights exists if a person infected with influenza is seated close to a susceptible individual. For these reasons, influenza should be considered a travel-related infection, and influenza vaccine should be recommended to travelers.

Other Vaccines

According to the CDC, anthrax vaccine is not recommended for travelers. A killed bacterial vaccine for plague exists, but the dosing schedule is long and protection is uncertain. An alternative for select persons at risk (e.g., field biologists) for plague is a daily 100-mg dose of doxycycline, which can double as protection against malaria. The protective efficacy of this regimen against plague is inferred from treatment recommendations.

ROUTINE VACCINES

"Routine" immunizations are those customarily given in childhood and then updated in adult life, regardless of travel. Visits to travel medicine clinics afford opportunities to update immunizations through booster doses of routine vaccines.

The routine vaccines currently recommended in childhood include those against tetanus, diphtheria, pertussis, measles, mumps, rubella, varicella, polio, *Haemophilus influenzae* type b (Hib), hepatitis A/B, pneumococcus (PCV), and rotavirus. Routine immunization schedules for children, including nuanced changes in routine schedules for traveling children, can be found in the CDC's Yellow Book.

50 Drowning and Cold-Water Immersion

The World Health Organization (WHO) estimates that unintentional drowning accounts for more than 500,000 deaths worldwide every year. Drowning is the leading cause of death in males 5 to 14 years of age. Definitions of drowning have been unclear in the past. WHO produced standard definitions that are used in this chapter; drowning is considered a process and not an outcome. Other water-related conditions that do not primarily involve the airway and respiratory system are considered submersion injuries rather than drowning.

Drowning: Respiratory impairment from submersion or immersion in liquid

Drowning with death: Drowning that results in fatality

Drowning with morbidity: Drowning injury that does not result in death (avoid historical terms such as *near drowning* and *wet or dry drowning*)

Drowning without morbidity

Immersion: Body entry into a liquid medium

Submersion: Entry into a liquid medium where the body—particularly the head—is below the surface

PATHOPHYSIOLOGY OF DROWNING

After gasping occurs, the initial struggle is sometimes followed by laryngospasm to protect the lower airways from liquid in the upper airways (i.e., nares, oropharynx, larynx). Laryngospasm may limit the amount of water aspirated and occurs in an estimated 7% to 10% of drowning cases, but all patients likely aspirate at least a small amount of liquid. Particularly during cold-water drowning, the initial event is accompanied by a drive to hyperventilate caused by stimulation of thermal skin receptors, in addition to increasing hypoxemia. Eventually the outcomes of breath-holding are hypoventilation, hypercapnia, respiratory acidosis, and hypoxemia. As breath-holding attempts are overwhelmed, respiration is involuntary. Loss of consciousness and cardiopulmonary arrest follow.

COLD-WATER IMMERSION
Cold Shock Response

- The cold shock response is the most common cause of drowning in cold water.
- Immediately on immersion, uncontrollable gasping lasts 1 to 3 minutes, which results in aspiration of water unless the head is kept above surface.

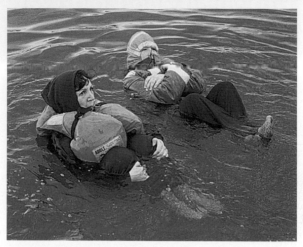

FIGURE 50.1   Heat Escape Lessening Posture (HELP). (Courtesy Alan Steinman, MD.)

- Sudden skin cooling results in increased peripheral vascular resistance of superficial blood vessels.
- Heart rate and cardiac output increase; outpouring of catecholamines may lead to fatal dysrhythmias.
- Cooling of the periphery decreases nerve conduction, and muscle control becomes difficult, making self-rescue virtually impossible.
- Priority for self-rescue is to maintain the head above water, assuming the heat escape lessening position (HELP; Fig. 50.1), if possible.
- If two or more persons are in the water, the huddle position (Fig. 50.2) is recommended to lessen total body heat loss.
- Because children become hypothermic much more quickly than do adults, they should be placed in the middle of the huddle.
- Drawstrings should be tightened in clothing to decrease the flow of cold water within clothing layers.
- In cold water a person may consider whether to stay in place to conserve heat or swim to safety. Note that at 45 to 90 minutes, swim failure may occur as a result of continued reduction of core body temperature causing loss of gross motor function. The average person can swim approximately 800 m (2625 ft) in 10°C (50°F) water while wearing a personal flotation device before swim failure and death occur.

On-Scene Rescue and Patient Management
Hypothermia may offer a protective benefit and prolong the time after which resuscitation can still be successful. There are case reports in which patients survived after 40 minutes of submersion in cold water with complete or nearly complete neurologic recovery.

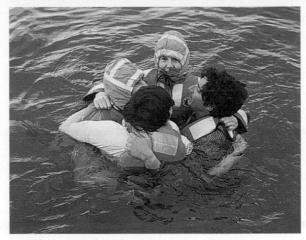

FIGURE 50.2   Huddle Technique. (Courtesy Alan Steinman, MD.)

Rescue attempts must always take into consideration the safety of rescuers to avoid creating additional victims. General guidelines for rescue and patient management are as follows:

- Safety devices should be used to tow the patient, or life preservers should be thrown to people in trouble in the water before a human responder enters the water.
- Anticipate cervical spine fracture or a significant head injury if trauma (e.g., diving or fall) is suspected.
- Evaluate for hypoglycemia (with or without diabetes), seizure disorder, and acute myocardial infarction as potential causes of drowning.
- Initiate resuscitation (see later).
- If rapid extrication from water is not feasible, institute in-water rescue breathing and maintain the patient in a vertical position to minimize the potential for vomiting and further aspiration of water and emesis (Fig. 50.3).
- After the patient is out of the water, initiate basic life support.
- Use ABC (airway, breathing, and circulation) rather than CAB sequence, because cardiac arrest in drowning is almost always due to hypoxia.
- Begin with five rescue breaths; then follow routine basic life support procedures with 30 compressions to 2 ventilations.
- Cardiopulmonary resuscitation (CPR) with compressions only is not recommended in drowning.
- Emesis is common during drowning resuscitation; do not attempt to expel water by abdominal thrust or head-down position, which only increase emesis and interfere with adequate ventilation.
- If the patient is breathing but unconscious, use the recovery position.

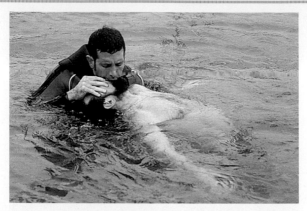

FIGURE 50.3   Mouth-to-Mouth Ventilation in the Water Is Difficult in the Best of Circumstances. (Courtesy Alan Steinman, MD.)

- Transport to an emergency facility with ongoing CPR unless resuscitation is determined futile (see later) or successful.

DROWNING CLASSIFICATIONS AND GENERAL TREATMENT
The Asymptomatic Patient: Grades 0 and 1
Patients who have been rescued from the water and who are alert, with a clear chest examination to auscultation, no respiratory distress, and with or without coughing may not need further medical care but still present a dilemma. Patients may leave the scene only to suffer complications later that are caused by acute lung injury. Any person with shortness of breath may have mild hypoxemia and should be treated as a symptomatic patient. Patients who are treated and released at the scene should be advised that respiratory symptoms can develop up to 24 hours later and should seek emergency treatment immediately after the development of such symptoms.

Hypothermia is often difficult to ascertain at the scene, so it may be prudent to have the person evaluated, even if only briefly, at a medical facility. Conscious and cooperative patients should be protected against hypothermia with passive warming techniques, protected from the wind, and offered dry clothes and blankets. If the person remains asymptomatic with normal vital signs and stable arterial oxygen saturation (if testing is available) on ambient air for 10 to 15 minutes, then it is unlikely that he or she will require further medical care.

The Symptomatic Patient: Grades 2, 3, and 4
All submersion patients requiring intervention or resuscitation or showing signs of distress (e.g., anxiety, tachypnea, dyspnea, syncope,

persistent cough, presence of foam in the mouth or nose, changes in vital signs) should be evacuated or transported to a hospital or another health care facility for evaluation.

Protection of the airway to ensure oxygenation and ventilation is the first priority. Maintaining perfusion to reverse the metabolic consequences of acidosis is a close second. The airway should be protected from aspiration by placing the patient in a lateral recumbent (i.e., recovery) position if possible. Vomiting is common with submersion incidents, and aspiration can worsen lung injury. Measures should be taken to prevent hypothermia and shivering. Rescuers must maintain vigilance and treat cardiac dysrhythmias that may arise as a result of hypoxemia. The management actions listed in Table 50.1 can then be considered. If cervical spine injury is suspected, use an extrication collar and an immobilization device. Routine cervical spine immobilization is unnecessary and should be reserved for patients with a known or suspected significant mechanism of injury.

The Patient in Respiratory or Cardiopulmonary Arrest: Grades 5 and 6

Initiation of immediate ventilatory support and early CPR, if indicated, results in a better prognosis and outcomes. Initiation of chest compressions while the patient remains in the water is ineffective, delays extrication, and may further endanger the patient and rescuer. Alternatively, rescue breathing should be initiated as soon as the subject's airway can be opened, even if in the water (see Fig. 50.3).

When the individual is out of the water, supplemental oxygen should be initiated as soon as possible. If the patient is spontaneously breathing, and a nonrebreathing mask, portable positive end-expiratory pressure (PEEP) valve, or portable continuous positive airway pressure (CPAP) device is available, oxygen should be delivered at a high flow rate (i.e., 10 to 15 L/min). A CPAP mask should be used cautiously if there is any concern about vomiting or loss of airway protective reflexes.

Maneuvers to empty the lungs of fluid, including abdominal thrusts, are not recommended. Gastric distention can interfere with ventilation by increasing intra-abdominal pressure. In such instances, gastric decompression by nasogastric tube is recommended. Digital or visual examination for foreign bodies should be done, and if foreign bodies are present, they should be removed with a swipe or grasp of the fingers.

Should vomiting occur, roll the patient onto his or her side or turn his or her head to the side and remove the vomitus with a cloth or finger-sweep maneuver. If spinal injury is of concern, the patient should be logrolled, maintaining linear alignment of the head, neck, and torso. Because most beaches, riverbanks, boat ramps, and other waterway access points are sloped, patients should be placed perpendicular to the incline so that head and feet are level. When the subject is out of the water and airway and breathing

Table 50.1 Prehospital Management and Classification of Drowning Patients

GRADE	The Asymptomatic Patient		The Symptomatic Patient				The Patient in Respiratory or Cardiopulmonary Arrest
	0	1	2	3	4	5	6
Mortality (%)	0	0	0.6	5.2	19	44	93
Pulmonary exam	No cough or dyspnea	Normal auscultation with cough	Rales, small amount of foam	Acute pulmonary edema	Acute pulmonary edema	Respiratory arrest	Cardiopulmonary arrest
Cardiovascular	Radial pulses	Radial pulses	Radial pulses	Radial pulses	Hypotension	Hypotension	
On-scene management	Release at scene	Rest, rewarm, reassure, and release	O$_2$ via nasal cannula; observe for 6-24 hr	O$_2$ via NRB ACLS	O$_2$ via NRB ACLS	Load and go	
Transport	No	No	Transport or observation	Yes	Rapid	Rapid	
En-route management			Vital signs	Vital signs	Possible ETT and manage pressure	ACLS	
Hospital			ED or overnight observation	Admission for observation	ICU	ICU	ICU

ACLS, Advanced cardiac life support; ED, emergency department; ETT, endotracheal tube; ICU, Intensive care unit; NRB, nonrebreather mask.
Courtesy Justin Sempsrott, MD. Modified from Szpilman D: Near-drowning and drowning classification: A proposal to stratify mortality based on the analysis of 1831 cases, Chest 112:660, 1997.

are addressed, the presence or absence of adequate circulation should be ascertained. In cases of hypothermia or hypotension, a pulse may be difficult to identify. If ventilation or cardiac function is impaired, chest compressions should be initiated as soon as the patient is removed from the water. For patients who are more than 1 year old, an automated external defibrillator may be used to evaluate heart rhythm. If the field rescue team is capable of advanced life support, cardiac monitoring, and intravenous or intraosseous access, fluids and medications should be administered according to advanced life support protocols. Basic life support or advanced cardiac life support should continue until the patient's core body temperature is more than 30°C (86°F). See Table 50.1 for a classification scheme for drowning field assessment and management.

Prognosis and Termination of Resuscitation

Declaring a patient dead from drowning is complicated by the fact that many of the most dramatic and physiologically unexpected recoveries from cardiac arrest have been in young patients after cold-water drowning. The duration of submersion, water temperature, patient core body temperature, and any cardiac electrical or echocardiographic activity should be considered before the declaration of death. If there is any uncertainty, then resuscitation should be continued until the patient is rewarmed to 30°C to 35°C (86°F to 95°F). Functional recovery with minimal neurologic impairment occurs in approximately 17% of those who require resuscitation in the emergency department. In a wilderness setting without access to EMS transportation, standards for field pronouncement of death include patients who have had more than 25 to 30 minutes of CPR with no return of vital signs.

Factors known to be useful for predicting outcomes in drowning are listed in Box 50.1. In the absence of profound hypothermia, the neurologic status of a patient on admission to the emergency

---

BOX 50.1   Prognostic Signs in Submersion Incidents

Good
Alert on admission
Hypothermic
Brief submersion time
On-scene basic or advanced life support (probably most important)
Good response to initial resuscitation measures

Poor
Fixed, dilated pupils in emergency department
Submerged longer than 5 min
No resuscitation attempts for more than 10 min
Preexisting chronic disease
Arterial pH ≤7.10
Coma on admission to emergency department

BOX 50.2   Strategies to Prevent Drowning

- Watch children. Toddlers are at greatest risk for drowning. Never leave small children unsupervised near water in which they might drown.
- Fence in all pools and swimming areas. Maintain the water level in a pool as high as possible to allow a person who reaches the edge to pull himself or herself out.
- Teach children to swim, but be advised that such teaching does not "drown-proof" a child. In other words, never let a small child out of your sight when he or she is near the water, even if the child knows how to swim. In a drowning situation, children may not have the body strength, judgment, or emotional reserve to allow self-rescue. Furthermore, new swimmers and children may have a false sense of security and take undue risks after being taught how to swim.
- Inflatable doughnuts, water wings, and pool rafts are not sufficiently effective safety devices to allow adults to leave children unsupervised.
- Never place nonswimmers in high-risk situations: small sailboats, whitewater rafts, inflatable kayaks, and the like. Do not allow nonswimmers to operate jet boats.
- In times of high surf and dangerous currents, stay out of the water. Know how to exit a rip tide.
- When boating or rafting, always wear a properly rated life vest with a snug fit and a head flotation collar. In a kayak or raft traversing white water, wear a proper helmet.
- Do not mix alcohol and water sports.
- Know your limits. Feats of endurance and demonstrations of bravado in dangerous rapids or surf are particularly risky.
- Be prepared for a flash flood. In times of unusually heavy rainfall, stay away from natural streambeds, arroyos, and other drainage channels. Use a map to determine your elevation, and stay off low ground or the very bottom of a hill. Know where the high ground is and how to get there in a hurry. Absolutely avoid flooded areas and unnecessary stream and river crossings. Do not attempt to cross a flowing stream where the water is above your knees. Abandon a stalled vehicle in a flood area.

department is of paramount importance for predicting survival with intact neurologic function. Persons who are alert when admitted seldom die.

PREVENTION

Prevention strategies are effective and crucial to the planning of any expedition near water (Box 50.2).

51

Scuba Diving–Related Disorders

Disorders related to scuba diving include those caused by environmental exposure (see Chapters 3 and 50), dysbarism, nitrogen narcosis, contaminated breathing gas, decompression sickness (DCS), and hazardous marine life (see Chapters 52 and 53; Box 51.1).

DYSBARISM

Dysbarism encompasses all the pathologic changes caused by altered environmental pressure. At sea level, atmospheric pressure is 760 mm Hg (14.7 psi), or 1 atmosphere (atm). Each 10-m (32.8-ft) descent under water increases the pressure by 1 atm. Gas in enclosed spaces obeys Boyle's law, which states that the pressure of a given quantity of gas when its temperature remains unchanged varies inversely with its volume.

BAROTRAUMA OF DESCENT

Mask Barotrauma

An air space is present between the face and the glass of a scuba (self-contained underwater breathing apparatus) diving mask. If nasal exhalations do not maintain air pressure within this space during descent, the volume of air contracts, creating negative pressure. This leads to capillary rupture, which is potentially dangerous after keratotomy because of the slow healing rate of corneal incisions.

Signs and Symptoms

- Skin ecchymoses in mask pattern
- Subconjunctival hemorrhage similar to strangulation injury
- Hyphema (rare)

Treatment

1. No treatment is necessary (unless hyphema is present) because the manifestations are self-limited.
2. Cold compresses can be used for analgesia.
3. Orbital hemorrhage is a rare complication and associated with diplopia, proptosis, and visual loss. Prompt referral should be made for magnetic resonance imaging and ophthalmologic care. Recompression therapy is not indicated.

Sinus Barotrauma

Sinus barotrauma, or "sinus squeeze," results from inability to inflate a paranasal sinus during descent, at which time contraction of the trapped air creates a relative vacuum. This damages the sinus wall

BOX 51.1 Medical Problems of Scuba Divers

Problems Related to Environmental Exposure
Motion sickness
Drowning
Hypothermia
Heat illness
Sunburn
Phototoxic and photoallergic reactions
Irritant and other dermatitis
Infectious diseases
Mechanical trauma

Disorders Related to Diving
Barotrauma
Arterial gas embolism
Decompression sickness
Dysbaric osteonecrosis
Dysbaric retinopathy
Immersion pulmonary edema
Shallow water blackout

Problems Related to Breathing Gas
Inert gas narcosis
Hypoxia
Oxygen toxicity
Hypercapnia
Carbon monoxide poisoning
Lipoid pneumonitis

Problems Related to Hazardous Marine Life (See Chapters 52 and 53)
Miscellaneous Problems
Hyperventilation
Hearing loss
Carotid sinus-related blackout
Panic and other psychological problems

mucosa, which ultimately hemorrhages. Less often, a "reverse sinus squeeze" can occur on ascent in the water because the expanding air cannot be vented from the sinus. The frontal sinus, followed by the maxillary sinus, is most commonly affected by barotrauma. With maxillary sinus involvement, the diver often experiences pain in the maxillary teeth caused by compression of the posterior superior branch of the fifth cranial nerve, which runs along the base of the maxillary sinus

Signs and Symptoms
- Pain in and over the affected sinus, with radiation like that seen with sinusitis (e.g., into the upper teeth with maxillary involvement)

- May be accompanied by epistaxis
- May develop bacterial sinusitis

Treatment

1. Give oral and topical decongestants (mucosal vasoconstrictors), such as pseudoephedrine and oxymetazoline.
2. Administer an analgesic as appropriate.
3. If an episode of sinus squeeze has occurred, particularly with epistaxis, and the patient subsequently develops symptoms of sinusitis (pain, fever, tenderness over the affected sinus, nasal discharge), administer an antibiotic, such as amoxicillin/clavulanate or azithromycin.

External Auditory Canal Barotrauma

A tight-fitting wet suit hood, earplugs, exostoses, or cerumen impaction can trap air in the external auditory canal. On descent, this air contracts in the enclosed space between the tympanic membrane and the (occluded) external opening of the ear.

Signs and Symptoms

- Pain, swelling, erythema, and petechiae or hemorrhagic blebs (bullae) of external ear canal wall
- Hemorrhage
- In severe cases, tympanic membrane rupturing outward

Treatment

1. If a remediable occlusion exists, correct it.
2. If inflammation of the external canal occurs without tympanic membrane rupture, instill eardrops suitable for the treatment of otitis externa (a fluoroquinolone combined with steroid) for 2 to 3 days.
3. If the tympanic membrane is perforated, seek otolaryngologic evaluation. Do not allow further diving until the membrane has healed. Instill fluoroquinolone otic drops for 2 to 3 days.
4. Do not incise bullae.

Middle Ear Barotrauma

If air cannot enter the middle ear via the (contracted or blocked) eustachian tube during an underwater descent, the existing air in the middle ear space contracts, creating a relative vacuum and pulling the tympanic membrane inward (Fig. 51.1).

Signs and Symptoms

- Initially, slight pain that progresses to severe pain with further underwater descent
- Hemorrhage in the tympanic membrane; ranges from erythema over the malleus to gross blood throughout the tympanic membrane; blood around the mouth and nose and hearing loss also possible
- If the tympanic membrane ruptures:

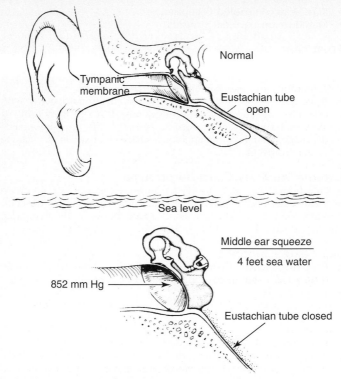

FIGURE 51.1   Middle Ear Trauma. Symptoms include feeling of "fullness" and pain caused by stretching of tympanic membrane.

- Sudden severe pain, accompanied by vertigo as water rushes into the middle ear
- Total hearing loss in the affected ear

Treatment

1. Before tympanic membrane rupture, administer an oral decongestant and a long-acting topical decongestant nasal spray, such as oxymetazoline. In a severe case, if the tympanic membrane is intact, a short course of prednisone (50 mg PO, tapered over 7 days) may be helpful. An antihistamine may be administered if there is an allergic component.
2. Repeated gentle autoinflation of the middle ear by use of the Valsalva or Frenzel maneuver may help displace any collection of middle ear fluid through the eustachian tube.
3. For tympanic membrane rupture, administer an antibiotic, such as amoxicillin/clavulanate, for 7 days. In addition, administer

fluoroquinolone otic drops. Suspend all diving activities until the tympanic membrane is fully healed or has been surgically repaired and eustachian tube function allows easy autoinflation.

Inner Ear Barotrauma

A serious but relatively unusual form of aural barotrauma is inner ear barotrauma in the form of labyrinthine window rupture. This is the most serious form of aural barotrauma because of possible injury to the cochleovestibular system, which may lead to permanent deafness or vestibular dysfunction.

Signs and Symptoms

- Tinnitus
- Vertigo
- Hearing loss
- Feeling of fullness or "blockage"
- Nausea and vomiting
- Nystagmus
- Pallor
- Diaphoresis
- Disorientation
- Ataxia

Treatment

1. Symptoms usually improve with time
2. Bed rest
3. Elevate head to 30 degrees
4. Avoid strenuous activity or straining
5. Good prognosis of recovery in 3 to 12 weeks
6. Deterioration of hearing, worsening vestibular symptoms, or persistent significant vestibular symptoms after a few days heralds the need for detailed otolaryngologic evaluation and possible surgical exploration and fistula closure.

Dental Barotrauma

Dental barotrauma, or barodontalgia (tooth squeeze), is caused by entrapped gas in the interior of a tooth or in the structures surrounding a tooth. The confined gas develops either positive or negative pressure relative to the ambient pressure, which places force on the surrounding sensitive dental structures.

Signs and Symptoms

- Tooth pain, with normal referral pathways
- Expulsion of a filling or crown; "exploding" or cracked tooth
- Imploded tooth

Treatment

1. Supply symptomatic and supportive therapy for the specific type of dental trauma.
2. Administer an analgesic.

Lung Squeeze

Lung squeeze is observed in a breath-hold diver who descends to a depth at which total lung volume is reduced to less than residual volume, which causes transpulmonic pressure to exceed intraalveolar pressure. This causes transudation of fluid or blood (from rupture of pulmonary capillaries) into the alveoli.

Signs and Symptoms
- Shortness of breath, cough, hemoptysis
- In severe cases, pulmonary edema

Treatment
1. Administer oxygen, 5 to 15 L/min, by nonrebreather mask.
2. Suspend all diving activities.

BAROTRAUMA OF ASCENT

Reverse Sinus or Ear Barotrauma (Reverse Squeeze)

The sinuses and ears are subject to barotrauma during ascent as well as descent. As the ambient pressure drops, the volume of the gas within the sinus or ear cavities expands, causing pain and tissue damage if not released. Gas pressure can exceed intravascular pressure in adjacent tissue, causing local ischemia. In the sinuses, a cyst or polyp can act as a one-way valve; air enters the sinus as the diver descends but cannot escape as the diver ascends. Signs, symptoms, and treatment are the same as with sinus and ear barotrauma of descent.

Facial Baroparesis (Alternobaric Facial Palsy)

The seventh cranial nerve courses through the middle ear and mastoid process via a bony channel. Parts of the nerve may be directly exposed to middle ear pressures through a defect in the canal wall. During ascent, if the eustachian tube mucosa is swollen due to irritation, infection, or allergy, middle ear pressure may exceed capillary pressure supplying the facial nerve and cause ischemic neurapraxia.

Signs and Symptoms
- Ear fullness and pain after surfacing
- Facial palsy
- Difficulty closing eye on the affected side

Treatment
1. Toynbee maneuver to release middle ear overpressure
2. Oral and topical decongestants
3. Persistent and severe symptoms may be treated with myringotomy to prevent permanent damage.

Gastrointestinal Barotrauma

Expanding intestinal gas can become trapped in the gastrointestinal tract during ascent and cause gastrointestinal barotrauma. Divers with gastrointestinal barotrauma typically complain of abdominal fullness, colicky abdominal pain, belching, and flatulence. Gastrointestinal barotrauma is most often self-remedied by elimination of the excess gas. Hyperbaric treatment may be necessary in very rare, severe cases.

Pulmonary Barotrauma

Pulmonary barotrauma of ascent results from expansion of gas trapped in the lungs, which ruptures alveoli or is forced across the pulmonary capillary membrane.

Signs and Symptoms

- History of rapid and uncontrolled ascent to the surface before onset of symptoms; history of breath-holding during ascent
- Pneumomediastinum: gradually increasing hoarseness or "brassy" voice, neck fullness, and/or substernal chest pain several hours after diving
- Subcutaneous emphysema (crepitus)
- In severe cases, chest pain, dyspnea, bloody sputum, dysphagia
- Syncope
- Pneumothorax
  - Pleuritic chest pain, breathlessness, dyspnea
  - With tension pneumothorax, progressive respiratory difficulty, cyanosis, distended neck veins, hyperresonant chest percussion, tracheal shift, absent or diminished breath sounds

Treatment

1. For pneumomediastinum, administer supplemental oxygen, 5 to 15 L/min, by nonrebreather mask. Have the patient rest.
2. For pneumothorax, administer supplemental oxygen, 5 to 15 L/min, by nonrebreather mask.
   a. Observe the patient closely for worsening condition.
   b. Be prepared to insert a thoracostomy (chest) tube or a decompression catheter with flutter valve.

Arterial Gas Embolism

Arterial gas embolism (AGE) results from air bubbles entering the pulmonary venous circulation from ruptured alveoli. These gas bubbles travel into the heart, from where they may be distributed to the coronary and carotid arteries. Arterial gas embolism typically develops immediately after a diver surfaces. Approximately 4% of divers who suffer AGE die immediately, presenting with sudden loss of consciousness, pulselessness, and apnea.

Signs and Symptoms

Sudden loss of consciousness upon surfacing from a dive should be considered an indication of air embolism until proved otherwise. There is a broad differential diagnosis for unconsciousness in divers (Box 51.2).

- Cardiac: chest pain related to myocardial ischemia, arrhythmias, or cardiac arrest
- Neurologic

BOX 51.2   Causes of Unconsciousness in Divers

Breath-Hold Divers
Underwater hypoxemia after hyperventilation before the dive
  (shallow water blackout)
Drowning

Divers Using Compressed-Gas Equipment
Hypoxic breathing gas
Contaminated breathing gas (e.g., carbon monoxide)
Equipment failure or empty breathing tank
Drowning
Inert gas narcosis
Oxygen toxicity
Pulmonary barotrauma with arterial gas embolism

Divers Using Rebreathing Equipment
Carbon dioxide toxicity
Oxygen toxicity
Hypoxia

- Possibly confusing pattern, because showers of bubbles randomly embolize the cerebral circulation
- Manifestations are often typical of an acute stroke (cerebrovascular accident), although hemiplegia is infrequent.
- Most often observed signs: loss of consciousness, monoplegia or asymmetric multiplegia, focal paralysis, paresthesias or other sensory disturbances, convulsions, aphasia, confusion, blindness or other visual field defects, vertigo, dizziness, headache
- Sharply circumscribed areas of glossal pallor (rare)

Treatment

1. Transport the patient for recompression treatment in a hyperbaric (oxygen) chamber.
   a. If an aircraft is used, do not expose the patient to significant cabin altitude. Ideally the aircraft will be pressurized to sea level.
   b. In an unpressurized aircraft, maintain the flying altitude as low as possible, not to exceed 305 m (1000 ft) above sea level.
2. Contact the Diver's Alert Network (DAN) to assist with locating the nearest hyperbaric chamber and coordinating resources.
   a. DAN hotline number is 919-684-9111.
   b. Maintain the patient in a supine position.
3. Administer oxygen at 15 L/min by nonrebreather mask.
4. Begin an intravenous infusion of isotonic solution to maintain urine output at 1 to 2 mL/kg/hr.
5. Current evidence does not support the use of IV lidocaine as an adjunct to recompression treatment for AGE.

NITROGEN NARCOSIS

Nitrogen narcosis is development of intoxication as an anesthetic effect as the partial pressure of nitrogen in inspired compressed air increases with depth.

Signs and Symptoms

- Usually becomes apparent at depths between 21 and 31 m (68.9 and 101.7 ft)
- Light-headedness, loss of fine sensory discrimination, giddiness, euphoria
- Progressively worsening symptoms at greater depths
  - When deeper than 46 m (150.9 ft): severe intoxication, manifested by increasingly poor judgment and impaired reasoning, overconfidence, and slowed reflexes
  - At depths of 76 to 91 m (249.3 to 298.6 ft): auditory and visual hallucinations, feeling of impending blackout
  - By 122 m (400.3 ft): loss of consciousness

Treatment

Have the patient safely ascend to a shallower depth until symptoms resolve.

OXYGEN TOXICITY

Oxygen toxicity in divers can affect either the CNS or pulmonary system. Inspired high PO_2 occurs in diving by breathing oxygen-enriched gas mixtures that are commonly used for mixed-gas "technical" diving. The most common clinical manifestation of pulmonary oxygen toxicity is substernal discomfort during inhalation. Reduction of inspired PO_2 to 0.21 to 0.5 ATA usually results in prompt relief. CNS symptoms may include diaphoresis, nausea, muscle or limb jerking, tunnel vision, diaphragmatic flutter, and/ or seizures.

CONTAMINATED BREATHING GAS

The pressurized air within a scuba tank may be contaminated with oil or carbon monoxide.

Signs and Symptoms

- With oil contamination: cough, shortness of breath, oily taste in mouth
- With carbon monoxide contamination: headache, nausea, dizziness during the dive
  - Examination at the surface: lethargy, mental dullness, non-specific neurologic deficits
  - May be confused with those accompanying DCS (see next) or air embolism (see earlier)

Treatment

Administer oxygen, 5 to 15 L/min, by nonrebreather mask.

DECOMPRESSION SICKNESS

DCS is caused by formation of bubbles of inert gas (typically nitrogen) within the intravascular and extravascular spaces after a reduction in ambient pressure. Symptoms of DCS are often catego rized into type I and type II, with type I referring to mild forms of DCS (cutaneous, lymphatic, and musculoskeletal) and type II including neurologic and other serious forms. Some investigators have advocated use of the term type III DCS to refer to combined arterial gas embolism and DCS with neurologic symptoms.

Signs and Symptoms
- Symptoms are highly variable (Table 51.1), neurologic and musculoskeletal systems are most often affected.
- Symptoms developing in the first hour after surfacing from a dive, with some patients noticing symptoms within 6 hours after diving; rarely, symptoms not noted until 24 to 48 hours after diving

Treatment
1. Transport the patient for recompression treatment in a hyperbaric (oxygen) chamber.
   a. If an aircraft is used, do not expose the patient to significant cabin altitude. Ideally, the aircraft will be pressurized to sea level.
   b. In an unpressurized aircraft, maintain the flying altitude as low as possible, not to exceed 305 m (1000 ft) above sea level.
2. Contact the DAN to assist with locating the closest hyperbaric chamber and coordinating resources.
   a. DAN hotline number is 919-684-9111.
   b. Maintain the patient in a supine position.
3. Administer oxygen at 10 L/min by nonrebreather mask.
4. Begin an intravenous infusion of isotonic solution to maintain urine output at 1 to 2 mL/kg/hr.

Although experimental proof of their efficacy is lacking, high-dose parenteral corticosteroids were widely used in the past as an adjunct to recompression treatment of both neurologic DCS and AGE. Nonsteroidal anti-inflammatory drugs (NSAIDs) and aspirin are not routinely recommended as adjuncts for treatment of DCS.

FLYING AFTER DIVING

Flying too soon after diving can seriously jeopardize safety, leading to development of DCS during or after the flight because of the reduced atmospheric pressure present in most commercial aircraft.
- Observe a minimum surface interval of 12 hours between the last dive and flying in a commercial jet.
- Divers who make daily, multiple dives for several days or who make dives that require decompression stops are advised to

Table 51.1 Common Symptoms and Signs of Decompression Sickness

CONDITION	SYMPTOMS	SIGNS
Musculoskeletal decompression sickness, limb bends	Severe joint pain, single joint or multiple joints involved, paresthesia or dysesthesia around the joint, lymphedema (uncommon)	Tenderness, which may be temporarily relieved by local pressure with a blood pressure cuff; pain worsened by movement of the joint
Neurologic decompression sickness		
Spinal cord	Back pain, girdling abdominal pain, extremity heaviness or weakness, paralysis, paresthesia of extremities, fecal incontinence, urine retention	Hyperesthesia or hypoesthesia, paresis, anal sphincter weakness, loss of bulbocavernosus reflex, urinary bladder distention
Brain	Visual loss, scotomata, headache, dysphasia, confusion	Visual field deficit, spotty motor or sensory deficits, disorientation or mental dullness
Fatigue	Profound generalized heaviness or fatigue	May precede signs of other forms
Cutaneous manifestations	Intense pruritus	No visible signs, mottling, local or generalized hyperemia, or marbled skin (cutis marmorata)
"Chokes"	Dyspnea, substernal pain that is worsened on deep inhalation, nonproductive cough	Cyanosis, tachypnea, tachycardia
Vasomotor decompression sickness (decompression shock)	Weakness, sweating, unconsciousness	Hypotension, tachycardia, pallor, mottling, hemoconcentration, decreased urine output
Inner ear (vestibular) decompression sickness	Tinnitus, vertigo, nausea, vomiting	Ataxia, possible nystagmus and positive Romberg test, acute sensorineural hearing loss

attempt to attain an interval of at least 18 hours between diving and flying. However, it is prudent to extend the interval to 24 hours or longer to minimize the risk for DCS.

ABSOLUTE CONTRAINDICATIONS FOR DIVING

The following conditions are felt to be absolute contraindications for diving:

- History of spontaneous pneumothorax
- Acute asthma with abnormal pulmonary function
- Cystic or cavitary lung disease
- Obstructive or restrictive lung disease
- Seizure disorder
- Atrial septal defect
- Symptomatic coronary artery disease
- Chronic perforated tympanic membrane
- Chronic inability to equalize sinus and/or middle ear
- Intraorbital gas
- Pregnancy
- Sickle cell disease
- Meniere disease

52

Injuries From Nonvenomous Aquatic Animals

Sharks, barracuda, moray eels, needlefish, and coral present typical dangers of wounds and infections to persons venturing into the ocean. The injuries range from bites or stings to cuts, impalements, and abrasions.

GENERAL TREATMENT
Wound Management

1. If the bill or spine of an animal is seen to be lodged in the patient and has penetrated deeply into the chest, abdomen, neck, femoral region, or popliteal space and may have violated a critical blood vessel or the heart, it should be managed as would be a weapon of impalement (e.g., a knife). In this case, the impaling object should be left in place if possible and secured from motion until the patient is brought to a controlled operating room environment where emergency surgery can be performed to guide its extraction and control bleeding that may occur upon its removal.

2. Irrigate all wounds with a sterile diluent, preferably normal saline (NS) solution. Seawater is not recommended because it carries a hypothetical risk for infection. Use disinfected potable or tap water if NS solution is not available.

   a. Note that proper irrigation technique involves using a 19-gauge needle or 18-gauge plastic IV catheter attached to a syringe to deliver a pressure of 10 to 20 psi.

   b. Flush a minimum of 100 to 250 mL of irrigant through each wound.

   c. If the wound was caused by a stingray, stonefish, scorpion fish, or lionfish, warm the irrigant to 45°C (113°F; see Chapter 53).

3. Add an antiseptic to the irrigation fluid. Add concentrated povidone-iodine solution (not "scrub") to the irrigant to achieve a final concentration of 1% to 5%. Allow a contact time of 1 to 5 minutes. After irrigation with the antiseptic-containing solution, thoroughly irrigate the wound with unadulterated NS solution.

4. With a coral cut or abrasion, scrub the area to remove debris that cannot be irrigated from the wound.

5. Remove any crushed or devitalized tissue using sharp dissection.

6. In the field, perform wound closure using the technique that is least constrictive and therefore less prone to trap bacteria, which could initiate a wound infection. From an infection risk perspective, unless wound preparation equivalent to that achieved in a hospital is undertaken, it is often better to approximate the wound edges with adhesive strips or loosely placed sutures

than to perform a tight approximation of the margins (see Chapter 20).
7. At the earliest sign of wound infection, release sufficient fasteners to allow prompt and thorough drainage from the wound. Initiate antibiotic therapy.
8. Administer appropriate tetanus prophylaxis.

Antibiotic Therapy

The following recommendations are based on the malignant potential of soft tissue infections caused by *Vibrio* (sea water) or *Aeromonas* (natural freshwater) species.
1. Be aware that minor abrasions or lacerations (e.g., coral cuts, superficial sea urchin puncture wounds) do not require prophylactic antibiotics in a person with normal immunity. However, for persons who are chronically ill (e.g., diabetes, hemophilia, thalassemia), are immunologically impaired (e.g., leukemia, AIDS, chemotherapy, prolonged corticosteroid therapy), or have serious liver disease (e.g., hepatitis, cirrhosis, hemochromatosis), particularly those with elevated serum iron levels, immediately begin a regimen of oral ciprofloxacin, trimethoprim/sulfamethoxazole (co-trimoxazole), or tetracycline/doxycycline. Note that penicillin, ampicillin, amoxicillin, and erythromycin are not acceptable alternatives. Although other quinolones have not been extensively tested against *Vibrio* species, they may be useful alternatives.
2. Note that the appearance of an infection indicates the need for prompt débridement and antibiotic therapy. If an infection develops, choose antibiotic coverage that will also be efficacious against *Staphylococcus* and *Streptococcus* species. Vancomycin is recommended in the event of methicillin resistance.
3. From an infection perspective, consider the following as serious injuries: large lacerations, extensive or deep burns, deep puncture wounds, and a retained foreign body.
   a. These injuries may be caused by shark, barracuda or other fish bites, stingray spine wounds, impalement by a fish bill, any spine puncture that enters a joint space, and full-thickness coral cuts.
   b. If the patient will require hospitalization for any of these serious injuries and intravenous antibiotics are accessible, the recommended drugs for prophylaxis include gentamicin, tobramycin, amikacin, and trimethoprim-sulfamethoxazole. Cefoperazone, cefotaxime, and ceftazidime may not be effective; if they are used, they should be combined with another agent listed or with tetracycline.
4. Manage infected wounds with antibiotics as noted earlier, with consideration of adding imipenem-cilastatin or meropenem for severe, progressive infections and sepsis.
5. If a wound infection is minor and has the appearance of a classic erysipeloid reaction (*Erysipelothrix rhusiopathiae*; see Plate 34), penicillin, cephalexin, or ciprofloxacin should be administered.

INJURIES CAUSED BY SHARKS AND BARRACUDA
Treatment
1. Control active hemorrhage with pressure if possible. If necessary, ligate large disrupted vessels.
2. Insert at least two large-bore intravenous lines. Obtain intraosseous access as needed.
3. Keep the patient well oxygenated and warm.
4. Transport the patient to a proper emergency facility equipped to handle major trauma and appropriate surgical management of the wounds.
5. If the wound is more than minor, administer a prophylactic antibiotic (see earlier).
6. Manage abrasions caused by contact with shark skin as if they were second-degree burns. Cleanse the wound thoroughly; then apply a thin layer of mupirocin (Bactroban) or bacitracin ointment, or silver sulfadiazine cream under a sterile dressing.

Prevention of Shark Attacks
1. Avoid shark-inhabited water, particularly at dawn, dusk, and night.
2. Do not swim through schools of bait fish in the presence of sharks.
3. Do not enter waters posted with shark warnings.
4. Do not wander into the ocean too far from shore.
5. Do not swim with animals (e.g., dogs or horses) in shark-inhabited waters.
6. Photograph hazardous sharks from within the confines of a protective cage.
7. Swimmers should remain in groups.
8. Avoid turbid water, drop-offs, deep channels, inlets, mouths of rivers, and sanitation waste outlets.
9. Do not swim in waters frequented by recreational or commercial fishers.
10. Do not swim in water that has been recently churned up by a storm.
11. Be alert when crossing sandbars.
12. Do not enter the water with an open wound, particularly if it is bleeding.
13. Do not dive during menses (controversial).
14. Do not wear flashy metal objects.
15. Do not dive or swim in the presence of spear fishermen. Do not carry captured fish. Tether captured fish at a sufficient distance from divers.
16. Be alert when schools of fish behave in an erratic manner or when pods of porpoises cluster more tightly or head toward shore.
17. Do not tease or corner a shark.
18. Do not splash on the surface or create a commotion in the water.

19. If a shark appears in shallow water, swimmers should leave the water with slow, purposeful movements, facing the shark if possible and avoiding erratic behavior that could be interpreted as distress.

MORAY EEL INJURY

Morays are forceful and vicious biters that can inflict severe puncture wounds with their narrow and vise-like jaws, which are equipped with long, sharp, retrorse, and fang-like teeth.

Treatment

1. Explore each wound to locate any retained teeth.
2. Irrigate each wound copiously.
3. Because the risk for infection is high, do not suture any puncture wound unless it is necessary temporarily to control hemorrhage.
4. If the wound is extensive and more linear in configuration (resembling a dog bite), débride the wound edges and loosely approximate them with nonabsorbable sutures or staples.
5. Administer a prophylactic antibiotic (see earlier).

SEA LION BITE

"Seal finger" follows a bite wound from a seal or sea lion or from contact of even a minor skin wound with the animal's mouth or pelt. The signs and symptoms include an incubation period of 1 to 15 (typically 4) days, followed by painful swelling of the digit, with or without joint involvement. Severe pain may precede the appearance of the initial furuncle, swelling, or stiffness. As the lesion worsens, the skin becomes taut and shiny and the entire hand may swell and take on a brownish-violet hue (see Plate 35). *Mycoplasma* species may be the inciting pathogens. The treatment is tetracycline 1.5 g PO initially, followed by 500 mg PO q6h for 4 to 6 weeks. Fluoroquinolone or macrolide antibiotics may be useful if tetracycline is not available.

NEEDLEFISH INJURY AND OTHER IMPALEMENTS

The pointed snout (teeth) of a needlefish that leaps from the water can penetrate into a human victim, creating a stab wound with a residual foreign body (the fish). Other fishes, such as sailfish and marlin, may also impale human victims.

Signs and Symptoms

Stab wound that may contain a foreign body

Treatment

1. If the bill or spine of an animal is seen to be lodged in the patient and has penetrated deeply into the chest, abdomen, neck, femoral region, or popliteal space, and may have violated a critical blood vessel or the heart, it should be managed as would be a weapon of impalement (e.g., a knife). In this case, the impaling object should be left in place if possible and

secured from motion until the patient is brought to a controlled operating room environment where emergency surgery can be performed to guide its extraction and control bleeding that may occur upon its removal.

2. Be aware that the major risk is wound infection caused by the retained organic material. Another risk is vascular injury.

3. Cleanse the wound thoroughly; then débride and dress it.

4. If the wound is more than superficial, administer a prophylactic antibiotic (see earlier). If the distal circulation is impeded, undertake immediate evacuation.

CORAL CUTS AND ABRASIONS
Signs and Symptoms
- Initial reactions: stinging pain, erythema, pruritus
- Break in skin surrounded within minutes by erythematous wheal, which fades over 1 to 2 hours
- Red, raised welts and local pruritus accompanied by low-grade fever and malaise, known as "coral poisoning"
- Progresses to cellulitis with ulceration and tissue sloughing
- Healing over 3 to 6 weeks, with prolonged morbidity
- Lymphangitis and reactive bursitis also seen

Treatment
1. Promptly and vigorously scrub the wound with soap and water, and then irrigate copiously to remove all foreign material.

2. If the wound is difficult to scrub and clean, hydrogen peroxide may be used to try to bubble out tiny particles of organic material deposited from the surface of the coral. Follow with a thorough NS solution or tap water irrigation.

3. If a stinging sensation is prominent, be aware that envenomation may have occurred. Briefly rinse the area with diluted (half-strength or 2.5%) household vinegar to diminish discomfort. Follow with a thorough NS solution or tap water irrigation.

4. If a coral-induced laceration is severe, close it with adhesive strips rather than sutures, if possible, because the margins of the wound are likely to become inflamed and necrotic. Be aware that serial débridement may become necessary.

5. To achieve a bed of healing tissue, apply twice-daily, sterile, wet-to-dry dressings using NS solution or a dilute antiseptic (e.g., povidone-iodine 1% to 5%). Alternatively, use a nontoxic topical antiseptic ointment (e.g., bacitracin, mupirocin, polymyxin B-bacitracin-neomycin) sparingly and cover the wound with a nonadherent dressing.

6. Be aware that despite the best efforts at primary irrigation and decontamination, the wound may heal slowly, with moderate to severe soft tissue inflammation and ulcer formation. Débride all devitalized tissue regularly using sharp dissection. Continue this regimen until healthy granulation tissue is formed.

7. Treat any wound that appears infected with an antibiotic (see earlier).

Interactions with various forms of marine life can result in stings and puncture wounds that lead to envenomation or anaphylactic reactions.

ANAPHYLAXIS

For signs, symptoms, and treatment of anaphylactic reactions, see Chapter 26.

REACTION TO SPONGES

Sponges (see Plate 36) are stationary animals that attach to the sea floor or coral beds. Embedded in their connective tissue matrices are spicules of silicon dioxide or calcium carbonate. Other chemical toxins and secondary coelenterate (stinging) inhabitants contribute to the skin irritation and systemic manifestations that result from dermal contact.

Signs and Symptoms

- *Within a few hours after contact:* burning and itching of the skin, sometimes progressing to local joint swelling and stiffness, soft tissue edema, and blistering
  - Skin becoming mottled or purpuric in appearance
  - If untreated, subsidence of minor reaction in 3 to 7 days; major reaction may require weeks to resolve
- *With involvement of large areas of skin:* fever, chills, malaise, dizziness, nausea, muscle cramps, and formication
  - Bullae becoming purulent
  - Surface skin desquamation after 10 days

Treatment

1. Gently dry the skin.
2. To remove embedded microscopic spicules, apply sticky adhesive tape, a commercial facial peel, or a thin layer of rubber cement; then peel away the adherent spicules.
3. Apply a 5% acetic acid (vinegar) soak for 10 to 30 minutes three or four times a day. If vinegar is not available, use isopropyl alcohol 40%. Do not use a topical steroid preparation as the primary (initial) decontaminant because this may worsen the reaction.
4. After decontamination and at least two vinegar applications, use a mild antiinflammatory cream (e.g., hydrocortisone or triamcinolone) to soothe the skin.

5. If the allergic component is mild, apply a topical steroid preparation. If the allergic component is severe, as manifested by weeping, crusting, and vesiculation, administer a systemic corticosteroid (e.g., prednisone, 60 to 100 mg, tapered over 14 days).
6. Perform frequent follow-up wound checks because significant infections sometimes develop. Culture infected wounds and administer antibiotics (see Chapter 52).
7. Erythema multiforme or dyshidrotic eczema may be treated with oral prednisone, 60 to 100 mg, tapered over 2 to 3 weeks.

Prevention
1. Ensure that all divers and net handlers wear proper gloves.
2. Do not allow sponges to be broken, crumbled, or crushed with bare hands.
3. Be aware that dried sponges may remain toxic.

JELLYFISH STINGS (ALSO FIRE CORAL, HYDROIDS, AND ANEMONES)
These creatures sting with a variation of the microscopic stinging cell, the nematocyst, which is stimulated to fire its venom-bearing injector into the victim by physical contact, hypotonicity, or chemical stimulation. An encounter with a single long-tentacle can simultaneously trigger hundreds of thousands of stinging cells.

Signs and Symptoms
- *Skin irritation:* stinging, pruritus, paresthesias, burning, throbbing, redness, tentacle prints, impression patterns (see Plate 37), blistering, local edema, petechial hemorrhages, skin ulceration, necrosis, and secondary infection
- *Neurologic:* malaise, headache, aphonia, diminished touch and temperature sensation, vertigo, ataxia, spastic or flaccid paralysis, mononeuritis multiplex, parasympathetic dysautonomia, plexopathy, peripheral nerve palsy, delirium, loss of consciousness, and coma
- *Cardiovascular:* anaphylaxis, hemolysis, hypotension, small artery spasm, bradycardia, tachycardia, congestive heart failure, and ventricular fibrillation
- *Respiratory:* rhinitis, bronchospasm, laryngeal edema, dyspnea, cyanosis, pulmonary edema, and respiratory failure
- *Musculoskeletal:* abdominal rigidity, myalgias, muscle cramps/ spasm, arthralgia, and arthritis
- *Gastrointestinal:* nausea, vomiting, diarrhea, dysphagia, hypersalivation, and thirst
- *Ocular:* conjunctivitis, chemosis, corneal ulcer, iridocyclitis, elevated intraocular pressure, and lacrimation
- *Other:* chills, fever, acute renal failure, and nightmares

Treatment

1. For systemic reactions:
   a. Maintain the airway and administer oxygen.
   b. Obtain intravenous access. Administer lactated Ringer's solution or normal saline solution to support the blood pressure to at least 90 mm Hg systolic.
   c. Treat anaphylaxis if present (see Chapter 26).
   d. If the sting is from the box jellyfish *(Chironex fleckeri)* (see Plates 38 and 39) or severe and from the sea wasp *(Chirop-salmus quadrigatus)*, consider immediate administration of *C. fleckeri* antivenom. Administer this in a dose of one ampule (20,000 units per ampule) IV diluted 1:5 to 1:10 in isotonic crystalloid. A large sting in an adult may require the initial administration of two ampules. Alternatively, administer this in a dose of three ampules intramuscularly into the thigh. Antivenom administration may be repeated once or twice every 2 to 4 hours until there is no further worsening of the reaction (skin discoloration, pain, or systemic effects).
   e. If the sting is from the Irukandji *(Carukia barnesi)*, hypertension from catecholamine stimulation may be severe. If necessary, administer an α-adrenergic blocking agent (phentolamine, 5 mg IV initially, followed by an infusion of up to 10 mg/hr). Magnesium sulfate (loading dose 10 mmol = 2.5 g = 20 mEq followed by an infusion of 5 mmol/hr) might be helpful.
   f. Authorities no longer recommend the pressure immobilization technique to treat a box jellyfish sting or any other jellyfish sting.
2. For dermatitis:
   a. If possible, apply a topical decontaminant immediately (described in step d, later). If more than 1 or 2 minutes will elapse before the application of the decontaminant, rinse the wound with seawater. Do not rinse gently with freshwater; if freshwater is to be used, the stream must be forceful (e.g., jet stream from a shower or hose).
   b. Hot packs or showers to tolerance (45°C [113°F]) may be more effective than dry, (nonmoist), cold (insulated ice) packs.
   c. Do not rub or abrade the wound.
   d. If these have been done, apply a topical decontaminant. The efficacy may vary depending on the stinging species.
      • Acetic acid 5% (vinegar) is the decontaminant of choice with a box jellyfish *(C. fleckeri)* sting.
      • For other stings, diminish the pain using vinegar, isopropyl (rubbing) alcohol 40%, sodium bicarbonate (baking soda), papain (papaya latex or nonseasoned meat tenderizer, the latter in a brief [<15 minutes] application), or lidocaine. Other substances that may be effective include sugar or olive oil, or lemon or lime juice. Household ammonia may irritate skin and is not recommended. Urinating on the sting is generally not helpful. A sting from the Australian

Physalia physalis, a recently differentiated species, should not be doused with vinegar.
- Do not apply a solvent (e.g., formalin, ether, gasoline).
- Perfume, aftershave, or high-proof liquor may worsen the skin reaction.

  e. After decontamination, remove the adherent nematocysts. Apply shaving cream or a paste of soap or baking soda, flour, or talc, and shave the area with a razor or other sharp edge.
  f. Apply a local anesthetic ointment or mild steroid preparation to soothe the skin.
  g. If the reaction is severe, administer a systemic corticosteroid (e.g., prednisone, 60 to 100 mg, tapered over 14 days).
  h. Pain control may require narcotic administration (see Chapter 24).
  i. Inspect the wound regularly for ulceration and the onset of infection.
  j. Administer tetanus prophylaxis.
3. If the eye is involved, it should be anesthetized with proparacaine 0.5% and irrigated to 100 to 250 mL of normal saline to remove foreign matter. Slit lamp examination and fluorescein staining to identify corneal defects are recommended.

Prevention
1. Give all jellyfish a wide berth when swimming or diving.
2. Wear a "stinger suit" when immersed in jellyfish-infested water.
3. When diving, scan for surface concentrations of stinging animals.
4. If "stinger enclosures" are present, do not venture beyond their confines.
5. Consider the use of a topical skin protective preparation such as Safe Sea (jellyfish-safe sunblock).

SEA BATHER'S ERUPTION
Sea bather's eruption, commonly misnomered "sea lice," predominantly involves covered areas of the body and has been attributed to stings from the microscopic larvae of certain jellyfish and anemones.

Signs and Symptoms
- Stinging of the skin while still in the water or immediately on exiting; may be intensified by the application of fresh water
- Skin redness, papules (see Plate 40), urticaria, and blisters minutes to 12 hours after exposure
  - Most common areas: buttocks, genitals, and under breasts (women)
  - Individual lesions resembling insect bites
  - Also seen under bathing caps and swim fins and along the edge of the cuffs of wet suits
- Fever, chills, headache, fatigue, malaise, vomiting, conjunctivitis, and urethritis

Treatment

1. Apply a topical decontaminant. Acetic acid 5% (vinegar) seems to be less effective than papain. Otherwise, scrub thoroughly with soap and water. A lidocaine-containing preparation may be helpful.
2. After decontamination, apply calamine lotion with 1% menthol to control itching. A high-potency topical corticosteroid preparation may be of benefit.
3. If the reaction is severe, administer a systemic corticosteroid (e.g., prednisone, 60 to 100 mg, tapered over 14 days).

STARFISH PUNCTURE

The most common venomous starfish (Fig. 53.1) have glandular tissue interspersed underneath the epidermis that covers the rigid spines, which may attain a length of 4 to 6 cm (1.6 to 2.4 inches). The envenomation occurs when a spine punctures the skin.

Signs and Symptoms

- Intense pain, bleeding, local soft tissue edema
- With multiple stings: paresthesias, nausea, vomiting, lymphadenopathy, muscular paralysis

Treatment

1. Immerse the wound in nonscalding, hot water to tolerance (45°C [113°F]) for 30 to 90 minutes or until there is significant pain relief.
2. Remove any obvious spine fragments. Do not attempt to crush remaining fragments.
3. Observe closely for subsequent wound infection.
4. Consider prophylactic antibiotics (see Chapter 52).

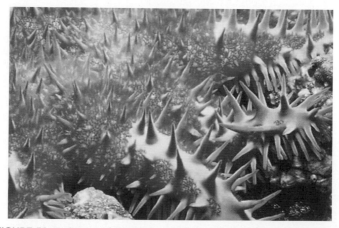

FIGURE 53.1   **Spines of the Crown-of-Thorns Starfish** (*Acanthaster planci*). (Courtesy Paul Auerbach, MD.)

SEA URCHIN SPINE PUNCTURE OR ENVENOMATION BY PEDICELLARIAE

Sea urchins envenom their victims in one of two ways: (1) puncture wound by sharp, venom-bearing spine(s), or (2) inoculation of venom via the venom gland in the base of flower-like, stalked pincer organs (globiferous pedicellariae) (Fig. 53.2).

Signs and Symptoms

- Intense pain, burning, local muscle aching, erythema, soft tissue edema, and black or purple tattoos (see Plate 41) at the sites of spine punctures
- Malaise, weakness, arthralgias, aphonia, dizziness, syncope, generalized muscular paralysis, respiratory distress, and hypotension

Treatment

1. Immerse the wound in nonscalding, hot water to tolerance (45°C [113°F]) for 30 to 90 minutes or until there is significant pain relief.
2. Remove any obvious spine fragments. Do not attempt to crush remaining fragments. If spines are felt to remain within the patient near a joint, splint the affected limb.
3. Dark (typically gray or blue) discoloration in the skin at the puncture sites may not be retained spines. This may be spine dye leached from the spines. Do not dig into the skin attempting to locate a spine. If a spine is not easily felt from the surface,

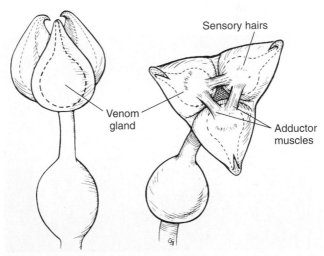

FIGURE 53.2 **Globiferous Pedicellariae of Sea Urchin Used to Hold and Envenom Prey.**

wait 24 hours to see if the dye is absorbed and the marking disappears. This usually means that a spine is not present.
4. If pedicellariae are attached, apply shaving foam and scrape them away with a razor.
5. Observe closely for subsequent wound infection.
6. Consider prophylactic antibiotics (see Chapter 52).

SEA CUCUMBER IRRITATION

Sea cucumbers are worm- or sausage-shaped bottom feeders (Fig. 53.3). They produce in their body walls a visceral cantharidin-like toxin that is concentrated in tentacular organs that can be projected and extended anally when the animal mounts a defense.

Signs and Symptoms
- Contact dermatitis when the tentacular organs contact the skin
- Corneal and conjunctival irritation from contact with the tentacles or high concentrations of the toxin
- Toxin is a potent cardiac glycoside and may cause severe illness or death if ingested

Treatment
1. Wash the skin with soap and water.
2. Because sea cucumbers may feed on stinging cells of jellyfish, initial skin detoxication should include topical application of 5% acetic acid (vinegar), papain, or 40% isopropyl alcohol.
3. If the eye is involved, it should be anesthetized with proparacaine 0.5% and irrigated with 100 to 250 mL of normal saline to remove foreign matter. Slit lamp examination and fluorescein staining are recommended to identify corneal defects.

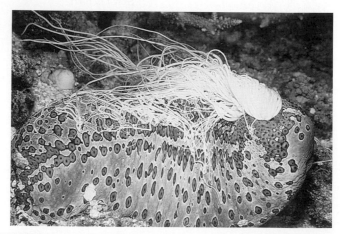

FIGURE 53.3 **Extruded Tentacular Organs of Cuvier From Within a Sea Cucumber.** (Courtesy Paul Auerbach, MD.)

BRISTLEWORM IRRITATION

Certain segmented marine worms have chitinous bristles arranged in soft rows around the body (see Plate 42). These are dislodged into the human victim when a worm is handled.

Signs and Symptoms
- Burning sensation, raised red urticarial rash, papular dermatitis, soft tissue edema, and pruritus

Treatment
1. Remove all large visible bristles using forceps.
2. Dry the skin gently.
3. To remove embedded spines, apply sticky adhesive tape, a commercial facial peel, or a thin layer of rubber cement; then peel away the adherent spines.
4. Apply acetic acid 5% (vinegar), isopropyl alcohol 40%, or a paste of unseasoned meat tenderizer for 10 to 15 minutes to achieve pain relief.
5. Apply a thin layer of a topical corticosteroid preparation.
6. If the reaction is severe, administer a systemic corticosteroid (e.g., prednisone, 60 to 100 mg, tapered over 14 days).

CONE SHELL (SNAIL) STING

These cone-shaped shelled mollusks intoxicate their victims by injecting rapid-acting venom by means of a detachable, dart-like radular tooth (Fig. 53.4).

Signs and Symptoms
- Mild sting (puncture) that resembles a bee or wasp sting
- Alternative initial symptoms: localized ischemia, cyanosis, numbness in the area around the wound

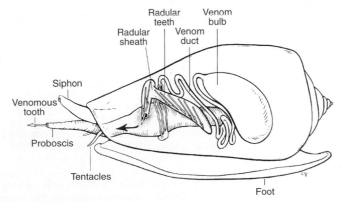

FIGURE 53.4 Venom Apparatus of Cone Shell.

- More serious envenomations: paresthesias at wound site, which become perioral and then generalized
- Dysphagia, nausea, syncope, weakness, areflexia, aphonia, diplopia, blurred vision, pruritus, disseminated intravascular coagulation, generalized muscular paralysis leading to respiratory failure, cardiac failure, and coma

Treatment

1. Apply the pressure immobilization technique for venom sequestration (see Chapter 37): If practical by virtue of the sting's location, place a cloth or gauze pad 6 to 8 cm (2.4 to 3.1 inches) by 2 cm (0.8 inch) thick directly over the sting, and hold it firmly in place using a circumferential bandage 15 to 18 cm (5.9 to 7 inches) wide, applied at lymphatic-venous occlusive pressure. If the cloth or gauze pad is not available, a rolled bandage may be used alone.
   a. Do not occlude the arterial circulation, as determined by the detection of arterial pulsations and proper capillary refill.
   b. Splint the limb, and do not release the bandage until after the patient has been brought to proper medical attention and you are prepared to provide systemic support, or after 24 hours.
   c. Check frequently that swelling beneath the bandage has not compromised the arterial circulation.

BLUE-RINGED OCTOPUS BITE

The blue-ringed octopus bite injects its victim with a venom containing tetrodotoxin, a paralytic agent that blocks peripheral nerve conduction.

Signs and Symptoms

- *Local reaction:* one or two puncture wounds characterized by minimal discomfort, described as minor ache, slight stinging, or pulsating sensation
  - Occasionally, initial numbness at the site, followed in 5 to 10 minutes by discomfort that may spread to involve the entire limb, persisting for up to 6 hours
  - Within 30 minutes: redness, swelling, tenderness, heat, and pruritus
  - Most common local tissue reaction: absence of symptoms, small spot of blood, or tiny blanched area
- *Within 10 to 15 minutes:* oral and facial numbness, followed rapidly by diplopia, blurred vision, aphonia, dysphagia, ataxia, myoclonus, weakness, sense of detachment, nausea, vomiting, flaccid muscular paralysis, and respiratory failure

Treatment

1. Apply the pressure immobilization technique for venom sequestration (see Chapter 37 and earlier Treatment section for cone shell sting).
2. Be prepared to assist ventilations. Administer oxygen.

STINGRAY SPINE PUNCTURE

The venom organ of stingrays consists of one to four venomous stings (spines) on the dorsum of the whip-like caudal appendage. The cartilaginous spine(s) is covered with venom glands and an epidermal sheath. When the spine(s) enters the victim, the sheath is disrupted and venom extruded, so the wound is both a puncture/laceration and an envenomation.

Signs and Symptoms

- Immediate local intense pain with central radiation, soft tissue edema, and dusky (ischemic) discoloration with surrounding erythema
- Rapid (hours to days) fat and muscle hemorrhage and necrosis
- Weakness, nausea, vomiting, diarrhea, diaphoresis, vertigo, tachycardia, headache, syncope, seizures, inguinal or axillary pain, muscle cramps, fasciculations, generalized edema (with truncal wounds), paralysis, hypotension, and arrhythmias

Treatment

1. Immerse the wound in nonscalding hot water to tolerance (45°C [113°F]) for 30 to 90 minutes or until there is significant pain relief. No reason exists to add ammonia, magnesium sulfate, potassium permanganate, or a solvent to the soaking solution. Do not immerse the wound in ice water.
2. Remove any obvious spine fragments. This may be done during the hot water soak. However, if the spine is seen to be lodged in the patient and has penetrated deeply into the chest, abdomen, or neck, and may have violated a critical blood vessel of the heart, it should be managed as a weapon of impalement (e.g., knife) would be. In this case the spine should be left in place (if possible) and secured from motion until the patient is brought to a controlled operating room environment where emergency surgery can be performed to guide extraction of the spine and control bleeding that may occur on its removal.
3. Administer appropriate pain medications. Consider local or regional anesthetic administration.
4. Administer prophylactic antibiotics if the wound is more than minor or if the patient is immunocompromised (see Chapter 52).
5. Do not suture the wound closed unless bleeding cannot be controlled with pressure or this wound closure method is necessary for evacuation.

SCORPION FISH SPINE PUNCTURE

Scorpion fish (Fig. 53.5), lionfish (Fig. 53.6), and stonefish (Fig. 53.7) envenom their victims using dorsal, anal, and pelvic spines, which are erected as a defense mechanism (Fig. 53.8). Other venomous fish that sting in a manner similar to scorpion fish include the Atlantic toadfish, European ratfish, rabbitfishes, stargazers, and leatherbacks. Other marine fishes carry spines that envenom to a lesser degree.

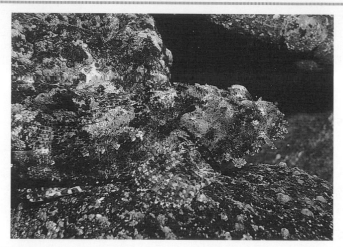

FIGURE 53.5   Scorpion Fish Assuming the Coloration of Its Surroundings.
(Courtesy Paul Auerbach, MD.)

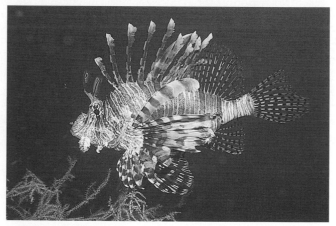

FIGURE 53.6   Adult Lionfish. (Courtesy Paul Auerbach, MD.)

Signs and Symptoms

The severity of the envenomation depends on the number and type of stings, the species, the amount of venom released, and the age and underlying health of the victim. In general, the severity is considered to be stonefish > scorpion fish > lionfish.

- Immediate, intense pain with central radiation
  - If untreated, pain peaking at 60 to 90 minutes and persisting for 6 to 12 hours (stonefish)

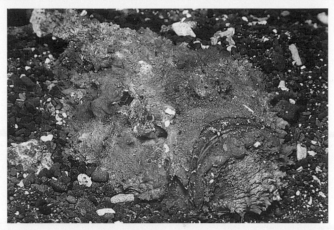

FIGURE 53.7 The Deadly Stonefish *(Synanceja horrida).* (Courtesy Paul Auerbach, MD.)

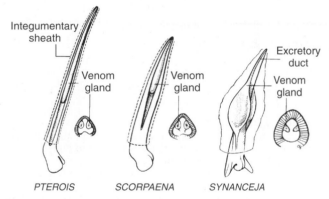

FIGURE 53.8 Lionfish, Scorpion Fish, and Stonefish Spines With Associated Venom Glands.

- Stonefish pain possibly severe enough to cause delirium and persisting at high levels for days
- Wound and surrounding area initially ischemic and then cyanotic, with more broadly surrounding areas of erythema, edema, and warmth
  - Vesicles possible
  - Tissue sloughing within 48 hours
- Anxiety, headache, tremors, maculopapular rash, nausea, vomiting, diarrhea, abdominal pain, diaphoresis, pallor, restlessness, delirium, seizures, limb paralysis, peripheral neuropathy, lymphangitis, arthritis, fever, hypertension, respiratory distress,

pulmonary edema, bradycardia, tachycardia, atrioventricular block, ventricular fibrillation, congestive heart failure, syncope, and hypotension

Treatment

1. Immerse the wound in nonscalding hot water to tolerance (45°C [113°F]) for 30 to 90 minutes or until significant pain relief occurs. No reason exists to add ammonia, magnesium sulfate, potassium permanganate, or a solvent to the soaking solution. Do not immerse the wound in ice water.
2. Remove any obvious spine fragments. This may be done during the hot water soak.
3. Administer appropriate pain medications. Consider local or regional anesthetic administration.
4. Administer prophylactic antibiotics if the wound is more than minor or the patient is immunocompromised (see Chapter 52).
5. Give stonefish antivenom in cases of severe systemic reaction from stings of *Synanceja* species. The antivenom is supplied in ampules containing 2 mL (2000 units) of hyperimmune horse serum, with one vial neutralizing one or two significant punctures. Anticipate anaphylaxis associated with the administration of an antivenom product.

CATFISH SPINE STING

The most frequent stinger is the freshwater catfish; the marine coral catfish has also been reported to sting humans. The venom apparatus consists of dorsal and pectoral fin spines. Some catfish generate skin secretions that are toxic.

Signs and Symptoms

- Instantaneous stinging, throbbing, or scalding pain with central radiation; normally, pain subsiding within 30 to 60 minutes, but possibly lasting up to 48 hours
- Area around the wound ischemic, with central pallor that grows cyanotic before the onset of erythema and edema
- Local muscle spasm, diaphoresis, fasciculations, weakness, syncope, hypotension, and respiratory distress

Treatment

1. Immerse the wound in nonscalding hot water to tolerance (45°C [113°F]) for 30 to 90 minutes or until significant pain relief occurs. No reason exists to add ammonia, magnesium sulfate, potassium permanganate, or a solvent to the soaking solution. Do not immerse the wound in ice water.
2. Remove any obvious spine fragments. This may be done during the hot water soak.
3. Administer appropriate pain medications. Consider local or regional anesthetic administration.
4. Administer prophylactic antibiotics if the wound is more than minor or the patient is immunocompromised (see Chapter 52).

5. Be aware that tiny Amazonian catfishes swim up the human urethra and are not easily dislodged. Ingestion of a large quantity of ascorbic acid (vitamin C), which is then excreted in the urine, may soften the spines and allow the fish to be "passed."

WEEVER FISH SPINE STING

The weever fish is the most venomous fish of the temperate zone. It is found in the Mediterranean Sea, eastern Atlantic Ocean, and European coastal areas. The venom apparatus consists of dorsal and opercular spines associated with venom glands.

Signs and Symptoms

- Instantaneous burning, scalding, or crushing pain with central radiation
  - Peak of pain at 30 minutes with subsidence within 24 hours, but can last for days
  - Possibly of an intensity sufficient to induce irrational behavior and syncope
- Little bleeding at puncture wound site; often appears pale and edematous initially
  - Over 6 to 12 hours, wound becoming red, ecchymotic, and warm
  - Increasing edema for 7 to 10 days, causing the entire limb to become swollen
- Headache, delirium, aphonia, fever, chills, dyspnea, diaphoresis, cyanosis, nausea, vomiting, seizures, syncope, hypotension, and cardiac arrhythmias

Treatment

1. Immerse the wound in nonscalding hot water to tolerance (45°C [113°F]) for 30 to 90 minutes or until significant pain relief occurs. No reason exists to add ammonia, magnesium sulfate, potassium permanganate, or a solvent to the soaking solution. Do not immerse the wound in ice water.
2. Remove any obvious spine fragments. This may be done during the hot water soak.
3. Administer appropriate pain medications. Consider local or regional anesthetic administration.
4. Administer prophylactic antibiotics if the wound is more than minor or the patient is immunocompromised (see Chapter 52).

SEA SNAKE BITE

Sea snakes have a venom apparatus consisting of two to four maxillary fangs and a pair of associated venom glands. Most bites do not result in envenomation.

Signs and Symptoms

- Onset potentially delayed by up to 8 hours
- No appreciable local reaction to a sea snake bite other than the initial pricking sensation

- Initially, euphoria, malaise, or anxiety
- Over 30 to 60 minutes, classic muscle aching and stiffness (particularly of the bitten extremity and neck muscles), along with dysarthria and sialorrhea
- Within 3 to 6 hours, moderate to severe pain with passive movements of the neck, trunk, and limbs
- Ascending flaccid or spastic paralysis, beginning in lower extremities
- Nausea, vomiting, myoclonus, muscle spasm, ophthalmoplegia, ptosis, dilated and poorly reactive pupils, facial paralysis, and trismus
- In severe cases, skin cool and cyanotic, loss of vision, and possible coma

Treatment

1. Apply the pressure immobilization technique for venom sequestration (see Chapter 37).
2. Be prepared to assist ventilations. Administer oxygen.
3. With any evidence of envenomation, give polyvalent sea snake antivenom. The minimum effective adult dosage is 1 ampule (1000 units). The patient may require 3 to 10 ampules depending on the severity of the envenomation. Anticipate anaphylaxis associated with the administration of an antivenom product. Tiger snake antivenom is no longer recommended for use if sea snake antivenom is unavailable.

Toxidromes associated with seafood that may be encountered in the wilderness are ciguatera fish poisoning, clupeotoxin fish poisoning, scombroid fish poisoning, tetrodotoxin fish poisoning, paralytic shellfish poisoning (PSP), diarrhetic shellfish poisoning, *Vibrio* fish poisoning, anisakiasis, domoic acid intoxication, gempylotoxism, botulism, and *Pfiesteria* syndrome.

CIGUATERA FISH POISONING
Ciguatera fish toxins are carried by more than 400 species of bottom-feeding reef fishes. The most frequently affected fish are the jacks, snappers, triggerfishes, and barracudas. Others include mullet, moray eels, porgies, wrasses, parrotfishes, and surgeonfishes. All toxins to date have been unaffected by freeze-drying, heat, cold, and gastric acid, and none has any effect on the odor, color, or taste of the fish. The free algae dinoflagellate *Gambierdiscus toxicus* is responsible for producing ciguatoxins. Other dinoflagellates may generate toxins that play a role in ciguatera syndrome. The toxic fish is generally unremarkable in taste and smell.

Signs and Symptoms
- Onset is possible within 15 to 30 minutes of ingestion and generally within 1 to 3 hours; increasing severity over ensuing 4 to 6 hours; almost all victims develop symptoms by 24 hours
- Abdominal pain, nausea, vomiting, and diarrhea usually occur 3 to 6 hours after ingestion and possibly persist for 48 hours
- Headache, metallic taste, chills, paresthesias (particularly of the extremities and circumoral region), pruritus (particularly of the palms and soles after a delay of 2 to 5 days), tongue and throat numbness or burning, sensation of "carbonation" during swallowing, odontalgia or dental dysesthesias, sensation of loose teeth, dysphagia, dysuria, dyspnea, weakness, fatigue, tremor, fasciculations, athetosis, meningismus, aphonia, ataxia, vertigo, pain and weakness in the lower extremities, visual blurring, transient blindness, hyporeflexia, seizures, nasal congestion and dryness, conjunctivitis, maculopapular rash, skin vesiculations, dermatographia, sialorrhea, diaphoresis, arthralgias, myalgias (particularly in the lower back and thighs), painful ejaculation with urethritis, insomnia, bradycardia, hypotension, central respiratory failure, and coma
- Tachycardia and hypertension are possible
- More severe reactions in persons previously stricken with the poisoning

- Pathognomonic symptom: reversal of hot and cold tactile perception, which may result from generalized thermal hypersensitivity or paresthesias
- Pruritus exacerbated by anything that increases skin temperature (blood flow), such as exercise or alcohol consumption
- If parrotfish ingested, possible second phase, showing locomotor ataxia, dysmetria, and resting or kinetic tremor

Treatment

1. Be aware that therapy is supportive and based on symptoms.
2. Control nausea and vomiting with an antiemetic (prochlorperazine, 2.5 mg IV; ondansetron, 4 mg IV or PO dissolving tablet; or promethazine, 25 mg IM).
3. Control hypotension with intravenous crystalloid volume replacement or oral rehydration if tolerated.
4. For arrhythmias, heart block, hypotension, or severe neurologic symptoms, administer mannitol (20% solution), 1 g/kg IV over 45 to 60 minutes during the acute phase (days 1 to 5). This therapy is not consistently proven to be beneficial.
5. Bradyarrhythmias or excess cholinergic stimulation may respond to atropine (0.5 mg IV, up to 2 mg).
6. For pruritus, administer hydroxyzine, 25 mg PO q6–8h. Cool showers may help. Amitriptyline, 25 mg PO q12h, may relieve pruritus and dysesthesias, as well as emotional depression.
7. Nifedipine (begin with 10 mg PO q8h) has been used to relieve headache.
8. In the recovery phase, avoid ingestion of fish, fish sauces, shellfish, shellfish sauces, alcoholic beverages, and nuts and nut oils.

CLUPEOTOXIN FISH POISONING

Clupeotoxin fish poisoning involves plankton-feeding fish, which ingest planktonic blue-green algae and surface dinoflagellates. These include herrings, sardines, anchovies, tarpons, bonefishes, and deep-sea slickheads. The poison does not impart any unusual appearance, odor, or flavor to the fish.

Signs and Symptoms

- Onset is abrupt, within 30 to 60 minutes of ingestion
- Initially, marked metallic taste, xerostomia, nausea, vomiting, diarrhea, and abdominal pain
- Next symptoms: chills, headache, diaphoresis, severe paresthesias, muscle cramps, vertigo, malaise, tachycardia, peripheral cyanosis, and hypotension
- Death can occur within 15 minutes of onset of symptoms

Treatment

1. Therapy is supportive and based on symptoms.
2. Because of the severe nature of the intoxication, early gastric emptying is desirable. However, the affliction is so unusual that the victim may die before the diagnosis is suspected.

SCOMBROID FISH POISONING

Scombroid fish (dark fleshed; predominantly tuna) and some non-scombroid fish (e.g., Hawaiian dolphin, or mahimahi) are affected with this toxin. L-Histidine within muscle tissue is decarboxylated to form histamine and similar compounds. Thus, the poisoning is also known as *pseudoallergic* fish poisoning. Affected fish typically have a sharply metallic or peppery taste. However, they may be normal in appearance, color, and flavor. Not all persons who eat a contaminated fish become ill, possibly because of an uneven distribution of histamine within the fish. The toxin is not destroyed by cooking.

Signs and Symptoms
- Onset within 15 to 90 minutes of ingestion
- Flushing (sharply demarcated, exacerbated by ultraviolet exposure, particularly of the face, neck, and upper trunk), sensation of warmth without elevated core temperature, conjunctival hyperemia, pruritus, urticaria, angioneurotic edema, bronchospasm, nausea, vomiting, diarrhea, epigastric pain, abdominal cramps, dysphagia, headache, thirst, pharyngitis, burning of the gingivae, palpitations, tachycardia, dizziness, hypotension, localized numbness of the oropharynx, and rare arrhythmias
- If untreated, resolution of symptoms generally within 8 to 12 hours
- Reaction much more severe in a person who is concurrently ingesting isoniazid

Treatment
1. Administer an antihistamine (diphenhydramine, 25 to 50 mg PO or IV; cimetidine, 300 mg, or ranitidine, 50 mg IV). Alternatives are nizatidine, 150 mg PO, or famotidine, 20 mg PO. Combination therapy with both a histamine₁ receptor antagonist and a histamine₂ receptor antagonist may be more effective than either alone.
2. If the patient is severely ill with facial swelling indicative of an airway obstruction, hypotension, or significant bronchospasm, treat as for an allergic reaction with epinephrine and inhaled bronchodilators in addition to antihistamines (see Chapter 26). Corticosteroids are of no proven benefit for scombroid in the absence of anaphylaxis.
3. Control nausea and vomiting that do not remit after antihistamine administration with an antiemetic (prochlorperazine, 2.5 mg IV; promethazine, 25 mg IM; or ondansetron 4 mg IV or PO dissolving tablet).
4. Treat persistent headache with acetaminophen or an antihistamine (such as cimetidine).

Prevention
1. Make sure that all captured fish are gutted, cooled, and refrigerated or placed on ice or frozen immediately.

2. Do not consume fish that has been handled improperly or carries the odor of ammonia. Fresh fish generally has a sheen or oily rainbow appearance; avoid "dull" fish or those that do not smell fresh.

TETRODOTOXIN FISH POISONING

Tetrodotoxin is a potent nonprotein poison that interferes with central and peripheral neuromuscular transmission. It is found in pufferfish (blowfish, globefish, swellfish, toadfish, balloonfish), and porcupine fish. "Puffers" are prepared as delicacies (fugu) and when ingested may cause paresthesias, a sensation of "floating," flushing of the skin, generalized warmth, and mild weakness with euphoria. The toxin is concentrated in the liver, viscera, gonads, and skin of the fish.

Signs and Symptoms

- Onset possibly as rapid as 10 minutes or delayed for up to 4 hours; usually occurs within 30 minutes of ingestion; death may occur within 20 minutes
- Initial symptoms: oral (lips and tongue) paresthesias, lightheadedness, and then general paresthesias
- Rapidly developing symptoms: hypersalivation, diaphoresis, lethargy, headache, nausea, vomiting, diarrhea, abdominal pain, weakness, ataxia, incoordination, tremor, paralysis, cyanosis, aphonia, dysphagia, seizures, bradycardia, dyspnea, bronchorrhea, bronchospasm, respiratory failure, coma, hypotension, and coagulopathy
- Gastrointestinal symptoms may be severe and include nausea, vomiting, diarrhea, and abdominal pain
- Miosis progressing to mydriasis with poor papillary light reflex
- When mechanical ventilation maintained and no anoxic brain injury present, full mentation maintained with total flaccid paralysis

Treatment

1. Be aware that the toxin is stable in gastric acid and partially inactivated in alkaline solutions.
2. Secure the airway, and administer oxygen.
3. Perform gastric lavage with 2 L of 2% sodium bicarbonate in 200-mL aliquots, followed by placement of 50 to 100 g of activated charcoal in 70% sorbitol solution (or 30 g of "highly activated" charcoal in sorbitol).
4. Further therapy is supportive and based on symptoms. Atropine may be used to treat bradycardia. Pressors that are α-agonists, such as phenylephrine or norepinephrine, may be effective to treat hypotension, taking care to first ensure adequate fluid resuscitation. Cholinesterase inhibitors, such as edrophonium and neostigmine, have met with varying success.

PARALYTIC SHELLFISH POISONING

PSP is induced by ingesting toxic filter-feeding (on certain dino-flagellates) organisms, such as clams, oysters, scallops, mussels, chitons, limpets, murex, starfish, and sand crabs. The toxins that cause PSP are water soluble, and stable in heat and gastric acid. They inhibit neuromuscular transmission. The phytoplankton genera that are implicated as the origins of PSP toxin are *Alexandrium*, *Gymnodinium*, *Pyrodinium*, and *Protogonyaulax*, among others.

Signs and Symptoms

- Within minutes (usually 30 to 60) to a few hours after ingestion of contaminated shellfish, onset of intraoral and perioral paresthesias, notably of the lips, tongue, and gums, which progress rapidly to involve the neck and distal extremities; early onset of vertigo
- Tingling or burning sensation that becomes numbness
- Gastroenteritis in only 25% of victims
- Light-headedness, sensation of "floating," disequilibrium, inco-ordination, weakness, hyperreflexia, incoherence, dysarthria, sialorrhea, dysphagia, dysphonia, thirst, diarrhea, abdominal pain, nausea, vomiting, nystagmus, dysmetria, headache, diaphoresis, loss of vision, sensation of loose teeth, chest pain, and tachycardia
- Flaccid paralysis and respiratory insufficiency 2 to 12 hours after ingestion
- Unless there is a period of anoxia, the patient is often awake and alert, although paralyzed

Treatment

1. Secure the airway and administer oxygen.
2. Do not induce emesis. If the airway is secure, perform gastric lavage with 2 L of 2% sodium bicarbonate in 200-mL aliquots, followed by placement of 50 to 100 g of activated charcoal in 70% sorbitol solution (or 30 g of "highly activated" charcoal in sorbitol).
3. Further therapy is supportive and based on symptoms. Hemoperfusion has met with varying success.

DIARRHETIC SHELLFISH POISONING

Diarrhetic shellfish poisoning is a rapid-onset illness with gastrointestinal symptoms, which although they are severe, are self-limited. It is caused by ingestion of shellfish contaminated with dinoflagellates belonging to the genus *Dinophysis* or *Prorocentrum*.

Signs and Symptoms

Onset within 30 minutes to 2 hours: diarrhea, nausea, vomiting, abdominal pain, and chills; rarely, symptoms are delayed by up to 12 hours; symptoms resolve after 2 to 3 days

Treatment
Therapy is symptomatic and supportive, with focus on hydration and antiemetics.

VIBRIO FISH POISONING
Vibrio organisms can cause gastroenteric disease and soft tissue infections, particularly in immunocompromised hosts. The most common vector is raw oysters, shrimp, or fish. Although some variation in clinical presentation exists depending on the particular *Vibrio* species (e.g., *vulnificus, parahaemolyticus, mimicus*), a general description of the signs and symptoms and an approach to therapy will suffice for the initiation of field therapy. Persons particularly prone to septicemia and rapid demise are those with elevated serum iron levels, achlorhydria, chronic liver disease, diabetes, human immunodeficiency virus infection, alcoholism, cancer, and various forms of immunosuppression.

Signs and Symptoms
- Gastroenteric manifestations
  - Ingestion of raw or partially cooked seafood products followed in 6 to 76 hours by explosive diarrhea, nausea, vomiting, headache, abdominal pain, fever, chills, and prostration in the case of *V. parahaemolyticus*. This is not likely to be the case with *V. vulnificus*.
  - Blood in stools
  - Hypotension initially secondary to dehydration and then, in immunocompromised individuals, sepsis
- Soft tissue infection
  - Ingestion of raw or partially cooked seafood products or direct skin (wound) contact with ocean water followed in 12 to 48 hours by skin erythema, vesiculation, and hemorrhagic or contused-appearing bullae, progressing rapidly to necrotizing fasciitis and tissue necrosis *(V. vulnificus)*
  - Hypotension secondary to sepsis

Treatment
1. Treat dehydration and hypotension with intravenous crystalloid fluid replacement.
2. Administer an appropriate antibiotic as soon as a *Vibrio* infection is suspected.
   a. Appropriate antibiotics for sepsis include doxycycline (100 mg IV q12h), ceftazidime (2 g IV q8h), or ciprofloxacin (400 mg IV q12h). Other antibiotics that have been suggested include trimethoprim/sulfamethoxazole, ciprofloxacin, tetracycline, carbenicillin, chloramphenicol, tobramycin, gentamicin, imipenem/cilastatin, meropenem, and many third-generation cephalosporins. A course of oral ciprofloxacin, trimethoprim/sulfamethoxazole, or doxycycline may shorten the course of severe gastroenteritis.

b. For information about antibiotic prophylaxis for marine-acquired wounds, see Chapter 52.

ANISAKIASIS

Anisakiasis is caused by penetration of the *Anisakis* or *Phocanema* nematode larva through the gastric mucosa. The nematode originates from the muscle tissue of raw fish.

Signs and Symptoms

- Within 1 hour of ingestion of raw fish: severe epigastric pain, nausea, and vomiting, mimicking an acute abdomen
  - If the worm does not implant, it may be coughed up, vomited, or defecated, usually within 48 hours of the meal
  - If the worm is felt in the oropharynx or esophagus, there is a "tingling throat" sensation
- Intestinal anisakiasis more often delayed in onset (up to 7 days after ingestion) and marked by abdominal pain, nausea, vomiting, diarrhea, and fever

Treatment

Unfortunately, no effective field treatment exists. Until the worm is rejected or endoscopically removed, give symptomatic therapy (e.g., an antacid). Albendazole, 200 mg PO bid for 3 days, has been recommended but is of questionable efficacy.

Prevention

Eat only cooked (60°C [140°F]) or previously frozen (to −20°C [−4°F]) fish. Candling is an inadequate method of surveillance, particularly in dark-fleshed fish. Smoking (kippering), marinating, pickling, brining, and salting may not kill the worms. Fish should be gutted as soon as possible after they are caught.

DOMOIC ACID INTOXICATION (AMNESTIC SHELLFISH POISONING)

Shellfish, particularly certain species of mussels and razor clams, which have concentrated domoic acid (glutamate agonist) generate in humans a syndrome of amnestic shellfish poisoning.

Signs and Symptoms

- Initial symptoms of nausea, vomiting, abdominal cramps, and diarrhea 1 to 24 hours after ingestion
- In 15 minutes to 38 hours (median 5 hours) after ingestion of contaminated shellfish, rapid onset of arousal, confusion, disorientation, and memory loss
- Severe headache, hiccups, arrhythmias, hypotension, seizures, ophthalmoplegia, hemiparesis, mutism, grimacing, agitation, emotional lability, coma, copious bronchial secretions, and pulmonary edema

Treatment
1. Therapy is supportive and based on symptoms.
2. For seizures, administer a potent rapid-acting anticonvulsant such as diazepam.

GEMPYLOTOXIC FISH POISONING
Gempylotoxic fishes are the pelagic mackerels, which produce an oil with a pronounced purgative effect. The "toxin" is contained in both musculature and bones.

Signs and Symptoms
- Within 30 to 60 minutes of ingestion: abdominal cramping, bloating, mild nausea, and diarrhea
- Fever, bloody or foul-smelling stools, or protracted vomiting suggests infectious gastroenteritis

Treatment
1. Therapy is supportive and based on symptoms.
2. Antimotility agents are not recommended unless the diarrhea is debilitating because inhibition of peristalsis may increase the duration of the disorder.

HAFF DISEASE
Haff disease is a syndrome characterized by severe muscle pain and rhabdomyolysis 6 to 21 hours after consuming fish. Most cases in the United States are associated with eating buffalo fish or crawfish, bottom-feeding species found in the Mississippi River and its tributaries. The toxin is unidentified.

Signs and Symptoms
- Muscle pain and tenderness, rigidity, weakness, and rhabdomyolysis
- Tachycardia, hypertension, tachypnea, and hypothermia.

Treatment
Aggressive intravenous hydration and diuretics to prevent renal failure from myoglobin toxicity.

BOTULISM
Botulism is a paralytic disease caused by the potent natural toxins of *Clostridium botulinum*. Seafood-related botulism can be caused by raw, parboiled, salt-cured, or fermented meats from marine mammals or fish products. Toxin types A, B, and E predominate.

Signs and Symptoms
- Within 12 to 36 hours of ingestion: nausea, vomiting, abdominal pain, and diarrhea, followed by dry mouth, dysphonia (hoarseness), difficulty swallowing, facial weakness, ptosis, nonreactive or sluggishly reactive pupils, mydriasis, blurred or double vision, descending symmetric muscular weakness leading to paralysis, and bulbar and respiratory paralysis

Treatment

1. Provide ventilatory support.
2. Consider a cathartic if airway is maintained.
3. Administer equine trivalent antitoxin A, B, and E as soon as possible. Initial dose is 10 mL (one vial) every 2 to 4 hours for three to five doses or longer if symptoms persist. Anticipate an anaphylactic reaction to antitoxin.

PFIESTERIA (POSSIBLE ESTUARY-ASSOCIATED) SYNDROME

Pfiesteria piscicida is a toxic dinoflagellate that inhabits estuarine and coastal waters of the eastern United States and has been associated with fish kills and possibly with human illness. The route of exposure is unknown, although it is thought to be either by prolonged direct skin contact with toxin-laden water or via aerosols after breathing air over areas where fish are dying.

Signs and Symptoms
Headache, erythematous and edematous skin papules on the trunk or extremities, muscle cramps, eye irritation, upper respiratory irritation, and neuropsychologic symptoms (forgetfulness, difficulties with learning)

Treatment
1. Therapy is symptomatic and supportive.
2. Empiric-based recommendations state that cholestyramine may be effective in patients with persistent syndromes.

AZASPIRACID SHELLFISH POISONING
Azaspiracid shellfish poisoning was first described in the Netherlands after an outbreak of severe vomiting and diarrhea from ingestion of mussels from Ireland. The toxin is a heat-stable compound(s).

Signs and Symptoms
Appear within hours of ingestion and include nausea, vomiting, severe diarrhea, and stomach cramps; illness persists for 2 to 3 days without any long-term effects

Treatment
Therapy is symptomatic and supportive, with focus on hydration and antiemetics.

ANEMONE POISONING
Anemone poisoning is from ingestion of the green or brown anemones *Radianthus paumotensis* or *Rhodactis howesii* (Matamalu samasama) in the South Pacific. This may be accidental or intentional.

Signs and Symptoms

Altered mental status within 30 minutes, often immediately: agitation, confusion, delirium leading to coma; other symptoms include fever, seizures, myalgias, abdominal pain, respiratory failure, hypotension, and death

Treatment

Therapy is symptomatic and supportive, with attention to blood pressure management and airway support.

Aquatic Skin Disorders

Among the disorders acquired in water that affect the skin are various dermatoses, cutaneous larva migrans, infections, sensitivity to diving equipment, pseudomonal folliculitis, and otitis externa.

DISORDERS
SARGASSUM ALGAL DERMATITIS
Signs and Symptoms
- Skin erythema, urticarial papular pruritus

Treatment
1. Promptly wash with soap and water to remove toxins.
2. Treat a mild to moderate reaction with antihistamines and a topical medium-potency corticosteroid preparation (Table 55.1).
3. Treat a severe reaction with PO prednisone, 60 to 100 mg for adults and 1 mg/kg for children, with a 2-week taper.

SEA CUCUMBER DERMATITIS
Signs and Symptoms
- Skin erythema, pain, and pruritus

Treatment
1. Promptly wash with soap and water to remove toxins.
2. Treat a mild to moderate reaction with a topical low- or medium-potency corticosteroid preparation (see Table 55.1).
3. Treat a severe reaction with PO prednisone, 60 to 100 mg for adults and 1 mg/kg for children, with a 2-week taper.

SEA MOSS DERMATITIS (DOGGER BANK ITCH)
Sea moss dermatitis is caused by a plant *(Fragilaria striatula)* or sea chervils (genus *Alcyonidium*), which appear in seaweed-like animal colonies (mosses or "mats"), usually drawn up within fishing nets.

Signs and Symptoms
- Irritation, first appearing on the hands and forearms (see Plate 43)
- Recurrent exposures are more severe, characterized by vesiculated and edematous eruption of the hands, arms, legs, and face

Table 55.1	Potency Ranking of Topical Steroids		
POTENCY	**BRAND**	**GENERIC**	**SIZES**
Super high	Temovate cream, ointment 0.05%,	Clobetasol propionate	15, 30, 45, 60 g
	Psorcon ointment	Diflorasone diacetate	15, 30, 60 g
Medium	Westcort cream 0.2%	Hydrocortisone valerate	15, 45, 60 g
	Locoid cream 0.1%	Hydrocortisone butyrate	15, 45 g
Low	Aclovate cream, ointment 0.05%	Alclometasone dipropionate	15, 45, 60 g
	DesOwen cream, lotion 0.05%	Desonide	15, 60, 118 mL

These topical steroids must be applied twice daily. However, the application rate can vary upwards to a maximum of three to four times per day according to the prescriber's discretion.

Treatment
1. Treat as for mild poison oak dermatitis (see Chapter 40).
    a. Depending on the severity of the reaction, apply calamine lotion or a topical medium- or high-potency corticosteroid preparation.
    b. Give an oral antihistamine to help control itching.
2. Treat a severe reaction with PO prednisone, 60 to 100 mg for adults and 1 mg/kg for children, with a 2-week taper.

SEAWEED DERMATITIS
Seaweed dermatitis is almost always secondary to irritation from contact with algae. For instance, the stinging seaweed *Microcoleus lyngbyaceus* (also known as *Lyngbya majuscula*) is green or olive colored, drab, and finely filamentous. The typical patient does not remove a wet bathing suit for a time after leaving the water.

Signs and Symptoms
- In minutes to hours after exposure, a pruritic, burning, moist, and erythematous rash developing in bathing suit distribution, followed by bullous escharotic desquamation in the genital, perineal, and perianal regions (see Plate 44)
- Lymphadenopathy, pustular folliculitis, and local infections
- Oral and ocular mucous membrane irritation, facial rash, conjunctivitis

Treatment
1. Wash the skin vigorously and copiously with soap and water to remove algal fragments.

2. Apply three sequential brief rinses with isopropyl alcohol 40%.
3. Apply a topical corticosteroid preparation. This may need to be medium to high potency.
4. Treat a severe reaction with PO prednisone, 60 to 100 mg for adults and 1 mg/kg for children, with a 2-week taper.
5. If necrosis is present, use sterile saline cleanses followed by white petroleum jelly or Hydrofera Blue bacteriostatic wound dressings.

PROTOTHECOSIS

The genus *Prototheca* consists of nonpigmented algae from the family Chlorellaceae. *Prototheca wickerhamii* and *Prototheca zopfii* are the most commonly isolated pathogens in human protothecosis. There may be an incubation period of weeks to months after inoculation into skin following exposure to contaminated water or soil.

Signs and Symptoms

- Superficial cutaneous lesions present as papulonodules or verrucous plaques with or without ulcerations. Bullous lesions or, rarely, eczematous and cellulitis-like lesions may occur (see Plate 45)
- Olecranon bursitis, with or without spontaneous drainage. A history of preceding trauma should suggest protothecosis
- Systemic infection may occur, particularly in immunosuppressed persons
- A case of esophageal protothecosis has been reported

In cases associated with a traumatic episode, the initial lesion is a nodule or tender red papule, which enlarges, becomes pustular, and ulcerates. There may be a purulent, malodorous, and blood-tinged discharge. Satellite lesions surround the primary lesion and may become confluent. Regional lymph nodes may develop metastatic granulomas. Diagnosis is made by tissue biopsy or culture.

Treatment

1. Localized lesions can be excised.
2. Topical medications are unsatisfactory.
3. Prolonged treatment with algaecidal agents, including ketoconazole, itraconazole, fluconazole, and miconazole, may inhibit or kill the organisms. Amphotericin B has been used successfully.

HUMAN PYTHIOSIS

The aquatic fungus-like organism *Pythium insidiosum* is a zoosporic plant pathogen and newly emerging human pathogen. It is found in tropical, subtropical, and temperate areas, preferentially in swampy environments. The zoospores encyst and form germ tubes, secreting an adhesive substance, cellulitic and macerating enzymes, and fungal products.

Signs and Symptoms
- Begins as a pustule at the site of inoculation (see Plate 46)
- Cellulitis and suppurative necrosis, usually of the lower extremities
- Can cause systemic arterial inflammation and occlusion

Treatment
Treatment is not well established. Antifungal medication, such as amphotericin B or itraconazole given for up to a year, has been attempted.

AQUAGENIC URTICARIA
Signs and Symptoms
- Urticaria on exposure to water of any temperature
- Eruption usually confined to the neck, upper trunk, and arms; the face, hands, legs, and feet are spared. (see Plate 47)

Treatment
1. Prevent or inhibit the reaction by applying petroleum ointment to the skin before water exposure.
2. Consider prophylaxis with an antihistamine 1 hour before exposure.
3. In persons with recurrent aquagenic urticaria, consider stanozolol 10 mg/day for symptom control.

AQUAGENIC PRURITUS
Signs and Symptoms
- Intense disabling itching without visible cutaneous changes on exposure to water of any temperature
- Reaction within minutes of exposure and lasting between 10 minutes and 2 hours
- Lack of concurrent skin disease or drug exposure
- Symptoms may occur only in areas exposed to water. Typically, the head, palms, soles, and mucosa are spared

Treatment
1. Alkalinization of water and application of petroleum ointment to the skin have had limited success.
2. Antihistamines may have limited success.

SCHISTOSOMIASIS (CERCARIAL DERMATITIS, "SWIMMER'S ITCH")

Swimmer's itch is caused by penetration of the epidermis by the cercariae of avian, rodent, or ungulate schistosomes. The cercariae are immature larval forms, usually microscopic, of the parasitic flatworms. Although penetration of cercariae may occur in the water, it usually occurs as the film of water evaporates on the skin. The eruption occurs primarily on exposed areas of the body.

Signs and Symptoms

- Initial symptom: prickling sensation (sometimes burning and itching sensations)
- Itching 4 to 60 minutes after the cercariae penetrate the skin, accompanied by erythema and mild edema
- Subsidence of the initial urticarial reaction over 60 minutes, leaving red macules that become papular and more pruritic over the next 10 to 15 hours; discrete and highly pruritic papules 3 to 5 mm (0.1 to 0.2 inch) in diameter are surrounded by a zone of erythema (see Plate 48)
- Vesicles, which may become pustules, frequently forming within 48 hours and possibly persisting for 7 to 14 days
- Peak inflammatory response within 3 days and subsidence slowly over 1 to 2 weeks

Treatment

1. Because the inflammatory response is self-limited, therapy is symptomatic.
2. In a mild case, apply isopropyl alcohol 40% or equal parts of isopropyl alcohol and calamine lotion to control the itching.
3. Oral antihistamines may be helpful.
4. For a severe case, give PO prednisone, 60 to 100 mg for adults and 1 mg/kg for children, with a 2-week taper.
5. Manage secondary bacterial infection, which is frequently caused by *Staphylococcus aureus* or *Streptococcus* species, with a topical antiseptic ointment (mupirocin, bacitracin) or a systemic antibiotic (e.g., erythromycin, dicloxacillin).

Prevention

Obtain some prevention by brisk rubbing with a rough, dry towel immediately on leaving the water to remove moisture that harbors the cercariae. Washing the skin with rubbing alcohol or soap and water is not effective.

SEA BATHER'S ERUPTION

See Chapter 53.

LEECHES

Leeches attach to the skin of the victim with jaws that allow the introduction of an anticoagulant, which causes moderate painless bleeding at the site of removal. Leeches feed until they are engorged, then fall off.

Signs and Symptoms

- In an unsensitized person: a freely bleeding wound that heals slowly
- In a sensitized person: urticarial, bullous, or necrotic reaction to the bite
- With rapid onset of bullae, necrosis, and sepsis, suspect *Aeromonas hydrophila* infection (see later)

Treatment

1. To remove a leech, use a gentle mechanical technique so as not to leave behind pieces of the teeth in the skin. A drop of any essential oil (volatile aroma compound derived from a plant) near the mouthpart causes rapid release. Do not apply brine, alcohol, or strong vinegar, or hold a flame near the site of attachment so the leech does not regurgitate and cause an infection. Do not rip the leech off the skin because its jaws may remain and induce intense inflammation.
2. After removal of the leech, inspect the wound closely for retained mouthparts.
3. Hasten hemostasis by the application of a styptic pencil, topical thrombin solution, oxidized regenerated cellulose absorbable hemostat, or "blood-stopper gauze" (e.g., QuikClot). Hold pressure for 15 minutes with any of these therapies.
4. Clean wounds several times daily with an antiseptic. Treat secondary infection with an antibiotic.

SEA "LOUSE" DERMATITIS

Sea "lice" are small, biting marine crustaceans often buried in the sandy bottom that attach to fish, feet, or hands.

Signs and Symptoms

* Immediate sharp pain, with noticeable punctate hemorrhage
* Injury resolving over 5 to 7 days

Treatment

1. Clean the acute wound with a brisk soap and water scrub or brief hydrogen peroxide application, then cover lightly with antiseptic ointment.
2. Inspect daily for secondary infection.

CUTANEOUS LARVA MIGRANS

Cutaneous larva migrans ("creeping eruption") is caused by the larvae of various nematode parasites for which humans are an abnormal final host. The larvae penetrate the epidermis but are unable to penetrate the dermis. The feet and buttocks are most often involved and show the superficial serpiginous tunnels.

Signs and Symptoms

* Thin, wandering, linear or serpiginous, raised, and tunnel-like lesion 2 to 3 mm (0.1 inch) in width (see Plate 49)
* Severe itching
* Creeping eruption as the larvae move a few millimeters to a few centimeters each day
* Older lesions that are dry and crusted

Treatment

1. Use cryotherapy with ethyl chloride for a mild infestation, topical 10% thiabendazole (crush two 0.5 g tablets and mix with 10 g

petrolatum) in a more refractory case, and oral thiabendazole (25 to 50 mg/kg) for 2 to 4 days in a more severe case. Alternative drugs are albendazole (400 mg/day PO for 7 days) or ivermectin (12 mg single dose).
2. Secondary infection may occur and require incision and drainage of pustules or furuncles, and the use of topical and systemic antibiotics.

SOAPFISH DERMATITIS
The soapfish (*Rypticus saponaceus*; Fig. 55.1) releases soapy mucus when handled or disturbed.

Signs and Symptoms
• Skin irritation with redness, itching, and mild swelling

Treatment
1. Apply cold compresses of Burow solution (aluminum acetate dissolved in water) to alleviate burning and itching.
2. For a severe case, apply a topical steroid preparation.

MYCOBACTERIUM MARINUM INFECTION
Infection occurs 2 to 3 weeks after exposure to fresh or salt water. *Mycobacterium marinum* invades skin through a preexisting skin lesion. Most lesions heal spontaneously within 2 to 3 years.

Signs and Symptoms
• Development of localized area of cellulitis 7 to 10 days after sustaining puncture wound or laceration, particularly of the cooler distal extremity; may progress to localized arthritis, bony erosion, formation of subcutaneous nodules, and superficial desquamation
• Development of red papule, nodule, or shallow ulceration within 3 to 4 weeks after inoculation. Nodules transform into hard, purple nodules, with scaling, ulceration, and verrucous appearance; may enlarge to 6 cm (2.4 inches) in diameter, although 1 to 2 cm (0.4 to 0.8 inch) is more common

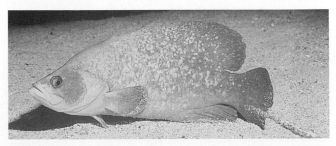

FIGURE 55.1   Soapfish *(Rypticus saponaceus)*. Skin contact with soapy mucus causes dermatitis. (Courtesy Carl Roessler.)

- New lesions developing in a pattern that resembles sporotrichosis, with dermal granulomas in linear distribution (see Plate 50) along the superficial lymphatics

Treatment
1. Administer clarithromycin, minocycline, doxycycline, amikacin, trimethoprim/sulfamethoxazole, or ethambutol plus rifampin as first-line therapy.
2. Subsequent treatment is determined by culture and drug sensitivity testing. Effective antibiotics have included minocycline, tetracycline, levofloxacin, azithromycin, amikacin, amoxicillin/clavulanate, and tuberculostatic drugs.
3. Therapy is continued for 1 to 2 months after clinical clearance. This may necessitate therapy for up to 4 to 6 months.

ERYSIPELOTHRIX RHUSIOPATHIAE INFECTION
Erysipelothrix rhusiopathiae, the causative agent of erysipeloid, enters the skin through a puncture wound or abrasion, usually on the finger or hand. It inhabits the exterior mucoid slime of fish.

Signs and Symptoms
- Appearance of violaceous, raised area within 1 to 7 days after inoculation
- Enlarged area, accompanied by pain and itching
- Low-grade fever, malaise
- Hallmark lesion: purplish skin irritation or paronychia, with edema and a small amount of purulent discharge
    - Surrounded by an area of relative central fading, which in turn is surrounded by centripetally advancing, raised, well-demarcated, and a marginated erythematous or violaceous ring (see Plate 34)
    - Lesion warm and tender, with progression up the dorsal edge of the finger into the web space, and descent along the adjoining finger
- Infection seldom affecting the palm; absence of pitting or suppuration
- Regional inflamed lymph nodes
- Malaise, fever
- Arthritis

Treatment
1. May be self-limited and resolve within 3 weeks. Antibiotic therapy facilitates resolution.
2. For skin involvement, administer penicillin VK (250 to 500 mg PO q6h), cephalexin (250 mg PO q6h), or ciprofloxacin (500 mg PO q12h) for 10 days. Erythromycin and trimethoprim-sulfamethoxazole are not recommended.
3. If arthritis is present, give IV aqueous penicillin G (2 to 4 million units q4h for 4 to 6 weeks).

CHROMOBACTERIUM VIOLACEUM INFECTION
This infection causes sepsis similar to that from melioidosis. The organism is found in water and soil.

Signs and Symptoms
- Inflammation of soft tissue with or without adenopathy
- Cellulitis followed by abscess formation
- May present as sepsis with fever, pneumonia, and spleen, liver, and lung abscesses

Treatment
Susceptible to fluoroquinolones, tetracycline, imipenem, aztreonam, and trimethoprim-sulfamethoxazole

SEAL FINGER
This is usually an infection of a digit after exposure to the skin or mucous membranes of a seal or sea lion, thought to be secondary to infection with strains of *Mycoplasma*.

Signs and Symptoms
- Swollen and painful digit, preceded by an inflammatory papule that develops into a nodule with swelling, purulence, and pain (see Plate 35)
- Stiff digit with occasional fever

Treatment
1. Tetracycline 1.5 g initial oral dose, followed by 500 mg PO q6h for 4 to 6 weeks

AEROMONAS HYDROPHILA INFECTION
Aeromonas hydrophila poses a threat to freshwater aquarists in the same manner that *Vibrio* species do to marine aquarists.

Signs and Symptoms
- Within 8 to 48 hours, wound (particularly of puncture variety) that becomes cellulitic, with erythema, edema, and purulent discharge (see Plate 51)
  - Most frequently affects the lower extremity
  - Appearance indistinguishable from streptococcal cellulitis
- Localized pain, lymphangitis, fever, chills
- Rapidly advancing, gas-forming soft tissue reaction, with bullae formation and necrotizing myositis, fasciitis, and osteonecrosis

Treatment
1. Administer an antibiotic such as chloramphenicol, gentamicin, tobramycin, tetracycline, trimethoprim/sulfamethoxazole (co-trimoxazole), ciprofloxacin, cefotaxime, ceftazidime, moxalactam, piperacillin-tazobactam, imipenem/cilastatin, or meropenem. Resistance to trimethoprim-sulfamethoxazole, aminoglycosides, and tetracycline has been reported.

2. For severe infection, administer IV antibiotics as soon as possible. Aggressive wound debridement may be necessary.

VIBRIO SPECIES INFECTION

For information on antibiotic prophylaxis against *Vibrio* spp. infection, see Chapter 52. For information on antibiotic therapy for established *Vibrio* spp. infection, see Chapters 52 and 54.

REACTIONS TO DIVING EQUIPMENT

Some chemical components in the plastic and rubber used to create masks and mouthpieces can cause irritant or allergic dermatitis.

Signs and Symptoms

- "Mask burn," which may appear as a reddish imprint of the mask on the face or a severe, vesicular, and weeping eruption
- Glossitis
- Redness and lichenification over exposed surfaces of the feet (contact with swim fins)

Treatment

1. Treat acute facial dermatitis with cool compresses of Burow's solution (aluminum acetate).
2. For a severe skin reaction, treat with an oral corticosteroid, specifically prednisone, 60 to 100 mg for adults and 1 mg/kg for children, with a 2-week taper.
3. For a serious intraoral reaction, use a twice-daily mouthwash of equal parts of antihistamine (diphenhydramine) elixir and magnesium salts (milk of magnesia). Coat individual sores twice daily and at bedtime with triamcinolone acetonide (0.1%) dental paste (Kenalog in Orabase) for 5 to 7 days.

PSEUDOMONAL FOLLICULITIS

Pseudomonas aeruginosa is the most common microbe causing skin disorders in occupational saturation divers and can occur after recreational use of diving suits. It is also a cause of folliculitis in occupants of heated recreational water sources.

Signs and Symptoms

- Follicular rash appearing within 48 hours of exposure, most pronounced in areas covered by a wet suit or bathing garment (see Plate 52), skin folds, trunk, buttocks, and proximal extremities
- Pruritus, mild pain, external otitis, conjunctivitis, tender breasts, enlarged and tender lymph nodes, fever, malaise

Treatment

1. May resolve spontaneously without therapy in 7 to 14 days.
2. Apply drying lotions, such as calamine, with or without oral antihistamines.

3. Treat local infection with antimicrobial ointment, such as poly-myxin B or gentamicin, until resolved.
4. Treat systemic infection with ciprofloxacin, levofloxacin, aztreo-nam, antipseudomonal cephalosporin, a carbapenem, or an aminoglycoside.

GREEN NAIL SYNDROME

Pseudomonas aeruginosa may cause greenish-black discoloration of the nail plate and paronychia.

Signs and Symptoms
- Onycholysis and bluish-green discoloration of the nail plate with or without paronychia

Treatment
1. Twice-a-day application of tobramycin ophthalmic solution or nadifloxacin cream.
2. An alternative therapy is repeated soaking with antiseptics such as diluted acetic acid solution or 0.1% octenidine dihydrochloride solution.
3. To reduce swelling and erythema of the paronychium, apply a topical corticosteroid cream or ointment, such as clobetasol.

OTITIS EXTERNA (SWIMMER'S EAR)

Otitis externa is inflammation and infection (often polymicrobial) of the external ear canal caused by constant moisture, warm body temperature, and introduction of microorganisms.

Signs and Symptoms
- Initial symptoms: itching, mild pain; rarely, decreased hearing
- Sensation of "fullness" in the affected ear
- Pain that worsens as the inflammation progresses until it is uncomfortable to push on the tragus or pull on the earlobe
- Severe infection: cellulitis, purulent discharge (see Plate 53), occlusion of the ear canal, cervical lymphadenopathy, headache, nausea, fever, and sepsis

Treatment
1. The most important topical therapy is reacidification and desic-cation of the ear canal, which can be accomplished with a 50:50 mixture of isopropyl alcohol 40% and acetic acid 5% (vinegar) or with Burow's solution (Domeboro: aluminum sulfate and calcium acetate).
2. Avoid oily solutions.
3. Administer appropriate pain medications.
4. For a mild infection (slight pain and discharge), use ear drops such as nonaqueous acetic acid (VoSol otic). Colistin sulfate has been recommended to combat *Pseudomonas*. Using acetic acid or acetic acid with hydrocortisone 1% (VoSol HC otic) avoids sensitization that may occur with neomycin-containing products.

5. If suppuration occurs, antibiotic ear drops, such as hydrocortisone 1%, polymyxin B, and neomycin (Cortisporin otic) or ofloxacin otic 0.3%, are indicated.
6. If the ear canal is so swollen that drops will not penetrate the debris, place a gauze or foam wick and keep it soaked with the topical solution for 24 to 72 hours.
7. If adenopathy, profuse purulent discharge, or fever is present, give oral co-trimoxazole, ciprofloxacin, or amoxicillin/clavulanate for 7 to 10 days.

Prevention

1. The most important preventive measure is to diminish moisture retention in the external ear canal.
2. Do not use cotton-tipped applicators to extract moisture because they can damage the ear canal lining or press cerumen deeply into the canal.
3. Acidifying and desiccating agents are effective prophylaxis.
4. Achieve prevention by briefly rinsing with common rubbing alcohol, vinegar, or a mixture of these after each entry into the water. Avoid petroleum jelly or other substances intended to form a watertight seal because they may act as a moist trap for debris.

This chapter addresses broad concepts of wilderness search and rescue (SAR); responders should evaluate their circumstances and seek specific training for the types of incidents they may encounter.

Not all rescuers need to be trained to the most advanced levels of wilderness operations, and individuals should always operate within the limits of their experience and training. Before attempting to respond to any rescue incident, responsible persons should ensure that every field team has the breadth and depth of experience to operate safely and make sound decisions. The safety of the rescuer(s) and rescue team should always be the first priority.

BASIC STAGES OF A SAR MISSION

- **Awareness**: notification is received by some means that an individual or group is in distress and/or requires assistance
- **Initial Action**: responsible authorities evaluate the information received and determine the degree of emergency. This can range from uncertainty about the safety of the party (e.g., overdue friends), to alertness of a possible problem (e.g., known incident with limited information), to distress (e.g., reasonable certainty that a party is threatened by grave and imminent danger and requires immediate assistance)
- **Planning:** develop a strategy for search and rescue and identify the resources needed to carry out the mission
- **Conclusion:** no one is in distress; rescue is concluded; debriefing and demobilization.

OVERVIEW

The following are essential for a safe and efficient SAR operation:

- Provide for the safety of rescuers and patients. This must include injury prevention from environmental and rescuer causes; providing water, shelter, food, and a mechanism for personal hygiene
- Communicate needs and changes during all phases of the operation. Call for backup at the earliest possible time. Ensure that rescuers are apprised of the activities and needs of others. Keep command, base of operations, medical control, and incoming rescuers informed. Communication is the most frequently missed or poorly managed aspect
- Locate and reach the patient with medical-rescue personnel and equipment. Implement organized and methodical procedures for finding the patient as soon as safety of rescuers and the patient has been ascertained

- Treat and monitor the patient during evacuation. Support basic personal hygiene and physiologic functions. Psychological support is essential. This may be as basic as verbal encouragement from a familiar and constant voice. Help the patient feel involved with the rescue by communicating as often as the situation permits.

PREPLANNING

- Before engaging in any type of technical rescue, responsible individuals should perform a risk assessment to identify necessary skills and capabilities
- The preplan should consider the types of terrain in the response area, people exposed to that terrain, types of accidents likely to occur, and available resources
- Exposed personnel must be specifically trained for terrain and environmental considerations commonly encountered in the theater of operation. For example, a rescuer responding to a fallen ice climber incident in the wilderness must be trained in both high-angle ice rescue and wilderness SAR
- Having wilderness skills enables rescuers to work independently of external support and resources in nonwilderness incidents. For example, self-sufficiency and ability to function with minimal external resources are beneficial when working in the aftermath of an earthquake, or when responding to a transmission tower incident far from a road.

Research the Location

- Review all geographic and medical concerns specific to the rescue location, identifying in advance any hazards that pose a threat
- Determine topography and potential evacuation routes before beginning travel
- Make certain that the location of cached equipment and supplies, and phone numbers for available rescue resources and local hospitals, are communicated to each member of the party.

Rescue Resources

- The outdoor recreation and rescue communities emphasize personal responsibility. If the group has the skills and technical abilities to accomplish self-rescue, the participants must know their limitations. If necessary, members must be capable and willing to mobilize organized rescue resources. Organized rescue is often more expeditious and mitigates the risk of rescue
- Rescuers not familiar with an environment or type of response should operate only under direct supervision and care of appropriately trained personnel. For example, placing an untrained person in a high-angle rope rescue situation to perform patient care endangers that person, the patient, and others involved in the operation
- Within the United States, law enforcement agencies are generally responsible for the command structure and direction of an

operation. Mutual aid contracts or interagency agreements may give certain agencies responsibility for specific incidents. When adventuring outside the United States, always discuss rescue issues (e.g., forms of payment, available resources, notification systems) with the foreign US embassy. In the United States, follow these guidelines:

- County sheriffs have jurisdiction in unincorporated county areas and in most Bureau of Land Management and US Forest Service lands
- City police have jurisdiction on city lands and, in some cases, adjacent watersheds.
- Fire districts and city fire departments may have jurisdiction over hazardous materials or urban SAR operations
- Emergency medical services (EMS) usually have jurisdiction over medical care of sick or injured persons, but may have limited backcountry travel and wilderness rescue capabilities
- The National Park Service has jurisdiction over its lands except where otherwise mandated

Support Services

Any single responsible agency may not have the most efficient means of conducting a rescue operation. It may delegate or request help from other groups that are more capable of performing the actual rescue, such as the following:

- Volunteer SAR and sheriff's SAR groups usually have responsibility and authority to conduct an operation
- Technically specialized volunteer teams, in addition to regular SAR teams, may be available and perhaps certified by national organizations. These organizations include the National Ski Patrol System, National Cave Rescue Commission, Mountain Rescue Association, and National Association for Search and Rescue
- Commercial enterprises or professional individuals or teams, even if they are not specifically certified, may be able to provide some benefit to an SAR mission. Such groups include mountain, river, and bicycle guides; commercial mine rescue teams; and military units.

Personal Preparation

Rescue operations are inherently dangerous. No amount of preparation can completely remove every danger. Rescue party members should possess personal skills specific to the terrain where they will operate.

Fitness

- Participate in a regular physical fitness program
- Psychological fitness:
  - Be prepared to put personal and team safety above patient outcomes
  - Be responsible for your personal safety

- Anticipate exposure to distressing and intense situations
- Because poor patient outcomes and other losses are possible on rescue missions, critical incident stress debriefing should occur.

General Safety Guidelines
- Use appropriate safety equipment for the environment
- Make sure that anchors are secure. Tie in anyone near an edge or precipice
- Make sure that helmets and eye protection are worn by persons at risk for falls or exposure to falling objects
- Wear personal flotation devices when performing rescues near or in the water
- Employ safety checks on all critical tasks and rescue system elements
- Practice using all technical-rigging systems before they are needed in an actual rescue operation
- Have backup systems available whenever possible

Training (Box 56.1)
Most rescue teams offer standardized training to educate eligible members in the basic skills they need to operate. Graduated levels of membership often designate promotion of responsibility after completion of advanced training. SAR and other rescue conferences offer additional opportunities to expand knowledge and skills. Attention should be placed on basic survival, navigation, thermo-regulation, water procurement and disinfection, and personal safety.

Personal Equipment
Most rescue teams have required and optional equipment lists relevant to the local environment and mission possibilities. This section provides only general considerations and guidelines.
- Rugged internal frame pack. Consider having both a smaller "hasty" or "24-hour" pack, and a larger pack for extended missions
- Appropriate footwear for the mission type; most commonly heavy leather boots or mountain boots
- Waterproof, breathable shell jacket and pants that are appropriate for local climates and anticipated weather conditions
- Layers of clothing to allow for ranges in temperature and exertion; use "water-compatible" materials (e.g., fleece, wool, polypropylene [Polypro]) that absorb less water and maintain loft and warmth
- Leather (durable) and weather-resistant shell gloves
- Sunglasses (with side shields or wrap-around) to minimize ultraviolet light and water exposure; goggles in winter
- Bivouac ("bivi") gear for unanticipated nights out
- Survival supplies (e.g., knife, garbage bags/bivi sack, duct tape, whistle, candles and fire starter, waterproof matches, flares, smoke signal, signal mirror) (Box 56.2)

BOX 56.1   Rescue Personnel and Training in the United States

- Most technical rescue personnel in the United States are climbers or skiers who add rescue techniques and medical training to their skills
- Foundational medical training on rescue teams can include: basic first aid, first responder, emergency medical technician, or paramedic. Some teams also incorporate registered nurses, advanced registered nurse practitioners, physician assistants, or physicians with wilderness medicine training
- A growing number of wilderness emergency medical technicians have been trained in the skills of extended patient care in the backcountry environment.

Key Skill Elements of Medical and Rescue Training for Wilderness Environments
- Thorough patient assessment and monitoring
- Technical skills and the authority to perform the following:
  - Airway management, including endotracheal intubation
  - Shock management, including IV/IO therapy
  - Use of pelvic stabilization device
  - Oxygen administration
  - Use of appropriate medications:
    - Epinephrine for anaphylaxis
    - Antibiotics for open fractures and significant soft tissue injury
    - Acetazolamide, nifedipine, sildenafil, dexamethasone and other drugs for acute high-altitude illnesses
- Pain medications for musculoskeletal trauma
- Field rewarming techniques
- Field reduction of fractures and dislocations
- Patient packaging and transportation skills

Key Skill Elements of Technical Training for Rescue Personnel in the United States
- Appropriate climbing, transportation, and navigation skills for terrain (rock, ice, snow, glacier, ocean)
- Radio communications skills and protocols
- Helicopter and fixed-wing protocols
- Training and expertise in the Incident Command System
- Swiftwater and ocean rescue (depending on environment)
- Hazardous materials awareness (depending on environment)

- Personal care items (e.g., prescription eyeglasses with lanyard, hygiene, personal first-aid kit that includes sunblock, insect repellent, blister care)
- Personal medications
- Self-evacuation and rescue equipment:
  - Tubular webbing (2.5 cm [1 in] in diameter) for improvised chest and seat harnesses, runners, anchors, etc.
  - Kernmantle climbing rope for lowering or raising if terrain is too steep or high for a simple climb up or down

---

BOX 56.2 Bivouac Kit

- Two large garbage bags (emergency shelter or rain gear), 3 m × 3 m (10 ft × 10 ft) sheet of plastic, and 30.5 m (100 ft) of parachute cord (shelter)
- Emergency space blanket (shelter, ground cloth)
- Stocking cap (warmth)
- Spare socks (warmth and can act as spare mittens)
- Cup with lid (to warm liquids)
- Drink mix containing sugar (e.g., hot chocolate, gelatin, Tang)
- Two plumber's candles (to warm water or start fire)
- Waterproof matches or lighter
- Knife
- Compass
- Whistle
- These items fit neatly into a small stuff sack that is 15.2 cm × 15.2 cm (6 in × 6 in) and weighs less than 0.5 kg (1 lb) when filled.

- Carabiners to improvise lowering (rappelling) or climbing devices on ropes
- Tubular webbing (2.5 cm) or 4-mm (0.2-in) rope for making improvised breaking devices (e.g., Prusik knot) for use with ropes and carabiners.

SEARCH AND RESCUE OPERATIONS
Sequence of Events in Backcountry Rescue (Box 56.3)
Making the Decision to Get Help

Before anyone leaves to seek assistance, the patient's companions should do the following:

1. Perform a physical examination.
2. Record vital signs if possible.
3. Determine level of consciousness.
4. Provide appropriate emergency care, which may entail moving the patient into a protective shelter.
5. Summarize patient information in a note that accompanies the individual(s) going for help.
6. Prepare a map depicting the patient's exact location and a list of other party members, noting their level of preparedness to endure the environmental conditions.
7. The individuals who are going for help should carry appropriate provisions.
8. Do not allow the leaving party to become a new set of patients. Plan and prepare for likely contingencies.

Locate Phase

- The first step in addressing any emergency is locating the subject or subjects

---

BOX 56.3   Sequence of Events in Backcountry Rescue

1. A patient becomes ill or injured.
2. The patient or party decides to ask for help.
3. Responsible agencies become aware of the need for help.
4. Responsible agencies take initial action and evaluate the critical information.
5. Planning occurs to develop an initial strategy and mobilize necessary resources.
6. Mission goes into "operations" phase:
   a. Location the patient
   b. Access scene and patient safety
   c. Stabilize life-threatening injuries and package for transport
   d. Transport the patient to safety
7. Conclude the mission; debrief and demobilize response teams.

- If the subject is easily found, rescuers can quickly move into the access phase. However, if locating the subject is difficult, this phase may turn into the crux of the SAR problem.

First Notice
Initial notification can occur by several means:
- Relatives who report an injury or missing person
- Witness to an incident
- Government agency reporting distress signals
- Bystanders who perceive a problem, or a caller to an emergency access number, such as 911

Once the initial notice is received, the individual taking the information must know what to do and whom next to call.

Planning Data and Their Uses
Information gathered at the onset of an incident initiates an ongoing investigation. It is used to determine the appropriate response and help predict how the subject or subjects might react to the situation.
- Name of the subject
- Situation that caused the problem
- Last known location of the subject
- Subject's physical and mental conditions
- Subject's plans (route of travel, camp sites, planned activities)
- Subject's communications (e.g., social media)
- Available resources
- Weather information (present and predicted)
- Geographic information
- History of similar incidents in the area

Once information is gathered, the urgency of the situation is assessed. This assessment ultimately determines the speed, level, and nature of any response, and may help determine whether a nonurgent or emergency response is needed.

Search Tactics

- During the initial (locate) phase of the incident, emphasis is on searching for the subject
- Indirect techniques (e.g., not requiring actual field searching) are usually quicker and easier to apply, so they are started first
  - Confining the search area to limit movement of the subject and others into and out of the area
  - Identifying and protecting the point last seen or the last known position
  - Attracting the attention of the subject if he or she is expected to be responsive
- Quick-response resources are usually begun in areas where early success is most likely
- Direct techniques include sending teams of searchers into an area to look for clues and the subject. In certain circumstances, drones may be helpful
- A fast, relatively low coverage search of high-probability, unbounded areas is called a *hasty search*. This type of search would be conducted at campsites, buildings, and other locations where the subject would likely be found
- High-coverage techniques, which are slow, highly systematic area searches, are used when the highest probability of detection is required.

Clues and Their Value

- Clues are discovered during the investigative and tactical phases of a search. Their importance cannot be overemphasized
- Clues may take the form of physical evidence, such as a footprint or discarded item, an eyewitness account, relayed message, or information gleaned from the investigation
- A person exudes scent in the form of dead skin cells, crushes or disturbs vegetation, and, when traveling, leaves marks on the ground or other physical evidence of passing
- Evidence is often discoverable if the appropriate resource(s) is applied in a coordinated, organized search effort.

Search Resources

Resources are defined as all personnel and equipment available or potentially available for assignment to support the search effort. Specific types of active tactics are categorized by the resource that performs them, such as dog teams, human trackers, ground search teams, and aircraft. Other common resources include management teams (e.g., overhead teams, public information officers), water-trained responders (e.g., river rescue, divers), cold weather responders (e.g., ice climbers, avalanche experts, ski patrollers), specialized vehicle responders (e.g., snowmobiles, four-wheel-drive trucks, all-terrain vehicles, mountain bikes, horses), and technical experts (e.g., communications experts, interviewers, chemists, rock climbers, physicians, cavers, drone handlers).

Dogs

- Dog teams are composed of a dog (occasionally more than one) and a human handler
- The dog uses scent to search for and follow a subject while the handler interprets signals from the dog and searches visually for evidence
- Three common categories are tracking, trailing, and air scenting dogs

Human Trackers

Human trackers use their visual senses to search for evidence left by a person in passing. In SAR, most trackers use a stride-based approach called the step-by-step method. This simple, methodical approach emphasizes finding every piece of possible evidence left by a subject. Its most important role is undoubtedly the ability to quickly determine the direction of travel of the subject and thus limit the search area.

Ground Search Teams

Hasty Teams

- A hasty team is an initial response team of well-trained, self-sufficient, and highly mobile searchers whose primary responsibility is to check out the areas (e.g., trails, roads, road heads, campsites, lakes, clearings) most likely to first produce the subject or clues
- Hasty teams should include two or three individuals who are knowledgeable about tracking
- Hasty teams should be clue oriented, familiar with the local terrain and dangers in the area, and completely self-sufficient
- Hasty teams should carry all the equipment they might need to assist themselves and the lost subject for at least 24 hours.

Grid Teams

- Grid searchers use a more systematic approach to searching. They usually examine a well-defined, often small, territory to discover evidence
- The classic approach to grid searching involves several individuals standing in a line, shoulder-to-shoulder, walking through an area in search of evidence or subjects
- When the subject of a search is a live person, searching in this thorough manner should be used only as a last resort, because it is slow and covers limited territory for the amount of time and resources utilized.

Aircraft and Drones

- Aircraft and drones serve the same purpose as grid searchers, only from a greater distance, at a greater speed, over a larger area, and usually with a lower level of thoroughness
- Within a search effort, aircraft can serve both as a tactical tool to look for clues and as transportation for personnel and equipment.

Search Planning Considerations

Search effectiveness also has been improved through the study of human behavior, statistics, probabilities, and leadership, and using good planning and management principles. Search planning is guided by two general considerations: where am I going to look for the lost or missing person (strategy), and how am I going to find this missing or lost person (tactics)? To be effective, modern searchers follow basic principles and techniques that include:

1. Respond urgently—search is an emergency.
2. Confine the search area.
3. Search for clues and the subject.
4. Search at night if the risk of darkness can be mitigated.
5. Search with a plan and in an organized manner.
6. Use grid searching (high coverage) as a last resort.

Search Theory

- Search theory aims to determine where and how to search by (1) quantifying the likelihood of a missing subject being in an area, and the likelihood of searchers finding the subject; and (2) offering tools with which one can estimate the chances of success of a search
- The chance that the missing person is in the search area is called *probability of containment* (POC) or, in the land search community, *probability of area* (POA)
- The conditional probability that a search resource will find the missing person, if he or she is indeed in the area being searched, is called *probability of detection* (POD)
- The product of these two important variables produces *probability of success* (POS) = (POA × POD).

Lost Subject Behavior

Many theories and publications on lost subject behavior help guide experienced search planners. Search personnel in possession of the following information can more accurately predict the subject's location:

1. Circumstances under which the person became lost.
2. Personality.
3. Terrain.
4. Weather.
5. Physical condition at time of becoming lost.
6. Known medical problems.

For instance, hikers travel about 2.3 times farther than do campers, and cross-country skiers breaking trail travel about 5.4 times farther than do cross-country skiers using groomed trails.

Access Phase

- After the subject is located, the search is over. Rescuers must now gain access to the subject to assess and treat injuries, evaluate the situation, and mitigate the problem. After rescuers

reach a subject, the situation and scene must be assessed (collectively known as the "scene size-up")
- The size-up consists of identifying hazards to the subject and rescuers, and then developing a strategy to deal with the problems
- Safety considerations for rescuers entering such a hostile and dangerous environment would certainly influence further actions and may well take priority over the rescue effort
- Accelerated rescue techniques may be required if the size-up indicates that the situation or environment is so hazardous that remaining on the scene poses an immediate threat to the subject.

Stabilization Phase (Box 56.4)
- The stabilization phase has three primary components: physical, medical, and emotional
- Once rescuers have access to the subject, the scene must be quickly evaluated, or sized up, for immediate physical hazards and threats from the environment
- Scene safety is an initial priority in the size-up, and risks to everyone must be weighed against the likely benefits
- Once the physical environment is stabilized, medical management can begin, beginning with a primary and secondary survey and progressing through treatment from basic to advanced life support
- The goal of medical stabilization is to prepare the subject for transport to a definitive care location, typically a hospital
- Emotional stabilization is necessary because an anxious victim is a hazard to rescuers and him/herself.

BOX 56.4   Patient Assessment

Primary Survey: Locating and Treating Life-Threatening Problems

A: Airway Management
- Ensure airway is open and patent
- Perform maneuvers to open airway if obstructed
- Place airway adjuncts (e.g., oral or nasal airway) if needed
- Consider endotracheal intubation for patients with a compromised airway and low Glasgow Coma Scale score

B: Breathing
- Assess the work and quality of breathing
- Evaluate for pneumothorax or major trauma to the chest wall
- Consider oxygen administration if available and appropriate
- Provide assisted ventilations as needed

C: Circulation
- Assess pulses for rate and quality
- Control major bleeding
- Place IV/IO access if available and indicated

Continued

BOX 56.4   Patient Assessment—cont'd

D: Disability
- Determine if conscious or unconscious
- Level of consciousness: AVPU (**a**wake, **v**erbal, **p**ainful, **u**nconscious) or Glasgow Coma Scale (see Appendix B)
- Evaluate pupillary function and extremity muscle strength, sensation, and tone
- Cervical spine stabilization (if indicated)

E: Environment
- Protect patient from the elements
- Keep patient warm and dry
- Place insulating material to protect from below and above

Secondary Survey: What Are All the Injuries or Illnesses and How Serious Are They?
Vital Signs: Indicate the Condition of the Patient
- Respiratory rate and effort
- Pulse rate and character
- Blood pressure: systolic/diastolic
- Level of consciousness: AVPU or Glasgow Coma Scale
- Tissue perfusion: skin color, temperature, and moisture
- Capillary refill (<2 sec)
- Temperature (via oral, esophageal, or rectal probe)

Patient Examination: Head-to-Toe Examination to Locate Injuries
SAMPLE History
- **S**igns and symptoms
- **A**llergies
- **M**edicines
- **P**ast medical history
- **L**ast in and out: food/drink and voiding
- **E**vents leading up

SOAP Note: To Record and Organize Patient Data
Subjective: age, gender, mechanism of injury, chief complaint, and SAMPLE history
Objective: vital signs, patient examination
Assessment: problem list
Plan: plan for each problem

Patient Reassessment
Subjective: Is the patient comfortable, too hot, too cold, hungry, thirsty, or in need of urination or defecation?
Objective:
- Vital signs: Are they stable?
- Patient examination: Recheck all dressings, bandages, and splints. Are they still controlling bleeding? Are they too tight or too loose? (Swelling limbs can cause bandages or splints to impede circulation, thereby resulting in ischemic injuries or worsening frostbite or snakebite.)

Assessment: Has the initial assessment changed?
Plan: Is the rate of evacuation still the same? Are there any changes in the care plan?

Transport Phase

In the fourth phase of SAR, the patient is "packaged" and moved to definitive care. The patient is optimally moved safely and efficiently while stabilization and assessment continue. While providing emergency care, part of the team is designated to be the evacuation team. The medical team leader should coordinate with the evacuation team about the patient's condition to determine how rapidly evacuation should occur.

- If speed is a consideration, weather conditions are reviewed and the availability of a helicopter-assisted rescue is determined
- If a helicopter is not an option, the fastest evacuation route is established
- If time or speed is not critical, the safest means of evacuation that is easiest on the patient and rescuers is defined
- It will take 1 to 2 hours for every mile to be covered by carryout, requiring six well-rested litter attendants for each mile
- Eventually the team reaches a trailhead and the patient is transferred to an ambulance for transport to a definitive care location.

Additional Patient Evacuation Considerations

Based on scene and patient assessments, evacuation may be divided into the following four methods:

- No evacuation. Definitive care is either not necessary or is available at the scene
- Assisted evacuation. Definitive therapy is necessary, but the patient is ambulatory and needs moderate support. Consider walking assists utilizing one or two rescuers
- Simple carries. The patient can sit, or the injuries allow positioning other than horizontal. Examples would include a patient with exhaustion and dehydration and an uncomplicated limb fracture
- Litter carries (see Chapter 57). The patient is unable to sit or injuries require a horizontal position. Examples would be a femoral fracture or spine immobilization. This type of transport usually requires a minimum of six rescuers. The longer the transport, the more necessary are additional party members. Depending on the terrain, this type of carry may present significant risk to patient and rescuers. Two general types of litters are found on rescues: commercial and improvised
- The most common commercial litter is the Stokes litter (wire, plastic, or fiberglass), which may be found with or without leg dividers; the latter is preferable because of flexible packaging configuration based on injuries
- Another commercial litter is the SKED, which is popular among SAR teams and the military because it is easily carried rolled up in its own backpack, slides easily, and has flotation capability. It is narrower than the Stokes litter and somewhat flexible. A short spine immobilization device is necessary if spinal injury is possible

- Other specialized litters, such as cave-evacuation litters, may be deployed in certain environments. One can construct improvised litters from the external frames of packs, saplings, or ropes (see Chapter 57).

Additional Litter Evacuation Considerations

- Litter packaging should provide patient comfort and protection from trauma and environmental impact. Secure the patient in the litter by attaching harnesses to side rails, using pretied foot loops hitched to rails or torso immobilizing devices (e.g., Kendrick Extrication Device [KED], or Oregon Spine Splint [OSS]), which may then be attached to the litter
- Monitor the patient. Protect the face from falling objects and passing branches. One can cover the head and face with a plexiglass (Lexan) shield or a helmet and goggles, or fashion a piece of closed-cell foam (Ensolite) for this. Package and adequately pad the patient to prevent pressure sores during prolonged transport. Protect the patient from insects with netting, repellent, or a secure outer wrap
- Environmental concerns relate primarily to temperature regulation and precipitation, but may include adverse weather events, including lightning. The goal is warmth without overheating. Immobility reduces heat production. Extra insulation and an external heat source may be necessary. In a cold environment, a double vapor barrier system may be necessary, with less insulation in a hot environment. A mixed system may be necessary in the high desert to allow venting of the package during the day and sealing at night. You can set up a double vapor barrier system as follows (see Fig. 3.1):
  - Place the outside vapor barrier on the ground first (e.g., the patient's tent fly or ground cloth)
  - Place the insulation layer(s), such as a sleeping bag or several blankets, on top
  - Strip the patient down to a base layer (or just skin), dry off, and place any instrumentation (e.g., blood pressure cuff, stethoscope, monitoring equipment, Foley catheter) properly
  - Cover the patient, and seal him or her in an inner vapor barrier (e.g., two garbage bags)
  - Place the patient in the insulation layer
  - Wrap the patient like a burrito with the outer vapor barrier
- Because the litter carry is strenuous and requires great focus, designate a route finder to find the most efficient trail. Choose a medical leader to direct patient monitoring and communication. Litter carries are best performed by at least six persons. Make sure the patient is level (or head up as indicated by injuries) and transported feet first. On level terrain with few obstructions, position extra rescuers behind the litter. Rotate the carriers through the three litter-carrying positions on one side until they

have finished their forward-most carry, and then have them rotate to the rear of the line on the opposite side. This allows for a change in sides to limit rescuer fatigue
- On terrain with short drops or obstructions, have extra rescuers place themselves in the forward direction of travel. This allows for a litter pass with rescuers in a stable, nonmoving position. When a rescuer has finished a pass, have the person move to the front of the line on the opposite side
- On steeper terrain, set up a simple belay using a tree wrap as the lowering device or an anchored lowering device such as a Munter hitch attached to a rock. Leave an extra length of rope, or "tag" line, at the head of the litter to tie off the litter and rescuers during belay transfers. Remind rescuers to lean downhill so that their legs are perpendicular to the hillside. Trying to stand upright usually results in feet slipping out from under the rescuer and dropping the litter.

Patient Evaluation and Treatment During Transport
Patient Communication and Monitoring
- Minimize the number of rescuers who are positioned directly over the patient's head. Limit the number of rescuers who communicate directly with the patient. This reduces perceived chaos and helps keep the patient oriented and calm
- Monitor oxygen saturation with pulse oximetry. Adequate circulation can be estimated by temporal or carotid artery pulses. Unless the patient's condition changes significantly, blood pressure probably does not need to be routinely measured
- Monitor blood pressure by placing a cuff over a flat-diaphragm stethoscope that is taped to the patient's upper arm. Run the cuff bulb, gauge, and stethoscope earpieces through a hole in the vapor barriers to the outside for easy access. Re-seal access holes with duct tape after placement
- Monitor respirations using a small pocket mirror or noting condensation on the face mask or in the endotracheal (ET) tube
- Obtain rectal temperature using an indoor/outdoor remote thermometer. Insert the "outdoor" probe into the rectum after covering with a lubricated finger cot, latex glove finger, or condom. The "indoor" reading reflects the patient's local environment. During the preplanning phase, test the thermometer's accuracy against glass thermometers in water of varying temperatures. Thermometry is an essential component of a double vapor barrier system because of the potential for raising the patient's core temperature
- Skin color, temperature, and moisture are difficult to monitor in a litter-packaged patient. Other vital signs, especially pulse rate, are used more frequently
- Mental status is extremely sensitive to perfusion changes. If the rescuers continuously interact with a conscious patient, they will perceive subtle changes.

Respiratory Guidelines
- Protect the airway
- The definitive airway is an ET tube. Neither oropharyngeal nor nasopharyngeal airways protect the trachea from upper airway bleeding or vomitus
- Improvise suction devices using a turkey baster or a 60-mL irrigating syringe with 1.5-cm (0.6-in) surgical tubing or an inverted nasal airway. A commercial device (V-VAC hand-powered suction unit) is compact and works well. Remember that gravity is readily available. A well-packaged patient can be quickly rolled to the side (rescue position) or tilted head-down without compromise of spinal alignment
- Remote ventilation systems, mouth-to-mask ventilation, or even a bag-valve-mask may be difficult to manipulate when a patient is packaged in a litter, being carried over steep or rough terrain, or transported in a confined space. For a patient needing ventilation, consider the following system:
  - Mask or ET tube (preferable). A mask can be taped to the face (with quick-release capability), or an anesthesia mask and rubber spider strapping may be used (airway must be constantly monitored)
  - One-way valve. This is placed in-line near the facemask to limit dead space. In cold weather, this may freeze from condensation, so always carry a spare valve inside your coat or pack
  - Oxygen
  - Ventilator tube
  - Bag-valve-mask
  - Commercial one-way valves, which can be purchased from most hospital respiratory therapy departments, may be taped to the ventilator tubing. The White Pulmonary Resuscitator is a commercial version of the improvised system.

Circulatory Considerations
- Because of weight and space restrictions, IV fluid therapy in the field is usually reserved for SAR teams or large expeditions
- IV fluids are typically infused by bolus during stops or when needed
- Do not leave any IV lines hanging during transport. They get in the way and are pulled out easily
- Blood pressure cuff and body weight methods of pressure infusion are usually inadequate for high-volume fluid replacement
- Pre-warm IV bags by carrying them inside your coat, and then protect lines from freezing by placing the fluids inside the litter package or your coat. Certain CamelBak and other commercial hydration units sometimes wrap tubing in foam to protect against freezing. To set up a non–gravity-feed field IV system, proceed through the following steps:
  - Invert the bag and squeeze out the air
  - Start the IV line using a saline lock and large-bore catheter

- Run in the amount of fluid desired using a pressure IV sleeve, with the quantity measured with the bag
- Disconnect the IV tubing from the saline lock and cap the needle
- Package the remaining fluids with the patient

Nervous System Considerations

- Vomiting is a classic sign of head injury. Monitor and protect the airway
- Apply padding around the patient when placed in a rescue litter or other carrying device wherever possible (without compromising spine immobilization) because compartment syndrome may be caused by inadequate padding
- Consider using a vacuum mattress system instead of a backboard for suspected spinal injuries.

Musculoskeletal System Considerations

- Pressure sores can be avoided by using adequate padding and periodically shifting the patient if possible
- Compartment syndrome from tissue edema is often overlooked because of the intensity of evacuation. Perform ongoing assessment of injured extremities
- When packaging for a long evacuation, place the patient's knees and elbows in slight flexion to achieve maximum comfort
- Continuously reevaluate for neurovascular compromise.

Gastrointestinal and Genitourinary Considerations

- Although the fasting status of patients who may require surgery is a consideration, hydration of the patient during the extended evacuation is more important. Persuade patients whose injuries or illness do not preclude fluids by mouth to take small sips of water. Encourage them to eat and drink regularly
- With proper double vapor barrier packaging and long transport delays unlikely, allow the patient to defecate or urinate freely inside the litter packaging. A proper or improvised diaper helps reduce discomfort. Rescue teams should carry diapers for patients if rescues have long anticipated transport times
- For the unconscious patient, insert a Foley catheter to allow for assessment of urine output. In a conscious male, one may use a condom catheter
- For the conscious patient, the litter can be inverted or stood on end for urination if the packaging arrangement allows. A bedpan or urinal can also be used
- Female patients may urinate into an improvised funnel made from an inverted pocket mask held against the perineum. Attach this to 1.5-cm (0.6-in) surgical tubing and drain it outside the litter. The Whiz Freedom or Lady J are manufactured devices that accomplish the same
- For defecation, a foam pad can be cut into the shape of a toilet seat (donutshaped), and placed over a hole dug into the ground

or snow (this method assumes the patient can be moved out of the litter). Constipation and fecal impaction may become problematic in the immobile and dehydrated patient. Adequate hydration is the best prevention.

Mission Termination Criteria
• Termination criteria should be identified and in place before the start of a search. Criteria should center on the probability of success weighed against the risk to rescuers.

Returning to Base
• Teams return to base to debrief and reorganize equipment in preparation for the next rescue.
• Problems should be discussed and managed in real time so that teams cooperate successfully, improve performance, and provide the best possible patient care during the current and subsequent rescues. A debrief immediately after the search is sometimes called a "hot wash."

ADDITIONAL RESCUE CONSIDERATIONS
Self-Rescue: Signaling
• Fire is an effective signaling method during darkness. The international distress signal is three fires in a triangle or in a straight line with about 25 m (82 ft) between fires. It is better to be able to maintain one signal fire if it is too difficult to keep three burning. Using a small campfire for a signal conserves fuel and energy. Keep a good supply of rapid-burning materials to throw on the fire quickly if needed. In hot and dry environmental conditions, take care to not start a wildland fire
• Make sure that smoke signals contrast to the surrounding area. Dark-colored smoke can be made with oil-soaked rags, rubber, plastic, or electrical insulation. Light-colored smoke can be made with green leaves, moss, ferns, or water sprinkled on the fire
• One can make a signal mirror from shiny metal or glass; this is probably the most effective method for signaling on a bright, sunny day. Extend your arm while sighting the reflection between thumb and forefinger on the outstretched arm. Slowly move the arm until an aircraft or vehicle comes into sight between your thumb and forefinger, and then move the reflection to signal the vehicle.

Rescue Communications
Emergency radio communications usually occur on the following bands:
• Common public safety bands:
  • Very high frequency (VHF), 32 to 50 MHz: good for two-way communication and paging; follows the terrain; susceptible to manmade and natural interference; uses more power and requires a long (45-cm [17.7-in]) antenna
    • VHF high band, 140 to 170 MHz: less distance; more line of sight; utilizes a short (15-cm [5.9-in]) antenna

- Ultrahigh frequency (UHF), 460 to 470 MHz or higher: least distance; more penetration of buildings; almost always needs repeaters; shortest (5-cm [2-in]) antenna
- Civilian radio bands
- Ham (amateur): many bands used; high power and good distance; phone patch and relay possible to Military Affiliate Radio System (MARS); emergency nets already in place (Radio Amateur Civil Emergency Service [RACES]); worldwide
- CB (citizens band): crowded high-frequency (HF) band with poor distance; heavy interference; common and inexpensive
- With cellular phones, it is important to know the location. The actual cell tower picking up the call may be many miles from your location, particularly if your location is at high altitude. Keep this in mind when placing a 911 call.

COSPAS-SARSAT

- The SARSAT (search and rescue satellite-aided tracking) system was developed in a joint effort by the United States, Canada, and France
- This system allows for transmission of a 406-MHz message of encoded position data acquired by beacons from global satellite navigation systems, such as global positioning system (GPS), using internal or external navigation receivers
- The system uses satellites to detect and locate emergency beacons carried by ships, aircraft, and individuals transmitting on 406 MHz
- When an emergency beacon is activated, the signal is received by a satellite and relayed to the nearest available ground station. The ground station, called a local user terminal, processes the signal and calculates the position from which it originated
- This position is transmitted to a mission control center, where it is joined with identification data and other information on that beacon, if the beacon has been registered with the National Oceanic and Atmospheric Administration (NOAA), which is required by law in the United States (see below)
- The mission control center transmits an alert message to the appropriate rescue coordination center (RCC), based primarily on the geographic location of the beacon
- New upgraded COSPAS-SARSAT assets are part of a system known as MEOSAR, for medium-altitude earth orbit search and rescue system.

Distress Radio Beacons

The most recognizable component of the SARSAT system is the distress radio beacon, also known as a *beacon*. There are generally three types of beacons used to transmit distress:

1. Emergency position-indicating radio beacons (EPIRBs) designed for maritime use.
2. Emergency locator transmitters (ELTs) designed for aviation use.
3. Personal locator beacons (PLBs) designed for use by individuals and land-based applications.

When turned on (automatically or manually), each transmits alert signals on specific frequencies intended to be received by COSPAS-SARSAT satellites.

Emergency Position-Indicating Radio Beacons (Marine EPIRBs)

There are several types of EPIRBs used for maritime applications. The U.S. Coast Guard website with information on EPIRBs is http://www.navcen.uscg.gov/?pageName=mtEpirb.

Emergency Locator Transmitters (Aviation Emergency Locator Transmitters)

Most aircraft operators are now mandated to carry an ELT. Although 121.5/243-MHz ELTs used by some aircraft may still be used, the COSPAS-SARSAT system ceased satellite processing of these beacons in 2009, and alerts from these devices (and from 121.5/243-MHz EPIRBs) are no longer acted upon unless detected by an overflying aircraft or ground-based receiver. Therefore, all ELT owners and users should replace their 121.5/243-MHz beacons with 406-MHz beacons as soon as possible and register their beacons with NOAA at beaconregistration.noaa.gov.

Personal Locator Beacons

- PLBs are portable units that operate in much the same way as EPIRBs or ELTs
- These beacons are designed to be carried by individuals instead of on a boat or aircraft
- Unlike ELTs and some EPIRBs, they can only be activated manually and operate exclusively on 406 MHz in the United States
- Like EPIRBs and ELTs, all PLBs also have a built-in, low-power homing beacon that transmits on 121.5 MHz. This allows rescue teams to homein on a beacon once the 406-MHz satellite system has put them within 3.2 to 4.8 km (2 to 3 miles)
- Some newer PLBs also allow GPS units to be integrated into the distress signal. This GPS-encoded position dramatically improves the location accuracy down to the level of 100 m (328 ft)
- PLB users should familiarize themselves with proper registration, testing, and operating procedures to prevent false activation, and avoid their use in nonemergency situations.

Satellite Communicators

- Technology now includes satellite communicators that can provide improved geographic location information, texting capabilities, and voice communications through low earth–orbit satellite networks with extensive global coverage
- The devices allow tracking by remote parties and much more

precise geographic location services, which could preclude or replace the need for activation of an emergency beacon, such as a PLB. DeLorme offers the inReach series of satellite communicators; SPOT offers the SPOT Gen3 satellite communicator; and Iridium offers a number of satellite-based options, including the Iridium GO!.

Knowledge, Skills, and Equipment Needed by Extended Rescue Teams

See Box 56.5.

BOX 56.5   Knowledge, Skills, and Equipment Needed by Extended Rescue Teams

Mountaineering Skills
- Understanding fabrics, clothing systems, and their seasonal variations
- Utilization and operation of personal protection equipment:
  - Helmets
  - Harnesses
  - Gloves
  - Boots
  - Goggles or sunglasses
  - Hearing protection
  - Backcountry equipment
- Utilization and operation of specialty equipment:
  - snowshoes/backcountry skis
  - crampons
  - ice axes
  - stoves
  - global positioning system/personal locator beacon devices
- Backcountry travel
- Route finding
- Navigation (e.g., map and compass, global positioning system)
- Survival skills
- Shelter and warmth; emergency bivouac kits
- Meal and nutrition planning
- Water procurement and disinfection
- Understanding how backcountry travel and rescue vary with different environments:
  - Alpine
  - Desert
  - Forest
  - Water (e.g., swamp, river, lake, ocean)
  - Tropics
  - High altitude

Continued

BOX 56.5 Knowledge, Skills, and Equipment Needed by Extended Rescue Teams—cont'd

- Low-impact camping and rescue work
- Basics of weather and weather forecasting
  - Principles of barometric pressure
  - Clouds and their significance in weather forecasting
  - Prevailing weather patterns in the rescue area
- Personal fitness

Mountain and Extended Emergency Medical Skills
- Medical team members should be trained to at least the Emergency Medical Technician level
- Training must include wilderness and extended emergency care procedures
- The Diploma in Mountain Medicine (DiMM) program, administered by the Wilderness Medical Society, provides an internationally recognized foundation for medical providers (paramedics, advanced practice providers, and physicians) to operate with wilderness rescue teams.

Topics of Extended Care Training and Principles Should Include the Following:
- Patient assessment
- Cardiopulmonary resuscitation
- Airway management, including endotracheal intubation and needle decompression for tension pneumothorax
- Shock and control of bleeding, including IV/IO therapy for fluid resuscitation
- Long-term wound care and prevention of infection
- Musculoskeletal injury management, including specific information about diagnosis and long-term management of the following:
  - Sprains and strains
  - Fractures, including how to reduce or realign angulated fractures
  - Stabilization and reduction of pelvic fractures
  - Diagnosis and reduction of dislocations
  - Management of compound fractures
  - Field amputation
  - Management of crush syndrome
- Management of chest injuries, including decompression of a tension pneumothorax using needle or tube thoracostomy
- Spinal cord injury diagnosis and management
- Head injury, including recognition and management of increasing intracranial pressure
- Management of environmental emergencies
- Hypothermia and frostbite, including use of IV/IO fluids
- Heatstroke and heat exhaustion, including use of IV/IO fluids
- Dehydration and nutrition, both acute and during evacuation
- Lightning injuries
- Animal attacks, insect bites, and reptile and marine envenomation, including anaphylactic reactions and use of epinephrine and antihistamines

> **BOX 56.5**   Knowledge, Skills, and Equipment Needed by
> Extended Rescue Teams—cont'd

- Contact dermatitis, such as that caused by poison ivy, poison oak, and poison sumac
- Sunburn and snowblindness
- High-altitude injuries, including acute mountain sickness, pulmonary edema, and cerebral edema
- Drowning
- Diagnosis and management of acute medical emergencies:
  - Chest pain (e.g., myocardial infarction, angina, costochondritis)
  - Shortness of breath (e.g., asthma, anaphylaxis, pneumothorax)
  - Seizures and cerebrovascular accidents
  - Acute abdomen (e.g., peritonitis, constipation, diarrhea)
  - Lower and upper urinary tract infections
  - Septic shock
- Patient lifting and handling techniques
- Improvised techniques (i.e., improvised litters and carries; see Chapter 57)
- Training involving the Incident Command System
- Blood-borne pathogens and infectious disease prevention
- Monitoring of bodily functions (i.e., hunger, thirst, and bodily waste management)
- General understanding and appreciation for the difference between urban (short-term) and wilderness (long-term) emergency care

Mountain and Extended Rescue Skills
Understanding equipment that is used in wilderness search and rescue operations, including its maintenance and care:
  - Ropes, slings, carabiners, harnesses, and helmets
  - Litters, litter harnesses, and haul systems
  - Litter patient packaging equipment
Basic radio communications:
  - Care and maintenance of communications equipment
  - Procedures and protocols
Basic helicopter operations and procedures:
  - Approaching a helicopter
  - Safety considerations
  - Landing zones
  - Haul techniques
  - Patient loading
Interagency relations
Basic understanding of search procedures
Basic understanding of rescue procedures
Basic understanding of the Incident Command System and its use in search and rescue management
How to care for and handle ropes

Continued

BOX 56.5   Knowledge, Skills, and Equipment Needed by Extended Rescue Teams—cont'd

Rappelling, belaying, and braking techniques

Knots:

- Figure-8
- Figure-8 follow-through
- Figure-8 on a bight
- Double figure-8
- Double fisherman's
- Prusik
- Tensionless hitch (i.e., round turn and two half hitches)
- Water knot
- Half hitch and full hitch
- Bowline
- Alpine butterfly
- Clove hitch
- Munter hitch

Specific rescue training:

- Water search
- Swiftwater safety and rescue
- Avalanche safety and rescue
- Technical or vertical (rock) safety and rescue
- Cave safety and rescue

Leadership

Leadership and "followship" training

Ability to use the Incident Command System

57 Improvised Litters and Carries

SCENE SIZE-UP

To select the best method for bringing a patient to definitive care, the rescuer must make a realistic assessment of several factors:

- Scene safety is the initial priority.
- The necessary evaluation, called the *scene size-up* (Box 57.1), involves a (usually hasty) determination of whether the patient, rescuer, or both are immediately threatened by the environment or situation.
- Proper immobilization and patient packaging are always preferable, but sometimes the risk for aggravating existing injuries is outweighed by immediate danger presented by the physical environment. In such a situation, the rescuer may choose to immediately move the patient to a place of safety before definitive care is provided or packaging is completed.
- Evacuation options are limited by three variables:
  - Number of rescuers
  - Fitness of rescuers
  - Technical ability of rescuers
- Carrying a patient, even over level ground, is an arduous task. At an altitude where walking requires great effort, carrying a patient may be impossible.
- Complex rescue scenarios requiring specially trained personnel and special equipment are called *technical rescues* and often involve dangerous environments, such as severe terrain, crevasses, avalanche chutes, caves, or swift water. To avoid becoming patients themselves, rescuers must realistically evaluate their abilities to perform these types of rescues.
- When a patient is transported on an improvised litter, especially over rough terrain, they should be kept in a comfortable position, with injured limbs elevated to limit pressure and movement.
- To splint the chest wall and allow full expansion of the unaffected lung, a patient with a chest injury generally should be positioned so that he or she is lying on the injured side (injured side "down") during transport.
- For a patient with a head injury, the head should be elevated slightly; and for a patient with dyspnea, pulmonary edema, or myocardial infarction, the upper body should be elevated. However, any patient positioning is superseded by the ability of rescuers to safely carry the victim without exhausting themselves.

BOX 57.1   Scene Size-Up Factors

What are the scope and magnitude of the overall situation?
Are there immediate life-threatening hazards?
What is the location, and how many patients are there?
What is the patient's condition? Is the patient able to assist
    rescuers?
  • No injury (able to walk unassisted)
  • Slight injury (able to walk unassisted)
  • Slight injury (assistance required to walk)
  • Major injury (requires considerable attention and assistance)
  • Deceased
Is there a need for technical rescue?
Is the scene readily accessible?
What rescue resources (including rescuers and equipment) are
    available?
How far must the patient (or patients) be transported?
Are ground or air transport assets available?

- Whenever possible, an unconscious patient with an unprotected airway should be positioned lying on his or her side ("rescue position") during transport to prevent aspiration.
- When time permits, practice constructing the improvised litter first and then use it to carry an uninjured person, to "work out the kinks."

DRAGS AND CARRIES

A drag or carry may be the best option when (1) a patient cannot move under his or her own power, (2) injuries will not be aggravated by the transport, (3) resources and time are limited, (4) the need for immediate transport outweighs the desire to apply standard care criteria, (5) travel distance is short, and (6) the terrain makes use of multiple rescuers or bulky equipment impractical. Spine injuries generally prohibit using drags or carries because the patient cannot be properly immobilized. Drags are particularly useful for patients who are unconscious or incapacitated and unable to assist their rescuer (or rescuers), but may be uncomfortable for conscious patients. When a drag is used, padding should be placed beneath the patient, especially when long distances are involved. The high fatigue rate of rescuers makes carries a less attractive option when long distances are involved.

Blanket Drag (Fig. 57.1A)

1. This can be performed on relatively smooth terrain by one or more rescuers rolling the patient onto a blanket, tarp, or large coat and then pulling it along the ground.
2. This simple technique is especially effective for rapidly moving a patient with a spinal injury to safety because the patient is pulled along the long axis of the body.

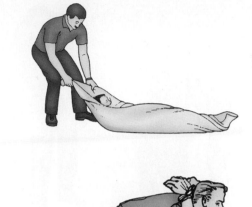

FIGURE 57.1 A, Blanket drag. **B,** Fireman's drag. Both techniques are intended to be used when expeditious transport over a short distance is required. (From Auerbach PS: *Medicine for the outdoors: The essential guide to emergency medical procedures and first aid,* ed 6, Philadelphia, 2016, Elsevier.)

Fireman's Drag (see Fig. 57.1B)
1. In an extreme circumstance, the "fireman's drag" can be used.
2. In this method, the rescuer places the bound wrists of the patient around his or her neck, shoulders, or both, and crawls to safety.

Fireman's Carry (Fig. 57.2)
Classic carry, but difficult for an untrained or smaller (than the patient) rescuer

Three-Person Wheelbarrow Carry (Fig. 57.3)
This system is extremely efficient and can be used for prolonged periods on relatively rough terrain. The patient places his or her arms over the shoulders of two rescuers standing side-by-side. The patient's legs are then placed over a third rescuer's shoulders. This system efficiently equalizes the weight of the patient.

Two-Hand Seat
1. Two carriers stand side by side. Each carrier grasps the other carrier's wrists with opposite hands (e.g., right to left).

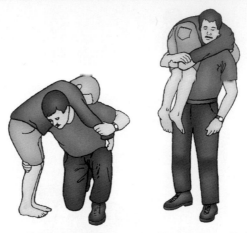

FIGURE 57.2 Classic Fireman's Carry: A Single-Rescuer Technique for Short-Distance Transport Only. The rescuer must use his or her legs, not a bent back, for lifting. (From Auerbach PS: *Medicine for the outdoors: The essential guide to emergency medical procedures and first aid*, ed 6, Philadelphia, 2016, Elsevier.)

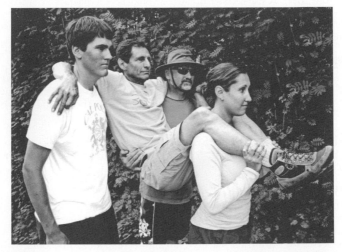

FIGURE 57.3 Three-Person Wheelbarrow Carry. The patient places his or her arms over two rescuers' shoulders (the rescuers stand side by side). The patient's legs are then placed over a third rescuer's shoulders.

2. The patient sits on the rescuers' joined forearms.
3. The carriers each maintain one free hand to place behind the back of the patient for support (support hands can be joined).
4. This system places great stress on the carriers' forearms and wrists.

Four-Hand Seat (Fig. 57.4)

1. Two carriers stand side-by-side. Each carrier grasps his or her own right forearm with the left hand, palms facing down.
2. Each carrier then grasps the forearm of the other with his or her free hand to form a square "forearm" seat.
3. The patient must support his/herself with a hand around the rescuer's back.

Ski Pole or Ice Axe Carry (Fig. 57.5)

1. Two carriers with backpacks stand side by side with four ski poles or joined ice axe shafts resting between them and the base of the pack straps.
2. The ski poles or ice axe shafts can be joined with cable ties, adhesive tape, duct tape, wire, or cord.
3. Because the rescuers must walk side-by-side, this technique requires wide-open, gentle terrain.
4. The patient sits on the padded poles or shaft with his or her arms over the carriers' shoulders.

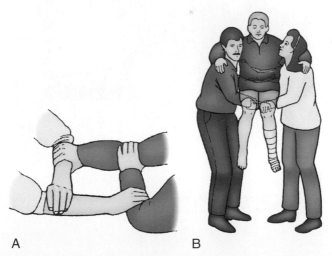

A   B

FIGURE 57.4 A, Four-hand seat used to carry a patient. In this technique, the upper body is not supported. **B,** Alternative four-hand seat that helps support the patient's back. (From Auerbach PS: *Medicine for the outdoors: The essential guide to first aid and medical emergencies*, ed 6, Philadelphia, 2016, Elsevier.)

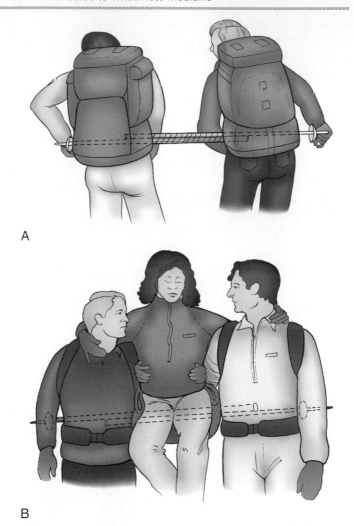

A

B

FIGURE 57.5   Ski pole seat. **(A)** Ski poles are anchored by the packs. **(B)** The patient is supported by the rescuers.

Split-Coil Seat ("Tragsitz") (Fig. 57.6)

1. The split-coil seat transport uses a coiled climbing rope to join the rescuer and patient together in a piggyback fashion (Fig. 57.7).
2. The patient must be able to support himself or herself to avoid falling back, or must be tied in.

Commercial Tragsitz Harness (Fig. 57.8)

A few commercial harnesses allow a lone rescuer and single patient to be raised or lowered together by a technical rescue system.

Two-Rescuer Split-Coil Seat (Fig. 57.9)

1. The two-rescuer split-coil seat is essentially the same as the split-coil Tragsitz transport, except that two rescuers split the coil over their shoulders.
2. The patient sits on the low point of the rope between the rescuers (Fig. 57.10). Each rescuer maintains a free hand to help support the patient.

Backpack Carry

1. A large backpack is modified by cutting leg holes in the base. The patient sits in the backpack as if it were a baby carrier.

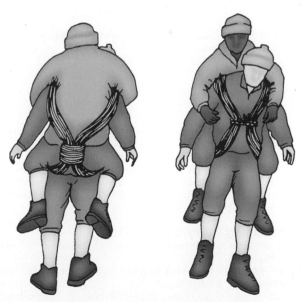

FIGURE 57.6   Single-Rescuer Split-Coil Carry. Note that the coil can be tied in front of the rescuer and the wrists of the patient can be bound and wrapped around the rescuer's neck for more stability.

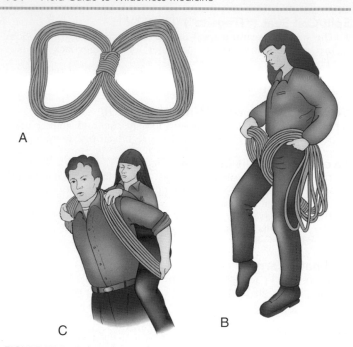

FIGURE 57.7   Split-coil seat. **A,** Rope coil is split. **B,** Patient climbs through rope. **C,** Rescuer hoists the sitting patient.

2. Some large internal frame packs incorporate a sleeping bag compartment in the lower portion of the pack that includes a compression panel. With this style of pack, the patient can sit on the suspended panel and place his or her legs through the unzipped lower section without damaging the pack; or the patient can sit on the internal sleeping bag compression panel without the need to cut holes.

Nylon Webbing Carry (Fig. 57.11)
1. Nylon webbing can be used to attach the patient to the rescuer like a backpack.
2. At least 4.6 to 6.1 m (15 to 20 ft) of nylon webbing is needed to construct this transport.
3. The center of the webbing is placed behind the patient and brought forward under the armpits. The webbing is then crossed and brought over the rescuer's shoulders, then down around the patient's thighs.

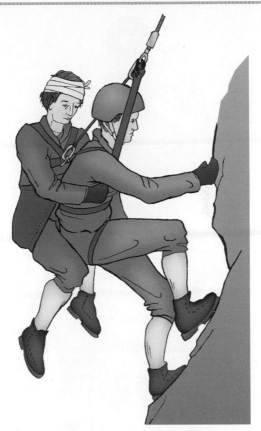

FIGURE 57.8 Tragsitz harness in use.

4. The webbing is finally brought forward and tied around the rescuer's waist. Additional padding is necessary for this system, especially around the posterior thighs of the patient.

Papoose-Style Sling
1. For carrying infants and small children, a papoose-style sling can easily be constructed by the rescuer tying a rectangular piece of material around his or her waist and neck to form a pouch.
2. The infant or child is then placed inside the pouch, which can be worn on the front or back of the rescuer's body.

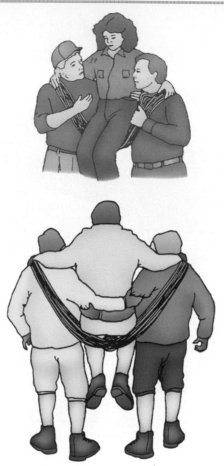

FIGURE 57.9   Two-rescuer split-coil seat.

LITTER IMPROVISATION
Litters (Nonrigid)
Nonrigid litter systems are best suited for transporting non–critically injured patients over moderate terrain. They should never be used for trauma patients with potential spine injuries.
1. When patients are transported in improvised litters, especially over rough terrain, they should be kept in a comfortable position, with injured limbs elevated to limit pressure and movement.
2. For a patient with a head injury, the head should be elevated slightly.

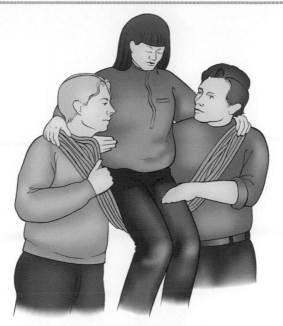

FIGURE 57.10 Two-Rescuer Split-Coil Seat. Balance could be improved by using a longer coil to carry the patient lower.

3. For patients with dyspnea, pulmonary edema, or myocardial infarction, the upper body should be elevated. Conversely, when the patient is in shock, the legs should be elevated and the knees slightly flexed.
4. Whenever possible, unconscious patients with unprotected airways should be positioned so that they are lying on their sides during transport to prevent aspiration.

Blanket Litter (Fig. 57.12)

1. A simple, nonrigid litter can be fabricated from two rigid poles, branches, or skis and a large blanket or tarp.
2. The blanket or tarp is wrapped around the skis or poles as many times as possible, and the poles are carried.
3. The blanket or tarp should not be simply draped over the poles, because this will not provide sufficient support and the patient will fall through. For easier carrying, the poles can be rigged to the base of backpacks.
4. Large external frame packs work best, but internal frame packs can be rigged to do the job.
5. Alternatively, a padded harness to support the litter can be made from a single piece of webbing, in a design like a nylon webbing carry.

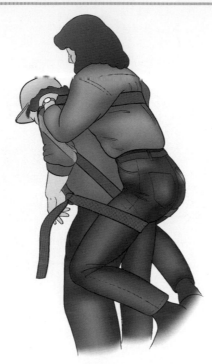

FIGURE 57.11 Webbing carry. Webbing crisscrosses in front of the patient's chest before passing over the shoulders of the rescuer.

6. An improvised blanket-type litter can be made from a heavy plastic tarpaulin, tent material, or large polyethylene bag (Fig. 57.13).
7. By wrapping the material around a rock, wadded sock, or glove and securing it with rope or twine, the rescuer can fashion handles in the corners and sides to facilitate carrying.
8. The advantage of this device is its simplicity, but it can be fragile, so care must be taken not to exceed the capabilities of the materials.
9. This type of nonrigid, "soft" litter can be dragged over snow, mud, or flat terrain, but should be generously padded, and extra clothing or blankets placed beneath the patient.

Tree Pole Litter
1. A tree pole litter is like the blanket litter.
2. In the tree pole litter, instead of a blanket or a tarp, the side poles are laced together with webbing or rope and then padded.
3. The poles may be fitted through pack frames to aid carrying.

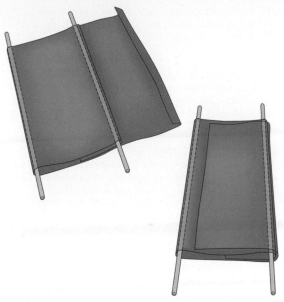

FIGURE 57.12   Improvising a stretcher from two rigid poles and a blanket or tarp.

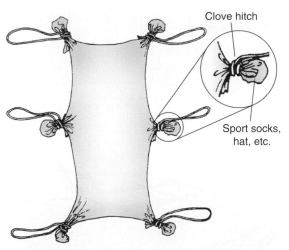

FIGURE 57.13   Improvised handled soft stretcher.

4. To give this litter more stability and to add tension to the lacing, the rescuer should fabricate a rectangle with rigid crossbars at both ends before lacing.

Parka Litter
1. Two or more parkas can be used to form a litter (Fig. 57.14)
2. Skis or branches are slipped through the sleeves of heavy parkas, and the parkas are zipped shut with the sleeves inside.
3. Ski edges should be taped first to prevent them from tearing through the parkas.

Internal Frame Pack Litter
1. The internal frame pack litter is constructed from two to three full-size internal frame backpacks, which must have lateral compression straps (day packs are suboptimal).
2. Slide poles or skis through the compression straps. The packs then act as a support surface for the patient.

Sledge (Fig. 57.15)
1. If long distances must be traveled or if pack animals are available, a litter may be constructed so that it can be dragged or slid along the ground like a sled.
2. The litter is fashioned out of two forked tree limbs, with one side of each fork broken off.
3. The limbs form a pair of sled-like runners that are lashed together with cross members to form a patient platform.

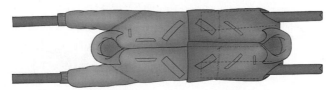

FIGURE 57.14   Parka litter. On the right the sleeves are zipped inside to reinforce the litter.

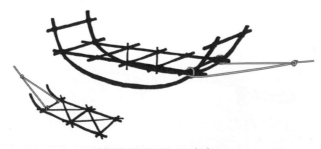

FIGURE 57.15   A sledge.

4. The sledge offers a solid platform for patient support and stabilization.
5. If sufficient effort is put into fashioning a smooth, curved leading edge to the runners, a sledge can be dragged easily over smooth ground, mud, ice, or snow.
6. Ropes can be attached to the front of the platform for hauling and to the rear for use as brakes when traveling downhill.

Life Jacket Litter

Life jackets can be placed over paddles or oars to create a makeshift nonrigid litter.

Rope Litter (Fig. 57.16)

1. On mountaineering trips, the classic rope litter can be used, but this system offers little back support and should never be used for patients with suspected spine injuries.
2. The rope is uncoiled and staked onto the ground with 16 180-degree bends (8 on each side of the rope center).
3. The rope bends should approximate the size of the finished litter.
4. The free rope ends are then used to clove hitch off each bend (leaving 5 cm [2 in] of bend to the outside of each clove hitch).

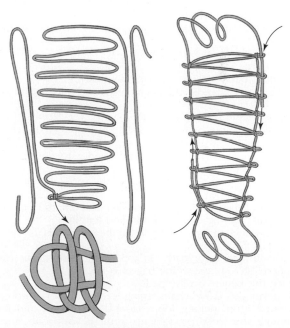

FIGURE 57.16   Rope litter.

5. The leftover rope is threaded through the loops at the outside of each clove hitch.
6. This gives the rescuers a continuous handhold and protects the bends from slipping through the clove hitches.
7. The rope ends are then tied off.
8. The litter is padded with packs, Therm-a-Rest pads, foam pads, or other cushioning materials.
9. This improvised litter is somewhat ungainly and requires six or more rescuers for an evacuation of any distance.
10. A rope litter can be tied to poles or skis to add lateral stability.

IMPROVISED RIGID LITTERS

It may be necessary to transport patients with certain injuries (i.e., spine injuries, unstable pelvis, or knee or hip dislocations) on a more rigid litter. The goal is not always long-distance evacuation. It is sometimes necessary to move severely injured patients a relatively short distance to a shelter, camp, or landing zone while awaiting formal rescue. Improvised litters should never be used for patients with suspected spine injuries unless no alternative exists for organized rescue.

Continuous Loop System (Daisy Chain Litter, Cocoon Wrap, Mummy Litter) (Fig. 57.17)

For the continuous loop system, the following items are necessary:
1. Long climbing or rescue rope
2. Large tarp
3. Sleeping pads (Ensolite or Therm-a-Rest)
4. Stiffeners (e.g., skis, poles, snowshoes, canoe paddles, tree branches)

To construct the continuous loop system:
1. Lay the rope out with even U-shaped loops as shown in Fig. 57.17A.
2. The midsection should be slightly wider to conform to the patient's width.
3. Tie a small loop at the foot end of the rope and place a tarp on the laid rope.
4. On top of the tarp, lay foam pads the full length of the system (the pads can be overlapped to add length).
5. Lay stiffeners on top of the pads in the same axis as the patient (see Fig. 57.17B).
6. Add multiple foam pads on top of the stiffeners, followed optionally with a sleeping bag (see Fig. 57.17C).
7. Place the patient on the pads.
8. To form the daisy chain, bring a single loop through the pre-tied loop, pulling loops toward the center and feeding through the loops brought up from the opposite side. It is important to take up rope slack continuously.

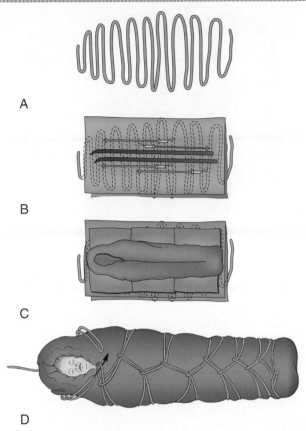

FIGURE 57.17 Continuous loop, or "mummy," litter made with a climbing rope. **A,** Rope is laid out with even U-shaped loops. **B,** Stiffeners, such as skis and poles, are placed underneath the patient to add structural rigidity. It is important to pad between the stiffeners and the patient. **C,** A sleeping bag may be used in addition to the foam pads. **D,** A loop of rope is brought over each shoulder and tied off (see text).

9. When the patient's armpits are reached, bring a loop over each shoulder and tie it off (or clip it off with a carabiner) (see Fig. 57.17D).
10. One excellent modification involves adding an inverted internal frame backpack. This can be incorporated with the padding and secured with the head end of the rope. The pack adds rigidity and padding, and the padded hip belt serves as an efficient head and neck immobilizer (Fig. 57.18).

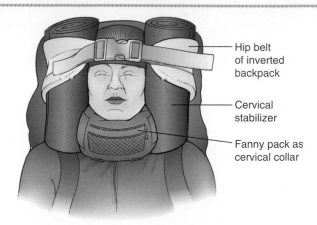

Hip belt
of inverted
backpack

Cervical
stabilizer

Fanny pack as
cervical collar

FIGURE 57.18   Inverted pack used as a spine board.

11. Although this type of litter offers improved support, strength, and thermal protection, careful thought must be given to the physical and psychological effects created by such a restrictive enclosure.

Backpack Frame Litters (Fig. 57.19)

1. Functional litters can be constructed from external frame backpacks.
2. Traditionally, two frames are used, but three or four frames (Fig. 57.20) make for a larger, more stable litter.
3. Cable ties or fiberglass strapping tape simplify this fabrication.
4. These litters can be reinforced with ice axes or ski poles.

Travois

1. A travois is a similar device that is less like a sled and more like a travel trailer (without wheels).
2. A travois is a V-shaped platform constructed of sturdy limbs or poles lashed together with cross members or connected with rope or netting.
3. The open end of the V is dragged along the ground, with the apex lashed to a pack animal or pulled by rescuers.
4. Although the travois can be dragged over rough terrain, the less smooth the ground, the more padding and support necessary for comfort and stabilization.
5. A long pole can be passed through the middle of the platform and used for lifting and stabilization by rescuers when rough terrain is encountered.

Kayak System

1. Properly modified, the kayak makes an ideal rigid, long-board improvised litter.

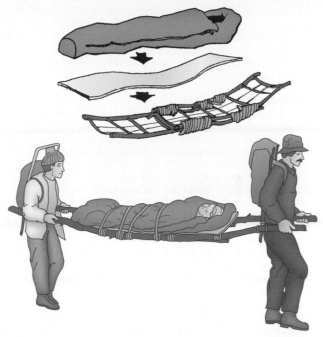

FIGURE 57.19 Backpack frame litter. Note that the sapling poles on the litter can be attached to the rescuer's backpack frames to help support the patient's weight.

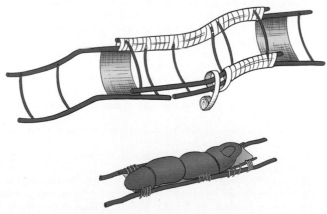

FIGURE 57.20 Backpack frame litter.

2. First, remove the seat along with sections of the upper deck if necessary.
3. A serrated river knife (or camp saw) makes this improvisation much easier.
4. Open deck canoes can be used almost as they are, after the flotation material has been removed.

Canoe System

1. Many rivers have railroad tracks that run parallel to the river canyon.
2. The tracks can be used to slide a canoe by placing the boat perpendicular to the tracks and pulling on both bow and stern lines.

Improvised Rescue Sled or Toboggan

A sled or toboggan can be constructed from one or more pairs of skis and poles that are lashed, wired, or screwed together. Many designs are possible. Improvised rescue sleds may be clumsy and often bog down hopelessly in deep snow. Nonetheless, they can be useful for transporting patients over short distances (to a more sheltered camp or to a more appropriate landing zone). They do not perform as well as commercial rescue sleds for more extensive transports.

1. To build an improvised rescue sled/toboggan, the rescuer needs a pair of skis (preferably the patient's) and two pairs of ski poles; three 0.6-m (2-ft) sticks (or ski pole sections); 24.4 m (80 ft) of nylon cord; and extra lengths of rope for sled hauling.
2. The skis are placed 0.6 m (2 ft) apart.
3. The first stick is used as the front crossbar and is lashed to the ski tips.
4. Alternately, holes can be drilled into the stick and ski tips with an awl, and bolts can be used to fasten them together.
5. The middle stick is lashed to the bindings.
6. One pair of ski poles is placed over the crossbars (baskets over the ski tips) and lashed down.
7. The second set of poles is lashed to the middle stick with baskets facing back toward the tails.
8. A third rear stick is placed on the tails of the skis and lashed to the poles. The lashings are not wrapped around the skis; the crossbar simply sits on the tails of the skis under the weight of the patient.
9. Nylon cord is then woven back and forth across the horizontal ski poles.
10. The hauling ropes are passed through the baskets on the front of the sled.
11. The ropes are then brought around the middle crossbar and back to the front crossbar. This rigging system reverses the direction of pull on the front crossbar, making it less likely to slip off the ski tips.

12. Another sled design includes a pre-drilled snow shovel incorporated into the front of the sled. A rigid backpack frame can also be used to reinforce the sled. This requires drilling holes into the ski tips and carrying a pre-drilled shovel. This system holds the skis in a wedge position and may offer slightly greater durability.

PATIENT PACKAGING

Patients on stretchers must be secured, or "packaged," before transport.

Packaging consists of the following:
- Stabilization
- Immobilization
- Preparation of a patient for transport

Physically strapping a patient into a litter is relatively easy, but making it comfortable and effective in terms of splinting can be a challenge.

The rescuer's goals are as follows:
1. Package the patient to avoid causing additional injury.
2. Ensure the patient's comfort and warmth.
3. Immobilize the patient's entire body in a way that allows continued assessment during transport.
4. Package the patient neatly so that the litter can be moved easily and safely.
5. Ensure that the patient is safe during transport by securing them within the litter and belaying the litter as needed. Generally, proper patient packaging must provide for physical protection and psychological comfort.
6. Once packaged in a carrying device, a patient feels helpless, so transport preparation must focus on alleviating anxiety and providing rock-solid security.
7. Rescuers must provide for the patient's ongoing safety, protection, comfort, medical stabilization, and psychological support.
8. Splinting and spinal immobilization are usually achieved by using a full or short backboard.
9. The patient is secured to the board, and then the patient (on the board) is placed into the litter.
10. When the immobilized patient is placed into the litter, adequate padding (e.g., blankets, towels, bulky clothing, sleeping bags) placed under and around them contributes to comfort and stability.
11. Avoid placing the legs in full extension at the knees; consider placing a small pad or cloth roll under the knees.
12. For long-duration evacuation, a "diaper" can be improvised with garbage bags, absorbable fleece, and duct tape around the patient's pelvis and genital area. This helps contain urine and feces, prevents the middle insulating layer from becoming wet, and facilitates changing the improvised diaper.

Improvised Short-Board Immobilization
Internal Frame Pack and Snow Shovel System

1. Some internal frame backpacks can be easily modified by inserting a snow shovel through the centerline attachment points (the shovel handgrip may need to be removed first).
2. The patient's head is taped to the lightly padded shovel (Fig. 57.21); the shovel blade serves as a head bed.
3. This system incorporates the remainder of the pack suspension as designed (i.e., shoulder and sternum straps with hip belt) and works well with other long-board designs, such as the continuous loop system (see earlier).

Inverted Pack System

1. An efficient short board can be made using an inverted internal or external frame backpack.
2. The padded hip belt provides a head bed, and the frame is used as a short board in conjunction with a rigid or semirigid cervical collar (see Fig. 57.18).
3. Turn the pack upside down, and lash the patient's shoulders and torso to the pack. Fasten the waist belt around the patient's head, as in the top section of a Kendrick extrication device.
4. The hip belt is typically too large to secure the head, but you can facilitate immobilization using bilateral Ensolite rolls.
5. Unlike the snow shovel system, this system requires that the patient be lashed to the splint.

Snowshoe System

A snowshoe can be made into a reliable short spine board (Fig. 57.22). Pad the snowshoe and rig it for attachment to the patient as shown.

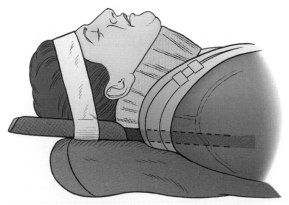

FIGURE 57.21   Head immobilized on a padded shovel.

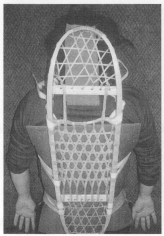 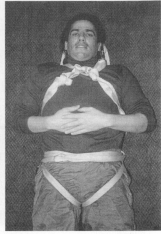

FIGURE 57.22 Improvised snowshoe short board. A well-padded snowshoe is pre-rigged with webbing and attached to the patient as shown. This system also can be used in conjunction with long-board systems, such as the continuous loop system.

During Transport

1. During transport, patients like to have something in their hands to grasp, to have pressure applied to the bottom of their feet by a footplate or webbing, and to be able to see what is happening around them.
2. Because patients are vulnerable to falling debris when packaged in a litter, especially in a horizontal high-angle configuration, a cover of some type should be used to protect them. A blanket or tarpaulin works well as a cover to protect most of the body, but a helmet and face shield (or goggles) are also recommended to protect the head and face.
3. Alternatively, a commercially available litter shield can be used and allows easy access to the airway, head, and neck (Fig. 57.23).
4. Remember also that the conscious patient desires an unobstructed view of his or her surroundings.

Securing a Patient Within the Litter

Carrying a patient in the wilderness often requires that the litter be tilted, angled, placed on end, or even inverted. In these situations, the patient must remain effectively immobilized and securely attached to the litter, the immobilizing device within the litter, and any supporting rope secured to avoid snagging. Poor attachment can cause patient shifting, exacerbation of injuries, or complete failure of the rescue system. Manufacturers have taken several approaches to securing a patient within the litter.

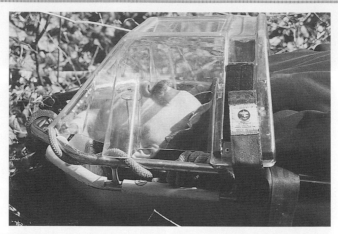

FIGURE 57.23 The CMC Litter Shield protects the patient from falling debris, while allowing access to the head and face. Litter shields also can be improvised.

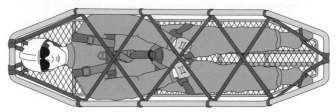

FIGURE 57.24 One 10-m (30-ft) web or rope can be used to secure a patient into a litter.

1. Most integrate a retention or harness system directly into the litter.
2. A few require external straps to secure the patient to the device.
3. Many users suggest that an independent harness be attached directly to the patient to provide a secondary attachment point in case there is failure of any link in the attachment chain.
4. When a harness is not available, tubular webbing, strips of sturdy material, or rope can be used to secure the patient.
5. One approach uses tubular webbing slings in a figure-8 at the pelvis and shoulders to prevent the patient from sliding lengthwise in the litter. A 10-m (32.8-ft) piece of 5-cm (2-in) webbing or rescue rope can be used to achieve the same goal (Fig. 57.24).
6. The rope or web is laced back and forth between the rails of the litter in a diamond pattern until the patient is entirely covered and secure.

7. Such a technique also easily incorporates a protective cover and support of the patient's feet.
8. For high-angle evacuation, be certain the patient is also secured via a harness (commercial or improvised) to the litter.
9. Regardless of the techniques and equipment used, frequently check vital signs (i.e., distal pulses and capillary refill) during transport to help ensure that strapping does not obstruct circulation.

Carrying a Loaded Litter
High Angle or Vertical

- An evacuation is defined as high angle or vertical when the weight of the stretcher and tenders (stretcher attendants) is primarily supported by a rope and the angle of the rope is 60 degrees or greater.
- This type of situation is often encountered when a rescue is performed on a cliff or overhang, or over the side of a structure, and usually requires only one or two tenders.
- In high-angle rescue, most often the stretcher is used in the horizontal position, to allow only one tender and to keep the patient supine and comfortable.
- When the packaged patient and stretcher must be moved through a narrow passage or when falling rock is a danger, the stretcher may be positioned vertically.

Low Angle

- In a scree or low-angle evacuation, the slope is not as steep, and the tenders support more of the weight of the stretcher, but a rope system is still necessary to help move the load. In this type of rescue, more tenders (usually four to six) are required and the rope is attached to the head of the stretcher.
- The head of the litter is kept uphill during a low-angle rescue.

Nontechnical Evacuation

- In a nontechnical evacuation, tenders completely support the weight of the stretcher during the carry.
- Generally, the terrain dictates the type of evacuation. If the stretcher can be carried without support from a rope, it is a nontechnical evacuation.
- If rope is necessary to support the load or to move the stretcher, it is either a low- or high-angle evacuation, depending on the angle of the slope.

CARRYING A LITTER IN THE WILDERNESS

- It takes at least six rescuers to carry a patient in a litter a short distance (0.4 km [0.25 mile] or less) over relatively flat terrain.
- With six rescuers, four can carry the litter while the other two clear the area in the direction of travel and assist in difficult spots.

- Depending on the terrain and weight of the patient, all six rescuers may be necessary to safely carry the litter any distance.
- If the travel distance is longer, many more rescuers are required (Fig. 57.25).

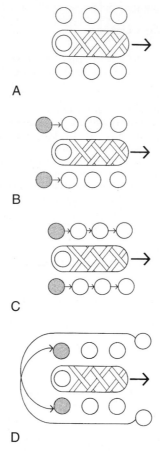

FIGURE 57.25   Litter-carrying sequence. **A,** Six rescuers are usually required to carry a litter, but may need relief over long distances (farther than 0.25 mile). **B,** Relief rescuers can rotate into position while the litter is in motion by approaching from the rear. As relief rescuers move forward **(C)**, the forwardmost rescuers can release the litter (peel out) and move to the rear **(D)**. Rescuers in the rear can rotate sides so that they can alternate carrying arms. Carrying straps (webbing) can also be used to distribute the load over the rescuers' shoulders. In most cases, the litter is carried feet first with a medical attendant at the head monitoring airway, breathing, level of consciousness, and so forth.

Because aeromedical transport involves medical care delivered in a hostile environment, the patient and crew are at risk for injury or death in the event of a mishap. Flight crew training must emphasize safety. A helicopter mountain rescue operation is a high-risk endeavor for the pilot and crew, as well as for the patient. Dangerous mistakes are easy to make around working helicopters. Therefore, aeromedical transport is not always the proper choice for rescue. Any decision to use aeromedical resources must be weighed against the lower risk associated with ground-based rescue or evacuation. One should consider the severity of the patient's condition, desired level of out-of-hospital care, access to ground transportation, weather conditions for helicopter flight, and whether local receiving hospitals have the capacity to land helicopters. Specific medical conditions may be more appropriate for aeromedical transport (Box 58.1).

COMMON AEROMEDICAL TRANSPORT PROBLEMS
Pretransport Preparation
- Once the decision is made to transport a patient by air and the appropriate aeromedical service is contacted, preparations must be made to ensure safety and comfort and to aid the flight crew in patient care.
- To minimize delays, pretransport preparations should be made for patients of acute trauma (Box 58.2).

Patient Comfort
Many factors can contribute to patient discomfort during a flight, including: motion, vibration, noise, temperature variations, dry air, changes in atmospheric pressure, confinement to a limited position or backboard, and fear of flying. Steps should be taken to educate the patient on what to expect and to address comfort needs as much as possible. Eye and ear protection should always be provided.

Patient Movement
- Patient handling and movement can contribute to morbidity and mortality in unstable patients.
- All transported patients should be adequately secured to the stretcher with safety straps to prevent sudden shifting of position or movement of a secured fracture.
- During transport from the ground to the aircraft cabin, attempts should be made to limit sudden pitching of the stretcher.

BOX 58.1   Medical Conditions That May Require Aeromedical Evacuation

- Acute neurologic, vascular, surgical, or cardiac emergencies requiring time-sensitive intervention
- Critical conditions in patients with compromised hemodynamic or respiratory function
- Critical conditions in obstetric patients whose time of transfer must be minimized to prevent complications in the patient or fetus
- Critical conditions in neonatal or pediatric patients with compromised hemodynamic or respiratory function, metabolic acidosis more than 2 hours after delivery, or sepsis or meningitis
- Electrolyte disturbances and toxic exposures requiring immediate lifesaving intervention
- Organ failure requiring transplantation
- Conditions requiring treatment in a hyperbaric oxygen unit
- Burns requiring treatment in a burn treatment center
- Any injury that is potentially threatening to life or limb, including penetrating eye injuries

Data from Teichman PG, Donchin Y, Kot RJ: International aeromedical evacuation. *N Engl J Med* 356:262, 2007.

BOX 58.2   Pretransport Preparations

Scene Response
- Airway secured
- Appropriate spinal precautions as needed
- Two large-bore intravenous lines
- Landing zone selected and secured

Interhospital Transport
- Airway secured
- Appropriate spinal precautions as needed
- Two large-bore intravenous lines
- Tube thoracostomy for pneumothorax/hemothorax
- Bladder catheterization (if not contraindicated)
- Nasogastric catheterization (if not contraindicated)
- Lactated Ringer's or normal saline solution hanging
- Typed and crossmatched blood if available
- Extremity fractures splinted (traction splinting for femur fractures)
- Copies of all available field and emergency department records and laboratory results, including a description of the mechanism of injury

- U.S. Department of Transportation guidelines recommend design of cabin access such that no more than 30 degrees of roll and 45 degrees of pitch may occur to the patient-occupied stretcher during loading.
- The stretcher should be adequately attached to the floor.
- Motion sickness in the patient may be treated with an antiemetic such as ondansetron (4 to 8 mg PO or IV), promethazine (25 mg PO, IV, or IM), or prochlorperazine (5 to 10 mg PO, IV, or IM).
- Transdermal scopolamine patches are useful for prolonged flights and do not require parenteral or oral administration. Scopolamine's antiemetic effects are not always uniform and may not occur until 4 to 6 hours after the application of a patch. Patches may best be used to decrease motion sickness in the flight crew because they are nonsedating.
- A novel approach to prevention of airsickness that does not induce excessive sedation is to give 25 mg of promethazine orally along with 200 mg of caffeine.

Oxygen Availability for Flight

- In general, enough oxygen should be provided for the flight, plus a 30- to 45-minute reserve.
- Sufficient oxygen should be carried to allow for ground handling time at either end.
- The amount of oxygen required can be obtained by multiplying the desired flow rate in liters per minute (L/min) by the total duration of transport, including patient loading and unloading.
- Table 58.1 lists the capacities of various types of oxygen tanks and their respective weights.
- Some portable ventilators have a gas-driven logic circuit that requires additional air or oxygen. Electrically powered ventilators have a lower requirement for oxygen but carry the additional need for a power inverter.

Table 58.1   Aluminum Oxygen Tank Specifications and Approximate Endurance

CYLINDER SIZE	EMPTY WEIGHT (KG)	CAPACITY (L)	Duration (min)	
			AT 2 L/MIN	AT 6 L/MIN
C	1.7	248*	124	41
D	2.3	414*	207	69
E	3.4	682*	341	113
H	38.7	7506†	3753	1251

*Fill pressure of 139 bar (2016 psi).
†Fill pressure 153 bar (2219 psi).
From Luxfer Gas Cylinders. http://www.luxfercylinders.com/products.

- Most patients are transported with oxygen supplied by nasal cannula (1 to 6 L/min). A single E-sized oxygen cylinder is adequate for short flights, although backup cylinders are usually carried.
- Patients intubated and maintained on 100% oxygen, as well as those ventilated on long flights, will quickly exceed the capacity of an E cylinder; several E cylinders or an H cylinder will be required.

Noise
- Noise can be avoided with hearing protectors, which are devices like headphones but without internal speakers.
- Inexpensive hearing protectors are available as moldable foam earplugs. In some cases, headphones may be used in the awake patient if the crew wants the patient to be able to communicate on the intercom system.

Cold
- For winter and cold weather operations, remember that rotor wash can produce wind speeds of 80 mph under the rotor.
- Always adequately dress or protect the patient from freezing rotor wash when loading under power ("hot loading") or for winch or short-haul operations (patient outside the aircraft).
- Use goggles to protect from blowing snow, along with full head and hand protection.

Eye Protection
- Serious eye injuries can result from debris blown into the air.
- When a patient is loaded onto or off a helicopter with the rotors turning, the patient's eyes must be protected.
- The eyes must be protected even if the patient is unconscious.
- Lightweight skydiver goggles ("boogie goggles") or ski goggles are effective and inexpensive.
- Taping temporary patches over the eyes is also effective.

Respiratory Distress
- Patients with respiratory disease or distress should have immediately treatable conditions addressed before takeoff.
- Endotracheal (ET) intubation is essential if airway patency is threatened or if adequate oxygenation cannot be maintained with supplemental oxygen.
- It is better to err on the side of caution when deciding about a patient's airway.
- During flight, it is easier to treat restlessness in an intubated patient than airway obstruction or apnea in a nonintubated patient.
- Nearly all patients should receive supplemental oxygen.
- Fraction of inspired oxygen (Fio_2) should be increased with increasing cabin altitude to maintain a stable partial pressure of oxygen (Po_2).

- When oxygen saturation monitoring is unavailable and pre-transport arterial oxygen content unknown, 100% oxygen may be administered throughout the flight to ensure adequate oxygenation.
- Patients with chronic lung disease who are prone to hypercapnia may undergo deterioration in condition if the hypoxic drive is eliminated. In these patients, the least oxygen necessary to maintain saturation above 90% is advisable.
- Close in-flight monitoring is essential, preferably by continuous pulse oximetry. Portable end-tidal CO_2 monitoring is now relatively easy to accomplish and should be used for intubated/ventilated patients whenever possible.
- Altitude changes may affect ET cuff volume, so cuff pressure must be checked frequently.
- If any other air-bladder devices (e.g., cuffed tracheostomy tubes, laryngeal mask airways, air splints) are present on the patient, they must also be adjusted during flight to avoid increased volume/pressure problems. Check these frequently.

Transport of Dive-Related Injuries (e.g., Decompression Sickness, Arterial Gas Embolism)

- Aircraft selection is crucial because the stricken diver should not be exposed to a significantly lower atmospheric pressure in the aircraft.
- Ideally, transport only by pressurized aircraft.
- For nonpressurized aircraft (i.e., helicopter), the flight altitude must be maintained as low as possible, not to exceed 305 m (1000 ft) above sea level, if possible.

Cardiopulmonary Resuscitation and Cardiac Defibrillation

- Cardiopulmonary resuscitation (CPR) in an aircraft is difficult. The rescuers must perform several tasks simultaneously while ventilating the lungs or compressing the chest, all in a physically confining space.
- There should be no concern with airborne defibrillation if all electronic navigational equipment on the aircraft has a common ground, as mandated by Federal Aviation Administration (FAA) standards.
- Despite cramped quarters and sensitive electrical equipment, defibrillation can be safely performed in all types of aircraft currently used for emergency transport using standard precautions routinely used during defibrillation on the ground.
- In the interest of safety, it is best to notify the pilot before performing defibrillation.

Patient Combativeness

- Patients may be combative to the point that they pose a threat to the safety of the flight and crew.

- An uncontrollable patient may cause sudden shifts in aircraft balance or may strike a crew member, or important flight instruments or equipment.
- Any combative patient should be properly restrained in advance.
- If sedation is necessary, document a thorough neurologic examination before administering medication.
- Useful sedative-hypnotic agents include diazepam (5 to 10 mg IV) or a shorter-acting agent such as midazolam (2 to 5 mg IV or IM).
- Paralyzing agents, such as pancuronium, vecuronium, and succinylcholine, have the advantage of not altering the sensorium, but they require airway control with ET intubation. In addition, it is humane to sedate a patient who is paralyzed to facilitate intubation and transport.

Endotracheal Intubation
- ET intubation may be difficult to perform while airborne, especially in a confining cabin, and should be done before departure if possible. This is especially true in trauma patients with head injuries and in burn patients who have carbonaceous sputum or hoarseness.
- Special techniques are available to supplement standard methods of intubation, including ET tubes with controllable tips, intubating laryngeal mask airways, and digital intubation. Video laryngoscopy has been shown to be effective in the air medical environment and is now being used by many transport teams.
- Sedation and/or pharmacologic paralysis may be necessary.
- Induction of paralysis before intubation in the aeromedical setting is controversial. Besides the need for a surgical airway if intubation is unsuccessful, concerns exist about cervical spine manipulation during intubation in the paralyzed patient, unrecognized esophageal intubation in a nonbreathing patient, and the relative contraindications to the use of paralyzing agents in certain patients. Determination of paralysis before ET intubation is made by the crew and medical control physicians, considering all relevant factors, including safety of the patient and crew in flight.
- Shorter-acting nondepolarizing paralytic agents (e.g., mivacurium) may have advantages, but they have not yet been thoroughly validated in the aeromedical setting.
- As with any critical airway intervention, there must always be a backup plan if ET intubation fails. Blind airway devices, such as a laryngeal mask airway or King LT airway device, or other salvage airway device with which the crew is comfortable, should always be available.
- In some flight programs, nonphysician crew members are taught to perform emergency cricothyrotomy. Although occasionally lifesaving, this procedure is often difficult to perform and should be undertaken only as a final method to secure an emergency airway.

Thrombolysis

Air transport of patients with acute myocardial infarction may involve thrombolytic therapy. Bleeding is the major adverse effect of thrombolysis. However, helicopter transport of patients with acute myocardial infarction after initiation of thrombolysis is without a clinically significant increase in bleeding complications compared to ground-based evacuation.

FLIGHT SAFETY

The pilot is ultimately responsible for the safety of the aircraft's occupants and trained not only to operate the aircraft skillfully and safely but also to provide necessary safety instructions and guidance to crew members and passengers. Safety practices vary depending on the type of aircraft, but include common guidelines. All medical personnel involved in loading and unloading patients from helicopters should be aware of the following safety concepts.

Approaching the Aircraft
Helicopters (Fig. 58.1 and Box 58.3)

- Approach helicopters with turning rotor blades only from the front and sides and only while under pilot observation.
- Give the tail rotor a wide berth, especially on helicopters with rear doors. The tail rotor is invisible when in operation.
- If on a slope, approach from the downhill side.
- Station a crew member in a safe position to direct approaching individuals away from the tail rotor.
- When the situation permits, shut down the helicopter's engines completely before patient loading and unloading.
- Approach the helicopter in a crouched position to minimize the risk for contact with the rotor blades should a sudden gust of wind or movement of the aircraft cause them to dip.
- Loose clothing, equipment, and debris should be secured.

Fixed-Wing Aircraft

- Fixed-wing aircraft should be approached with similar precautions regarding propellers.
- This is especially important in aircraft with access doors in front of the wing and engine nacelles.
- Engine shutdown on the side of entry enhances safety of loading and unloading.

Safety Belt Use

- Use of safety belts (preferably with shoulder harnesses, especially in helicopters) is an important safety measure. Certain patient care activities (e.g., ET intubation, CPR) may be impossible to perform with safety belts secured.
- Design and selection of aircraft and interior configurations should allow maximal access to the patient with the crew members properly restrained.

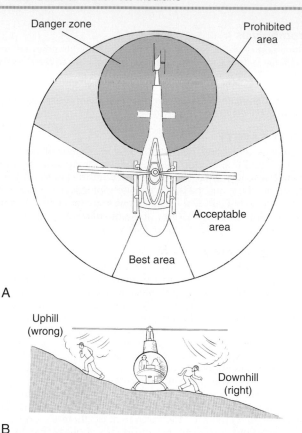

A

B

FIGURE 58.1 Helicopter Safety. A, Safe approach zones. **B,** Proper way to approach or depart from a helicopter.

BOX 58.3   Steps in Helicopter Safety

- Approach and depart downhill
- Use crouched position
- Approach after approval from pilot
- Await direction of flight crew
- Secure area of people and debris
- Do not shine lights toward aircraft
- Use tag line to prevent spinning of hoist
- Ground the hoist line to prevent electric shock

- Throughout the flight, the crew members and patient should remain restrained as much as possible in smooth air and always in rough air.
- Movement inside the cabin affects aircraft balance. An aircraft loaded near its aft center-of-gravity limit may exceed its limits if a crew member moves to a new position within the cabin.
- Changes in position should be preceded by consultation with the pilot.
- Light aircraft are sensitive to turbulent air, and appropriate precautions must be taken to avoid being injured from sudden motion.

Proper Use of Aircraft Equipment

- Crew members must be familiar with all aircraft equipment they may be required to operate in flight or during an emergency. This includes aircraft doors, fire extinguisher, communications equipment, emergency locator transmitters (ELTs), oxygen equipment, and electrical outlets.
- The crew must be familiar with emergency shutdown procedures.
- Before takeoff, door security must be confirmed by a crew member familiar with the operation of the door.

In-Flight Obstacle Reporting

- An extra pair of eyes can be invaluable to a pilot in a busy airspace or on a scene approach complicated by trees and electrical or phone wires.
- If during flight you observe anything of which the pilot may not be aware, such as air traffic, point it out. Most pilots appreciate the "heads-up" even when these factors seem obvious.
- Primarily important in visual flight conditions, assistance with obstacle identification can enhance safety of the mission; however, a flight should not occur under conditions in which obstacle reporting by a crew member is essential to safety, because the person must then divide attention between patient care and obstacle reporting.

Flight Crew–Ground Coordination

- Flight crew members must be able to communicate with ground units during the landing phase to ensure adequate scene preparation.
- Enthusiastic rescue personnel or curious onlookers may approach the aircraft in a hazardous manner.
- Crew may be required to perform crowd control while on the ground. This requires directing individuals away from the rotor blades, propellers, or other hazardous equipment.
- If loading or unloading the patient while the rotors or propellers are still turning ("hot loading" or "hot off-loading") is necessary, special precautions must be undertaken for ground crews, the flight crew, and the patient.

Emergency Procedures

All crew members should memorize and routinely practice emergency procedures that address in-flight fires, electrical failures, loss of pressurization, engine failure, emergency landing with and without power, precautionary landing away from an airport, and other in-flight emergencies.

Survival

- An emergency or precautionary landing away from an airport necessitates survival before rescue.
- Under adverse environmental conditions and with injured patients, survival may depend on specific actions by the crew.
- The crew should be proficient in emergency egress from the aircraft, including escape after crashes and water landings, especially in helicopters.
- After water landings, helicopters usually roll inverted and sink rapidly. Helicopter "dunker" training is required for all military helicopter crews and should be practiced by any crew involved in over-water operations.
- All crew members should be trained in the use of emergency signaling devices, such as ELTs, flares, signal fires, and ground emergency signals.
- Survival skills taught to all crew members include advanced first aid, building emergency shelters, fire starting, and obtaining water and food from the environment.

Landing Zone Operations

- The ideal helicopter landing zone (HLZ, or simply LZ) is a wide, flat, clear area with no obstacles during approach or departure.
- Vertical landings and takeoffs can be accomplished, but it is safer for the helicopter to make a gradual descent while flying forward.
- Higher altitudes and higher temperatures require larger landing zones.
- The center of the landing zone can be marked with a V, with the apex pointing into the prevailing wind.
- The FAA recommends that the HLZ be marked at night with a "box and one" configuration (Fig. 58.2). Each corner of the HLZ is marked with a light or flare, with a fifth flare outside the box indicating the wind direction. Any obstacles can be marked with brightly colored, properly secured clothing.
- Landing zones should be at least 100 × 100 ft in dimension with less than 5 degrees of slope. Poor weather, obstacles, or larger helicopters may require a larger HLZ.
- The condition of the ground (e.g., loose snow, dust, gravel) should be communicated to the pilot before the final approach.
- Before the helicopter lands, all loose clothing and equipment should be secured.
- During approach, no personnel or vehicles should move on or near the landing zone.

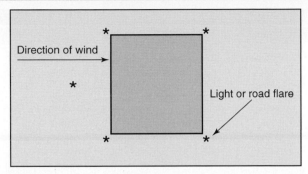

FIGURE 58.2 A "box and one" temporary helicopter landing zone (HLZ). A light (illumination), piece of light-colored clothing, or flare is placed at each corner of the HLZ. A fifth light, flare, or piece of light-colored clothing is placed 5 to 10 m (16.4 to 32.8 ft) outside the square directly upwind, showing the pilot the wind direction. All lights, flares, or clothing should be firmly attached to the ground to prevent them from being blown away by rotor wash.

- Once the helicopter is on the ground, it must be approached only from the front and side under direct observation of the pilot.
- The aft portion of the aircraft and areas around the tail rotor must always be avoided. Some helicopters have rear doors for loading and unloading patients, and ground personnel should await direction from the crew before approaching the rear area. A safety person should be assigned to prevent anyone from inadvertently walking toward the tail rotor.
- If the ground is uneven or sloped, all personnel should approach and depart the helicopter on the downslope side.
- It is safest to load the patient into the helicopter with the engines off and rotors stopped ("cold load").
- If the patient must be loaded with the engines on and blades turning ("hot load"), eye and ear protection should be worn by all personnel and patients approaching the helicopter.
- Once the patient is loaded, all persons should leave the landing zone, take cover, and stay in place until the helicopter has departed.
- It is best to be off to the side, not directly in the takeoff path.
- If you have a radio and know your frequency, inform the flight crew at the time of dispatch. You can more easily direct them into the HLZ and warn of potential hazards. Wires are almost impossible to see during daytime and virtually invisible at night.

Ground-to-Air Signaling

- It is best to have radio communication between the ground party and helicopter crew. If this is not possible, hand signals may be necessary.
- Standard hand signals are used by military rescue personnel for communication between a deployed rescue swimmer and the

Table 58.2 Swimmer to Helicopter and Ground-to-Air Signals	
INTENTION	**ACTION**
Deploy medical kit	Arms above head, wrists crossed
Situation okay	Thumbs up
Lower rescue cable with rescue device	Arm extended overhead, fist clenched
Lower rescue cable without rescue device	Climbing-rope motion with hands
Helicopter move in/out	Wave in/out with both hands
Cease operations	Slashing motion across throat
Deploy litter	Hands cupped, then arms outstretched
Personnel secured, hoist rescue device	Vigorously shake hoist cable or thumbs up with vigorous up motion with arm
Team recall	Circle arm over head with fingers skyward

helicopter (Table 58.2). These same signals can be used while on land.
- To acknowledge the signals, the hoist operator gives a "thumbs up" or the pilot flashes the rotating beacon. It is best to coordinate these signals with flight crew before rescue.

Using a Ground Guide

Note: Using a ground guide to "marshal" a helicopter into a tight or crowded HLZ using hand signals is a difficult and dangerous procedure and should be attempted only by personnel specifically trained in this procedure. The pilot also must have been specifically trained in this procedure and know that the ground guide is competent to guide the aircraft to the ground.

1. A ground guide individual should wear eye protection and keep their back to the wind, because helicopters take off and land into the wind.
2. If a ground guide for the HLZ is to be used, the person designated to be the ground guide should initially stand in the middle of the HLZ.
3. Once the helicopter is in sight, the ground guide should hold both arms over their head (daytime) or hold two flashlights over their head (night operations).
4. Once the pilot has identified the HLZ, the ground guide should move out of the HLZ in the upwind direction.

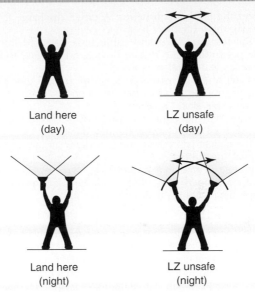

Land here
(day)

LZ unsafe
(day)

Land here
(night)

LZ unsafe
(night)

FIGURE 58.3   Ground Guide Hand Signals. The ground guide should stand in the middle of the helicopter landing zone (HLZ) with arms raised over his or her head (the "safe to land" signal) until the pilot has seen the HLZ. The ground guide should then immediately exit the HLZ heading upwind at least 5 to 10 m (16.4 to 32.8 ft) outside the marked HLZ and maintain the "safe to land" signal. If at any time the ground guide sees a danger or unsafe condition around or within the HLZ, he or she should immediately give the wave-off signal and continue this signal until the helicopter has aborted the approach/landing. *LZ,* Landing zone.

5. The guide should continue to give the "safe to land" signal from well outside the HLZ until the aircraft has landed.
6. No persons should be in the HLZ or moving toward the HLZ during landing.
7. If at any time during the helicopter's approach the ground guide sees any unsafe condition in the HLZ or surrounding area, he or she should immediately give a "wave off" signal (Fig. 58.3).

Hoist Operations

If a helicopter is not able to land and has a rescue hoist installed, hoist operations may be the only means to evacuate the patient. In most circumstances a helicopter crew member rides the hoist down to the site to rig the patient into the rescue device and to oversee the hoist operation, using the following guidelines:

1. Do not touch the hoist, rescue device, or cable until after it has touched the ground (or water). A helicopter can build up a powerful static electricity charge that will be grounded through

whatever the hoist first touches. A direct discharge to humans can knock them off their feet.

2. Once the rescue device and cable have touched the ground, put the patient into the rescue device, taking care to keep the hoist cable clear of all persons.

3. Do not allow the hoist cable to loop around any person or around the rescue device, because serious injury is possible when the cable slack is taken up.

4. Make sure that the patient is properly secured in the rescue device, with all safety straps tightened.

5. When the patient is secured, move away from the rescue device and signal "up cable."

6. If the rescue device is a basket (e.g., Stokes) litter, use a tag line with a properly installed weak link to prevent the litter from spinning during the hoist.

Night Operations

- Night helicopter rescue operations are considerably more dangerous than daylight operations. It is preferable to delay helicopter insertion or extraction operations until daylight.
- The landing zone should be clearly marked and the pilot allowed to make the approach. All personnel should stay clear of the landing zone until the pilot has made a safe landing.
- Persons approaching the landing zone should have a small light or reflective material attached to outer clothing so it can be clearly seen.
- A minimum number of people should approach the helicopter, and a safety observer is mandatory to keep the ground team together and clear of the tail rotor and rotor blades.
- The landing zone should be as large as possible, preferably at least 50% larger than a daylight landing zone.
- Any obstacles should be clearly marked with light-colored streamers, small lights, or even light-colored clothing.
- The landing zone can be illuminated with flashlights at the corners, with another flashlight at the center point. These flashlights should be pointed at the ground, not into the air; flashlights pointed at the helicopter during landing and takeoff may distract or momentarily blind the crew. If flashlights are not available, chemical light sticks can be used. Although small fires have been used to illuminate the edges of the landing zone, the scattered burning embers are fire hazards, so this technique is not recommended.
- Because crew members may be using night vision equipment, lights must never be flashed at the helicopter. Even the amount of white light from a small flashlight may be sufficient to overload night vision equipment, functionally blinding the crew.

Dispatch and Communications

- The dispatch center is the focal point for communications during aeromedical transport operations.

- Dispatchers receive incoming requests for service; obtain necessary information relative to the launch decision; coordinate interactions between essential parties; "scramble" the flight crew; assemble and maintain necessary information regarding destination, weather, local telephone numbers and frequencies; follow flight progress; input data into the system database; and communicate with ground emergency medical services (EMS) units and hospitals.
- Communication may occur through a combination of methods: land telephone lines into a dispatch switchboard, hospital-EMS net transceiver, discrete frequency transceiver (communications with aircraft), or walkie-talkie radios.
- Familiarity with the EMS system and EMS communications is essential for successful dispatch.
- Flight following is an important part of aeromedical safety and involves tracking the position of the aircraft during a mission by plotting the location according to reports at 10- to 15-minute intervals from the pilot. If an accident or in-flight emergency occurs, the dispatcher is soon aware and can initiate search and rescue to a precise location, which enhances the chances for survival.

APPROPRIATE USE OF AEROMEDICAL SERVICES

- Aeromedical transport combines skilled treatment and stabilization capability with rapid access to definitive care, but not without risk and at a financial cost approximately four times that of ground transport.
- The comparative risk of aeromedical transport must be placed in perspective against the risk for patient death from less timely ground transport with limited medical capability en route.
- In isolated rural or wilderness locations, a helicopter may be the only means of expedient access.
- Prolonged patient extrication allows time for a helicopter to arrive at the scene, decreasing total transport time and thereby increasing the advantages of helicopter transport.
- Patient comfort must be considered, especially during long transports in turbulent air. Although a helicopter moves in three dimensions, fore and aft acceleration is usually steady, without the starting and stopping motions present during ground transport. However, helicopters typically travel within 914 m (3000 ft) of the ground's surface and are more subject to turbulence than are high-flying fixed-wing aircraft.
- The decision to transport a patient by air requires judgment and realistic appraisal of risks. A patient should be transported by air only if he or she is so ill that this method of transport is necessary; if ground transport is unavailable, delayed, or unable to reach the patient; or if aeromedical transport would reduce the risk for death by permitting more rapid access to definitive care, providing greater medical skill en route, or both.

59 Survival

The term *survival* means "to continue to live or exist" and implies the presence of adverse conditions that make this more difficult. Survival scenarios frequently accompany wilderness medical events.

COLD WEATHER SURVIVAL
Shelter

Anyone who spends time in the wilderness should practice construction of emergency survival shelters. In a cold environment, a shelter becomes an extension of the microclimate of still, warm air created from body heat and trapped by insulated clothing. All shelters need adequate ventilation, which is especially important to consider when building a snow shelter.

Choosing the type of survival shelter to build depends on why the shelter is necessary and the availability of resources.

A properly designed shelter should permit easy and rapid construction with simple tools and give good protection from adverse elements. The type and size of shelter also depend on the presence or absence of snow and its depth, on natural features of the landscape, and on whether firewood or a stove and fuel are available. If external heat cannot be provided, a shelter must be small, waterproof, and windproof to preserve body heat.

General guidelines and considerations for choosing a location for a shelter include the following:

- Is the shelter needed solely for warmth or also for protection from wind and snow?
- Where should the shelter be built?
- What are the avalanche or rock-fall risks in the area?
- Avoid exposed windy ridges.
- Avoid any areas at risk for flooding (drainages, dry riverbeds).
- Avoid low-lying areas, such as basins that tend to collect the colder night air.
- A timbered area provides protection from foul weather, but can also block the sun.
- Select a shelter site where there is access to water.
- In windy conditions, a shelter should be built with the entrance at 90 degrees to the prevailing winds.
- Shelters can be built in small caves or indentations in a rock outcropping, in a "tree well," or under downed trees.
- Environmental resources that can be used for building and insulating a shelter include small trees, branches, thick grass, or leaf piles.

- Snow is a good insulator because it traps the warmed air generated by body heat; however, direct contact with snow must be avoided.
- An insulation barrier between the snow and an individual can be created by using equipment, such as a closed cell foam pad or backpack, or it can be created by piling up small tree branches and boughs.
- The insulation layer, if using tree boughs, should be 25.4 to 30.5 cm (10 to 12 in) thick to allow for compression when sitting or lying on this layer.

TYPES OF SHELTERS
Constructed Shelters
Tarpaulins
1. Cut open a 3- to 4-mil (1 mil = 0.0254 mm [0.001 in]) large, heavy-duty plastic bag to form a tarp.
2. Fifty feet of cordage is also needed.
3. A tarp can be rigged into either a lean-to or an A-frame shelter. In cold weather, an A-frame provides the best method for retaining heated air.
4. Tie cordage between two trees situated approximately 3 m (10 ft) apart. The tree at the entrance end should be a large tree if a fire is going to be made (see later). If there is a slight slope to the terrain, the head end of the shelter should be uphill.
5. Tie the foot end of the cord 45.2 to 61 cm (18 to 24 in) above the ground.
6. Tie the head end of the cord 1.1 to 1.2 m (3.5 to 4 ft) above the ground.
7. Fold the tarp in half over the cord, and secure both ends to the cord.
8. Ideally, place the foot end next to a large tree, which offers a natural closure for that end of the shelter.
9. Secure the edges of the sides of the tarp to the ground by tying them to rocks or other trees.
10. To prevent heat from escaping along the edges of the A-frame, the sides should have an overlapping flap on the ground that can be secured with dirt, snow, or rocks.
11. Close the foot end to prevent heat escape.
12. Leave the front end, or entrance, open if a fire is going to be built.
13. If there will be no fire, the entrance can be at least partially closed off by stacking a backpack or tree branches in the opening.
14. Insulate the sides of the constructed shelter by thatching brush, branches, or broad leaves (e.g., the first layer is placed at ground level, with each successive layer overlapping the one below it).

Plastic Bag Shelters (Fig. 59.1)

Large, heavy-grade (3 to 4 mil) orange plastic 208.2-L (55-gallon) drum liners make good short-term emergency shelters. Alternatively, heavy-duty trash bags can be used.

1. Cut an opening in the bottom end of the bag that is just large enough for your head, and then pass the bag over your head so that your face is at the opening.
2. When creating the hole, cut the plastic at 90 degrees to the fold to reduce the likelihood of the bag tearing along the seam.
3. A second bag, pulled over the legs, used in conjunction with the system described above, will form a one-person survival shelter.

Tube Tents (Fig. 59.2)

- Tube tents are inexpensive polypropylene sleeves that are 2.4 m (8 ft) long and provide a tubular shelter that is 0.9 to 1.5 m (3 to 5 ft) high, depending on the brand.
- A tube tent can be pulled over the body to provide a quick shelter or pitched as a "pup tent." To do this, find two anchors (e.g., rocks, trees) that are the proper distance apart, tie a line to one of them, spread the tent out along the length of the line, run the line through it, and then tie off the other end of the line. The height of the line should be such that the tent can be spread out to accommodate the occupant.
- To avoid ripping, the tent plastic should be 3 to 4 mm thick.
- Tube tents can be improvised from two plastic 208.2-L (55-gallon) drum liners, which are 3 to 4 mm thick, or from large,

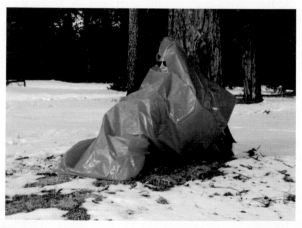

FIGURE 59.1   Example of two large plastic bags used to form a one-person survival shelter. (Courtesy Peter Kummerfeldt.)

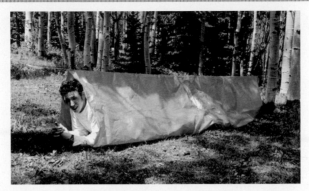

FIGURE 59.2   Two large plastic bags can be taped together in tandem and used with a line to form a tube tent. (Courtesy Peter Kummerfeldt.)

heavy-grade household trash bags by opening the closed end of one bag, sliding it into the open end of the second bag, and then duct taping the bags together.

Tents and Bivouac Sacks

- Tents are generally comfortable and dry, but in very cold weather they are not as warm as snow shelters.
- Tents are preferable to snow shelters at mild temperatures, during damp snow conditions at temperatures above freezing, or when the snow cover is minimal.
- Bivouac sacks are carried by climbers on long alpine-style climbs or for emergencies. They are usually made of Gore-Tex or waterproof fabric and hold one or two persons. They pack small, are lightweight, and can easily be carried for an emergency shelter on any trip into the backcountry.
- Many modern packs have extensions, so when used with a cagoule or mountain parka, form acceptable bivouac sacks. The cagoule is donned, and the backpack is pulled on the feet and legs, extending the top of the pack as high up the body as it can be placed.

Natural Shelters

- Caves and alcoves under overhangs are good shelters and can be improved by building barrier walls with rocks, snow blocks, or brush to protect from wind.
- In deep snow, large fallen logs and bent-over evergreens frequently have hollows underneath them that can be used as small snow caves.
- Cone-shaped depressions around the trunks of evergreens (tree wells) can be improved by digging them out and roofing them over with evergreen branches or a tarp (Fig. 59.3).

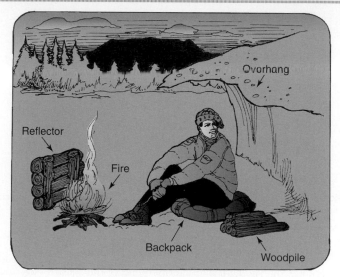

FIGURE 59.3   Natural shelter.

SNOW SHELTERS
Snow Trenches (Figs. 59.4 and 59.5)
A snow trench is the easiest and quickest survival snow shelter and the one least likely to leave the diggers wet. If a shovel, large tarp, structural support items (skis, poles, trees), and a small fire, candle, or stove are available, a trench can be created that is as comfortable as a snow cave. It is easiest to dig a trench in a flat area. However, if the snow is deep enough, it can be dug out on an incline, keeping the trench itself level.

1. If possible, dig all the way to the ground. If the snow is too deep to dig to the ground, dig to a depth of 0.9 m (3 ft). If the snow is not deep enough, pile snow up around all four sides of the trench to make walls, until the total depth of the trench is 0.9 m (3 ft).
2. The trench width should be just slightly wider and 0.6 to 0.9 m (2 to 3 ft) longer than the person(s) that will be lying in the shelter. The additional length allows for a fire pit at one end of the shelter.
3. Ski poles, skis, or long tree branches are placed perpendicular to the length of the trench.
4. The trench is then covered with a tarp, leaving one end open for the entrance.
5. Secure the tarp on all sides by packing the edges into the snow.
6. Gently toss snow on top of the reinforced tarp to provide insulation to the shelter.
7. The snow pack on top should be 20.3 cm (8 in) or more.

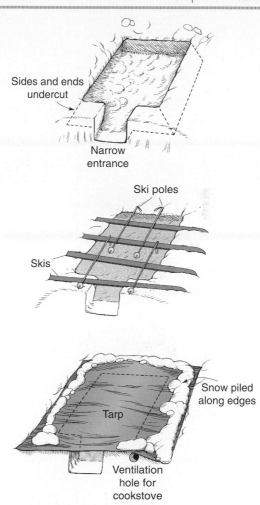

Sides and ends undercut

Narrow entrance

Ski poles

Skis

Snow piled along edges

Tarp

Ventilation hole for cookstove

FIGURE 59.4 Three-person snow trench.

8. The object is to keep the maximal amount of snow around and over the trench for optimal insulation.
9. If the trench is going to be wide enough to accommodate more than one person, the entrance should still be only wide enough for one person to pass through at a time. A narrow entrance is easier to close off and helps contain heat within the shelter.
10. A barrier can be created at the entrance by stacking backpacks or snow blocks, or hanging a tarp across the opening.

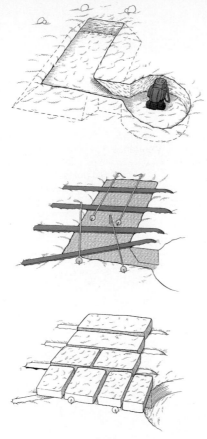

FIGURE 59.5 Above-timberline snow trench.

11. When the entrance is closed, a small votive-size candle or stove and the occupants' body heat will raise the interior temperature to −4° to −1°C (24.8° to 30.2°F).
12. Higher temperatures should be avoided so that clothing and bedding will not become wet from melting snow.
13. Ventilation is necessary to prevent build-up of carbon monoxide within the shelter.
14. Anywhere that deep snow has been wind packed, as happens above timberline, the trench can be roofed with snow blocks.
15. The blocks are cut to a width of 45.2 to 50.8 cm (18 to 20 in), a depth of 10.2 cm (4 in), and a length equal to the length of the snow saw.

16. They are then laid horizontally for a narrow trench or vertically for a wider trench, set as an A-frame, or laid on skis (see Fig. 59.5).
17. Any spaces between the blocks are chinked with snow.

Snow Caves (Fig. 59.6)

A shovel is the best item to use when digging a snow cave, although small snow caves large enough for one person can be dug with a ski or cooking pot. The optimum site is a large snowdrift, often found on the lee side of a small hill; areas in avalanche zones must be avoided.

1. Ski poles, skis, or tree branches are poked in the snowdrift to a depth of 45.2 cm (18 in) around the area that will be the outside walls of the cave.
2. The entrance is dug just large enough to crawl through and is angled upward toward the sleeping chamber (see Fig. 59.6).
3. After the entrance is dug with the shovel, the digger crawls inside, lies supine, and uses the shovel to excavate the chamber, which should be large enough for a stove and the number of occupants requiring shelter.
4. The snow is removed from the walls inside the shelter until the ends of the ski poles, skis, or tree branches are met. This ensures that the snow cave walls maintain a depth of 45.2 cm (18 in), necessary to prevent collapse of the walls.
5. Because diggers tend to become wet, water-resistant or water-proof jackets and pants should be worn.
6. Pine branches or other natural materials can be used to cover the floor if a sleeping pad is not available.
7. The entrance to the snow cave can be blocked off using backpacks or blocks of snow.
8. If the group is large and there are several people available to dig out the cave, a larger entrance can be created, providing room for multiple diggers to excavate the interior.
9. The disadvantage is the larger opening that needs to be closed to maintain warmth inside the snow cave.
10. The cooking area for the snow cave can be in the entrance area outside the cave itself.
11. If cooking is going to be done inside the cave, a ventilation hole as large as a ski pole basket must be cut in the roof over the cooking area to provide adequate ventilation.
12. A snow cave large enough for two persons takes several hours to dig and therefore is not the primary choice of shelter in an emergency. It can be built after a faster-improvised shelter is provided for the safety and well-being of the group.

Quinzhee (Snow Dome)

A quinzhee is an artificially created pile of snow that is dug out to create a snow cave. It is an alternative method available when

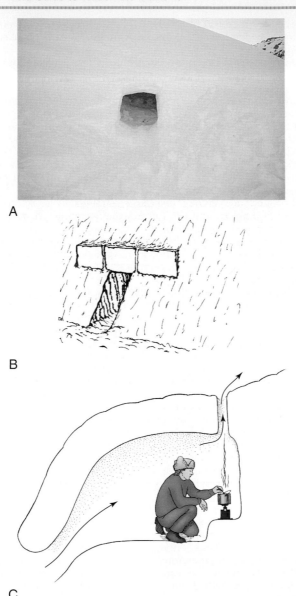

A

B

C

FIGURE 59.6   A, Snow cave entrance. **B,** Snow cave partly closed with snow blocks. **C,** Interior of snow cave.

a snow cave is desired and a natural snowdrift cannot be located, as occurs when the ground is flat or the snow cover is shallow.

1. The snow is piled into a large dome 1.8 to 2.1 m (6 to 7 ft) in height and width and left to harden for a few hours. The waiting time allows the snow crystals to adequately consolidate so that the dome will not collapse when it is excavated.
2. After the settling time, the dome is dug out in the same method as described earlier for the snow cave.
3. Sticks can be used as spacers; walls should be 25.4 to 30.5 cm (10 to 12 in) thick.
4. A low entrance is dug on one side, and from there the interior is carved out to make a dome-shaped room that is large enough to sleep three or four people.
5. The sleeping platform should be higher than the entrance.
6. Another method is to make a "form" (i.e., a pile of vegetation or equipment), cover this form with snow, allow the snow to set, and then open one end and remove the form.
7. A ventilation hole is cut in the roof over the stove.

Igloos (Fig. 59.7)

Igloos are the most comfortable arctic shelters, but require time, experience, and engineering skill. They are not recommended for the novice, but may be worth the effort if the party will be stranded for any length of time.

1. An igloo requires one, or ideally two, snow saws and snow that is well packed and easy to cut into multiple uniform blocks.
2. This type of packed snow is found in wind-blown, treeless areas.
3. Packed, consolidated snow can be created by stamping a large area of snow and letting it settle and harden for several hours.
4. To mark the diameter of the igloo, a ski pole is held by the handle and the body turned so that the pole basket makes a large circle. This will outline the base of an igloo suitable for three people. The first snow blocks are cut from inside the circle. This will lower the floor so that fewer blocks are required for the dome.
5. At least two persons are needed for this project: one to cut and carry the blocks and the other inside the igloo to lay the blocks.
6. The blocks should be about 45.2 cm (18 in) wide, 76.2 cm (30 in) long, and 20.3 cm (8 in) thick.
7. They are laid in a circle leaning in 20 to 30 degrees toward the center of the igloo, with the sides trimmed for a snug fit.
8. The tops of the first few blocks in the first circle are beveled so that a continuous line of blocks is placed down, with the first few blocks of each succeeding circle cocked upward (see Fig. 59.7A).

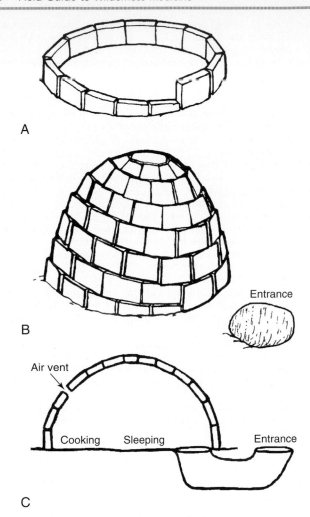

FIGURE 59.7   A to **C,** Stages of igloo construction.

9. A common error is to not lean the blocks inward enough, resulting in an open tower instead of a dome.
10. Gaps between the blocks are caulked with snow.
11. The dome should be 1.5 to 1.8 m (5 to 6 ft) high inside and can be closed with a single capstone of snow.
12. The entrance is dug as a tunnel underneath rather than through the edge of the igloo, preventing warm air from escaping (see Fig. 59.7B and C).

FIRE
Fire Building

The ability to build a fire under adverse conditions is an essential skill that should be practiced by persons who engage in outdoor activities. One needs about 10 armloads of wood logs to keep a fire burning all night. The area in which to build a fire should be carefully chosen so that the fire can provide warmth to the shelter and not create danger of spreading to the surrounding area.

Mandatory equipment for starting a fire includes the following:
- A heat source (e.g., spark from a striker)
- Tinder

Three other helpful items for fire preparation are as follows:
1. Solid-shank, nonfolding knife with a 10.2- to 15.2-cm (4- to 6-in) blade.
2. Waterproof/windproof matches. Windproof matches have longer and fatter heads than do normal matches. These matches can be difficult to light under benign conditions and almost impossible in adverse weather. Some brands are better than others. Experiment before your trips (Fig. 59.8). (Note: All of the matches that are currently available were tested under field conditions, and REI Stormproof Matches proved to be the most reliable for starting fires under adverse weather conditions, and are particularly effective in windy and wet conditions.)
3. Match containers. The ability to light a match is tied directly to the condition of the matchbox, most of which are made from cardboard or thin wood, with striking pads along each side. Neither of these materials is particularly durable, and both tend to disintegrate quickly when wet. For this reason, matches should be protected in a container that is waterproof, easy to open with one hand, and easy to find if dropped. Do not take it for granted that a match case is as waterproof as claimed; be sure to test it. These also make perfect containers for storing fire starter (i.e., petroleum jelly-saturated cotton balls) (Fig. 59.9).

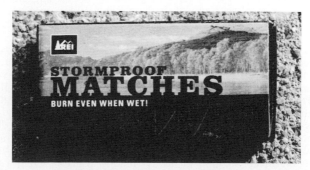

FIGURE 59.8 REI Stormproof Matches.

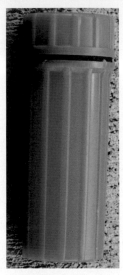

FIGURE 59.9   Orange military-style match case.

A **heat source** can be thought of as a spark to start the fire.
- Matches or lighters are the easiest way to create the spark.
- However, in adverse conditions in wilderness environments, matches and lighters do not always work and are not reliable 100% of the time.
- The heat source that is always reliable is a metal match. Like a regular match, it needs to strike against something. A knife blade, when scraped briskly against a metal match, readily produces a shower of very hot sparks that can be used to ignite tinder.
- Other strikers similar in appearance to a 5.1-cm (2-in) piece of hacksaw blade are often packaged with a metal match.
- A metal match and striker are the perfect fire-starting tools for a survival scenario, because they will work in any weather condition, at any altitude, and last for 10,000 or more strikes (Fig. 59.10).
- Metal matches are a composite of several different types of metals heated and molded into a round or rectangular bar.
- This molded metal is usually joined to a piece of wood or a magnesium bar, which then acts as a handle for the match.

Tinder is any type of flammable material that ignites instantly when spread out and a spark is applied.
- Natural tinder includes dry grass and leaves, dry pine needles, inner bark of birch trees, shavings from dry sticks, and pitch wood (or "fat wood").
- Natural materials are not always readily available when a fire is necessary.
- Tinder should be carried in a survival kit.

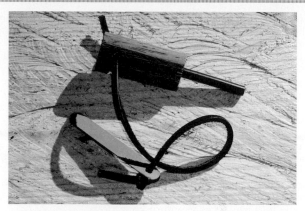

FIGURE 59.10 Metal match with a hacksaw blade scraper.

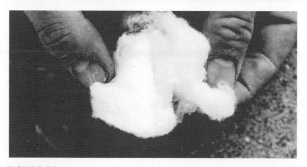

FIGURE 59.11 Smearing petroleum jelly into a cotton ball disk.

- The most practical tinder for this purpose is a cotton ball generously saturated with petroleum jelly (Vaseline) that is prepared and placed in a container before leaving home (Fig. 59.11).
- Small screw-top containers the size of a film canister can hold 8 to 12 cotton balls, depending on the size of the cotton ball. Commercial match containers also work well for this purpose.
  Kindling and fuel are necessary to maintain the fire.
- Kindling is small to medium pieces of wood, usually sections of small dead branches or larger branches that have been split lengthwise with a knife or ax.
- In a wet environment, standing dead wood is preferable to wood lying on the ground, and wood that has lost its bark to wood with bark, because both will be drier and less rotten than the alternatives.
  Fuel is the largest material, usually branches and sections of dead tree trunks several inches or more in diameter.
- Several times more fuel than the predicted need should be collected.

- Long, dead sections of trees can be shortened by first laying them across a fire. When they burn through, two shorter sections result.
- Fires generally should be kept small to conserve wood, to allow them to be approached more closely, and to be able to easily extinguish the flames should the wind pick up and threaten the safety of having a fire.
- Firewood for the kindling and fuel must be gathered and prepared before lighting the fire.
- It is helpful to stack the wood by the designated fire site, arranging it into piles according to size, beginning with pine needle kindling, progressing to pencil size, then thumb size, and then up to wrist and arm size.
- Wood that is too big will not burn as efficiently unless the fire is very hot.
- Some logs can be split with a knife or ax.
- If a knife is used, the knife blade is placed on the end of a piece of wood. Another log or rock is used to hammer the knife until a piece of the log splits off.
- The fuel supply should be protected from rain and snow.
- The fire needs a platform and a brace to protect it from the natural earth contact surface (snow or grasses).
- The platform can be as simple as several logs of similar diameter laid side by side.
- The brace is laid perpendicular to the platform logs.
- Wind direction needs to be considered when placing the brace.
- The brace should be placed parallel to the direction of the wind.
- The fire can also be built behind a rock or log.
- In a snow environment, if possible, dig to the ground to build the fire.
- If the snow is too deep and it is not possible to dig to the ground, build the fire on the platform on the snow.

Fire Starting

Once the fire site is chosen, the platform is prepared, and the wood for fuel is gathered, split, and arranged, it is time to light the fire. A petroleum jelly-impregnated cotton ball is spread out to enable air to reach the fibers and is placed on the platform. The metal match is positioned next to the cotton ball, which allows the spark from the striker to fall onto the cotton ball. Once the cotton ball is ignited, the pine needle-size kindling is then placed on the burning cotton ball to allow the kindling to catch on fire. Large pieces of kindling are then added. Fuel is added after the kindling is burning well. Too much smoke from a fire indicates the fire is not getting enough air and the fuel should be spread out, allowing for better airflow.

- A fire should be built in such a way that heat reflects onto the occupant, regardless of the type of shelter. If the shelter is a natural cave or underneath a rock overhang, the fire should be 1.5 to 1.8 m (5 to 6 ft) from the back of the shelter. A reflector wall of logs or stones on the opposite side of the fire should be constructed. The occupant should sit between the fire and the back of the shelter (see Fig. 59.3).

- For an A-frame type of shelter, the fire is built in the 0.9- to 1.2-m (3- to 4-ft) space between the entrance and the large tree. If reflective material is available, it is secured to the tree. This fire is a small fire and needs to be monitored always.
- Fires can be built in tree wells but should not be positioned under snow-laden branches. Fires can be built on a platform at the entrance of a trench. The entrance area needs to be large enough to allow ingress and egress from the trench without risk of encountering the fire.
- All fires should be observed and carefully controlled. It is imperative that water, sand, dirt, or snow be readily available should the fire need to be immediately extinguished.

Additional Concepts and Fire-Building Tips

- When the ground is wet, it is advisable to assemble a platform of sticks to protect the tinder.
- If tinder is placed directly on wet ground, it tends to absorb moisture from soil that may make it more difficult to light. There is no practical way for a survivor to build a fire on top of snow. Try to locate an area where the snow is shallow enough to scrape it away down to ground level.
- Wind has a dramatic effect on fire-building efforts. To provide the best chance of having tinder ignite and continue to burn, place a log that is about 25.4 to 30.5 cm (10 to 12 in) long and 10.2 cm (4 in) in diameter along the windward side of the platform. Place the tinder in the lee of the log, where it is protected from the wind.
- When trying to build a fire in rainy conditions or when snow is falling, find a sheltered area or erect a temporary roof over the fire site to shelter the tinder until the larger fuel is burning.
- Before lighting the tinder, everything must be ready. A very common mistake made by those who are inexperienced is igniting tinder and then having to scramble to find kindling to add to the rapidly burning tinder before it burns out.
- With everything ready to build out the fire, place the tinder on the platform in the lee of the windbreak, and ignite it (Fig. 59.12).
- As soon as the tinder is burning, place a handful of the smallest fuel directly over the flames, with one end of the twig bundle resting on the log brace (Fig. 59.13); this will work well only if you have resisted the urge to break the twigs into overly short pieces.
- The fuel should be broken into lengths that are 25.4 to 30.5 cm (10 to 12 in) long. Resting one end of the twigs on the brace ensures that good airflow is maintained and that the tinder is not smothered when additional fuel is added.
- If it appears that more oxygen is needed, lift up one end of the brace to allow more oxygen to flow to the core of the fire.

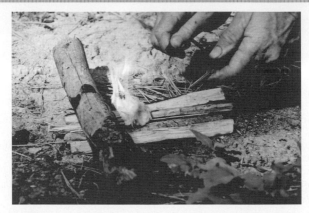

FIGURE 59.12   Cotton ball saturated with petroleum jelly being lit with a metal match.

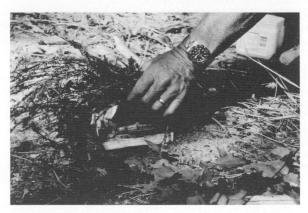

FIGURE 59.13   Placing the first handful of twigs over a burning cotton ball.

- As the twigs begin to burn and flames appear through the first layer of fuel, lay a second handful of twigs at a 90-degree angle over the first layer (Fig. 59.14).
- As the flames appear above this layer, place another handful of slightly larger twigs on the fire, again at a 90-degree angle to the previous layer. (Fig. 59.15). This process continues until the larger fuel has been added and until the fire will sustain itself without the immediate attention of the person building it.
- Your fire-building success with the use of this method is contingent on the use of tinder that produces a lot of heat, that is well ventilated, and that graduates step by step from the smallest twigs to the largest sizes of fuel (Fig. 59.16).

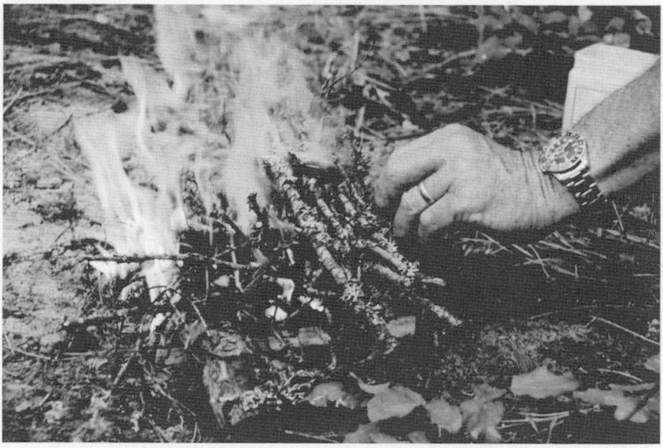

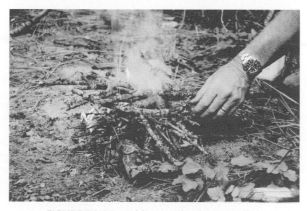

FIGURE 59.14 Placing a second handful of twigs over a burning cotton ball.

FIGURE 59.15 Adding another layer to a fire.

FOOD

Although most persons in a survival situation worry more about food than anything else, food is usually less important than are shelter and water because a person can survive for weeks without food, even in cold weather. Bare ridges, high mountains above timberline, and dense evergreen forests are difficult places to find wild food, even in summer. Success is more likely on river and stream banks, on lakeshores, in margins of forests, and in natural clearings. In most cases the amount of wild food found by an untrained individual will not provide enough calories to replenish the energy expended in searching for it. Therefore, it is important to carry extra food for emergencies.

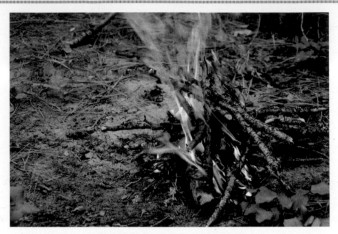

FIGURE 59.16   Self-sustaining fire.

WATER

- A human can survive 3 to 5 days without water. Because about 800 mL (27.1 oz) of water per day are contained in food and 300 mL (10.1 oz) produced by metabolism, a minimum daily intake of 1200 mL (40.6 oz) is necessary in a temperate climate at sea level to avoid dehydration.
- In a hot, dry climate, at high altitude, or with exertion, insensible losses and sweating increase considerably, so fluid intake should be increased proportionally.
- Whenever open water is encountered, individuals should drink their fill of disinfected water and then top off all water bottles.
- Almost all surface water should be considered contaminated by animal or human wastes, except for small streams descending from untracked snowfields; springs erupting from underground; or high, uninhabited areas.
- If survival forces you to drink from a stagnant or muddy pool, remember that it is always better to drink dirty water than to die of dehydration. Let water filled with particulates settle, and then strain it through a cloth.
- Water can be disinfected by heat, filtration, ultraviolet light or addition of chemicals (see Chapter 45).
- Rainwater can be collected by spreading out a survival tarp and channeling it into a container.
- On a sunny day in a snow environment, snow can be spread on a dark plastic sheet to melt and then be channeled into a container.
- On cloudy days, in subfreezing temperatures, and in locations above the snow line where liquid water is difficult to find, snow or ice must be melted to obtain water. This requires a metal pot (which should be included in every survival kit), fire-starting equipment, and wood for fuel.

- If it is possible to melt the snow and heat the water, enough snow should be melted to provide water for rehydration and to fill a water bottle. The water bottle is placed in the bottom of the sleeping bag to keep it from freezing and is ready for drinking during the night or the next day.
- Melting ice or hard snow is more efficient than melting light, powdery snow.
- Melting enough snow to maintain hydration in harsh winter environments requires a significant amount of vigilance.
- Enough snow should be melted to provide everyone with at least one or two 1-liter water bottles for the day.
  Several general guidelines apply when water supplies are limited:
- Overexertion is avoided, and energy expenditure is kept to a minimum.
- Do not drink seawater, alcohol, or urine.
- Food intake should be kept to a minimum (i.e., do not overeat).
- You may eat snow or ice, but only if hypothermia is not a risk. There is significant heat loss when melting snow in one's mouth.

EMERGENCY SNOW TRAVEL

Travel in deep snow is almost impossible without skis or snowshoes.

1. Emergency snowshoes (Fig. 59.17A) can be made from poles that are 1.8 m (6 ft) long, 1.9 to 2.5 cm (0.75 to 1 in) thick at

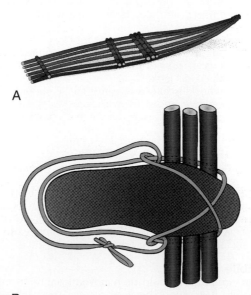

A

B

FIGURE 59.17 **A,** Emergency snowshoe. **B,** Detail of snowshoe binding.

the base, and 0.64 cm (0.25 in) thick at the tip, and sticks 1.9 cm (0.75 in) thick and 25.4 cm (10 in) long.

2. Snowshoes require 12 long poles and 12 short sticks. For each snowshoe, 6 long poles are placed side by side on the ground, and the middle point of the poles is marked.

3. One short stick is lashed crosswise to the tail (base) of the poles, and three short sticks are lashed side by side just forward of the midpoint of the poles where the toe of the boot will rest.

4. Two sticks are lashed where the heel of the boot will strike the snowshoe. The tips of the six poles are tied together.

5. Each binding (see Fig. 59.17B) is made of a continuous length (about 1.8 m [6 ft]) of nylon cord, preferably braided, because it will eventually fray.

6. The midpoint of the cord is positioned at the back of the boot above the bulge of the heel.

7. Each end of the cord is run under the three side-by-side short sticks at the side of the boot, then up and across the boot toe so that it crosses the other end on top of the toe, forming an X.

8. Then, each end is looped around the cord running along the opposite side of the boot, and the ends are brought around the back of the boot heel.

9. The cord is pulled tight around the boot, and the ends are tied together at the lateral side of the heel.

10. When walking, the tip of the snowshoe should rise, the boot heel should rise, and the boot sole should remain on the snowshoe.

11. Snow travelers should avoid stepping close to trees (because of funnel-shaped tree wells around tree trunks), large rocks (because of weak snow or moats around them), and overhanging stream banks.

12. A person who falls into a stream or lake should roll repeatedly in powdery snow to wick the water from clothing, brushing the snow off each time. A fire completes the drying process.

STALLED OR WRECKED VEHICLE

Persons stranded in an automobile or a downed airplane can often survive using the equipment in the vehicle. Usually the survivors should stay with the vehicle rather than go for help because a vehicle is much more visible to rescuers than is a person. Floor mats and upholstery can be used for insulation, but it is much better to have a vehicle survival kit containing extra clothing, blankets, and gear listed in Appendix P.

Automobile

- Survival equipment should be removed from the trunk as soon as possible if it cannot be accessed via the back seat of the automobile.

- The marooned driver should tie brightly colored flagging tape to the antenna and at night should leave the inside dome light on to be seen by snowplow drivers and rescuers. Headlights consume too much battery current.
- If there are people only in the front seat of the car, a space blanket is duct-taped to the back of the front seat, cutting in half the amount of space in the car that needs to be heated via body heat or the candle.
- One 36-hour candle is placed on the dashboard and lit. Although variation occurs depending on the air tightness of the vehicle and the outside air temperature, a candle can raise the interior temperature above freezing.
- A window should be cracked 2.5 to 5.1 cm (1 to 2 in) to prevent build-up of carbon monoxide.
- Reusable carbon monoxide detectors are available and can be carried in the survival kit.
- Running the motor and heater for a couple of minutes each hour has its disadvantages. Someone will need to regularly get out of the automobile to check if the exhaust pipe is free of snow. In doing so, too much heat from the interior of the car is lost, negating the benefit of running the engine and heater.

Airplane

- In most circumstances, it is advisable to remain with the aircraft.
- Sizeable parts from the aircraft can be used for the shell of a shelter.
- Because aircraft often do not provide sufficient insulation, a fire is optimal for providing warmth in a cold environment.
- Cloth and stuffing from the seats and life vests can be used for insulation.
- Seat belts can be cut away from the aircraft, clipped together, and used for rope.
- Any accessible baggage should be investigated for useful supplies.
- Creating a signal in clear weather is important.
  - The area of the crash site should be made visible from the air.
  - Anything of color and contrast that will help to identify the site should be tied to trees around the area or laid out in a large X on the ground.
  - Words can be stomped in snow and then lined with tree branches.
  - Rocks can be arranged to form SOS or HELP.
  - A smoke signal can be made by white or black smoke from a fire. Black smoke can be created by burning a chunk of tire, gasoline, or oil.
  - Dried wood creates white smoke.
  - The color of smoke desired depends on the environment.
  - Black smoke is preferred in contrast with snow.

- Oil and gasoline are more safely ignited when poured over a container full of dirt or sand.

HOT WEATHER/DESERT SURVIVAL

The body adapts to heat by increasing the blood volume, dilating skin blood vessels, and improving cardiac efficiency to carry more heat from the body core to the shell. The process of acclimatization takes about 10 days, during which the subject begins to perspire at a lower temperature, the volume of perspiration increases, and the perspiration contains fewer electrolytes (see Chapter 5). The following discussion emphasizes survival in a desert environment.

Practical Methods for Adjusting to Hot Weather

- Heat loss can be increased by exposing the maximum amount of skin to the circulating air. This should be done only when in the shade; when in the sun, skin should be completely protected by clothing.
- Wearing clothing when exposed to hot sun also reduces water loss by reducing sweating.
- Because heat loss and sweating may be impaired by sunscreens, a good compromise is to cover the face and hands with sunscreen and to wear a long-sleeved shirt and long trousers of tightly woven, loose-fitting, and light-colored (preferably white) cotton.
- Consider special clothing with an SPF of 30 or greater (e.g., Solumbra). T-shirts have an SPF of only 5 to 9.
- If desired, ventilation holes can be cut at the axillae and groin.
- Optimal hydration maintains blood volume and shell circulation and supports the sweating mechanism.
- Enough water must be carried or be available in the field. Water bottles may be wrapped with clothing to insulate them and be buried in the backpack.
- The layer principle of clothing is recommended in the desert, as well as in cold weather. Layers can be taken off during the heat of the day and added at night when the dry desert air cools rapidly.
- Because high winds and sandstorms occur frequently in desert areas, a wind-resistant parka and pants are desirable; because rains occasionally occur as well, the garments should also be water repellent.
- Because of its high thermal conductivity, poor insulating ability, and good wicking ability, cotton—which is avoided in cold weather—is a reasonable fabric for hot weather clothing.
- Clothing should be loose to promote air circulation.
- Before exposure to prolonged or strenuous hot weather exertion, individuals should allow time for acclimatization.
- A hat with a wide brim or a Foreign Legion-style cap with a neck protector and ventilation holes in the crown is recommended.
- A neck protector can be improvised from a large bandanna by placing it on the head with the point just above the forehead,

bringing the two tails around in front of the ears, tying them under the chin, and then replacing the hat.

- Be aware that gullies and other dry watercourses can be the sites of flash floods.
- A sun shelter can be made by suspending a tarp from brush or cacti or by laying the tarp on a framework of poles.
- Travelers who become stranded in a vehicle should lie under it, not in it.
- Because desert air is much cooler a foot above or a few inches below the ground surface, the desert traveler should lie on a platform or in a scooped-out depression rather than directly on the ground.
- Sturdy hiking or climbing boots should be worn to protect the feet, not only from the hot ground but also from sharp rocks, the spines of cacti, and snakes.
- Rest periods should be taken in the shade rather than in the direct sun.
- High-quality sunglasses should be used to protect the eyes; if necessary, sunglasses can be improvised from a piece of cardboard or wood with a narrow slit cut for each eye.
- Body heat production can be minimized by avoiding muscular exertion during periods of high heat and humidity. Persons should travel only early in the morning, late in the evening, or at night.

DESERT WATER PROCUREMENT

Table 59.1 shows the expected days of survival in the desert in relation to the amount of water available.

1. Waterholes and oases are rare in deserts. They occasionally may be located by watching the behavior of animals and birds, which travel toward water at dawn and dusk.
2. Animal trails tend to lead to water and may be joined by other trails and become wider as they approach it.
3. Birds may circle before landing at a waterhole, especially in the morning. A pool of water with no animal tracks or droppings may be poisonous.
4. Muddy and dirty water should be filtered through cloth, and all water should be treated chemically or by filtration or boiling before drinking (see Chapter 45).
5. Persons should not drink urine, or water from a vehicle radiator.
6. A device often mentioned for producing potable water is a solar still (Fig. 59.18). Be advised that water output may be negligible if vegetation is desiccated.
   a. The materials needed include a 1.8 × 1.8 m (6 × 6 ft) piece of sturdy, clear plastic sheeting (preferably reinforced with duct tape in the center), a shovel, a 1.8- to 2.4-m (6- to 8-ft) piece of surgical tubing, a 1-L (1-quart) plastic bowl, duct tape, and a knife.

Table 59.1 Expected Days of Survival at Various Environmental Temperatures and With Varying Amounts of Available Water						
	MAXIMUM DAILY TEMPERATURE IN SHADE (°F)	Available Water Per Person (U.S. Quarts)				
		0	1	2	4	10
No walking	120	2	2	2	2.5	3
	110	3	3	3.5	4	5
	100	5	5.5	6	7	9.5
	90	7	8	9	10.5	15
	80	9	10	11	13	19
	70	10	11	12	14	20.5
	60	10	11	12	14	21
	50	10	11	12	14.5	21
Walking at night and resting thereafter	120	1	2	2	2.5	3
	110	2	2	2.5	3	3.5
	100	3	3.5	3.5	4.5	5.5
	90	5	5.5	5.5	6.5	8
	80	7	7.5	8	9.5	11.5
	70	7.5	8	9	10.5	13.5
	60	8	8.5	9	11	14
	50	8	8.5	9	11	14

From Adolph EF et al.: *Physiology of man in the desert*, New York, 1947, Interscience.

b. A cone-shaped hole about 1.1 m (3.5 ft) in diameter and 45.2 to 50.8 cm (18 to 20 in) deep should be dug in a low area where water would stand the longest after rain.
c. With the surgical tubing taped securely to its bottom, the bowl is placed in the center of the hole.
d. The plastic sheet is positioned loosely on top of the hole and weighted with a fist-sized rock in the center so that it sags into a cone whose apex is just above the bowl.
e. Crushed desert vegetation, preferably barrel and saguaro cactus parts, is placed inside the hole to provide additional moisture.
f. Unknown or possibly poisonous plants are avoided.
g. Dirt and rocks are piled around the rim on top of the plastic sheet to seal the edges of the hole (see Fig. 59.18).

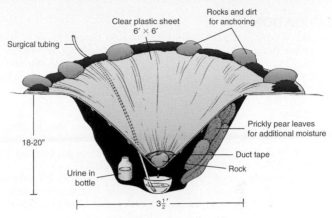

Surgical tubing

Clear plastic sheet 6′ × 6′

Rocks and dirt for anchoring

Prickly pear leaves for additional moisture

Duct tape

Rock

Urine in bottle

18-20"

$3\frac{1}{2}'$

FIGURE 59.18 Solar still.

h. Urine can be placed inside the hole in an open container.
i. Contaminated surface water can also be purified inside a solar still, but water from a vehicle radiator should not be used because the glycols will distill along with the water.
j. The still is not opened once it starts operating.
k. Optimally it will produce 0.5 to 1 L (1 pint to 1 quart) of water per 24 hours without added urine or vegetation and up to 3.8 L (4 quarts) with these present.
l. The surgical tubing is used to suck water from the bowl periodically as it collects.
7. If vegetation is plentiful, another type of solar still can be made from a large, clear plastic bag:
   a. On a slope, a hole several feet in diameter is dug with a crater-like rim surrounded by a moat that drains downhill into a small hole.
   b. The bag is centered on the large hole with its edges over the moat and its mouth downhill at the small hole.
   c. An upright stick is placed inside the bag in the middle and clean rocks along the crater rim inside the bag to keep the bag anchored and ballooned out.
   d. Duct tape reinforces the bag where the stick tents it. After the bag is filled with vegetation, its mouth is tied shut.
   e. The vegetation should not touch the sides of the bag or spill into the part of the bag that is over the moat.
   f. The warmth of the sun causes water to evaporate from the vegetation and condense on the inside of the bag, run down into the part of the bag that is over the moat, run downhill toward the mouth of the bag, and collect in the part of the bag's neck that is in the small hole.
   g. Survivors open the mouth of the bag and pour out the water as needed.

NAVIGATION

Anyone venturing into the wilderness should be proficient in basic navigation skills. It is outside the scope of this book to endeavor to teach map and compass or global positioning system (GPS) navigation. The following are a few simple suggestions on safety and what should be carried into the wilderness.

Compass

- Even if in a familiar area, backcountry travelers should always carry a compass, map, and altimeter.
- The best type of compass for the layperson is an orienteering compass that adjusts for magnetic declination.
- It is important to note that not all compasses work all over the world. Many compasses purchased in the northern hemisphere will not work south of the equator. A compass that works any place in the world is called a "global compass."
- The compass is always followed even if at odds with "gut feelings" about direction.
- Some navigation experts recommend carrying two compasses. The second compass can be part of a GPS unit, a watch, or another regular compass. That way, if there is concern about a compass not working, it can be checked against the other compass.

Topographic Maps

- Topographic maps in a 1:24,000 to 1:50,000 scale are the best maps to use for land navigation.
- The 1:24,000 scale provides more terrain detail than a 1:50,000 scale.
- Topographic maps are available at most outdoor stores in both the 7.5- and 15-minute series.

Global Positioning System

- GPS units are small electronic devices that can mark a traveler's position by receiving signals from satellites.
- Although very useful and a worthy adjunct to navigation, it is important to note that they should never be relied on as the only source for navigation.
- Drawbacks include the fact that they are battery dependent, they require at least three satellites to mark a position, and the satellite system is provided by the US government.
- The government is at liberty to "take away" access to GPS information at any time and without warning.
- GPS also requires some prior practice to accurately translate output into a position on a map.
- The backcountry traveler should be expert with map and compass and not rely solely on a GPS unit for navigation safety.

WEATHER

- Blue sky, a few cirrus or cumulus clouds, cold temperatures, low to medium winds, and a steady or dropping altimeter are predictors of good weather.
- A lowering cloud pattern (cirrus followed by cirrostratus, altostratus, and nimbostratus), rising temperatures, wind freshening and shifting to blow from the southeast or south, and an altimeter rise of 152.4 to 243.8 m (500 to 800 ft) indicate a possibly severe winter storm.
- Building cumulus congestus clouds changing to cumulonimbus clouds indicate probable thunderstorms and possible hail. A thunderstorm is often immediately preceded by a rush of cold air (gust front).
- Signs that a severe winter storm is abating include clouds thinning, cloud bases rising, temperature falling, altimeter dropping (i.e., pressure rising), and winds shifting to originate from the north or northwest.

GENERAL ASPECTS OF SURVIVAL
Injured Team Member

- A person with a minor injury or illness should be encouraged to self-evacuate, accompanied by at least one healthy party member.
- When a person with a severe injury or illness needs to be evacuated, the party must decide whether to use the resources at hand or to send for help.
- The decision will depend on the weather, party size, training, available equipment, distance, type of terrain involved, type of injury or illness, patient's condition, and availability of local search and rescue groups, helicopters, and other assistance.
- Unless the weather is excellent, the party strong and well equipped, the route short and easy, and the patient comfortable and stable, the best course of action generally is to make a comfortable camp and send the strongest party members for help.
- A written note should include each patient's name, gender, age, type of injury or illness, current condition, and emergency care; the party's resources and location (preferably map coordinates); and names, addresses, and telephone numbers of relatives.
- The patient who must be left alone should have an adequate supply of food, fuel, and water.

As soon as you realize that you are lost, do the following:

1. Stop, sit down in a sheltered place, calmly go over the situation, and make an inventory of your survival equipment and other resources.
2. If it is cold or becoming dark, start a fire and eat if you have food.

3. Take out your map or draw a sketch of your route and location based on natural features.
4. Unless you know your location and can reach safety before dark, prepare a camp and wait until morning.
5. Do not allow yourself to be influenced by a desire to keep others from worrying or the need to be at work or keep an appointment.
6. Your life is more important than anyone else's peace of mind.
7. If you are alone and unquestionably lost, and especially if injured, you must decide whether to wait for rescue or attempt to walk out under your own power.
8. Almost always, it is better to use the time to prepare a snug shelter and conserve strength if rescue is possible.
9. If you decide to leave, mark the site with a cairn or bright-colored material, such as surveyor's tape; leave a note at the site with information about your condition, equipment, and direction of travel; and then mark your trail.
10. These actions will aid rescuers and enable you to return to the site if necessary. Travel should never be attempted in severe weather, desert daytime heat, or deep snow without snowshoes or skis.
11. If no chance of rescue exists, prepare as best as possible, wait for good weather, and then travel in the most logical direction.

SIGNALING

- Besides radios, cell phones, and other electronic equipment, signaling devices are either auditory or visual.
- Three of anything is a universal distress signal: three whistle blasts, three shots, three fires, or three columns of smoke.
- The most effective auditory device is a whistle. Blowing a whistle is less tiring than shouting, and the distinctive sound carries farther than a human voice.
- A very effective visual ground-to-air signal device is a glass signal mirror, which can be seen up to 16.1 km (10 miles) away, but requires sunlight.
- Smoke is easily seen by day, and a fire or flashlight is visible at night. On a cloudy day, black smoke is more visible than white; the reverse is true on a sunny day.
- Black smoke can be produced by burning parts of a vehicle, such as rubber or oil and white smoke, by adding green leaves or a small amount of water to the fire (see Airplane, earlier).
- Ground signals (e.g., SOS, HELP) should be as large as possible—at least 0.9 m (3 ft) wide and 5.5 m (18 ft) long—and should contain straight lines and square corners, which are not found in nature.
- They can be tramped out in dirt or on grass or can be made from brush or logs. In snow, the depressions can be filled with vegetation to increase contrast.

- Many pilots do not know the traditional 18 international ground-to-air emergency signals, so remember the following two:
  - (X) I require medical assistance
  - (↑) Am proceeding in this direction
- When using cell phones, radios, and other electronic devices, persons should move out of valleys and gullies to higher elevations if possible.
- Operational pay phones in campgrounds closed for the season or other facilities can be used to call for help.
- Most will allow 9-1-1 or another emergency number to be dialed without payment, but carrying the right change and memorizing your telephone credit card number are recommended.

Practice Before You Really Need To Use Them.

TERMINOLOGY

The most practical way to select a knot is to first evaluate what role that knot is expected to perform. The following knots are addressed based on function:

- Stopper knot—a knot tied at the end of a rope to keep something from slipping off the rope (e.g., figure 8 knot)
- End-of-line knot—a knot used to form a loop or other construction in the end of a rope to anchor, tie in, or attach the rope to something (e.g., double-bowline knot)
- Midline knot—a knot used to form a loop in the middle of the rope for clipping into, grasping, or bypassing a piece of damaged rope (e.g., butterfly knot)
- Knots to join two ropes—a knot used to connect two ropes of equal or unequal diameter (e.g., double fisherman's bend)
- Safety knot—a final knot tied into the tail of the rope after the original knot is tied to keep the original knot from deforming or unraveling (e.g., barrel knot)
- Hitch—a knot that is tied around something, which conforms to the shape of the object around which it is tied and that does not keep its shape when the object around which it is tied is removed (e.g., Prusik hitch)
- Tied loop—a knot that forms a fixed eye or loop in the end of a rope (e.g., bowline knot)

ANATOMY OF A KNOT

- The working end of the rope is the section used to tie or rig the knot.
- The standing part of the rope is the section not actively used to form the knot or rigging.
- The running end of the rope is the free end.
- A line is a rope in use.
- A bight of rope is formed when the rope takes a U-turn on itself so that the running end and standing end run parallel to each other. The U portion, where the rope bends, is referred to as the *bight.*
- A loop of rope is made by crossing a portion of the standing end over or under the running end. Note that a loop, unlike a bight, closes. Many knots that form a loop from a bight in the standing part of the rope are named *something on a bight*, such as *figure 8 on a bight.*

- The tail of a rope is the (usually) short, unused length of rope that is left over once the knot is tied.
  Examples of knots are presented in Figs. 60.1 to 60.24.

Stopper Knots (Figs. 60.1 and 60.2)

A stopper knot is typically tied into the end of a rope to prevent the rope from exiting the system (e.g., tying a stopper on the end of a rappel line to prevent the rappeller from rappelling off the end).

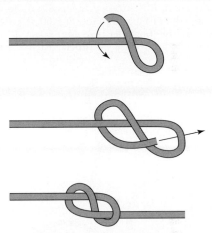

FIGURE 60.1   Figure 8 stopper knot.

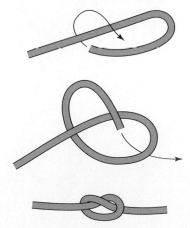

FIGURE 60.2   Overhand stopper knot.

End-of-Line Knots (Figs. 60.3 to 60.6)

These knots form a loop or bight in the end of the rope. The bight can then be used to attach the rope to something (e.g., an anchor).

The **double bowline** (see Fig. 60.4) is preferred for rescue over the less secure single bowline (see Fig. 60.3)

A figure 8 on a bight (see Fig. 60.5) creates a preformed loop, so it will function only if you can clip into the loop (e.g., with a carabiner).

The **figure 8 on a bight** is probably the single knot every potential rescue worker should know. Climbers and rescue personnel across the world use it. It is strong and easy to undo when loaded. It can be tied directly into a bight (see Fig. 60.5), or it may be tied as a retrace (or follow-through) (see Fig. 60.6). It is easy to tell when it has been tied correctly by quick visual inspection.

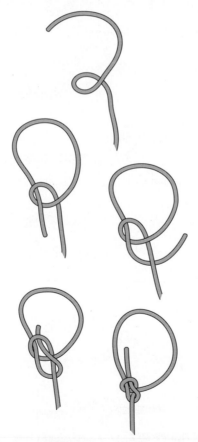

FIGURE 60.3   Bowline.

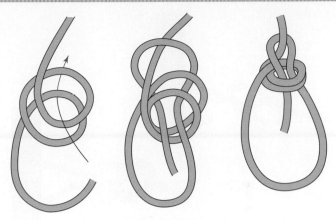

FIGURE 60.4   Double-Bowline.

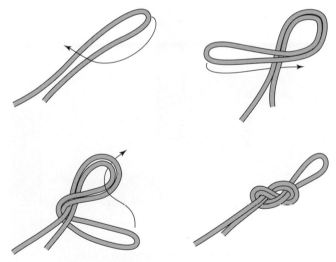

FIGURE 60.5   Figure 8 on a bight.

Midline Knots

These knots are used to form loops in the middle of a rope. They are used for clipping into, grasping, or bypassing a piece of damaged rope. A **figure 8 on a bight** may be used (see Fig. 60.5). In addition, the following knots can be used:

Butterfly knot (Fig. 60.7)
Overhand on a bight (Fig. 60.8)
Bowline on a bight (Fig. 60.9)

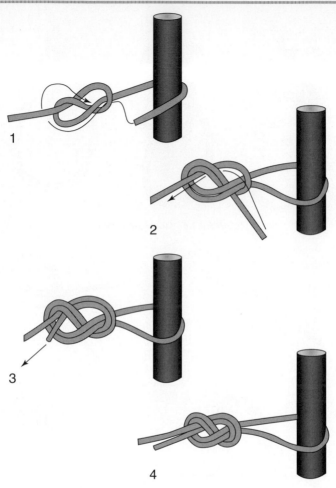

FIGURE 60.6 Retrace figure 8 on a bight.

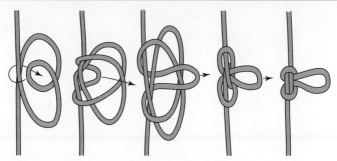

FIGURE 60.7   Butterfly knot.

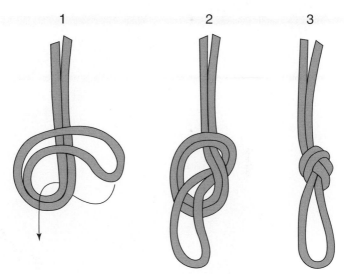

FIGURE 60.8   Overhand on a bight.

Knots to Join Two Ropes

The overhand bend (Fig. 60.10) is functional, simple, and easy to tie but not secure enough for rescue.

The **double fisherman's bend** (Fig. 60.11) is an excellent knot for joining ropes of equal diameter.

The **double-sheet bend** (Fig. 60.12) is an excellent knot for joining ropes of unequal diameter.

The **single-sheet bend** (Fig. 60.13) is less secure than the double-sheet bend.

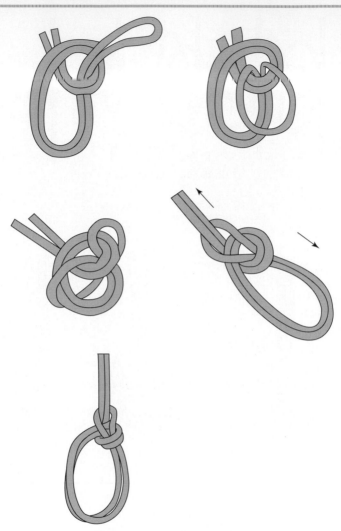

FIGURE 60.9   Bowline on a Bight.

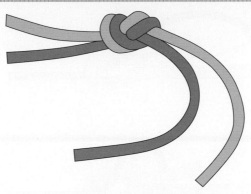

FIGURE 60.10 Overhand bend.

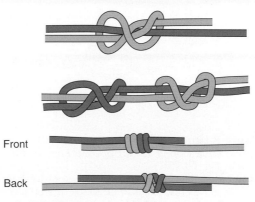

Front

Back

FIGURE 60.11 Double fisherman's bend.

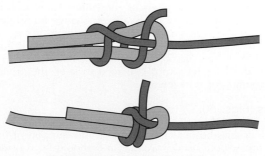

FIGURE 60.12 Double-sheet bend.

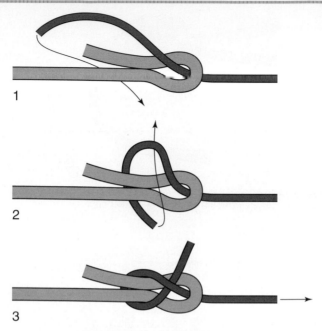

FIGURE 60.13 Single-sheet bend.

The **figure 8 bend** (Fig. 60.14) is a reasonable choice if tied with the rope ends exiting from opposite ends of the bend. Do not tie it as in Fig. 60.15.

The **ring bend** (Fig. 60.16) is the ideal knot for joining flat or tubular webbing. It is also used to tie loops of webbing (runners).

Knot Safety

Every knot should be checked (preferably by someone other than the person who tied it) to ensure that it is tied properly, and it should be monitored at intervals thereafter. Many knots have a tendency to loosen, and some can even change form (e.g., into a slipknot).

A safety knot can help prevent mishaps. A safety knot is an overhand knot (see Fig. 60.2) tied into the tail of the rope after a knot is tied. The safety knot is placed to keep the original knot from deforming or unraveling.

Hitches (Figs. 60.17 to 60.20)

Hitching is a method of tying a rope around itself or an object in such a way that the object is integral to the support of the hitch. Hitches are seldom used in rescue and should be considered for use only by a skilled technician, because there may be severe

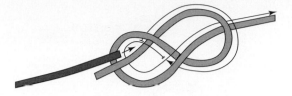

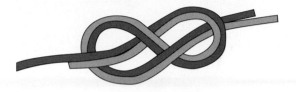

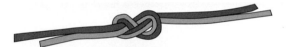

FIGURE 60.14   Figure 8 bend.

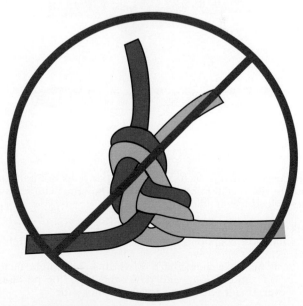

FIGURE 60.15   Incorrectly tied figure 8 bend.

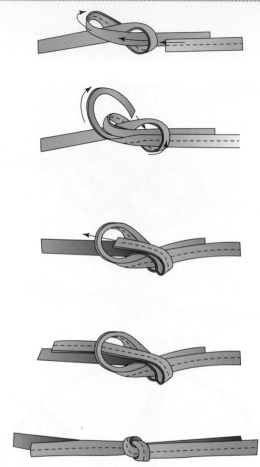

FIGURE 60.16   Ring bend (tape knot, web knot, water knot).

consequences when a hitch comes untied or does not perform as intended. Disintegration of a hitch results in immediate release of whatever load it is holding.

Prusik Hitch

One of the most commonly used hitches is the **Prusik hitch** (see Fig. 60.17).

- A Prusik hitch is a sliding hitch by which a cord can be attached to a rope and slid up and down the rope for positioning. However, under tension, the hitch will not slide.

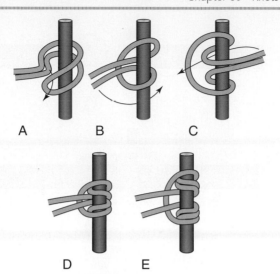

A   B   C

D   E

FIGURE 60.17   Prusik hitch. **A** to **C,** Tying sequence for the Prusik knot. **D,** Two-wrap Prusik knot. **E,** Three-wrap Prusik knot.

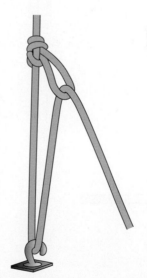

FIGURE 60.18   Trucker's hitch.

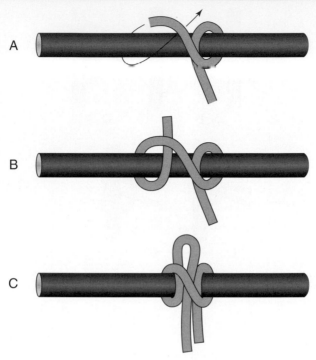

FIGURE 60.19 A and **B,** Clove hitch. **C,** Clove hitch with draw loop for temporary attachment.

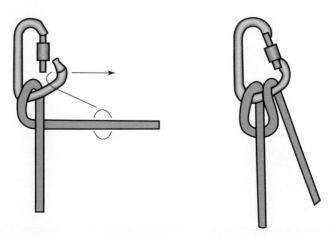

FIGURE 60.20   Munter hitch.

- A Prusik hitch is created by tying a length of cordage into a loop by means of a double fisherman's bend.
- Wrapping the loop around the main rope and through its own loop two or three times and then pulling it tight forms the hitch.

Trucker's Hitch
A handy hitch, known as a **trucker's hitch,** is useful for pulling cord or webbing tight across something (e.g., a load in the bed of a pickup truck, hence the name) or securing a patient snugly into a litter (see Fig. 60.18).

Clove Hitch
Another common hitch used in climbing and rescue applications is the **clove hitch** (see Fig. 60.19).
- This hitch can be useful when trying to shorten the distance between two objects, such as the climber's belay and the climber or the litter rail and the rescuer.
- It is also useful in some lashing techniques but can tend to roll loose.

Munter Hitch
Another type of hitch, called the **Munter hitch** or Italian hitch (see Fig. 60.20), can be used around a carabiner or pole to add friction to a system, as in a belay. This hitch is particularly useful because it effectively adds friction regardless of the direction in which the rope is moving.

Care should be taken when using the hitch around a carabiner because there can be a tendency for the moving rope to slip through the gate of the carabiner, rendering the hitch useless.

Additional Knots and Hitches
See Figs. 60.21 to 60.24.

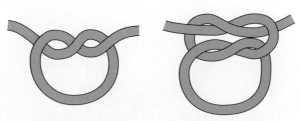

FIGURE 60.21   Reef Knot, or Square Knot.

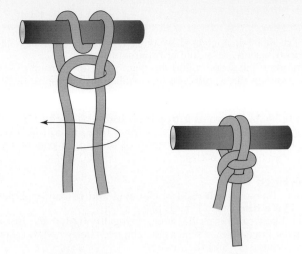

FIGURE 60.22 Round turn and two half-hitches.

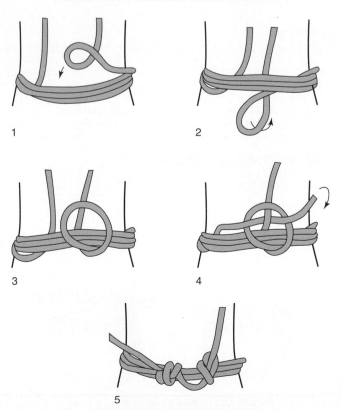

1

2

3

4

5

FIGURE 60.23 Bowline on a Coil.

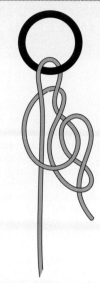

FIGURE 60.24 Halter hitch.

61 Wilderness Medical Kits

Organizing the medical equipment for an expedition requires an enormous amount of planning and forethought. No matter how much equipment is hauled in, one cannot possibly prepare for every conceivable illness or accident. The variables on any expedition or wilderness excursion are complex, making generic advice on "what to take" difficult without an operational context. Major considerations should include the following:

- Environmental extremes of the trip (e.g., arctic, high altitude, tropical, desert)
- Time of year (e.g., climatic conditions) and disease conditions
- Specific endemic diseases
- Medical expertise of the intended user
- Medical expertise of other trip members
- Total number of expedition members, including ancillary staff (e.g., porters, local guides, expedition staff)
- Duration of trip
- Age and sex of participants
- Known preexisting medical problems of the group
- Distance from definitive medical care
- Availability of communications (e.g., cell phones, radios, satellite phones, telemedicine capability)
- Availability and time frame of rescue
- Medical kit weight and volume limitations
- Responsibility for local health care

MEDICAL KITS
Design
- The wilderness medical kit should be well organized in a protective and convenient carrying case or pouch. For backpacking, trekking, or hiking, a nylon or Cordura organizer bag is optimal.
- Clear vinyl compartments protect components from dirt, moisture, and insects and keep items from falling out when the kit is turned on its side or upside down.
- In aquatic environments, store the kit in a waterproof dry bag or watertight container, such as a Pelican or OtterBox case. Inside, seal items in resealable plastic bags with "zippers" (e.g., Ziploc) because moisture will invariably make its way into any container.
- Some medicines may need to be stored outside of the main kit to ensure protection from extreme temperatures. Capsules and suppositories melt when exposed to temperatures above 37°C

(98.6°F), and many liquid medicines (e.g., insulin) become useless after freezing.
* Commercially produced kits are available, either prestocked or unfilled.
* Fragile items and injectable medications can be carried in small, portable plastic containers (e.g., Tupperware).

Organization
Medical supplies can be divided into four categories: personal kits, group kit, medical devices and medications, and specialized equipment for environmental and recreational hazards. The size and complexity of the medical kit depend on the amount of equipment required, duration of trip, and number of team members. For smaller trips, a single person can carry a moderately sized comprehensive medical kit for the group. For longer expeditions, or expeditions with many participants, larger kits may be divided into several smaller kits for individual members to carry.

Personal Kit
Each trip member should be responsible for and carry a personal kit. This avoids constant disruption of the group kit. Personal kits are variable but should include commonly used items. A personal kit might contain the following:
* Nonnarcotic analgesics and/or nonsteroidal anti-inflammatory drugs
* Throat lozenges or hard candy
* Sunscreen and lip protection
* Water disinfection equipment or chemicals
* Blister care
* Duct tape
* Minor wound care (e.g., bandages [Band-Aids])
* Insect repellent
* Malaria prophylaxis (if risk exists)
* Vitamins
* Personal medications (for preexisting problems)
* Copy of identification
* Personal hygiene materials
* Ear plugs (sleep hygiene)

Comprehensive Group Medical Kit
The group medical kit should be carefully constructed to meet the likely needs of the entire group. The contents of the group medical kit will vary greatly depending on the environment, risks and hazards, and skill level of the medical provider. In general the group kit should contain the following:
* Medical guidebooks (electronic or print) and Internet sources if available
* Comprehensive first-aid kit (Box 61.1)

BOX 61.1   Contents of a Comprehensive Community Medical Kit*

Wound and Trauma Management
Liquid soap
Alcohol based gel (e.g., Purell) for hands
Sterile nitrile gloves
Nonsterile gloves
Splash shield and face protection
Syringes (2, 5, 10, 20, or 30, and 60 cc [mL])
Large- and small-gauge hypodermic needles (e.g., 18 and 25
    gauge)
Sterile irrigation saline
Morgan eye lenses
Alcohol pads
Antiseptic towelettes
Povidone-iodine 10% solution (Betadine) or chlorhexidine
    (Hibiclens)
Wound closure strips (Steri-Strips)
Tincture of benzoin (or Mastisol)
Tissue glue for wound closure (2-octyl cyanoacrylate [Dermabond])
Suture materials (2-0, 4-0 nylon or silk with cutting needle; 3-0
    Vicryl with tapered needle)
Disposable skin stapler and remover
Silver nitrate sticks
Esmarch bandage, 3 × 36 in
Disposable scalpels with No. 11 or 15 blade
Hot and cold packs
Tactical tourniquet
10 × 10 cm (4 × 4 in) sterile dressing pads
15 × 27 cm (5 × 9 in) sterile dressing pads
9-cm (3-in) sterile gauze bandage
Cotton-tipped applicators
Nonadherent sterile dressing
Xeroform and petroleum jelly (Vaseline) gauze burn dressings
Elastic bandage wraps with Velcro closures
Adhesive cloth tape
Adhesive porous paper tape (1.3 cm [0.5 in])
Gauze roll (11.4 cm × 3.7 m [4.5 in × 4 yd])
Adhesive bandages (Band-Aids)
Tegaderm
Eye pad and eye shield
Moleskin, Blist-O-Ban, and silver duct tape
SAM Splints (15 × 110 cm [4.4 × 36 in])
Aluminum finger splints
Kendrick (or improvised) femoral traction device
Traction splint (e.g., Kendrick, Slishman)
Rescue harness
Triangular (cravat) bandage and safety pins
Head lamp
Hemostats and or needle drivers (Spencer Wells)
Trauma shears
Surgical scissors

BOX 61.1   Contents of a Comprehensive Community Medical Kit*—cont'd

Toothed and nontoothed forceps
Chlorhexidine surgical scrub brushes
Surgicel Nu-Knit, QuickClot
Plastic finger
Cotton pledgets
Nasal balloon device
Absorbable nasal packing
Urinary catheter, 14 Fr (catheter bag and tubing)
Absorbable nasal packing

Medications
Select medication listed in Table 61.1 (tailored to anticipated conditions and trip duration, party size, and available space)

Miscellaneous Items
Waterproof flashlight and matches
Signal mirror/dental mirror and whistle
Plastic resealable bags (e.g., whirlpacks)
Permanent markers (e.g., Sharpie)
Notebook and record-keeping supplies (waterproof, depending on environment)
Adhesive labels
Pill bottles and cotton balls
Nail clippers
Steel sewing needles, paper clips, and safety pins
Forceps for removal of splinters and ticks
Pocket knife or multitool knife
Trauma shears
Eyelet scissors
Silver duct tape
Tongue depressors
Chemical ice packs and heating packs
Sun hats and high-SPF sunscreen and lip balm
Emergency blanket (e.g., Space blanket, Pro Tech)
N,N-diethyl-*m*-toluamide–containing insect repellent (e.g., REI Jungle Juice 100)
Contact lens solution and case
Digital thermometers
Commercially made oral rehydration powder packs[†]

Equipment
Diagnostic instruments: see Table 61.3
Specialized equipment: see Box 61.3

Dental and Ear-Nose-Throat Supplies
Oil of cloves (eugenol), 3.5 mL; combine with calcium hydroxide powder to make temporary fillings
Calcium hydroxide powder or putty
Cavit (7 g)

Continued

BOX 61.1   Contents of a Comprehensive Community Medical
Kit*—cont'd

Intermediate restorative material
Express Putty
Wooden spatulas for mixing and applying
Paraffin (dental wax) stick
Dental floss
Dental mirror
Cotton rolls and pellets
Ear curettes (consider for trips with aquatic activity)
Ear wicks (consider for trips with aquatic activity)

*This is intended to serve as a list of potential equipment that ultimately must be tailored to the specific details of the proposed trip itinerary.
†Recommend purchase of commercially made oral rehydration salts (ORS) in line with current World Health Organization guidelines (equimolar glucose:sodium and 200–310 mOsm/L). *Oral Rehydration Salts: Production of the new ORS*, Geneva, 2006, WHO Press. http://apps.who.int/iris/bitstream/10665/69227/1/WHO_FCH_CAH_06.1.pdf?ua=1&ua=1.

- Priority first aid equipment, supplies, and medications (see Appendix G)
- Appropriate prescription medications for general illness (Tables 61.1 and 61.2)
- Antimicrobial considerations (see Appendix H)
- Advanced devices for the medically trained (Box 61.2), including portable diagnostic instruments for wilderness travel (Table 61.3)
- Indicated equipment based on recreational and environmental hazards (Box 61.3)
- Wilderness pediatric medical kit considerations (see Appendix Q)
- Wilderness ophthalmology medical kit considerations (Appendix I)
- Wilderness gynecology medical kit considerations (see Table 31.1)

GENERAL GUIDELINES FOR EXPEDITION DRUGS
- When possible, choose medications with low side-effect profiles.
- Choose medications with few contraindications (e.g., amoxicillin/clavulanate is contraindicated in penicillin-allergic patients).
- When possible, choose medications that have multiple indications (e.g., drugs like diphenhydramine and prednisone have many uses).
- Choose medications that have favorable dosing schedules (e.g., once a day). Compliance will markedly improve, and the weight and volume of the medical kit will be greatly reduced.

Text continued on p. 849

Table 61.1 Select Medications for Wilderness Travel*

DRUG	FORMULATION	SELECT INDICATIONS	COMMENTS
Analgesics**			
Acetaminophen (Tylenol, paracetamol, APAP [acetyl-para-aminophenol])	500-1000 mg PO tabs	Analgesia, fever reduction	Although OTC, this drug can have significant analgesic effects, especially when used in combination with NSAIDs, or with opiates for moderate to severe pain. Caution in patients with history of liver disease or alcoholism. Overdose can be life threatening. Many flu remedies contain acetaminophen and should be accounted for in total daily dose calculations. Paracetamol is metabolized to acetaminophen.
Ibuprofen† (Advil, Motrin)	200 mg PO tabs	Analgesia, antiinflammatory	When no contraindications, NSAIDS should be considered in combination with acetaminophen for mild to moderate pain and with opiates if necessary for moderate to severe pain. This is not to be used if GI bleeding, pregnancy, chronic kidney disease, or severe dehydration is present. NSAIDs may help prevent acute mountain sickness. Caution with total daily dose and prolonged use.

Continued

Table 61.1   Select Medications for Wilderness Travel*—cont'd

DRUG	FORMULATION	SELECT INDICATIONS	COMMENTS
Acetylsalicylic acid† (Aspirin, Bayer, Ecotrin)	325-500 mg PO tabs	Analgesia	This is not to be used if significant bleeding is present. Can be used for antiplatelet effect in suspected ACS (preferably chewed, non-enteric coated tabs). May be administered PR.
Hydrocodone and acetaminophen** (Vicodin, Lortab, Norco)	5 to 10 mg/325 mg PO tabs, dose limited by total daily acetaminophen dose	Analgesia	As with all opiates, may cause severe constipation. Given concern for inadvertent acetaminophen toxicity, would recommend hydrocodone or oxycodone preparations without acetaminophen. Given hydrocodone's reclassification as Schedule 1 and variable metabolism, oxycodone may be considered as a more reliable analgesic.
Oxycodone**	5 mg PO tabs	Analgesia	As with many opioids, significant nausea, especially when taken without food. Monitor for constipation. May cause impaired reaction time, balance, and wakefulness.
Tramadol** (Ultram)	50 mg PO tabs	Analgesia	Use caution, because may cause CNS depression and impair reaction time, balance, and wakefulness. May increase risk of seizures, especially in patients taking several drugs, including SSRIs, TCAs, and MAOIs. Multiple interactions.

| Bupivacaine (Marcaine, Sensorcaine) | 0.25% solution, maximum SC dose of 2.5 mg/kg | Advanced-tier local or regional anesthesia | Use with caution on the feet, because such use may allow further skin damage to go unnoticed. Hypotension and dysrhythmias can occur at toxic doses. IV injection can be fatal. Perineural injections may be effective for tooth pain and extremity fractures, and effects may last up to 10 hours. Soak gauze with this drug for topical and dental applications. |
| Lidocaine (Xylocaine) | 1%-2% solution for injection with or without epinephrine; maximum SC dose of 4.5 mg/kg without epinephrine, up to 7 mg/kg with epinephrine | Local anesthesia | Conventional teaching is that lidocaine with epinephrine should not be used when injecting distal extremities (i.e., fingers, nose, penis, toes, ears) because of potential for vascular compromise. Consider bringing multiple small vials; repeat use of single vials is not recommended. Local anesthetic of choice for minor procedures because of fast onset and relatively wide therapeutic window. This short-acting agent (relative to bupivacaine) may be used as an antiarrhythmic in ACLS. Toxic doses may result in seizure or cardiac arrest. |

Continued

Table 61.1	Select Medications for Wilderness Travel*—cont'd		
DRUG	**FORMULATION**	**SELECT INDICATIONS**	**COMMENTS**
Lidocaine jelly 2%	Apply to skin as needed or 30 min before procedure; 5 mL packages	Analgesia, prophylaxis for catheter insertion	Use with caution; it may allow further skin damage to go unnoticed.
Tetracaine	0.5% solution for eye drops	Analgesia for procedures	Should not be used if etiology of injury and expert consultation unavailable, because it can worsen injury.
Morphine sulfate**	20 mg IV/IM vial	Advanced-tier analgesia	Morphine may cause nausea, vomiting, rash (histamine release), hypotension, sedation, and apnea. Administer it with an antiemetic as a precaution.
Ketamine**	50 mg/mL, 5-10 mL vial IV (alternate dosing for IM and PO available)	Advanced-tier analgesia	Anticipate increased oral secretions and potential for hallucinations. May consider premedication with antisialagogue (glycopyrrolate, scopolamine) and sedative (midazolam). Can be used only by qualified and experienced providers to achieve sedation for surgical procedures or control of severe pain with relatively less respiratory depression than opiates.
Naloxone (Narcan)	0.4-2 mg SC, IM, IV, or by endotracheal tube	Opioid overdose	Naloxone may precipitate opioid withdrawal among chronic opioid users. Rare adverse effects include pulmonary edema and seizure.

Pentazocine** (Talwin)	50 mg PO tabs	Opioid agonist-antagonist	Pentazocine still has abuse potential. IV/IM formulations also available.
Capsaicin ointment†	2 g tube	Topical analgesic for osteoarthritis	Prolonged use may result in burns. Adjunct or alternative when NSAIDs or PO medications contraindicated.
Antimicrobials			
Albendazole (Albenza)	200 mg PO tabs	Anthelmintic with broad range of activity against neurocysticercosis, echinococcosis, ascariasis, hookworm, and trichuriasis	Not to be used by pregnant patients or by children <2 years old. Consider expert consultation before administration because significant contraindications exist.
Amoxicillin/clavulanic acid (Augmentin)	875 mg/125 mg PO tabs	Animal bites, oral infections, skin and soft tissue infections, severe acute otitis media, and tonsillopharyngitis	Contraindicated in patients with penicillin allergy. Can be used in conjunction with clindamycin for suspected polymicrobial anaerobic pulmonary infections (aspiration pneumonia).
Artemether/lumefantrine (Coartem, Riamet)	20 mg artemether, 120 mg lumefantrine PO tabs	Malaria (Plasmodium falciparum) treatment in chloroquine-resistant areas (check CDC.gov for guidelines)	Can be used for malaria treatment, although significant side effects and contraindications exist. Use caution when purchasing in certain regions because significant quality differences may exist between manufacturers.

Continued

Table 61.1   Select Medications for Wilderness Travel*—cont'd

DRUG	FORMULATION	SELECT INDICATIONS	COMMENTS
Artesunate	60 mg ampule for IV or IM	Severe malaria (*P. falciparum*) treatment in chloroquine-resistant areas (check CDC. gov for guidelines)	Can be used for malaria treatment, although significant side effects and contraindications exist. May not be able to purchase in certain regions.
Atovaquone/proguanil (Malarone)	250 mg/100 mg PO tabs	Severe malaria prophylaxis and treatment in chloroquine-resistant areas (check CDC. gov for guidelines)	Use with caution in a patient with severe GI upset. This is not to be used for complicated or cerebral malaria.
Azithromycin (Zithromax)	250 mg PO tabs	Pneumonia, otitis media, tonsillopharyngitis, gonococcal infection, bacterial sinusitis, traveler's diarrhea	May cause nausea, vomiting, and QT prolongation. Single 1000 mg dose may be more effective for traveler's diarrhea than divided dosing.
Bacitracin† (ointment)	28 g, 120 g, or 454 g tube	Topical infection prevention	Can cause allergic reactions. Clear affected area before application. Many potential alternatives.
Cefazolin (Ancef, Kefzol)	1 g vials IM/IV‡	Soft tissue infection, uncomplicated cystitis, crush injuries, open fractures	Penicillin allergy is a risk factor for cephalosporin allergy.
Ceftriaxone (Rocephin)	1 g vials, powder for reconstitution IM/IV‡	Pneumonia, meningitis, gonorrhea, intraabdominal infection, pyelonephritis, sepsis	Third-generation cephalosporin. Penicillin allergy is a risk factor for cephalosporin allergy.

Cephalexin (Keflex)	500 mg PO tabs	Superficial, soft tissue infection, streptococcal pharyngitis, uncomplicated cystitis	First-generation cephalosporin. Penicillin allergy is a risk factor for cephalosporin allergy.
Chloroquine (Aralen)	500 mg PO tabs	For severe malaria prophylaxis or treatment in chloroquine-sensitive areas (check CDC. gov for guidelines)	May cause nausea and diarrhea. Significant contraindications, including caution in patients with preexisting auditory problems, G6PD deficiency, psoriasis, or seizure disorder.
Ciprofloxacin (Cipro)	250-750 mg PO tabs	Traveler's diarrhea, cystitis, pneumonia, intraabdominal infection, prostatitis, sinusitis, typhoid fever, meningitis prophylaxis (off-label use)	Fluoroquinolones are not recommended for patients <16 years old because of the risk for cartilage injury and tendinopathies. Do not give with calcium containing foods or antacids (chelates quinolones). Avoid in patients receiving concurrent corticosteroids.
Ciprofloxacin otic solution (Cetraxal)	0.2% solution, formulations with dexamethasone available	Acute otitis externa; formulation for ophthalmic applications is 0.3%	May need ear wick for administration. Warm bottle in hand before administration to avoid adverse response. Pseudomonal resistance can occur.
Clindamycin (Cleocin)	150-450 mg PO tabs	Anaerobic infections; severe soft tissue infection (off-label use), toxic shock syndrome, pelvic inflammatory disease	May be useful for suspected MRSA soft tissue infections.

Continued

Table 61.1 Select Medications for Wilderness Travel*—cont'd

DRUG	FORMULATION	SELECT INDICATIONS	COMMENTS
Doxycycline (Vibramycin)	100 mg PO tabs	Severe malaria prophylaxis, Lyme disease, Vibrio cholerae, Chlamydia, pneumonia, bronchitis, tick-borne rickettsial disease; may be useful for unidentified infections from marine environment	Not recommended for patients <8 years old because of teeth staining. Inactivated by calcium-containing products (food and antacids). Causes significant photosensitivity and pill esophagitis (remain upright at least 30 min after ingesting with full glass of water). Expired doxycycline is considered dangerously nephrotoxic.
Erythromycin	3.5 g tube, 0.5% ointment	Bacterial conjunctivitis, uncomplicated corneal abrasion	Consider antipseudomonal coverage (quinolone drops) if contact lens wearer.
Fluconazole (Diflucan)	150 mg PO tabs	Vaginal and oropharyngeal candidiasis; coccidioidomycosis, dermatophyte (tinea) infections	Liver toxicity may occur. May be required for female patients taking concurrent antibiotics. Topical antifungals may be sufficient for tinea infections when available.
Ivermectin (Stromectol)	3 mg tabs PO (dosing in mcg/kg, usual dose 150-200 mcg/kg)	Scabies and lice (off-label use); onchocerciasis and strongyloidiasis; cutaneous larval migrans (Ancylostoma braziliense or Ancylostoma caninum); activity against Wuchereria bancrofti, Brugia malayi, Mansonella ozzardi, and Loa loa, although not first-line therapy.	Multiple doses are not well evaluated in patients with severe liver disease. Ivermectin is often more practical and effective than topical treatment for scabies (95% effective if given in two doses).[49] May not be necessary to bring, depending on travel conditions and geography.

Drug	Form	Indications	Comments
Levofloxacin (Levaquin)	500 mg or 750 mg PO tabs	Intraabdominal infections, pneumonia, cystitis, traveler's diarrhea (off-label use)	In the absence of ileus, same bioavailability when given PO as IV. Tendon inflammation and rupture (e.g., Achilles tendon, rotator cuff, biceps) are significant concerns. Avoid concurrent calcium-containing foods and medications. Ciprofloxacin can often be considered an alternative. Avoid in patients taking corticosteroids.
Mefloquine (Lariam)	250 mg PO tabs	Chloroquine-resistant malaria prophylaxis and treatment (check CDC.gov for guidelines)	Dosed weekly for prophylaxis. Do not prescribe to patients with prior adverse reactions to mefloquine, which may include hallucinations and night terrors. Caution in patients with significant psychiatric history.
Metronidazole (Flagyl)	500 mg PO tabs	Suspected giardiasis; severe diarrhea or diarrhea with fever, blood, or leukocytes	Alcohol consumption may cause a disulfiram-like reaction. The use of metronidazole may increase the toxicity of lithium, phenytoin, and anticoagulants.
Moxifloxacin (Moxeza)	0.5% optic solution, 3 mL bottle	Bacterial conjunctivitis, corneal ulceration	Not first-line therapy for bacterial conjunctivitis (due to emerging resistance) unless contact lens wearer, because of high incidence of Pseudomonas infection

Continued

Table 61.1 Select Medications for Wilderness Travel*—cont'd

DRUG	FORMULATION	SELECT INDICATIONS	COMMENTS
Penicillin V (Pen-Vee)	500 mg PO tabs	Dental infections, streptococcal pharyngitis	Multiple broad-spectrum alternatives may be more appropriate for wilderness travel.
Permethrin (Elimite)	60 g tube, 5% cream	Scabies and head lice	See Ivermectin above and discussion of permethrin-impregnated apparel in text.
Praziquantel (Biltricide)	600 mg (scored) PO tabs	Schistosomiasis, intestinal tapeworms, cysticercosis	Limited or no activity in acute exposure (larval stage). Consider inclusion in medical kit only if prolonged (>21 day) travel to endemic regions.
Quinine (Qualaquin)	650 mg PO tabs	Malaria treatment (P. falciparum) in chloroquine-resistant areas (check CDC. gov for guidelines)	Quinine may prolong the CT interval. An IV form is available if patient unable to tolerate PO route. Additional concurrent therapy may be required (e.g., doxycycline)
Rabies vaccine (RVA, RabAvert)	1 mL IM (vials)‡	Postexposure and pre-exposure rabies treatment	Dosing varies based on prior vaccination history. Wound cleansing and possibly immunoglobulin (at separate IM site) also required for postexposure prophylaxis.
Rabies immune globulin (Imogam, BayRab)	20 units/kg	Postexposure rabies treatment	Local wound infiltration with immune globulin, and remainder of dose given IM at a site remote to vaccine site. Consider inclusion in medical kit based on risk.

Trimethoprim-sulfamethoxazole (Bactrim, Septra)	160 mg/800 mg tab PO tabs	Cystitis, traveler's diarrhea, soft tissue infections	Caution in patients with chronic kidney disease or sulfa allergy.
Vancomycin	1 g vial IV‡	Meningitis, sepsis, suspected MRSA infection	Can cause profound hemodynamic instability with rapid administration. Only to be used by experienced personnel. For consideration by well-equipped trips staffed by qualified personnel.
Cardiovascular			
Amiodarone	450 mg/9 mL vial	Antiarrhythmic in ACLS	Multiple contraindications and adverse reactions, including hemodynamic collapse and fatal arrhythmia with administration. Only to be considered by expeditions with advanced medical support.
Acetylsalicylic acid† (Aspirin, Bayer, Ecotrin)	325 mg PO tabs	ACS, analgesia, antiinflammatory	Increased risk for GI bleeding and other bleeding diatheses. Preferably chewed when used for ACS. Can be given PR.
Atropine	1 mg/mL vial	Symptomatic bradycardia, ACLS	This drug causes tachycardia and stool and urinary retention.
Clonidine (Catapres)	0.1 mg PO tabs	Hypertension	Clonidine may cause drowsiness and dizziness. Can lead to rebound hypertension.

Continued

Table 61.1 Select Medications for Wilderness Travel*—cont'd

DRUG	FORMULATION	SELECT INDICATIONS	COMMENTS
Enoxaparin (Lovenox)	80 mg/0.8 mL prefilled syringes; subcutaneous administration only; weight-based dosing differs by indication	ACS, pulmonary embolism, deep vein thrombosis	Significant risk of bleeding.
Lidocaine	10 mL 2% vial, IV	Antiarrhythmic in ACLS	Potential for significant cardiac and neurotoxicity.
Metoprolol tartrate (Lopressor)	25 mg PO tabs	SVT and ACS	May impair exercise tolerance; may cause bronchospasm and unstable bradycardia.
Epinephrine	1 mL, 0.3 mg IM q 10-15 min for anaphylaxis; 10-300 mcg IV for anaphylaxis; 1 mg q 3-5 min for cardiac arrest	Anaphylactic reaction, hypotension, cardiac arrest, severe asthma, ACLS	Special consideration must be given to appropriate dosing, dilution, and route of administration, which vary considerably between indications. Advanced training and licensure required.
Epinephrine autoinjector (EpiPen)	0.3 mg single-dose autoinjector	Anaphylactic reaction	Inject into an extremity large muscle group (usually anterolateral thigh). Requires pretrip training. Requirement for all travelers with history of anaphylaxis. EpiPen Jr. (lower dose) may be required based on weight of travelers.

Nitroglycerin (Nitrostat, Nitrolingual)	0.4 mg sublingual tabs, or inhaler, 400 mcg/spray	Angina, select exacerbations of congestive heart failure	Relief of chest pain with nitroglycerin does not identify the pain as being cardiac in origin. Nitroglycerin is heat and light sensitive with a short shelf life. May cause hypotension and potentially life-threatening interactions with phosphodiesterase inhibitors, such as those used for erectile dysfunction (e.g., Viagra, Cialis, Levitra, Silagra).
Oxygen	Titrate to effect	Respiratory distress, ACS, decompression sickness, traumatic head injury, inhalational injury	Oxygen tanks are explosive, heavy, and bulky. Oxygen storage requires special attention and regular maintenance. Can be problematic if traveling by air.
Neurologic			
Alprazolam** (Xanax)	0.25-0.5 mg PO tabs	Insomnia, anxiety	Causes sedation and can lead to respiratory compromise. Potential for abuse and withdrawal.
Clonazepam** (Klonopin)	0.25-0.5 mg PO tabs	Insomnia, anxiety	Causes sedation and can lead to respiratory compromise. Potential for abuse and withdrawal.
Dextroamphetamine (Dexedrine, Dextrostat)	5 mg PO tabs	Fatigue, difficulty concentrating	May cause nervousness, diarrhea, or loss of appetite.

Continued

Table 61.1 Select Medications for Wilderness Travel*—cont'd

DRUG	FORMULATION	SELECT INDICATIONS	COMMENTS
Diazepam** (Valium)	5 mg PO scored tabs	Anxiety, agitation, seizures	Causes sedation and can lead to respiratory compromise. Potential for abuse and withdrawal.
Dimenhydrinate† (Dramamine)	50 mg PO tabs	Antihistamine, motion sickness	Causes CNS depression.
Etomidate (Amidate)	20 or 40 mg vial, IV injection	Rapid-sequence intubation	To be used only by trained providers planning to intubate during emergencies. Can cause hemodynamic compromise by depressing sympathetic tone.
Haloperidol (Haldol)	5 mg/mL vial; IM, IV, PO formulations available	Agitation, mania, psychosis	Dystonic reactions may occur; treat these with diphenhydramine or benztropine (Cogentin). Can cause QT prolongation.
Lorazepam** (Ativan)	2 mg/mL IM/IV	Anxiety, agitation, seizures, alcohol withdrawal	Causes sedation and can lead to respiratory compromise. Potential for abuse and withdrawal.
Meclizine† (Antivert, Bonine)	25 mg PO tabs	Vertigo, motion sickness prophylaxis	Adverse reactions include CNS depression and blurred vision (which can impair reading and ability to perform procedures requiring fine dexterity).
Midazolam** (Versed)	10 mg/mL vial; oral syrup also available	Anxiety, procedural sedation	Must be secured as significant abuse potential and side effects.

Modafinil (Provigil)	100 mg PO tabs	Circadian rhythm disturbances, shift work (e.g., night watch), fatigue	Use with caution in patients with cardiovascular disease or a history of psychiatric disorders.
Olanzapine (Zyprexa)	10 mg PO tabs; SL/IM administration available	Agitation, mania, psychotic disorders	Can cause tardive dyskinesia, neuroleptic malignant syndrome, orthostatic hypotension, and hyperglycemia.
Scopolamine (Transderm Scop)	1.5 mg TD patch	Motion sickness prevention, antiemetic	Significant anticholinergic symptoms, including blurred vision, CNS depression, and dyshydrosis (which can impair sweating and thermoregulation).
Succinylcholine	200 mg vial	Rapid-sequence intubation	Consider inclusion in medical kit only if personnel present with advanced airway equipment, training, and licensure. Review potentially life-threatening contraindications before use.
Dermatologic			
Clotrimazole† (Lotrimin, Mycelex)	1% cream	Topical fungal infections	Multiple alternatives exist.
Hydrocortisone† (Cortaid, Hytone)	1% cream	Contact dermatitis	Hydrocortisone is not to be used to treat infections. Repeated use can cause skin atrophy, especially on face, genital area, and dorsum of hand.

Continued

Table 61.1 Select Medications for Wilderness Travel*—cont'd			
DRUG	**FORMULATION**	**SELECT INDICATIONS**	**COMMENTS**
Triamcinolone (Aristocort, Kenalog)	0.1% ointment	Contact dermatitis, severe itching	Triamcinolone is significantly more potent than hydrocortisone OTC, although requires prescription. It should not to be used to treat infectious rashes. Repeated use can cause skin atrophy, especially on face, genital area, and dorsum of hand. Numerous alternatives exist.
Mupirocin (Bactroban)	2% cream, 15 g or 30 g tube	Impetigo	MRSA coverage for superficial infections. Components of OTC triple-antibiotic ointments (bacitracin-neomycin-polymyxin B) may be inferior to mupirocin for impetigo.
Diphenhydramine† (Benadryl)	25-50 mg PO tabs	Seasonal allergies, allergic reactions, dystonic reactions	Causes significant impairment of psychomotor performance and cognitive function.
Metronidazole (Metrogel)	Vaginal 0.75% cream	Bacterial vaginosis	The formulation tends to separate at high temperatures; consider an oral formulation for more compact and stable transport.
Nystatin (Nyamyc)	Vaginal suppositories and creams	Vulvovaginal candidiasis, balanitis, localized skin infections	Creams and suppositories tend to melt in warm or hot environments. Fluconazole is more stable and can be taken as a single oral dose, but it belongs to Pregnancy Category C and requires prescription. Nystatin is very inexpensive.

Permethrin (Elimite, Nix)	5% cream	Scabies; head lice may be treated with a 1% permethrin rinse	This cream causes temporary stinging. Treatment may be repeated after 7 days for increased efficacy. Read notes on ivermectin adjunctive therapy.
Polymyxin B, bacitracin, and neomycin ointments† (Neosporin)	15 g packs	Lacerations, superficial skin infections	This is not a substitute for systemic antibiotics for soft tissue infections.
Silver sulfadiazine (Silvadene)	1% cream, 50 g tube	Burns, large soft tissue injuries, open fractures	Remove cream from a previous application before reapplying. This drug contains sulfa.
Tolnaftate† (Tinactin)	1% cream, gel, spray, or powder	Localized skin infections that are suspected of being fungal in origin	The safety profile is unknown for pregnancy.
Eye, Ear, Nose, and Throat Topical Medications§			
Artificial Tears†	10 mL container	Xerophthalmia (dry eyes)	Rule out foreign body, corneal abrasion, or other pathologies before use.
Cyclopentolate (AK-Pentolate, Cyclogyl)	1% drops, 5 mL container	Snowblindness (off-label use)	Decreases pain (photophobia) by decreasing ciliary muscle spasm. Not to be used for patients who need to walk or drive. It may cause acute angle-closure glaucoma. Scopolamine 0.25% and homatropine 2%-5% may be alternatives.

Continued

Table 61.1   Select Medications for Wilderness Travel*—cont'd

DRUG	FORMULATION	SELECT INDICATIONS	COMMENTS
Diclofenac	0.1% drops	Snowblindness	Consider using adjunct PO analgesic.
Dexamethasone, neomycin, and polymyxin ointment (Maxitrol)	Drops or ointment	Snowblindness, disabling allergic conjunctivitis	Cortisporin (neomycin, polymyxin, and hydrocortisone) may be interchangeable with Maxitrol for otic and ophthalmic irritation.
Erythromycin ophthalmic ointment (Ilotycin)	0.5% ointment, 3.5 g tube	Corneal abrasions or ulcerations	The ointment stays on the eye but blurs vision; it should be used at night or while resting. Multiple alternatives exist.
Gentamicin (Garamycin) or Tobramycin (Tobrex) drops	0.3% drops	Corneal abrasions or ulcerations in contact lens wearers	May cause chemical keratitis. Interchangeable with ofloxacin or ciprofloxacin drops in select indications.
Moxifloxacin (Vigamox)	0.5% drops	Bacterial keratitis	Fourth-generation fluoroquinolone with possibly less resistance than earlier generation meds. Increased cost.
Neomycin and polymyxin B sulfate and hydrocortisone otic suspension (Cortisporin Otic Suspension)	Neomycin 0.35%, polymyxin B 10,000 units/mL, hydrocortisone 0.5%	Otitis externa	Must avoid the use of topical aminoglycosides if tympanic membrane ruptured.

Ofloxacin (Floxin Otic)	0.3% otic solution	Otitis externa	Second-generation fluoroquinolone. Multiple alternatives exist. A wisp of cotton wool placed in the ear as a wick will draw medication into the ear canal.
Oxymetazoline (Afrin)	0.05% nasal spray	Congestion, epistaxis	This drug may be sprayed on a laceration to temporarily decrease bleeding. It causes rebound congestion with prolonged use.
Pilocarpine (Isopto Carpine)	2% drops	Acute angle-closure glaucoma	Only to be used by experienced and appropriately trained personnel.
Phenylephrine (Neo-Synephrine)	0.5%–2.5% drops	To induce mydriasis	Only to be used by experienced and appropriately trained personnel.
Polymyxin B and trimethoprim eye drops (Polytrim)	10000 units/mL solution	Corneal abrasions or ulcerations, snowblindness	Ointments can be used instead of drops, but these impair vision and should only be used when patients are resting or sleeping. Worsening eye irritation suggests chemical keratitis caused by medication.
Prednisolone	1% drops	Allergic keratitis, acute angle-closed glaucoma	Because steroids may worsen eye infections, they are typically prescribed only on advice from ophthalmologist.
Tetracaine	0.5% drops	See Analgesia section	
Timolol (Istalol)	0.5% drops	Acute angle-closure glaucoma	Significant side effects can occur; should be used only under expert consultation.

Continued

Table 61.1 Select Medications for Wilderness Travel*—cont'd

DRUG	FORMULATION	SELECT INDICATIONS	COMMENTS
Gastrointestinal			
Bismuth subsalicylate† (Pepto-Bismol, Kaopectate)	262 mg PO tabs	Abdominal pain, vomiting, diarrhea	With this drug, the stool and tongue may turn black; excessive intake can cause salicylate poisoning. May provide good GI prophylaxis from coliform infection if taken before meals.
Docusate sodium† (Colace)	100 mg PO tabs	Constipation	Docusate may cause diarrhea and abdominal cramping. Liquid form may also be useful for cerumen disimpaction.[43]
Famotidine† (Pepcid)	20 mg PO tabs	Peptic ulcer disease, dyspepsia	Decreased stomach pH may predispose patient to GI infections. Consider including one H₂ blocker, because this will have faster onset than PPI (even faster if combined with calcium carbonate and/or magnesium hydroxide).
Lactase† (Lactaid)	250 mg PO tabs	Lactose intolerance	Travelers with known lactose intolerance are advised to bring lactase. Transient lactose intolerance often develops after traveler's diarrhea.
Loperamide† (Imodium)	2 mg PO tabs	Diarrhea	Decreases symptoms in most cases of traveler's diarrhea, but has not been adequately studied for safety in patients with bloody diarrhea. Use contraindicated with certain diarrheal illnesses.

Meclizine† (Antivert)	25 mg PO tabs	Motion sickness, nausea	See Neurologic section.
Omeprazole† (Prilosec)	20 PO tabs	Peptic ulcer disease, dyspepsia	Decreased stomach pH may predispose patient to GI infections.
Ondansetron (Zofran)	8 mg PO tabs; 4 mg/2 mL vials	Nausea, vomiting	May cause QT prolongation; limited efficacy for motion sickness–induced nausea.
Promethazine (Phenergan)	25 mg PO tabs	Nausea, vomiting, motion-sickness	Especially effective for motion sickness. Acute dystonic reactions related to promethazine can be treated with diphenhydramine or benztropine. Do not use in pediatric patients. Black Box warnings exist.
Prochlorperazine (Compazine)	5 mg PO tabs; also available PR and as solution for injection, 5 mg/mL	Nausea, vomiting	Causes sedation and dystonia; is not for use in patients <2 years old. Acute dystonic reactions related to prochlorperazine can be treated with diphenhydramine or benztropine.
Senna† (Senokot)	8.6 mg PO tabs	Constipation	Constipation can be a significant challenge for many travelers, and care must be taken before severe constipation is mistaken for more serious illness.
Witch hazel pads† (Preparation H)	Package, 10 each	Hemorrhoids	Multiple alternative antihemorrhoidal medications exist.

Continued

Table 61.1   Select Medications for Wilderness Travel*—cont'd

DRUG	FORMULATION	SELECT INDICATIONS	COMMENTS
High Altitude			
Acetazolamide (Diamox)	250 mg PO tabs	Acute mountain sickness treatment and prevention, acute angle closure glaucoma	Acetazolamide is contraindicated for patients with sulfa allergy; it may cause vertigo, diuresis-induced hypovolemia, paresthesias, and taste changes.
Dexamethasone (Decadron)	10 mg/mL vial for IV administration	High-altitude cerebral edema, antiinflammatory for allergic reactions	Dexamethasone may cause agitation, mood disturbances, hypertension, and hyperglycemia. Takes hours to achieve maximal effect. One IV corticosteroid may be sufficient for the purposes of a medical kit; many alternatives exist.
Nifedipine (Procardia, Adalat)	30 mg PO tabs	High-altitude pulmonary edema	Do not give to patients who are hypotensive. Nifedipine can also be used to treat hypertension.
Sildenafil (Viagra)	50 mg PO tabs	May enhance cardiovascular performance at high altitude, but still experimental	May cause hypotension, headache, lightheadedness, and blue scotomata. Sildenafil is not for patients who are taking nitrates or who have a history of retinal disease.
Respiratory			
Albuterol inhaler (Ventolin, Proventil, Salbutamol)	90 mcg/puff metered-dose inhaler	Asthma exacerbation, COPD	Albuterol may cause tachycardia or provoke anxiety.

Beclomethasone (QVAR, Vanceril)	40 mcg/dose aerosol inhaler	Chronic asthma	This is one of the inhaled corticosteroids given for chronic asthma; it may have fewer systemic side effects than oral corticosteroids.
Diphenhydramine† (Benadryl)	25-50 mg PO tabs	Seasonal allergies, allergic reactions, dystonic reactions	Causes significant impairment of psychomotor performance and cognitive function.
Epinephrine (Primatene Mist)	0.22 mg/puff aerosolized	Asthma exacerbation, allergic reactions (airway edema), anecdotal use for symptomatic bradycardia	Use with caution in older adults and those with known coronary disease.
Fexofenadine† (Allegra)	60 mg PO tabs	Seasonal allergies, urticaria	Nonsedating antihistamine is useful for the treatment of nasal congestion and allergy-induced itching; it costs more than diphenhydramine, but CNS effects are less pronounced.
Promethazine/ codeine**	6.25/10/5 mL syrup PO	Persistent cough	This may be a good medication for acute gastroenteritis in adults, due to the combined antiemetic (promethazine) and antimotility actions (codeine). Black Box warnings exist.
Ipratropium (Atrovent)	18 mcg/puff inhaler	Asthma exacerbation, intranasal administration for treatment of URI symptoms	Ipratropium is not for patients with life-threatening soy or peanut allergies. Also available in combination with albuterol (e.g., Combivent).

Continued

Table 61.1 Select Medications for Wilderness Travel*—cont'd

DRUG	FORMULATION	SELECT INDICATIONS	COMMENTS
Loratadine† (Claritin)	10 mg PO tabs	Seasonal allergies, urticaria	Potentially less impairment in psychomotor performance and cognitive function than diphenhydramine, but may be less effective[5,40]
Phenylephrine†	10 mg PO tabs	Nasal congestion	Contraindicated in patients taking MAOI. Caution in patients with hypertension. Pseudoephedrine may be used as an alternative.
Prednisone (Deltasone, Pred-Pak)	5 mg PO tabs	Asthma exacerbation, allergic reactions, severe allergic contact dermatitis (poison ivy/oak)	Short-term side effects include insomnia and anxiety. Taper may be therapeutically beneficial, although rarely required when used in doses <50 mg daily for <5 days. Monitor for vaginal and oropharyngeal candidiasis.
Pseudoephedrine† (Sudafed)	30 mg PO tabs	Nasal congestion	May have significant cardiovascular and CNS effects.
Cetylpyridinium and benzocaine† (Cepacol)	20 PO lozenges	Sore throat	Acetaminophen and ibuprofen can be helpful adjunct to treating pharyngitis. Many alternative lozenges exist.
Miscellaneous Medications			
Oral glucose† (Glutose)	20 g PO tabs	Hypoglycemia	Hard candy or naturally sweetened fruit juice may be as effective.

Dextrose solution	50%, 25g/50 mL vial	Hypoglycemia	For advanced providers where IV access is possible.
Methylprednisone (Solu-Medrol)	1000 mg/vial‡	Anaphylaxis or severe asthma/ COPD exacerbation	Can be used as alternative to dexamethasone, hydrocortisone, or prednisone in select indications.
Hydrocortisone powder	100 mg/2 mL	Anaphylaxis or severe asthma/ COPD exacerbation	Can be used as alternative to dexamethasone, methylprednisone, or prednisone in select indications.

ACS, Acute coronary syndrome; *ACLS,* advanced cardiac life support; *CNS,* central nervous system; *COPD,* chronic obstructive pulmonary disease; *GI,* gastrointestinal; *IM,* intramuscular; *IV,* intravenous; *MAOIs,* monoamine oxidase inhibitors; *MRSA,* methicillin-resistant Staphylococcus aureus; *NSAIDs,* nonsteroidal antiinflammatory drugs; *CTC,* over the counter; *PO,* by mouth; *PPI,* proton pump inhibitor; *PR,* by rectum; *q,* every; *SC,* subcutaneous; *SL,* sublingual; *SSRIs,* selective serotonin reuptake inhibitors; *SVT,* supraventricular tachycardia; *TCAs,* tricyclic antidepressants; *TD,* transdermal; *URI,* upper respiratory tract infection.

*This table is intended to serve as a list of potentially useful medications for management of commonly encountered medical scenarios in the wilderness. The table should not be used as a treatment guide or as a substitute for manufacturer labels or information contained in the *Physicians' Desk Reference*. All medications listed here must be administered by personnel with appropriate training and licensure. Selection of medications to include in a first-aid kit must be tailored to the specifics of a trip including but not limited to the itinerary, number of travelers, preexisting medical conditions, potentially encountered conditions, and region of travel.

**Providers who bring opioids and other controlled/scheduled medications should do so only if appropriate licensure and training has been obtained. Nonphysician travelers must have a prescription from their personal physician and bring appropriate documentation while traveling. Laws for controlled substances are not universal, and traveling with certain medications may even be illegal in certain destination countries.

†Does not require a prescription in the United States.

‡Requires resuspension. Read package inserts to ensure adequate supply of solution. Usually a supply of any sterile IV fluid solution can work, although some medications may require sterile water to avoid precipitation.

§Caution with multiuse ophthalmic drop applicators because contamination can be source of bacterial keratitis.

Table 61.2   Indications for Antibiotic Treatment in Wilderness Travelers

Traveler's diarrhea: sensitivity to various antibiotics varies based on region and should be researched before departure (e.g., there is high resistance to ciprofloxacin by *Campylobacter* species in the Himalayan region and Southeast Asia)	Ciprofloxacin, 750 mg PO × 1, or azithromycin, 1 g PO × 1, if diarrhea is being treated within the first 24 hr. If treating diarrhea of >24 hr duration, then use azithromycin, 500 mg PO daily × 3 days, or ciprofloxacin, 750 mg PO q12h × 3 days. Antimotility agents should not be given in the setting of dysentery, fever, or other abnormal vital signs.
Diarrhea (suspected giardiasis)	Metronidazole, 250 mg PO q8h × 5 days
Diarrhea in pregnant women or children	Trimethoprim/sulfamethoxazole DS, 1 tab PO q12h × 3 days
Fungal infections (e.g., yeast vaginitis)	Fluconazole, 150 mg PO × 1
Lacerations from animal bites	Amoxicillin/clavulanic acid, 875/125 mg PO q12h × 3–5 days (this recommendation is controversial)
Lacerations with gross contamination or bone, tendon, or cartilage exposure	Cephalexin, 500 mg PO q6h × 5–7 days
Pneumonia	Doxycycline, 100 mg PO q12h × 7 days, or azithromycin, 500 mg PO on day 1 then 250 mg daily on days 2–5, or levofloxacin, 500 mg PO daily, or moxifloxacin, 400 mg PO daily
Sexually transmitted urethritis	Ciprofloxacin, 500 mg PO × 1 or cefixime, mg; and azithromycin, 1 g PO × 1, or doxycycline, 100 mg PO q12h × 7 days
Urinary tract infections	Ciprofloxacin, 500 mg PO q12h × 3 days
Appendicitis or other intraabdominal infection	Ciprofloxacin, 500 mg PO q12h and metronidazole, 500 mg PO q6h

PO, By mouth.

BOX 61.2 Advanced Devices for the Medically Trained Traveler*

Oral and nasopharyngeal airways
Bulb suction device
Self-inflating bag-mask ventilation device with pediatric/adult mask sizes
Oxygen supply (see text)
Laryngoscope (MacIntosh blade sizes 2, 3, 4, Miller 3)
Oral and nasogastric tubes, 14 Fr
Nasal cannula and nonrebreather face mask (if oxygen supply available)
Cricothyrotomy cannula or catheter (e.g., Abelson cannula) or prepackaged cricothyrotomy kit (e.g., Portex Cricothyroidotomy Kit, Nu-Trake cricothyrotomy device, Tactical CricKit)
Endotracheal tube (size 7.0 internal diameter and pediatric sizes when appropriate) and stylets
Laryngeal mask airway (LMA; sizes 3, 4, and 5)
King airway or combitube
Gum elastic bougie
Chest tube set, 32 Fr (practical only on major expeditions) with capability for formal or improvised water seal
Heimlich valve
Intravenous tubing with high-flow drip chamber and spike
Needles and syringes (for intravenous hydration and emergency injectables)
Intravenous catheters (assorted sizes 14, 16, 18, 20, and 22 gauge)
Sharps disposal device (biohazard disposal container)
Intravenous tourniquet
Intravenous fluid (normal saline, lactated Ringer's, or Plasma-Lyte)
Adjustable cervical collar
Automated external defibrillator (AED)
Surgical tools
Surgical or fine-dust masks, N95 mask when concern for tuberculosis (TB)

*Selection of the equipment listed here must be made at the discretion of the trip medical officer based on several factors, including level of training and space allotted for medical supplies.

Table 61.3 Portable Diagnostic Instruments for Wilderness Travel*	
DEVICE	**INDICATION**
Thermometer (e.g., ADTEMP 419 digital or other low-reading device)	Essential for evaluation of hypothermic and hyperthermic patients (e.g., infection, exposure).
Sphygmomanometer (blood pressure cuff)	Useful for accurate measurement of blood pressure, particularly in trauma patients and patients with tachycardia or altered mental status; may be used as an adjustable tourniquet. Ensure appropriate cuff sizes and stethoscope are also packed.
Stethoscope	Useful for auscultation of Korotkoff sounds for manual blood pressure measurement and for chest auscultation, particularly to evaluate for the presence of wheezing, pulmonary edema, or pneumothorax.
Precordial stethoscope	A precordial stethoscope with earpiece can be a useful and inexpensive tool for continuously monitoring heart rate and respiratory rate.
Urinalysis test strips (e.g., Clinitek)	Useful for evaluation of abdominal pain, urinary symptoms, ketosis, and hyperglycemia.
Chronometer (waterproof with second hand)	Useful for accurate measurement of heart rate and respiratory rate; also important when planning evacuations.
Urine pregnancy test (e.g., Baby Check, Midstream, SureStep, or one of many other generic and name brands)	Essential for evaluation of abdominal pain in women of childbearing age; a positive pregnancy test may raise the possibility of ectopic pregnancy, and immediate evacuation might be considered. These tests vary in sensitivity and may also produce false-positive results.
Pulse oximeter (e.g., Nonin)	Considerable variation exists in the quality of over-the-counter probes (https://www.ncbi.nlm.nih.gov/pubmed/27089002). Choosing a manufacturer who also makes FDA-approved (medical-grade) probes, ideally with plethysmography, is recommended (extra batteries likely needed). Keep in mind that most of these units do not feature alarms or capability to provide continuous monitoring.

Table 61.3   Portable Diagnostic Instruments for Wilderness Travel*—cont'd

DEVICE	INDICATION
Glucometer (e.g., Therasense)	Useful for routine diabetes management and for evaluation of ill-appearing diabetic individuals who may have too-low or too-high serum glucose levels.
Fluorescein dye strips	Necessary for diagnosis of corneal abrasions. The cobalt light source on an ophthalmoscope or a fluorescent light stick can be used to illuminate the fluorescein.
Magnifying glass	For foreign body identification and removal.
Otoscope	For foreign body or otalgia evaluation (infectious, inflammatory, and traumatic etiologies); consider a device with capability for pneumatic otoscopy. Do not forget specula (preferably reusable soft tips of varying sizes).
Ophthalmoscope	Devices with cobalt light filters when used in conjunction with fluorescein are especially useful for the diagnosis of corneal abrasions.
End-tidal carbon dioxide detector (e.g., Nellcor)	Colorimetric devices are available to help with confirmation of endotracheal tube placement, while quantitative digital devices remain expensive and not practical for many expeditions.
Rapid diagnostic tests	When traveling to endemic regions, purchase of rapid diagnostic kits can be useful when evaluating febrile illnesses. Several kits are available for malaria, dengue, and typhoid as well as other illnesses. These kits require a drop of blood on a test strip. Travelers must investigate sensitivity and specificity for specific manufacturers and types of organisms (e.g., *Plasmodium vivax* vs. *P. falciparum*) because this is an evolving technology, may not be FDA-approved, and usually is available for purchase at pharmacies in country of travel.

*Appropriate training is required for use of these devices.
FDA, US Food and Drug Administration.

BOX 61.3 Specialized Equipment for Environmental and Recreational Hazards

High Altitude
Gamow bag and accessories
Pulse oximeter
Oxygen canisters, nasal cannulas, face masks, oxygen tubing, and
    connections

Cold and Avalanche Exposure
External thermal stabilizer bag
Res-Q-Air
Hot Sac
Intravenous fluid warmer
Chemical warmers (e.g., Grabber)
Electric foot warmers (e.g., Hotronic)
Low-reading thermometer
Space thermal reflective survival bag
Adhesive climbing skins
Ice axe
Adjustable ski or probe pole
AvaLung avalanche vest
Avalanche beacon

Water Sports (Low Impact)
CPR microshield
Water disinfection equipment (i.e., filter, iodine or chlorine,
    SteriPEN)

Water Sports (High Impact)
Cervical spine immobilizer
Pelvic immobilizer (e.g., SAM pelvic sling)

Bicycling
All-terrain cyclist kit
Occlusive dressings

Tropical and Third-World Travel
Pressure immobilization equipment (for snakebite)
Permethrin-containing insect repellent
Mosquito nets
Oral rehydration electrolyte powder packs
Water disinfection equipment (i.e., filter, iodine or chlorine,
    SteriPEN)

Mountain Climbing and Hiking
Prefabricated splints and pelvic immobilizer (sling)
Slishman traction splint (not available in the United States)
Slishman rescue harness
Ankle brace (e.g., aircast)

- Carry enough medications to treat multiple persons over the course of the expedition.
- Consider drug storage and stability (see Appendix R).

Antibiotics

Prepare for the common infectious disease problems listed in Table 61.2 and by selecting appropriate antibiotics. Also see Appendix H for more discussion on antimicrobials.

WILDERNESS MEDICATIONS

- When assembling medicine kits for a group, always include copies of the manufacturer's package insert with each medicine.
- Table 61.1 lists commonly carried over-the-counter and prescription medications. This list is not comprehensive but provides options from which medical designees can choose based on their group needs.
- Many medications (e.g., atropine, epinephrine, dexamethasone, nifedipine, nitroglycerin) have significant systemic effects. Administration of these medications is usually directly managed or guided by physicians, nurses acting under the direction of a physician, or designated medical providers with appropriate training.
- Many emergencies can be managed by either oral or transdermal application of medicines.
- Intravenous medications are temperature-sensitive and fragile, expire quickly, and require monitoring of vital signs because of their potency and immediate onset of action.
- Opioid analgesics should be used to treat pain only if mild analgesics (e.g., ibuprofen, acetaminophen) are inadequate, mental status is clear, and respiratory distress is not present (unless it is due solely to discomfort).
- Any expedition carrying opioids should also carry a reversal agent (e.g., naloxone).
- Whenever possible, medicines should be purchased as tablets rather than capsules because of the tendency of capsules to break apart or dissolve.
- Under extremes of temperature, creams may become unusable; in such environments, oral medications are preferred.
- Purchasing medications on arrival may be necessary and save money. Many medications that require prescriptions for purchase in industrialized countries, including opioids, are available over the counter in developing countries.
- Many international medications do not contain the desired active ingredient or are adulterated with dangerous compounds. Travelers should make every effort to obtain medications from a reliable source.

WHAT MAKES CHILDREN DIFFERENT

- Medications and fluids must be calculated based on the weight of the child (Table 62.1). One should also be aware of normal ranges of vital signs according to age (Table 62.2).
- Children experience greater toxicity from envenomation because of the increased dose of venom per kilogram of weight.
- Children are more likely to have incomplete "greenstick" fractures or injuries involving the growth plates.
- Children are more susceptible to blunt chest and abdominal injuries due to their height and flexible ribs, which afford less protection of internal organs.
- Children experience greater exposure to environmental factors such as cold, heat, and solar radiation because they have a larger body surface area–to–mass ratio than do adults.
- Thermoregulation is less efficient in children, making them more susceptible to heat illness and hypothermia.
- Children can often maintain a normal blood pressure in the face of significant fluid or blood losses (30% to 40% of total blood volume).
- The airway of a child is more prone to obstruction due to its smaller size and conical shape.
- Children experience a greater number of infections than do adults.
- Children are at greater risk for dehydration than are adults.
- Small children tend to explore their environment with their hands and mouths.

Food and Drink

- Infants in their first 4 to 6 months require only breast milk or formula.
- Baby cereals can be carried conveniently in a dry form to be mixed with formula or breast milk.
- Dry cereals mixed with breast milk or formula have a higher nutritional value than ready-to-feed cereals in jars.
- Squeeze tubes of infant food are convenient for all but the shortest ventures.
- By age 9 to 12 months, many babies are eating finger foods.
- Any new food should be tested at home prior to travel to be certain the baby will accept it when away from home.
- Chronic iodine poisoning and neonatal goiter have been associated with prolonged ingestion of large amounts of iodine,

Table 62.1   Average Weight for Age

AGE (YR)	WEIGHT	
	kg	lb
1	10	22
3	15	33
6	20	44
8	25	55
9.5	30	66
11	35	77
13	45	100

From U.S. Centers for Disease Control and Prevention: *National Center for Health Statistics* (http://www.cdc.gov/nchs/).

Table 62.2   Age-Specific Resting Heart Rate and Respiratory Rate

AGE	HEART RATE (BEATS/MIN)	RESPIRATORY RATE (BREATHS/MIN)
0–5 mo	140 ± 40	40 ± 12
6–11 mo	135 ± 30	30 ± 10
1–2 yr	120 ± 30	25 ± 8
3–4 yr	110 ± 30	20 ± 6
5–7 yr	100 ± 20	16 ± 5
8–11 yr	90 ± 30	16 ± 4
12–15 yr	80 ± 20	16 ± 3

Mean rate, ± 2 standard deviations.

although small amounts ingested for short-duration water disinfection appear safe.
- Children 2 to 4 years old can choose from a diversity of nutritious snacks, such as raisins, granola bars, nuts, and cheese as their meals.

Equipment
- Most infants and young children will have to travel in child carriers for some or all the trip.
- Sleeping bags are available for infants and toddlers but should not be used for babies under the age of 1 year to avoid entanglement and possible suffocation.

- Children, including young infants, also need their own sleeping pads.
- Shoes for young children should protect their feet and allow for full range of movement.
- Older children (5 years old and older) may feel more engaged and independent if allowed to carry some of their own gear.
- The maximal weight of these packs should be 20% of the child's body weight until he or she has had significant backcountry experience and can comfortably carry more.

AGE-SPECIFIC EXPECTATIONS FOR WILDERNESS TRAVEL
See Table 62.3.

ENVIRONMENTAL ILLNESSES
Dehydration
Signs and Symptoms

Mild to moderate dehydration (5% to 10% weight loss)
- Irritability
- Sunken eyes
- Dry mucous membranes
- Thirst
- Dark urine
- Tachycardia

Severe dehydration (>10% weight loss)
- Lethargy
- Extremely sunken eyes
- Extremely dry mucous membranes
- Cool, mottled extremities
- Rapid thready pulse
- Tachypnea
- Absent tears
- No urine output

Treatment
1. Replace fluids and electrolytes.
   a. Oral rehydration with water and oral rehydration solution (ORS) is the most important treatment for dehydration in the backcountry. Simply drinking plain water is inadequate replacement.
   b. Gatorade can be used but should be diluted to half-strength with water.
   c. Add commercial ORS containing sodium chloride, 3.5 g; potassium chloride, 1.5 g; glucose, 20 g; and sodium bicarbonate, 2.5 g to 1 L (1 quart) of drinking water.
   d. Improvise an ORS by adding 5 mL (1 teaspoon) of table salt and 40 mL (8 teaspoons) of table sugar to 1 L (1 quart) of drinking (disinfected) water. A rice cereal–based rehydration

Table 62.3   Age-Specific Expectations for Wilderness Travel

AGE	EXPECTATION	SAFETY ISSUES
0–2 years	Distance traveled depends on how far an adult may go with child in carrier	Provide safe play area (e.g., tent floor, extra tarp laid out) for child; put bells on child's shoes; be aware that child may put things found outside in mouth
2–4 years	Child is at a difficult age; child can hike 1–2 miles on own and needs to stop every 15 min	Dress child in bright colors; give child a whistle to carry and teach child how to use it (three blows for "I'm lost")
5–7 years	Child can hike 1–3 hr/day and cover 3–4 miles over easy terrain; needs to rest every 30–45 min	Child carries a whistle; child can carry own pack with mini–first-aid kit, flashlight, garbage bag, and water
8–9 years	Child can hike a full day at an easy pace and cover 6–7 miles over variable terrain; if child is 1.2 m (>4 ft) tall, can use a framed pack	Same as for age 5–7 years, plus adult can teach child to use a map and find a route; preconditioning can be done by increasing maximal distances by <10%/week; watch for overuse injuries; keep weight of pack at <20% of child's body weight
10–12 years	Child can hike a full day at a moderate pace and cover 8–10 miles over variable terrain	Same as for age 8–9 years, plus child can expand role for route planning and can learn to use a compass
Teens	Teen can hike 8–12 miles or more at an adult pace; while growth spurt is occurring, there may be a decrease in teen's pace or distance hiked	Same as for age 10–12 years, plus teen can expand survival and wilderness first-aid knowledge

solution is made by adding 5 mL (1 teaspoon) of table salt and 50 g (1 cup) of rice cereal to 1 L (1 quart) of drinking (disinfected) water.

e. For rapid treatment of mild to moderate dehydration, 50 to 100 mL/kg (1 to 1.5 oz/lb) of ORS should be administered over the first 4-hour period, followed by maintenance fluid volumes (75 to 150 mL/kg/day or 1 to 2 oz/lb/day). An additional 10 mL/kg, or 4 oz, can be given for each diarrhea stool and 5 mL/kg, or 2 oz, for each episode of emesis. If vomiting develops, most children will still tolerate ORS if given small volumes (5 to 10 mL [1 to 2 teaspoons]) every 5 minutes. Severe dehydration requires prompt medical attention and administration of IV fluids for rehydration.

Hypothermia (See Chapter 3)

Children cool more rapidly than adults because of their proportionally larger body surface area and because they lack the knowledge and judgment to initiate responses that will maintain warmth in a cold environment.

Prevention

- Dress in layers.
- Avoid excessive perspiration.
- Use clothing that stays warm despite being wet (e.g., wool, synthetics, Gore-Tex).
- Maintain adequate hydration and nutrition to support metabolism.

Signs and Symptoms (Table 62.4)

- Ataxia.
- Altered mental status.
- Inappropriate remarks,
- Shivering is not a reliable marker of hypothermia in children.

Treatment

1. Remove any wet clothing and replace it with dry, insulating garments. Cover the child's head and neck.
2. If the child is alert, oral hydration with warm fluids containing glucose repletes glycogen and corrects dehydration, which frequently accompanies hypothermia.
3. Place the child in a sleeping bag with a normothermic person.
4. Place hot water bottles insulated to prevent burns at the axillae, neck, and groin.
5. If the child is alert, administer oral hydration with warm fluids containing glucose.

Hyperthermia (See Chapter 5)

Children generate more heat per kilogram and are less able to dissipate heat from the core to the periphery.

Table 62.4	Signs and Symptoms of Hypothermia	
RECTAL TEMPERATURE		**SIGNS AND SYMPTOMS**
Mild	33°C–35°C (91°F–95°F)	Sensation of cold, shivering, increased heart rate, progressive incoordination in hand movements, development of poor judgment
Moderate	28°C–32°C (82°F–90°F)	Loss of shivering, difficulty walking or following commands, inappropriate (for the outside temperature) undressing, increasing confusion, decreased arrhythmia threshold
Severe	<28°C (<82°F)	Rigid muscles, progressive loss of reflexes and voluntary motion, hypotension, bradycardia, hypoventilation, dilated pupils, increasing risk of fatal arrhythmias, looks as if death is imminent

Data from adult subjects.

Prevention
- Ensure adequate hydration.
- Offer fluids frequently.
- Dress in layers to avoid overheating.
- Modify exertional activity to accommodate heat acclimatization (it often takes 10 to 14 days for children to fully adapt).

Signs and Symptoms
- Early signs and symptoms include flushing, tachycardia, weakness, headache, and nausea.
- Late signs are confusion, ataxia, or any altered mental state.
- Sweating is either present or absent.
- Temperature is elevated.

Treatment
1. Remove the child from sources of heat and remove clothing.
2. Spray the child with warm water, and fan vigorously.
3. Place ice packs or cold compresses at the neck, axillae, scalp, and groin.
4. If the child is alert and not vomiting, administer oral fluids (see earlier).

High-Altitude Illness (See Chapter 1)
High-altitude illness can be viewed as a continuum from acute mountain sickness (AMS) to life-threatening conditions such as

high-altitude pulmonary edema (HAPE) and high-altitude cerebral edema (HACE). AMS usually develops within 24 hours of ascent.

Prevention
• Avoid abrupt ascent to a sleeping altitude higher than 3000 m (9843 ft).
• Spend two or three nights at 2500 to 3000 m (8202 to 9843 ft) before going higher.
• Avoid abrupt increases of greater than 500 m (1640 ft) in sleeping altitude per night.
• Provide acetazolamide prophylaxis (5 mg/kg/day, in two divided doses, up to a maximum daily dose of 250 mg started 24 hours before ascent and continued while at altitude) in children with a history of recurrent AMS despite graded ascent.

Signs and Symptoms
• Bitemporal throbbing headache.
• Anorexia.
• Nausea and vomiting.
• Dizziness, dyspnea on exertion, and fragmented sleep.
• Infants may display irritability, poor feeding, and sleep disturbance.
• Ataxia, altered mental state.

Treatment
1. Descend at least 500 to 1000 m (1640 to 3281 ft).
2. Administer acetaminophen for headache.
3. Ondansetron (Zofran) or promethazine (Phenergan) may be used to relieve nausea and vomiting. Dystonia in response to phenothiazines, such as promethazine, occurs disproportionately in young children, so ondansetron is preferred. Ondansetron is given orally at 0.1 to 0.15 mg/kg up to 4 mg every 4 hours; promethazine is given at 0.2 to 0.5 mg/kg/dose up to 25 mg every 6 hours, preferably per rectum.
4. Administer oxygen if available.
5. Administer acetazolamide 5 mg/kg/day divided q12h up to 250 mg/day if symptoms persist despite descent.
6. Administer dexamethasone 0.15 mg/kg/dose up to maximum dose of 4 mg IM/IV/PO q6h for children with deterioration of consciousness, truncal ataxia, or severe vomiting. The symptoms of high-altitude cerebral edema or high-altitude pulmonary edema demand immediate descent and possible evacuation.

Traveler's Diarrhea
Young children are at greater risk for traveler's diarrhea (TD) and its complications because of relatively poor hygiene, immature immune systems, lower gastric pH, more rapid gastric emptying, and difficulties with adequate hydration.

Prevention

- Careful selection and preparation of food and beverages can decrease the risk of acquiring TD.
- Washing hands thoroughly before eating decreases bacterial illness.
- Raw vegetables and salads should be avoided, meats and seafood well cooked, and fruits properly peeled.

Signs and Symptoms

- Greater than three unformed stools a day
- Fever
- Abdominal cramps
- Vomiting
- Blood or mucus in the stool

Treatment

1. Provide oral rehydration to correct dehydration and electrolyte losses (see earlier).
2. Give rice, bananas, and potatoes as supplements to ORS. Fats, dairy products, caffeine, and alcohol should be avoided.
3. If the patient is older than 3 years of age and does not have bloody diarrhea or fever, administer loperamide (Imodium). The dosage is 1 to 2 mg for the first dose followed by 1 to 2 mg after each loose stool with a maximum of 3 mg/day in 3- to 5-year-olds, 4 mg/d in 5- to 8-year-olds, and 6 mg/day in 8- to 12-year-olds.
4. In a severe case (fever, bloody stool, or abdominal distention), consider giving an antibiotic (azithromycin 10 mg/kg per day up to 500 mg/day for 3 days).
5. Consider using a probiotic agent such as *Lactobacillus acidophilus* for prevention and treatment. This is available over the counter with dosing of one tablet or capsule a day for children younger than 2 years of age and two capsules a day for children older than 2 years of age. Capsules can be opened and placed into food or drink for children unable or unwilling to take pills.

Medications

Most children can chew tablets once their first molars are present (15 months of age). Before that time, chewable medications or tablets can be crushed between two spoons and mixed with food. Liquid medications add excess weight and the potential for leaks; they should be carried in powder form only for children younger than 6 months of age. Medication can be camouflaged in a food such as instant pudding.

Emergency Veterinary Medicine

Animals may be used for support or companionship in the wilderness. Canines are often used in search and rescue, as well as disaster recovery teams. The ideal treatment is always to seek qualified veterinary care as soon as possible; the information in this chapter is intended to be useful when a veterinarian is not available.

Wild animals may stalk support animals. Wild (and occasionally domestic) animals are most likely to respond adversely if

- Approached too closely
- Handled improperly
- They are fearful for their lives
- Their young are approached too closely
- They are cornered or otherwise threatened
- They are protecting their territory
- They are breeding
- They are wounded or ill (diseased)
- They are being fed by hand

PRETRIP ANIMAL HEALTH CONSIDERATIONS

Carry proper health certificates of travel. Perform a proper pretrip examination. Condition and train animals for the expected environment and terrain. Do not travel with immature animals. Dogs should be at least 1 year old. Llamas and horses should be older than 3 years. Well-conditioned and trained horses, mules, burros, and dogs can carry approximately 30% of their body weight. Llamas usually carry only 25% of their body weight.

- For normal vital statistics of trek animals see Table 63.1.
- For equipment and supplies for large trek animals, see Box 63.1.
- For first-aid kit for canines, see Box 63.2.

HORSES, MULES, AND DONKEYS

A tetanus booster should have been given within the past year. Vaccinate against rabies if appropriate. Encephalomyelitis vaccine should be used in endemic areas. Determine internal parasite levels by fecal flotation, and use medication if needed to reduce the parasite burden. Feet should be trimmed and shod properly at least 2 weeks and not more than 4 weeks before a trek begins. Use sole pads if sharp rocky terrain is expected.

LLAMAS

Tetanus immunization should be current within the past 6 months. Other basic immunizations should include *Clostridium perfringens*

Table 63.1   Vital Statistics of Trek Animals

| ANIMAL | BODY WEIGHT | | HEART RATE (BEATS/MIN) | RESPIRATORY RATE (BREATHS/MIN) | BODY TEMPERATURE | | WEIGHT CARRIED BY WELL-CONDITIONED ANIMAL* | |
	kg	lb			°C	°F	kg	lb
Horse	360–540	800–1200	28–44	12–24	37.2–38.0	99.0–101.0	110–136	240–300
Mule	275–540	600–1200	28–44	12–24	37.2–38.0	99.0–101.0	82–136	180–300
Donkey	136–275	300–600	28–44	12–24	37.2–38.0	99.0–101.0	40–82	90–180
Llama	136–200	300–450	60–90	10–30	37.2–38.7	99.0–101.8	34–50	75–110
Dog	9–45	20–100	65–120	15–30	37.5–38.6	99.5–102.5	3–14	6–30
Camel	400–550	880–1200	40–50	5–12	36.4–42.0	97.5–107.6	225	500
Elephant	2300–3700	5000–8000	25–35	4–6	36.0–37.0	97.5–99.0	900	2000
Yak	1000	2200	60–80	12–36	37.8–39.2	100.5–102.5	235	550
Ox	499–1361	1000–3000	60–80	12–36	37.8–39.2	100.5–102.5	235	550

*Sustained trekking for 24 to 40 km (15 to 25 miles) per day on moderately difficult trails. The weight includes tack. Animals in training should be expected to carry only one-half to two-thirds of this weight.

BOX 63.1   Equipment and Supplies for Large Animals in the Wilderness

Lip twitch
Battery-operated hair clippers
Wire cutters
Hoof care equipment: hoof file, nail pullers, shoe pullers, hoof trimmers, hoof knife, hoof testers, clinch cutter, hammer
Topical disinfectant such as chlorhexidine gluconate 2% to 4% or povidone-iodine 5% scrub
Bandaging material: gauze pads, gauze roll, cast padding, nonadhesive dressing, adhesive tape, VetRap, Elastikon, fiberglass casting tape; splinting material (wood boards, PVC pipe)
Skin stapler and/or tissue glue
Suture material: monofilament and multifilament, absorbable and nonabsorbable, sizes, 3-0 to No. 2
Activated charcoal preparation (ToxiBan); must be administered via nasogastric (NG) tube
Sterile nonlatex surgical gloves
Lidocaine 2% with epinephrine
Sterile disposable syringes: 1 to 60 mL
Sterile needles: 22 to 18 gauge
IV catheter: 14 gauge
Sterile surgical pack
    Needle holders
    Thumb forceps
    Suture scissors
    Mayo scissors
    Metzenbaum scissors
    Hemostats
    Scalpel handle (no. 3)
    Scalpel blades (no. 10)
Tubing
    Silastic, 1-cm outside diameter, 10 cm (4 in.) long, for nasal tube
    Large-animal tracheostomy tube
    Large-animal stomach tube, 1-cm inside diameter, 300 cm (120 in.) long
    Funnel (plastic) to fit into stomach tube
Thermometer
Stethoscope
IV, Intravenous.

toxoid, types C and D, within the past 6 months and vaccinations against leptospirosis and rabies if entering an endemic area. Toenails should have been trimmed within the past 2 months. Ova levels should be checked, but usually treatment with an antihelmintic (ivermectin 0.2 mg/kg subcutaneously or fenbendazole 5 mg/kg orally) is desirable within the previous 2 months.

BOX 63.2   Canine First-Aid Kit

Information card containing veterinarian, emergency clinic, and
    national poison control numbers as well as the dog's weight for
    medical dosing to facilitate phone consultation
Commercial muzzle or length of fabric to improvise a muzzle
Hemostat
Thumb forceps (e.g., Brown-Adson forceps)
Battery-operated hair clipper
Wire cutter
Toenail clipper (canine)
Topical disinfectant, such as 2% to 4% chlorhexidine solution or 5%
    povidone-iodine solution
Bandaging material, such as gauze pads and rolls, cast padding,
    nonadhesive dressing, adhesive tape, VetRap, Elastikon,
    fiberglass casting tape
Skin stapler and/or tissue glue
Activated charcoal preparation (ToxiBan)
Sterile nonlatex examination gloves
Lidocaine 0.2% with sterile syringes and needles for injection
Apomorphine (3 mg/mL injectable given at a dose of 0.03 mg/kg
    IV) and 3% hydrogen peroxide for emesis induction
Prescription medications and dosages (see Table 63.4)
Properly fitted booties to protect feet
Pill gun if it is difficult to administer pills to your dog

DOGS

Immunize dogs against canine distemper, canine adenovirus,
leptospirosis, and rabies. Check for internal parasites and fleas.
Bathe with a pyrethrin insecticide–containing shampoo, and carry
a flea-tick-lice powder. Dogs should be on a heartworm preventive
medication if traveling in a mosquito-endemic area. Because external
parasites, particularly ticks, can be carriers of multiple diseases, a
flea and tick preventive (e.g., Frontline Plus with fipronil) is also
highly recommended and can be purchased from a veterinarian
before the trip.

Canine Physiology and Physical Examination
Temperature
- Dogs' temperatures are measured rectally.
- Normal range is approximately 37°C to 39°C (98.6 to 102.5°F).
  Exercising dogs may safely reach temperatures of 40.5°C (105°F),
  but a core body temperature higher than that risks inducing
  heatstroke.
- Dogs thermoregulate by panting rather than sweating, so
  any condition that affects their ability to pant effectively can
  impair their ability to cool themselves and predispose to heat
  stress.

Cardiac Evaluation
- Normal heart rate for adult dogs is 70 to 180 beats/min in small dogs and 60 to 140 beats/min in larger dogs.
- To evaluate rhythm, it is important to check an arterial pulse while auscultating the heart to verify that each heart sound is matched by a strong pulsation.

Mucous Membrane Color
- Normal mucous membranes in the dog should be pink and slightly moist.
- Anemia or vasoconstrictive shock can cause pale mucous membranes.
- Vasodilation from systemic inflammatory states and hyperthermia can cause red mucous membranes.
- Dry mucous membranes should raise suspicion for dehydration.

Capillary Refill Time
- Normal capillary refill time (CRT) in dogs is 1 to 2 seconds.
- Even recently deceased dogs can have a normal CRT, so this should be interpreted in relation to pulses, respiratory rate, gingiva color, and other clinical parameters.
- A CRT longer than 2 seconds indicates poor perfusion or peripheral vasoconstriction.

Pulse
- The easiest location to check a dog's pulse is in the femoral triangle of the groin just anterior to the proximal femur.
- The femoral pulse in most dogs is palpable down to a systolic blood pressure of approximately 60 mm Hg.
- The pedal pulse on the cranial aspect of the foot just below the hock (ankle) is generally palpable at a systolic pressure of 80 mm Hg, although the clinician's experience plays a major role in ability to appreciate the pulse at this location.
- Bounding pulses indicate a hyperdynamic state, whereas weak pulses correlate with decreased cardiac contractility, peripheral vasoconstriction, or decreased blood pressure.

Hydration Status
- In a hydrated dog, the skin can be gently pulled upward and when released immediately springs back into normal position.
- With mild to moderate dehydration, the skin returns to normal position more slowly; with severe dehydration, it may remain standing in a ridge.

EMERGENCY RESTRAINT
Know how to create a halter tie (Fig. 63.1) and a temporary rope halter (Fig. 63.2).

For horses, mules, and burros, if the animal is down and entangled in rope, wire, or bushes, approach it from its back and keep the head held down until it can be extricated. Stay out of reach of the

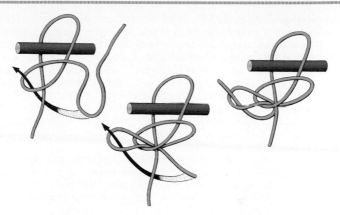

FIGURE 63.1 Sequence of steps to create a halter tie.

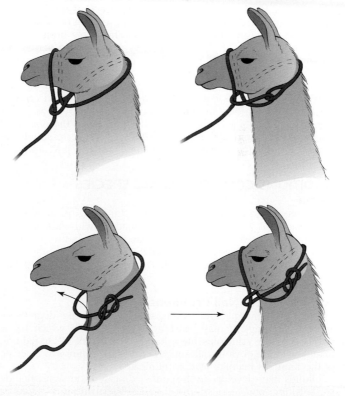

FIGURE 63.2 Temporary rope halters.

fore and hind limbs. If the animal is standing, stand close to the left shoulder. If examining the feet and legs of a standing animal, keep your head above the lower body line to avoid having the animal reach forward and strike with a rear limb. You can "ear" the animal by grasping one or both ears. Stand at the left shoulder and grasp the halter or lead rope with the left hand. Place the right hand palm down with the fingers together and the thumb extended, on top of the neck. Slide the hand up the neck until the thumb and fingers surround the base of the ear. Squeeze tightly, but do not twist the ear. Be prepared to move with the horse while maintaining a firm grip.

For llamas, one or two people should stand on the side opposite any limb to be lifted, or the animal should be placed next to a tree or large rock to prevent it from moving away. The limb should be firmly grasped. If a llama refuses to get up, the rear limbs may be pulled out behind it. If it still refuses to rise, an injury or illness should be suspected. Llamas can be "eared" in a manner like that used for horses. Control spitting by draping a cloth over the animal's nose and tucking the top around the nose piece of the halter.

For dogs, if a mild painful medical procedure must be performed, the head and mouth should be secured. The dog's body can be securely held against the handler's body by reaching across the back of the dog and grasping the base of the neck while pulling the opposite shoulder with the elbow toward the handler. The other hand should tuck the dog's head under the handler's arm. Alternatively, a muzzle can be constructed from a nylon cord or even a shoelace. A loop should be formed with an overhand knot on one side. The loop is placed over the muzzle of the dog, with the knot on top, and tightened. The ends of the loop should be wrapped around the muzzle, crossed beneath the jaw, and tied behind the ears.

CONDITIONS COMMON TO ALL SPECIES
Trauma
Hair or wool should be trimmed from the margins of wounds before treatment or suturing to prevent matting with exudate. The skin may be sutured with any suture material suitable for humans. Antibiotics are not necessary unless vital structures such as synovial or serosal membranes are exposed. Therapy for rope burns is like that for human burns.

Foot, Hoof, and Nail Problems
Foot and limb trauma are accompanied by varying degrees of lameness (limping). It may be difficult to establish which leg is painful, but the principles are like evaluation of such pain in humans, with the obvious differences of two extra limbs to evaluate and the animal's inability to communicate.

Cellulitis may develop on the limbs or body. The signs include heat, swelling, and redness, and they are the same in all species, as is therapy.

Therapy for foot injuries includes providing drainage of infected lesions, disinfection, and protection of exposed sensitive structures. Antibiotics are not indicated for most wounds unless a joint surface is exposed. It may be necessary to bandage the foot to provide protection while in camp and to fashion special shoes or boots to keep an animal functioning on the trail. Special booties are available commercially for dogs, but a temporary moccasin may be constructed from soft leather (such as the leather used by crafts people to make moccasins) or duct tape.

Hyperthermia (Heat Stress, Heat Exhaustion)
Clinical Signs
- Signs may vary according to species and the stage of hyperthermia, but all affected animals have increased heart and respiratory rates, usually accompanied by open-mouth breathing.
- Rectal temperatures may vary from 41.1°C to 43.3°C (106°F to 110°F).
- Horses, mules, burros, and llamas sweat in the early stages of hyperthermia, but sweating may cease if the animal becomes severely dehydrated.
- Sweating is evident in horses but imperceptible in llamas because most sweating occurs on the ventral abdomen in what is known as the *thermal window*, where the fibers are less dense and the fiber length is short.
- Dogs cool themselves by evaporation of respiratory fluids while panting. The mouth is held open, and the tongue lolls from the mouth. The respiratory rate increases from a normal of 30 breaths/min up to 200 to 400 breaths/min. Moisture may be observed dripping from the tongue. As dehydration intensifies, salivation and dripping may slow or cease.
- Hypotension causes hypoxemia of the brain, resulting in dullness, restlessness, and incoordination. Hypoxemia may lead to convulsions and collapse. The shift of blood from the gastrointestinal tract may cause decreased motility and the potential for ileus and tympany.
- Signs of colic in horses and llamas (kicking at the belly, looking back at the side, treading, attempting to lie down and roll) may be noted.

Treatment
1. Cessation of excessive muscular activity may be all that is necessary if hyperthermia is mild.
2. If streams or lakes are nearby, the animal can be walked into the water and water splashed on its underbelly.
3. Contingencies for hyperthermia are part of all plans for capture operations for wildlife translocation and reintroduction projects. Water is carried for cooling and IV fluids to deal with heat stress.
4. Cold water enemas are the most effective and rapid way to cool the body of a large animal. Caution should be used when

cooling a dog. The dog should be cooled to a rectal temperature of 39.4°C (103°F) within 30 to 60 minutes.
5. Overcooling or cooling too rapidly can be fatal.

Tick Paralysis
Clinical Signs
- Signs may not appear for 5 to 7 days following the tick bite. Initially there is paresis of the legs; progressing to unsteady gait; knuckling; ataxia; and, ultimately, flaccid paralysis of the hind limbs. Loss of motor function ascends cranially, causing paralysis of the fore limbs.
- Pain perception remains.
- Even with paralysis of the limbs, the animal is bright and alert and able to eat and drink if feed is placed within reach.
- Ultimately paralysis involves the neck, throat, and face, causing difficulties in chewing, swallowing, and breathing. Respiratory failure is the cause of death.

Diagnosis
The sequence of clinical signs is the only sure method of diagnosis unless the tick or ticks are found. That may be quite difficult on an animal the size of a horse. Differential diagnoses should include encephalitides, head or spinal trauma, and hyperthermia.

Management
1. No antidote is available for the toxin.
2. The offending tick or ticks must be removed, which may produce a dramatic response. Look in the lightly haired areas of the axillary space, perineum, and behind the ears if tick paralysis is suspected.

Skunk Odor Removal
In addition to the obvious odor, skunk musk is nauseating to some people and may also cause retching in dogs. If a person or pet is sprayed in the face, the musk is an irritant that causes conjunctivitis, keratitis, lacrimation, temporary impairment of vision, glossitis, slobbering, and foaming at the mouth.

Management of Odor Removal
1. Quick flushing of the face and eyes with copious quantities of cold water will restore vision and minimize persistent irritation.
2. If conjunctivitis persists, instill contact lens solution or a drop of olive oil into the conjunctival sac.
3. The objective of odor removal is to wash away the offending oily liquid and neutralize the compound.
4. Simple bathing will not eliminate the odor, which is pungent even in a remarkably dilute concentration.
5. One of the most effective oxidizing agents is a dilute solution of household bleach (Clorox); however, this may bleach

clothing and hair and is harsh on the skin of people and animals.

6. Skunk musk is alkaline, so mild acidic solutions may be at least partially effective and will reduce the pungency of the odor. Tomato juice, white vinegar, and ammonia in water have been described but may not eliminate the odor.

7. A formula that is mentioned most frequently is a combination of hydrogen peroxide (347 mL, 3%), water (1 cup [237 mL]), baking soda (sodium bicarbonate, ¼ cup [60 mL]), and a dish detergent (1 tablespoon [15 mL]).
   a. Mix the peroxide with the water and then add the baking soda and shampoo.
   b. Mix and pour into a squirt bottle/sprayer.
   c. This solution may be sprayed onto a dog or horse but should not be sprayed directly into the eyes or nose.
   d. The solution should be allowed to remain on the coat for 10 minutes while being worked into the coat with a gloved hand.

8. Washable clothing should be washed with a strong soap or heavy-duty detergent. In a permanent camp, items that cannot be washed (shoes, leather goods) may be buried in sandy soil for a few days. The soil will adsorb the odorous chemicals.

9. Several commercial products are available that have been formulated to eliminate the skunk odor:
   a. Neutroleum alpha is nontoxic and may be used on clothing and pets.
   b. Skunk-off is nontoxic and nonirritating, even to mucous membranes, and safe to use on pets and clothing.
   c. Odormute is available in granular form and easy to transport. It is nontoxic and may be applied to pets and clothing after being dissolved in water.
   d. Summer's Eve douche is an effective product to neutralize skunk spray odor.

All the products mentioned are for use on pets or fabric and not recommended for use directly on people. The trek physician is the only one qualified to make such a recommendation. However, washing with soap and copious amounts of cold water will wash away considerable musk.

Plant Poisoning
Certain highly toxic plants that grow in wilderness areas of the United States should be recognized as potentially harmful to pack animals (Table 63.2).

Lightning Strike
During an electrical storm, animals on the trek should be positioned in the safest environment possible, away from tall trees and exposed hills. Llamas may be encouraged to lie down in a small ravine or a depression or against a rock face, with the head tied close to the ground. A picket line stake may be used for the tie-down. Avoid tying an animal to a tree; using a small bush for a tie-down

Table 63.2	Poisonous Plants That May Affect Horses or Llamas on Trek					
COMMON NAME	SCIENTIFIC NAME	POISONOUS PRINCIPLE	SIGNS OF POISONING	HABITAT	SPECIES	THERAPY*
False hellebore, corn lily	Veratrum californicum	Alkaloids	Vomiting, salivation, convulsions, fast irregular pulse	High mountains, meadows	Llama	Symptomatic
Death camas, sandcorn	Zigadenus spp.	Alkaloids	Foaming at mouth, convulsions, ataxia, vomiting, fast weak pulse	Hillsides, fields, meadows, in spring of year	Horse, llama	Symptomatic
Water hemlock	Cicuta douglasii	Resin	Frothing at mouth, muscle twitching, convulsions, death in 15–30 min	Standing or running water, obligate aquatic	Horse, llama	Symptomatic
Nightshade	Solanum species	Alkaloidal glycoside, solanine	Vomiting, weakness, groaning	Ubiquitous	Horse, llama	Symptomatic
Jimsonweed	Datura stramonium	Alkaloid, atropine	Dry mucous membranes, dilated pupils, mania	Waste places	Horse, llama	Parasympathomimetics

Tobacco, tree tobacco	Nicotiana spp.	Alkaloid, nicotine	Stimulation of CNS, then depression; sweating, muscle twitching, convulsions	Waste places	Horse, llama	Symptomatic
Lupine, bluebonnet	Lupinus spp.	Alkaloid	CNS depression, dyspnea, muscle twitching, ataxia, frothing, convulsions	Ubiquitous	Horse, llama	Symptomatic
Dogbane, Indian hemp	Apocynum cannabinum	Cardioactive glycoside (similar to digitoxin)	Dyspnea, cardiac arrhythmias, agonal convulsions, vomiting, diarrhea	Ubiquitous	Horse, llama	Symptomatic
Oleander	Nerium oleander	Same as for dogbane	Same as for dogbane	Ornamental	Horse, llama	Symptomatic, gastrctomy
Castor bean	Ricinus communis	Ricin, water solution	Anaphylactic shock, diarrhea	Ornamental	Horse, llama	Treat for shock; fluids
Rhododendron	Rhododendron species	Andromedotoxin glycoside	Vomiting, colic, severe depression	Shrubs in meadows and moist places	Llama	Activated charcoal, time

*In most cases of poisoning from ingestion of poisonous plants, no specific antidote exists. Victims are treated symptomatically. The critical factor is to empty the digestive tract of the plant material with cathartics, parasympathomimetic stimulation, and enemas. Activated charcoal, given orally, may be of value.

CNS, Central nervous system.

may be a safer alternative. Horses are more difficult to deal with because it is impossible to get them to lie down unless they are specially trained to do so. Get them into a ravine, a depressed area, or near a rock face.

If the strike is witnessed and the heart has stopped beating, chest compression (cardiac massage) may be performed if it is determined that it is safe for a human to be in the open. With the animal in lateral recumbency, pull the fore limb as far cranially as possible and press on the chest wall just caudal to the triceps muscle. Cardiac massage may be required for several minutes.

Snakebite

Llamas and, to a lesser extent, young horses are curious animals and may stick their noses out to investigate strange animals in their area. Thus it is not uncommon for an animal to be struck on the nose. Leg bites may occur in any animal.

Clinical Signs

- Venom injection results in pronounced swelling in the bite, beginning 1 to 3 hours after the bite.
- The most serious consequence of being bitten on the nose is swelling that occludes the nostrils, making it virtually impossible for horses and llamas to breathe.
- Dogs are not obligate nasal breathers, but the effects of a bite may be more severe in them than in the larger animals.
- A rattlesnake bite on the nose is an emergency.

Management

1. A 10-cm (3.9-in.) segment of a flexible plastic tube 1 cm (0.4 in.) in diameter should be in the first aid kit of the trek. This should be inserted into a nostril before any swelling occurs.
2. The swelling will be in the nostril, and the tube will prevent occlusion of the nostril, providing a passage for air. It is not possible to insert a tube after the swelling has developed. If swelling has already developed, the only lifesaving procedure is a tracheotomy.
3. *Do not* attempt to cut the skin and suck out the venom with your mouth. This procedure is not effective.
4. The only specific treatment for pit viper envenomation is the administration of antivenom. The same product used for humans is used in animals.
5. One to three vials should be administered intravenously once signs of envenomation have appeared.

Choke

"Choke" in animals usually refers to lodging of food or other objects in the esophagus. The signs of choke may be alarming, but an animal will rarely die unless feed is regurgitated and inhaled into the lungs. Choke is most often caused by overly rapid ingestion of pellets and/or grain. Importantly, animals must be accustomed to any supplemental feed to be used on the trek. Ingestion may be slowed by placing rock pebbles in the container used to feed the animal, causing it to separate the rocks from the feed. Metallic or wooden objects will rarely be swallowed. Llamas and horses are too fastidious in their eating habits to consume such objects.

Retching is the principal sign of choke, as the animal attempts to dislodge the mass. Choked animals can breathe, but they are obviously in distress. Saliva may flow from the mouth, and the animal may cough up particles of the material (grain or pellets). It may be possible to feel a mass on the left side of the neck if the obstruction occurs in the cervical area. Peristaltic waves may be observed moving up and down the left side of the neck. The mass may lodge anywhere along the course of the esophagus, but generally it lies within the chest and is not visible externally.

Management

1. Water may be offered, but feed should be withheld until the problem has corrected itself.
2. Palpate along the lower neck to determine if a bulge is present. If so, gently massage it to determine if it can be moved.
3. Sometimes moderate exercise may cause the object to move toward the stomach.
4. In some cases, passage of a stomach tube and application of gentle pressure may push the mass into the stomach.
5. Medication (acepromazine, 0.05 mg/kg IV, or xylazine, 0.05 to 0.25 mg/kg IV for a llama and 1.1 mg/kg IV for a horse) may be necessary to relax esophageal spasm.

Wound Dressing and Bandaging

The principles of wound dressing are basically the same as for humans, to provide uniform pressure over a variably shaped surface.

The foot requires special consideration. When dressing a foot wound, make certain that the spaces between the digits of dogs or llamas are padded with cotton. The easiest bandage to apply is a Vetrap elastic bandage that conforms to the odd shape. If a severe foot wound occurs while trekking in the backcountry, additional protection may be necessary to allow the animal to continue the journey. A sheet of pliable leather of the type used to construct moccasins may be a useful addition to the veterinary medical kit. The dressed foot is placed in the center of the sheet, and then the leather is gathered up around the pastern and held in place by duct tape or another bandage, to form a roughly shaped boot.

Cardiopulmonary Resuscitation

Rescue Breathing

The procedure is different than that employed in humans because mouth-to-mouth breathing cannot be performed on an adult llama or horse. Mouth-to-mouth breathing could be performed on a dog by clamping the mouth and lips shut and breathing through the nostrils. A llama or horse should be placed in lateral recumbency, preferably on the right side. Stand at the animal's withers (top of the shoulder) and reach across the body to grasp and lift the arch of the rib cage. This maneuver will flatten the diaphragm and expand the chest, producing inspiration. Do not press in this same area to force expiration because this will put pressure on the stomach and possibly cause regurgitation. Instead, press over the heart area just above the elbow and caudal to the muscles of the upper limb. The rate for the horse or llama is 10 to 15 breaths per minute. Rescue breathing in the dog is performed by compressing the chest at the widest segment of the thorax at a rate of 20 to 30 breaths per minute.

Cardiac massage may be performed by placing the llama or horse on its right side if not already there. Have an assistant pull the upper foreleg forward and press the chest in the area vacated by pulling the leg forward. Kneel next to the bottom of the chest. Position the heels of both hands against the chest approximately 6 in (15.2 cm) above the sternum, with the fingers directed toward the spine. Press firmly with the arms held straight and release quickly. Repeat the movement every second. After 15 compressions, check for a pulse in the saphenous artery on the medial aspect of the stifle in a llama, or listen for the heartbeat with a stethoscope. After 15 heart compressions, administer five cycles of rescue breathing, as described previously. It is futile to continue cardiac massage if no oxygen is available to the heart or the general circulation. Massage must be continued until heartbeat returns and the animal begins to breathe, or when signs indicate that the animal is dead (pupils dilated, no response to touching the cornea).

For a dog, cardiac massage is performed in lateral recumbency in the type of dogs that are likely to be on a trek (a small dog or one that is round-chested is placed on its back and compression is exerted over the sternum).

West Nile Viral Encephalitis
Transmission is via mosquito bites (*Culex*, *Aedes*, *Anopheles* spp.) and possibly other blood-sucking insects. West Nile viral disease has recently become endemic in the United States.

Signs in Horses, Llamas, and Humans
The incubation period is 6 to 10 days. Although most infections are subclinical in horses and humans, 10% of affected individuals develop fever and the encephalitic signs of depression, ataxia, and paresis, particularly of the hind limbs. More advanced signs include head shaking, incessant chewing, paralysis of the lower lip or tongue, severe ataxia, ascending paralysis, and terminal recumbency.

Management
Two vaccines are approved for use in horses in the United States, but have also been used in camelids (West Nile-Innovator killed and Recombitek live). If a trek is planned for an area where West

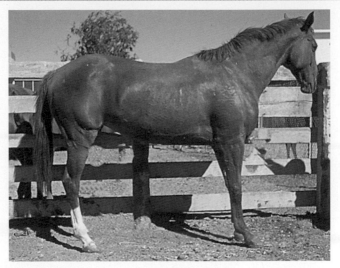

FIGURE 63.3   Stance of a Horse With Laminitis. Front and hind legs are extended forward.

Nile virus is endemic and when mosquitoes are prevalent, trek horses and llamas should be vaccinated (two injections 1 month apart).

UNIQUE DISORDERS OF HORSES, MULES, AND DONKEYS
Laminitis (Founder)
Clinical Signs
- Laminitis usually develops on both forefeet, but rear feet may also be affected in severe cases.
- The horse shifts its center of gravity to the hind limbs to minimize pressure on the forefeet, standing with the hind limbs forward under the body and the forelimbs extended in front of the body (Fig. 63.3).
- The feet are warm or hot to palpation, and there is a pounding digital artery pulse. The horse is reluctant to move.

Management
1. Prevention or minimizing the effects of the inciting causes of laminitis is vitally important.
2. Once clinical signs occur, the objectives of treatment are to eliminate the predisposing factors, decrease inflammation, and maintain or reestablish blood flow to the laminae.
3. If laminitis is the result of a digestive upset, it is imperative to administer a cathartic (magnesium sulfate [Epsom salts], 1 kg in 4 L of water via nasogastric tube).

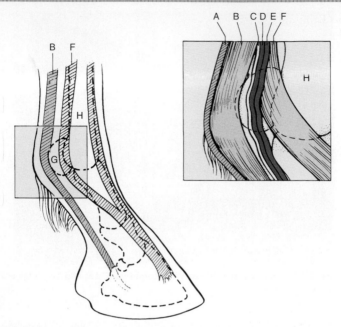

FIGURE 63.4 Diagram of the Anatomy of the Equine Fetlock. A, Skin. **B,** Flexor tendons. **C,** Volar nerve. **D,** Palmar digital artery. **E,** Digital vein. **F,** Suspensory ligament. **G,** Sesamoid bone. **H,** Metacarpal bone (cannon).

4. Phenylbutazone, 6 mg/kg IV daily, should be administered to relieve pain so that the horse will move.
5. Acepromazine maleate, 0.04 mg/kg IM every 6 hours, is used as a vasodilator to enhance blood flow to the laminae.
6. In acute laminitis, the feet are warm or hot, so the inclination would be to soak the feet in cold water. This is contraindicated because the goal is to increase circulation to the foot.
7. Mild exercise is an important aid in preventing damage to the laminae. The horse should be exercised slowly on soft ground for 10 to 15 minutes every hour for 12 to 24 hours, and then exercise should be stopped. Even slow walking may be quite painful.
8. A low volar nerve block relieves pain and inhibits vascular constriction within the foot. This is accomplished by palpating the pulsating artery on the posterolateral aspect of the fetlock (Fig. 63.4). The nerve lies posterior to the artery. With a 20- to 22-gauge needle, 3 mL of 2% lidocaine is injected over each nerve. It may be necessary to repeat nerve blocks two or three times daily for several days. Corticosteroids are contraindicated.

Saddle, Cinch, and Rigging Sores

If the lesion is rested and treated as inflamed tissue, complete healing may occur. However, if the saddle is reapplied, it will overlie a lump that is subject to abrasion. The injury can extend through the dermis, resulting in severe ulceration. Cinch and rigging sores are usually caused by friction, leading to blister formation.

Clinical Signs

Hot, tender swellings are the primary signs of acute saddle sores. The hair or epidermis may be rubbed off. General sensitivity over the back is usually caused by muscle soreness.

Treatment

1. Prevention is better than treatment. Proper pads or blankets must be selected for each horse.
2. Upon arrival at a rest area, the girth should be slowly loosened at intervals of 10 to 15 minutes to prevent rapid flow of blood into ischemic areas.
3. Once a sore has developed, the horse must be rested or the tack changed to eliminate pressure or friction on the lesion.
4. Holes are often cut in pads to accommodate a saddle sore, but spot pressure at the ring edge may be as detrimental as the original cause of the saddle sore. Keep tack cleaned and in good repair.
5. When the saddle is removed, cold water poured over the back for 15 minutes may minimize swelling.

Myopathy

Exertional myopathies of horses vary from simple muscle soreness, through the "tying up" syndrome (like charley horses in humans), to paralytic myoglobinuria (rhabdomyolysis, azoturia).

Clinical Signs

- Mild muscle soreness is characterized by alterations in gait that indicate muscle weakness.
- As severity increases, the gait becomes progressively altered until the horse is in obvious pain and reluctant to move.
- The horse has an anxious expression and may sweat excessively.
- Affected muscles are painful to palpation and may be swollen.
- Skin temperature over the muscle may be elevated.
- Myoglobinuria may be observed in moderate to severe cases and should prompt resting or treating the horse.

Treatment

1. Rest is paramount in all cases.
2. A rider may have difficulty differentiating the pain associated with myopathy from that seen with colic until the horse can lie down, look at its side, or kick at its belly). It is disastrous to force the severely myopathic horse to walk, as is done with a suspected case of colic.

3. If there is doubt, the horse should not be exercised.
4. Horses in inaccessible locations should not be walked out until all possible recovery has taken place.
5. Horses with mild muscle soreness may improve if walked slowly, but rest from ride exertion is the primary recommended therapy.

Dehydration
The horse must have an adequate amount (37.9 to 56.8 L [10 to 15 gallons]) of water each day during a trek.

Clinical Signs
- Signs of mild dehydration are low urine output, dry mouth, and mild loss of skin elasticity.
- More severe dehydration is characterized by marked loss of skin elasticity. The eyes become sunken. Weakness, fever, and a weak pulse may be observed.
- Sweating is not possible, even with elevated body temperature.
- Shock ensues if dehydration is left untreated.

Treatment
1. During 3 hours of hard work, a 450-kg (992.1-lb) horse may lose as much as 45 L (11.9 gallons) of fluid. The horse should be allowed to drink along the trail if water is available. Small amounts of cool but not cold water should be offered.
2. If the horse refuses to drink, gastric intubation may be indicated. Fluid is also absorbed from the colon; thus enemas (10 to 20 L [2.6 to 5.3 gallons] of water) are effective in rehydration.
3. Electrolyte replacement is encouraged, but for the usual case of dehydration it is not critical. Packaged electrolytes are available in veterinary supply shops.
4. Heat stress usually accompanies dehydration, so cooling (such as shade or a water bath) is important.
5. Administration of IV fluids, if available, is routine therapy.
  Camels are uniquely adapted to desert conditions. They can survive a week without water. Optimally a camel should be watered daily, just as are horses and llamas. Camels do not store water but conserve it by enduring a diurnal fluctuation of body temperature, from a normal 37.0°C (98.6°F) up to 42°C (107.6°F). The body acts as a heat sink during the heat of the day, thus conserving vital water that would otherwise be lost through evaporative cooling. During the cool desert night, the heat is dissipated by conduction. Camels can concentrate urine to a syrup consistency to avoid water loss through urination. Fecal pellets are passed that are dry enough to be used for fuel immediately following defecation.

Exhausted Horse Syndrome
The term *exhausted horse syndrome* (EHS) was coined to describe a complex metabolic disease occurring when horses are pushed beyond their endurance limits.

Clinical Signs

- Movements are lethargic, head held low.
- Facial grimacing and corneal glazing are present.
- Anorexia is typical, and frequently the horse is not inclined to drink even though dehydrated.
- Heart rate, respirations, and temperature are elevated. (Heart rates of 150 beats/min are not uncommon after a grueling climb. With 10 to 15 minutes of rest, the heart rate of a conditioned horse should drop below 60 beats/min, whereas tachycardia and tachypnea persist in the exhausted horse.) Auscultation of the thorax may reveal moist rales and, in extreme cases, frank pulmonary edema.
- Severe dehydration is the most consistent sign of EHS. (See signs described under Dehydration.)
- Horses suffering from EHS are prone to colic, which also may occur independently. (See later.)

Treatment

Rest, rehydration, and electrolyte supplementation are the keys to recovery.

Synchronous Diaphragmatic Flutter

Synchronous diaphragmatic flutter (SDF) is a clinical sign observed in endurance horses while on long-distance rides and may be seen on an expedition. SDF is defined as a spasmodic contraction of the diaphragm synchronous with the heartbeat. It is not life-threatening but indicates a mild to serious metabolic condition that may be or may become life-threatening. Overexertion with excessive sweating produces metabolic alterations. The development of SDF at any point on a trek should be ample reason to prevent the horse from going farther until the metabolic alteration is resolved.

Clinical Signs

SDF may develop after 32.2 to 48.3 km (20 to 30 mi) of riding. The primary sign is spasmodic contraction in the flank area. The "thump" is easily felt by light palpation in the flank area. A person who auscultates the heart while holding a hand over the dorsocaudal rib area can tell that diaphragmatic contraction is synchronous with the heartbeat. SDF may be the only clinical sign noted, or it may be part of EHS.

Treatment

Rest and rehydration are required.

Colic

Colic is the clinical manifestation of abdominal pain, usually the result of a gastrointestinal disorder. The most likely inciting causes on a trek are overeating of nonregular forages, ingestion of poisonous plants, or exhaustion.

Clinical Signs

Horses express colic by looking back at one side, stamping the feet, getting up and down, rolling, and pressing the head against trees or rocks. The pulse rate may exceed 100 beats/min with severe pain. The conjunctival membranes are congested and cyanotic.

Treatment

1. Mild obstructions may be relieved by hydration and administration of a cathartic.
2. Cold water enemas may stimulate sluggish intestinal peristalsis and relieve impaction of the small (terminal) colon.
3. For pain and spasms, give flunixin meglumine, 0.6 mg/kg IM bid.
4. Walk the horse to prevent it from lying down and rolling, which may result in torsion of the intestine.

UNIQUE PROBLEMS OF DOGS
Laryngeal Paralysis

This disease occurs in older medium- and large-breed dogs, particularly Labrador retrievers. The problem is due to degeneration of the recurrent laryngeal nerve that innervates the intrinsic muscles of the larynx.

Clinical Signs

- Respiratory stridor
- Hoarse bark
- Inability to thermoregulate effectively by panting. Because the animal cannot dissipate heat, heat stroke can result.

Treatment

Prevent and manage heat and exertional stress by keeping the dog cool and calm. If the dog is in extremis, endotracheal intubation or tracheostomy can be performed in addition to active cooling.

Gastric Dilatation and Volvulus ("Bloat")

Gastric dilatation and volvulus occur most commonly in older, large- and giant-breed dogs, particularly deep-chest breeds such as Great Danes. The stomach twists such that both the esophagus and pyloric outflow become occluded. The stomach distends with gas and stretches until it severely impedes blood flow, with resultant shock and gastric necrosis. This condition can be fatal within 6 hours of onset if untreated, and mortality rates are high even with appropriate treatment.

Clinical Signs

- Inability to swallow or to vomit; attempts to vomit produce only saliva
- Progressive distention of the abdomen
- Shock

Treatment

1. Arrange emergent evacuation for definitive surgical treatment.
2. Place an orogastric tube to decompress the stomach or, if unable, decompress the stomach with a large-bore IV catheter. This procedure should be attempted only in situations where veterinary care is not immediately available because of the risk of lacerating abdominal organs.
   a. The catheter is inserted about a hands' width behind the last rib in the center of the lateral body wall.
   b. The operator will hear and smell gas escaping if the procedure is successful.
   c. This can be repeated multiple times if necessary while the animal is being transported.

Porcupine Quills

When dogs are brought into porcupine country, the risk for an encounter is great. Some dogs fail to learn from experience and are repeatedly quilled. The dog must have physical contact with the porcupine for the tail to introduce the quills. The muzzle and face are the usual sites of penetration, and a dog can be blinded by perforation of the eye.

The quills should be extracted, ideally with a pair of pliers, because retrograde barbs on the quill foster migration and abscess formation.

The process is painful, and sedation with diazepam, 0.2 to 1 mg/kg IM or IV, is indicated.

Grass Awns

Numerous species of grass awns ("foxtails") may become attached to the dog's hair coat or lodged in the external ear canal, nasal passage, conjunctival sac, or interdigital space.

Signs depend on the location of the foreign body. When it is within the ear canal, the dog paws at its ear and shakes its head. The head may be held tilted. Exudate may flow from the ear. Awns in the nostril cause sneezing and nasal exudate. Awns in the conjunctival sac cause lacrimation, photophobia, and corneal edema and ulceration. The dog paws at the eye. Awn penetration between the digits and at other locations through the skin is more difficult to diagnose because the awn may be at some distance from the fistula.

Awns must be removed physically. Sedation, topical anesthesia, or both may be necessary. Although topical ophthalmic anesthetics are desirable in the eye, lidocaine may be used in an emergency. A pair of small alligator forceps is most suitable for reaching into otherwise inaccessible places. An otoscope may be necessary to visualize awns in the nostril or ear canal. Instillation of an antiseptic or antibiotic ointment after removal of the awn is desirable.

Stinging Nettle Poisoning

Stinging nettle (*Urtica* spp.) is common along streams and lakes in wilderness areas. Leaves and stems are covered by harsh hairs, some of which have tiny ball tips that break off just before penetration. The specialized hairs are hollow. A base gland produces histamines and acetylcholine, which are injected into the victim.

Short-haired dogs that move through patches of stinging nettle are at risk for poisoning from the cumulative effect of thousands of minute injections of acetylcholine. Weakness, dyspnea, and muscle tremors are characteristic of the action of acetylcholine on peripheral nerves. Parasympathomimetic effects include salivation, diarrhea, tachycardia, and pupillary dilation. Atropine sulfate, 0.04 mg/kg SC, is a specific treatment.

MEDICATION PROCEDURES
A list of medications and indications for their use is provided in Table 63.3 for trek animals and Table 63.4 specifically for dogs. In the horse, intramuscular injections are given in the neck or rump. Subcutaneous injections are given by lifting a fold of skin just cranial to the scapula. IV injections are given in the jugular vein, which is easily distended along the jugular groove on the ventral aspect of the neck.

In the llama, intramuscular injections are given in the relatively hairless area at the back of the upper rear leg; this is done by standing against the body in front of the rear limb while facing the rear and reaching around the back of the animal to give the injection. Subcutaneous injections are given in the relatively hairless area of the caudal abdomen, just in front of the rear limb or by lifting a fold of skin just cranial to the scapula.

In the dog, intramuscular injections may be administered in the triceps muscles caudal to the shoulder or in the muscle masses on the upper rear limb. Subcutaneous injections are made by lifting a fold of loose skin on the neck near the withers. IV administration is via the jugular vein or the cephalic vein. For the latter, an assistant grasps the limb at the elbow to occlude the vein, which courses on the dorsal aspect of the forearm. The vein is more visible if the hair is wetted down with water.

Administering Oral Medications
Most dogs will take pills if these are put inside tasty treats, such as butter, cheese, or any type of meat. If the wily dog can separate pills from food, then non–time-release pills can be crushed and mixed into the food. If the dog will not consume pills placed in any manner into food, the handler can grab the dog around the maxilla (upper jaw) with one hand, using the thumb and forefinger on either side of the maxilla and exerting pressure just behind the canine teeth, and use the other hand to pull down on the mandible (lower jaw). After the jaw is opened, the pill should be placed as far back on the tongue as possible, and then the mouth should be helped to close and the throat rubbed to encourage swallowing. Watch for several minutes afterward to ensure the dog does not regurgitate the pill.

Text continued on p. 887

Table 63.3 Medications for Trek Animals*

GENERIC NAME	TRADE NAME (COMPANY)	CONCENTRATION IN VIAL	ROUTE OF ADMINISTRATION	DOSAGE		INDICATION
				Horse	Llama	
Acepromazine maleate	PromAce (Boehringer Ingelheim)	10 mg/mL	IV, IM	0.02–0.05 mg/kg	Not indicated	Tranquilizer
Ampicillin sodium	Generic	—	IV	15–20 mg/kg qid	10–25 mg/kg tid	Infection
Charcoal (activated)	Generic	—	PO via NG intubation	0.5–1 g/kg	0.5–1 g/kg	Toxin ingestion
Dexamethasone	Azium (Schering-Plough)	2 mg/mL	IV, IM	0.02–0.05 mg/kg	0.1 mg/kg	Shock, severe nonseptic inflammation
Epinephrine	Generic	1:1000, 1 mg/mL	IV, IM	0.01–0.02 mg/kg	0.01 mg/kg	Anaphylaxis
Flunixin meglumine	Banamine (Merck Animal Health)	50 mg/mL	IV	1.1 mg/kg daily	1.1 mg/kg daily	Colic pain, inflammation, fever
Lidocaine	Generic	2%	SC, IM	<10 mL/100 lb	<10 mL/100 lb	Local anesthesia

Continued

Table 63.3 Medications for Trek Animals*—cont'd

GENERIC NAME	TRADE NAME (COMPANY)	CONCENTRATION IN VIAL	ROUTE OF ADMINISTRATION	DOSAGE		INDICATION
				Horse	Llama	
Penicillin G benzathine	Benzapen (Pfizer)	150,000 units/mL	IM	Not recommended	5000–15,000 U/kg q2d	Infection
Penicillin G procaine	Generic	300,000 IU/mL	IM	22,000 IU/kg bid	22,000 IU/kg bid	Infection
Phenylbutazone	Butazolidin (Schering-Plough)	200 mg/mL; 1-g/tablet	IV, PO	2.2–4.4 mg/kg bid	2.2–4.4 mg/kg daily	Pain, inflammation, fever
Trimethoprim/sulfadiazine	Tribrissen (Schering-Plough)	960-mg/tablet	PO	20–30 mg/kg bid	45 mg/kg bid	Infection
Xylazine	Rompun (Bayer)	100 mg/mL	IV, IM	0.2–0.6 mg/kg	0.2–0.3 mg/kg	Sedation

*Most veterinary-specific drugs are not listed. Doses for food animal species are not listed; such drugs should be administered as directed by a veterinarian. In the United States, drugs should be administered to food animals in accordance with the Animal Medicinal Drug Use Clarification Act (AMDUCA).
IM, Intramuscular; *IV,* intravenous; *NG,* nasogastric; *PO,* oral; *SC,* subcutaneous; *IU,* international units; *bid,* twice daily; *tid,* three times daily; *qid,* four times daily; *q2d,* every 2 days.

Table 63.4 Medications for Dogs*

GENERIC NAME	TRADE NAME (COMPANY)	CONCENTRATION IN VIAL	ROUTE OF ADMINISTRATION	DOG	INDICATION AND NOTES
Acepromazine maleate	PromAce (Fort Dodge)	10 mg/mL or tabs	IM, SC, PO	0.05–0.22 mg/kg PO, 0.55 to 1.1 mg/kg IV, IM, or SC	Tranquilizer
Amoxicillin	Generic	Tabs	PO	10–20 mg/kg q12h	Infections and Lyme disease
Ampicillin sodium	Generic	—	IM	10–30 mg/kg q6–8h	Infection
Apomorphine	Generic	Tabs, injectable	SC, IV, IM, or crushed tab placed in conjunctival sac	0.03 mg/kg IV, 0.04 mg/kg IM	For induction of emesis; rinse conjunctiva after emesis occurs
Aspirin-buffered and enteric-coated forms preferred	Generic		PO with food	10–20 mg/kg q12h	Canine-specific NSAIDs are safer and more effective; inhibit platelet function
Atropine sulfate	Generic	2 mg/mL	IM, SC	0.04 mg/kg	Bracycardia; antidote for blue-green algae or muscarinic mushroom intoxication

Continued

Table 63.4 Medications for Dogs*—cont'd

GENERIC NAME	TRADE NAME (COMPANY)	CONCENTRATION IN VIAL	ROUTE OF ADMINISTRATION	DOG	INDICATION AND NOTES
Azithromycin	Zithromax (Pfizer)	Concentration varies with reconstitution	PO	5–10 mg/kg qd for 3–5 days	Infections
Cephalexin	Generic, Keflex	250- and 500-mg capsules	PO	22 mg/kg bid-tid	Infections, skin
Charcoal (activated)	Generic	—	PO	1–4 g/kg as slurry with water	Toxin adsorbent
Ciprofloxacin	Generic	Tabs	PO	10–20 mg/kg qd	Infections
Clindamycin	Antirobe, Cleocin, generic	Tabs	PO	5–11 mg/kg q12h	Infections, abscesses, oral infections
Diazepam	Generic	5 mg/mL	IV, per rectum, intranasal	0.2–1 mg/kg IV, 2 mg/kg per rectum or intranasal for status epilepticus	Sedation or antiepileptic
Diphenhydramine	Generic	Tabs, injectable	PO, SC	2–4 mg/kg q8h	Allergic reactions, motion sickness

Doxycycline	Generic	Tabs	PO	3–5 mg/kg q12h (infection), 10 mg/kg q24h (Lyme disease)	Infecion, Lyme disease, ehrlichiosis, Rocky Mountain spotted fever
Famotidine	Pepcid	Tabs, injectable	PO, SC, IM	0.5 mg/kg q12h	Decreases gastric acidiry
Hydromorphone	Generic	Injectable	IM, IV, SC	0.05–0.2 mg/kg q2–6h	Pain control, sedation
Lidocaine	Generic	2%		As needed; do not exceed 8 mg/kg total dose	Loca anesthesia
Metoclopramide (Reglan)		Tablets, injectable	PO, SC, IM, IV	0.2–0.5 mg/kg q12h	Antiemetic, prokinetic
Metronidazole	Flagyl (Pharmacia)	Tabs	PO	15 mg/kg q12h	Antibacterial, antiprotozoal, and amebicidal agent
Misoprostol	Cytotec (Pfizer)	Tabs	PO	3 µg/kg q12h	Gastric ulcers, abortifacient
Morphine	Generic	Oral, injectable variable concentrations	IM, SC, IV	0.5–2 mg/kg IM, SC, or 0.1–0.2 IV q4h	Can cause histamine release particularly with IV injection

Continued

Table 63.4 Medications for Dogs*—cont'd

GENERIC NAME	TRADE NAME (COMPANY)	CONCENTRATION IN VIAL	ROUTE OF ADMINISTRATION	DOG	INDICATION AND NOTES
Nitenpyram	Capstar	Tabs	PO	Give per label directions	Very safe, effective over-the-counter flea adulticide; will not treat larvae or eggs
Omeprazole	Prilosec	Tabs	PO	0.5–1.0 mg/kg q24h	Gastric ulcers
Oxycodone	Generic	Tabs	PO	0.1–0.2 mg/kg q6–8h	Pain, sedation (not well studied in canines)
Prednisone	Generic	Tabs	PO	0.5–1 mg/kg q12–24h	Antiinflammatory
Trimethoprim/ sulfamethoxazole	Tribrissen (Schering-Plough)	Tabs	PO	15–30 mg/kg q12h	Infection
Tramadol	Ultram (Ortho-McNeil)	Tabs	PO	2–4 mg/kg q8h	Analgesic

*Many drugs and/or dosages are not evaluated and approved by the FDA and should be considered off-label usage.
IM, Intramuscular; IV, intravenous; NSAID, nonsteroidal anti-inflammatory drug; PO, oral; q12h, every 12 hr; q6–8h, every 6 to 8 hr; qd, once daily; bid, twice daily; tid, three times daily; qid, four times daily; SC, subcutaneous.

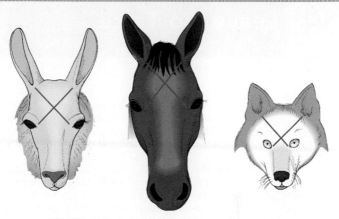

FIGURE 63.5   Location for euthanasia blow or shot.

If it is difficult or dangerous to open the dog's mouth, a pill gun can be used to deliver the pill to the back of the oral cavity. A plunger is depressed to release the pill. The mouth should be held closed until the dog swallows to minimize risk of regurgitation.

EUTHANASIA

Indications for euthanasia include the following:

- Compound and comminuted fractures of long bones
- Falling or sliding into inaccessible places from which the animal is unable to extricate itself or trek participants are unable to aid the animal
- Lacerations exposing abdominal or thoracic organs
- Head injuries resulting in persistent convulsions or coma
- Protracted colicky pain unrelieved by analgesics or mild catharsis

The expedition may carry a bottle of euthanasia solution, which must be given intravenously or intraperitoneally. If firearms are carried, a properly placed bullet to the head produces a fast and humane death.

For placement, the shooter stands in front of the animal's head and draws an imaginary line from the medial canthus of each eye to the base of the opposite ear. The shot should be aimed where those lines cross and approximately perpendicular to the contour of the forehead (Fig. 63.5). The tip of the barrel should be no more than 6 in. from the head. A heavy blow to the head at the same location is equally effective. The blow may be administered with the blunt edge of a single-bladed ax or hatchet. A large rock held in the hand may also be used. A less desirable but sometimes expedient method is to sever the jugular vein to allow exsanguination. This would be best used on an animal that is already unconscious.

Humanity's footprint exceeds the earth's regenerative capacity. Whether consuming irreplaceable resources, fouling the environment on a grand scale, or disrespecting recommended rules for waste disposal, humans frequently erode, weaken, and destroy their natural surroundings.

In order to preserve the wilderness environment, individuals should follow to the best of their abilities the following recommendations. These recommendations are made solely upon the basis of their environmental impact and not upon their monetary or economic impact or the desires or politics of individuals or nations.

- Use renewable energy sources. An example is a solar electricity-generating panel, rather than disposable batteries, when charging mobile personal devices, lights, and lanterns.
- Seek to consume less energy. For instance, use cold water in preference to water that is heated by consuming nonrenewable energy. A good alternative to burning wood or fossil fuel to heat water is a "solar shower," in which the rays of the sun can be passively harnessed to heat a container of water.
- Create shelters that take optimal advantage of natural protection from the elements and therefore do not require exogenous fuel consumption for warmth or ventilation.
- When it is necessary to harvest plants, replant similar vegetation if needed to create a net neutral biomass tally.
- Live sustainably. Learn which foods, clothing, and other consumables require the least water and energy consumption for their creation, and shift your habits and style preferences toward these.
- Favor transportation toward carbon-neutral or carbon-friendly conveyances.

SUSTAINABILITY IN THE WILDERNESS

The Leave No Trace Center for Outdoor Ethics (http://www.LNT.org) organization promotes sustainability in the wilderness. The principles espoused reflect a sense of stewardship and passion for and about the world, especially in untamed wilderness areas.

Seven copyrighted guidelines, adapted here for brevity, are the official principles of The Leave No Trace Center for Outdoor Ethics.

Plan Ahead and Prepare

- Before departing for an expedition, trip, or hike, research the environs and become familiar with the regulations for use.
- Acquire permits if needed.

- Limit party size or split the group if necessary to minimize impact. Hike and camp separately if necessary.
- Avoid high-use times on popular trails.
- Do not travel if poor conditions, as when a trail is muddy, would cause adverse impact.
- Use proper gear and plan meals to minimize waste. Repackage food before departure in reusable containers or plastic bags that can be easily packed out.
- Register at the trailhead or with the ranger.
- Be responsible and aware of personal and party limitations to minimize the chance of needing a rescue.
- Use a map and compass or global positioning system (GPS) to eliminate the need for rock cairns or markings on the trail that can mar the landscape.

Travel and Camp on Durable Surfaces
- Travel on surfaces that are resistant to impact. These include rocky outcroppings, sand, gravel, dry grasses, snow, and water.
- Stay on well-traveled trails and hike in the center of the trail in single file.
- Do not take shortcuts and injure terrain.
- When boating, launch the craft from a durable area and camp at least 200 ft (70 adult steps) from the waterfront.
- Use preestablished campsites rather than creating new campsites.
- When campsites are not apparent, try to disperse the impact rather than camping in a tight group.

Dispose of Waste Properly
- For human waste, use outhouses where available.
- If necessary to use a cathole, dig it 6 to 8 in (15 to 20 cm) deep, and choose a site far from water sources. Disguise the hole as much as possible.
- Bury toilet paper in the hole or pack it out. Do not burn it.
- Pack out feminine hygiene products.
- Treat pet waste the same as human waste.
- Urinate far from camps and trials. Aim to urinate on rocks or bare ground to discourage animals from eating tasty and salty urine-soaked foliage.
- On the water, use a portable toilet.
- Plan meals to minimize leftovers that are tempting for wildlife and potentially dangerous.
- Clean pots with hot water and a scant amount of soap and, after it has been strained to remove food particles, scatter the dishwater at least 200 ft (61 m) from any water source.

Leave What You Find
- Leave artifacts where they are found.
- Do not collect rocks or other portable objects.
- Take care to avoid transporting plant species from one location to another on pack animals, on boots, or in tire treads.

Minimize Campfire Impacts
- Avoid campfires unless they are essential for survival, comfort, or food preparation.
- If a campfire is unavoidable, use a fire ring.
- Gather wood that has fallen on the ground. Do not cut down plants for fuel.
- Terminate any campfire properly and completely to avoid igniting an uncontrolled grass fire or forest fire.
- For campfires on the beach, dig a shallow depression in the sand or gravel along the shoreline. Once the fire is cool, scatter the ashes and refill the depression.

Respect Wildlife
- Observe wildlife from a safe distance. Do not approach wildlife if you are not an expert.
- Avoid wildlife outright during mating season, nesting season, and when animals are rearing young.
- Do not come between an adult animal and its offspring.
- When traveling with pets, keep them under control.

Be Considerate of Other Visitors
- Be considerate of other visitors, natives, and native lands.
- Yield to other users on the trail.
- On encountering pack animals, step to the downhill side of the trail unless otherwise advised by an expert.
- Avoid loud talk, music, and other cacophony unless advised to make noise in order to warn away potentially dangerous animals.

SUSTAINABILITY IN SPECIAL ENVIRONMENTS
The Mountains
- Approach the route on an established trail, using a trail guide to minimize impact.
- Use removable protection and as little chalk as possible.
- Avoid "scrubbing" or "gardening" the route, removing vegetation only when necessary for safety reasons.
- Do not climb near archeologically sensitive sites or animal habitats.
- For feces removal, the preferred method (over smearing them on the rocks away from the route) is to pack them out in a "poop tube" constructed of polyvinyl chloride (PVC) pipe with a screw top that can be attached to the outside of a pack or haul sack.
- Defecate into small brown paper bags, add cat litter, place the bag into the tube, and then deposit the collection into a vault toilet or dumping station.

Snow
- Avoid skiing or camping near game trails or in areas with obvious animal activity.
- Campfires are not recommended.

- When camping, attempt to "fluff up" the trampled snow for the benefit of subsequent visitors.
- Do not leave visible "yellow snow" near well-traveled areas.
- Pack out all waste. Digging a cathole in the snow simply leaves the frozen trophy eventually to thaw on the exposed ground.

Water
- Do not litter or dump waste in the water or on the shore.
- Recreate when possible in the ocean intertidal zone.
- Camp in an established campsite above the ocean high-tide line.
- Tread on durable surfaces such as trails or rock.
- If fires are permitted and driftwood is available, build a campfire, if necessary, below ocean high tide.
- Urinate below the high-tide line away from fellow campers and tidal pools.
- Use a cathole above the ocean high-tide line or pack out feces.
- Launch and land watercraft on sand or gravel, avoiding dirt and vegetation.
- Do not approach marine wildlife.
- On rivers and freshwater, camp in the river's floodplain.
- Bury waste in a cathole at least 200 ft (61 m) from shore or pack it out.
- For large groups, use a toilet tank or other latrine.

Tundra
- Avoid trampling on summer tundra.
- Preserve the thin layer of ground-cover plants.
- Hike and camp only on durable surfaces.
- If trails are not available, travel on shallow streambeds or snow. As a last resort, walk on tundra grasses rather than on lichen beds.
- Do not hike in single file on tundra unless upon a durable surface.
- For waste disposal, do not dig a cathole. Rather, smear feces on a rock or pack them out.
- Do not create campfires.

Desert
- Remain on designated trails or durable surfaces (e.g., slickrock, gravel, sand washes) to avoid disturbing delicate biologic soil crusts.
- Camp on a durable surface or in an established campsite.
- Avoid campfires.
- Do not wander off the trail in search of water.
- Do not use precious water sources for bathing because soaps and body oils contaminate the environment.
- Catholes are the preferred method for waste disposal, but keep them 200 ft (61 m) from any water source.

GENERAL AVALANCHE INFORMATION

http://www.americanavalancheassociation.org

American Avalanche Association: The national professional association for avalanche workers in the United States maintains a website with information about the study, forecasting, control, and mitigation of snow avalanches.

http://www.avalanche.org

Avalanche.org: Avalanche.org provides global, high-level avalanche information to public and professional avalanche workers. It is also a direct link to regional US avalanche forecast centers for local avalanche conditions.

http://www.avalanche-center.org

The CyberSpace Avalanche Center: The avalanche center is a source of worldwide avalanche information, including news, conditions, forecasts, accidents, education, and forums.

http://www.fsavalanche.org

The US Forest Service National Avalanche Center: fsavalanche.org provides technology transfer and education for the US avalanche community.

http://www.avalanche.ca

Canadian Avalanche Centre: The Canadian Avalanche Centre provides Canadian-based reports, information, and conditions.

http://www.avalanches.org/eaws/en/main.php

European Avalanche Warning Service: Contains maps of participating avalanche centers throughout Europe with links to regional specific sites.

REGIONAL AVALANCHE INFORMATION

Twenty-four-hour regional avalanche information is available, generally from November through April, from the following Internet websites or recorded telephone messages.

Alaska

Alaska Avalanche Information Center: http://alaskasnow.org

Anchorage Avalanche Center: http://www.anchorageavalanche-center.org

Chugach National Forest Avalanche Information Center: http://www.cnfaic.org

California

Sierra Avalanche Center, Tahoe National Forrest: http://www.sierraavalanchecenter.org

Eastern Sierra Avalanche Center: http://www.esavalanche.org

Mount Shasta Avalanche Center: http://www.shastaavalanche.org

Colorado
Colorado Avalanche Information Center: http://avalanche.state.co.us

Idaho
Sawtooth National Forrest Avalanche Center: http://www.sawtoothavalanche.com

Montana
Gallatin National Forrest Avalanche Center: http://www.mtavalanche.com

Utah
Utah Avalanche Center: http://utahavalanchecenter.org

Washington and Oregon
Northwest Avalanche Center: http://www.nwac.us

Wyoming
Bridger-Teton National Forest Avalanche Center: http://www.jhavalanche.org/

Glasgow Coma Scale, Simplified Motor Score, and Other Measures of Responsiveness

Glasgow Coma Scale	
Eye Opening	
Spontaneous	4
To voice	3
To pain	2
None	1
Verbal Response	
Oriented	5
Confused	4
Inappropriate words	3
Incomprehensible words	2
None	1
Motor Response	
Obeys command	6
Localizes pain	5
Withdraw (pain)	4
Flexion (pain)	3
Extension (pain)	2
None	1
TOTAL:	

The Glasgow Coma Scale (GCS) is reputed to assess the degree of coma by determining the best motor, verbal, and eye-opening response to standardized stimuli. A GCS of 13 or less is often used to prompt transport to a trauma center. A GCS of 14 or less in persons ages 65 years or older ("elders") is likely a safer triage criterion for transport to a trauma center. It should be noted that the GCS was devised for repeated bedside assessment of state of consciousness, not for acute care decisions. It may be unreliable, difficult to remember, and suffer from subjective interpretation.

There are alternatives to the GCS for predicting outcomes after traumatic brain injury. These may also be used to assist in keeping track of a person's level of consciousness:

Simplified Motor Score
    Obeys commands
    Localizes pain
    Withdrawal or a lesser response to pain

AVPU
    A: **A**lert
    V: Responds to **v**erbal stimuli
    P: Responds to **p**ainful stimuli
    U: **U**nresponsive to all stimuli

ACDU
    A: **A**lert
    C: **C**onfused
    D: **D**rowsy
    U: **U**nresponsive

What is obvious is that when possible, the patient should be examined at a minimum for level of alertness, response to pain, and ability to understand instructions, follow commands, and speak. The purpose of any examination is to follow the patient over time to determine neurologic stability, deterioration, and improvement.

SCAT5©

SPORT CONCUSSION ASSESSMENT TOOL – 5TH EDITION
DEVELOPED BY THE CONCUSSION IN SPORT GROUP
FOR USE BY MEDICAL PROFESSIONALS ONLY

supported by

 FIFA®

Patient details

Name: _____

DOB: _____

Address: _____

ID number: _____

Examiner: _____

Date of Injury: _____ Time: _____

WHAT IS THE SCAT5?

The SCAT5 is a standardized tool for evaluating concussions designed for use by physicians and licensed healthcare professionals[1]. The SCAT5 cannot be performed correctly in less than 10 minutes.

If you are not a physician or licensed healthcare professional, please use the Concussion Recognition Tool 5 (CRT5). The SCAT5 is to be used for evaluating athletes aged 13 years and older. For children aged 12 years or younger, please use the Child SCAT5.

Preseason SCAT5 baseline testing can be useful for interpreting post-injury test scores, but is not required for that purpose. Detailed instructions for use of the SCAT5 are provided on page 7. Please read through these instructions carefully before testing the athlete. Brief verbal instructions for each test are given in italics. The only equipment required for the tester is a watch or timer.

This tool may be freely copied in its current form for distribution to individuals, teams, groups and organizations. It should not be altered in any way, re-branded or sold for commercial gain. Any revision, translation or reproduction in a digital form requires specific approval by the Concussion in Sport Group.

Recognise and Remove

A head impact by either a direct blow or indirect transmission of force can be associated with a serious and potentially fatal brain injury. If there are significant concerns, including any of the red flags listed in Box 1, then activation of emergency procedures and urgent transport to the nearest hospital should be arranged.

Key points

- Any athlete with suspected concussion should be REMOVED FROM PLAY, medically assessed and monitored for deterioration. No athlete diagnosed with concussion should be returned to play on the day of injury.

- If an athlete is suspected of having a concussion and medical personnel are not immediately available, the athlete should be referred to a medical facility for urgent assessment.

- Athletes with suspected concussion should not drink alcohol, use recreational drugs and should not drive a motor vehicle until cleared to do so by a medical professional.

- Concussion signs and symptoms evolve over time and it is important to consider repeat evaluation in the assessment of concussion.

- The diagnosis of a concussion is a clinical judgment, made by a medical professional. The SCAT5 should NOT be used by itself to make, or exclude, the diagnosis of concussion. An athlete may have a concussion even if their SCAT5 is "normal".

Remember:

- The basic principles of first aid (danger, response, airway, breathing, circulation) should be followed.

- Do not attempt to move the athlete (other than that required for airway management) unless trained to do so.

- Assessment for a spinal cord injury is a critical part of the initial on-field assessment.

- Do not remove a helmet or any other equipment unless trained to do so safely.

IMMEDIATE OR ON-FIELD ASSESSMENT

The following elements should be assessed for all athletes who are suspected of having a concussion prior to proceeding to the neurocognitive assessment and ideally should be done on-field after the first first aid / emergency care priorities are completed.

If any of the "Red Flags" or observable signs are noted after a direct or indirect blow to the head, the athlete should be immediately and safely removed from participation and evaluated by a physician or licensed healthcare professional.

Consideration of transportation to a medical facility should be at the discretion of the physician or licensed healthcare professional.

The GCS is important as a standard measure for all patients and can be done serially if necessary in the event of deterioration in conscious state. The Maddocks questions and cervical spine exam are critical steps of the immediate assessment; however, these do not need to be done serially.

STEP 1: RED FLAGS

RED FLAGS:

- **Neck pain or tenderness**
- **Double vision**
- **Weakness or tingling/ burning in arms or legs**
- **Severe or increasing headache**
- **Seizure or convulsion**
- **Loss of consciousness**
- **Deteriorating conscious state**
- **Vomiting**
- **Increasingly restless, agitated or combative**

STEP 2: OBSERVABLE SIGNS

Witnessed ☐   Observed on Video ☐

Lying motionless on the playing surface	Y	N
Balance / gait difficulties / motor incoordination: stumbling, slow / laboured movements	Y	N
Disorientation or confusion, or an inability to respond appropriately to questions	Y	N
Blank or vacant look	Y	N
Facial injury after head trauma	Y	N

STEP 3: MEMORY ASSESSMENT
MADDOCKS QUESTIONS[2]

"I am going to ask you a few questions, please listen carefully and give your best effort. First, tell me what happened?"

Mark Y for correct answer / N for incorrect

What venue are we at today?	Y	N
Which half is it now?	Y	N
Who scored last in this match?	Y	N
What team did you play last week / game?	Y	N
Did your team win the last game?	Y	N

Note: Appropriate sport-specific questions may be substituted.

Name: _____
DOB: _____
Address: _____
ID number: _____
Examiner: _____
Date: _____

STEP 4: EXAMINATION
GLASGOW COMA SCALE (GCS)[3]

Time of assessment			
Date of assessment			
Best eye response (E)			
No eye opening	1	1	1
Eye opening in response to pain	2	2	2
Eye opening to speech	3	3	3
Eyes opening spontaneously	4	4	4
Best verbal response (V)			
No verbal response	1	1	1
Incomprehensible sounds	2	2	2
Inappropriate words	3	3	3
Confused	4	4	4
Oriented	5	5	5
Best motor response (M)			
No motor response	1	1	1
Extension to pain	2	2	2
Abnormal flexion to pain	3	3	3
Flexion / Withdrawal to pain	4	4	4
Localizes to pain	5	5	5
Obeys commands	6	6	6
Glasgow Coma score (E + V + M)			

CERVICAL SPINE ASSESSMENT

Does the athlete report that their neck is pain free at rest?	Y	N
If there is NO neck pain at rest, does the athlete have a full range of ACTIVE pain free movement?	Y	N
Is the limb strength and sensation normal?	Y	N

In a patient who is not lucid or fully conscious, a cervical spine injury should be assumed until proven otherwise.

OFFICE OR OFF-FIELD ASSESSMENT

Please note that the neurocognitive assessment should be done in a distraction-free environment with the athlete in a resting state.

STEP 1: ATHLETE BACKGROUND

Sport / team / school: _____

Date / time of injury: _____

Years of education completed: _____

Age: _____

Gender: M / F / Other

Dominant hand: left / neither / right

How many diagnosed concussions has the
athlete had in the past?: _____

When was the most recent concussion?: _____

How long was the recovery (time to being cleared to play)
from the most recent concussion?: _____ (days)

Has the athlete ever been:

Hospitalized for a head injury?	Yes	No
Diagnosed / treated for headache disorder or migraines?	Yes	No
Diagnosed with a learning disability / dyslexia?	Yes	No
Diagnosed with ADD / ADHD?	Yes	No
Diagnosed with depression, anxiety or other psychiatric disorder?	Yes	No

Current medications? If yes, please list:

_____

_____

_____

_____

_____

_____

Name: _____

DOB: _____

Address: _____

ID number: _____

Examiner: _____

Date: _____

2

STEP 2: SYMPTOM EVALUATION

The athlete should be given the symptom form and asked to read this instruction paragraph out loud then complete the symptom scale. For the baseline assessment, the athlete should rate his/her symptoms based on how he/she typically feels and for the post injury assessment the athlete should rate their symptoms at this point in time.

Please Check: ☐ **Baseline** ☐ **Post-Injury**

Please hand the form to the athlete

	none	mild		moderate		severe	
Headache	0	1	2	3	4	5	6
"Pressure in head"	0	1	2	3	4	5	6
Neck Pain	0	1	2	3	4	5	6
Nausea or vomiting	0	1	2	3	4	5	6
Dizziness	0	1	2	3	4	5	6
Blurred vision	0	1	2	3	4	5	6
Balance problems	0	1	2	3	4	5	6
Sensitivity to light	0	1	2	3	4	5	6
Sensitivity to noise	0	1	2	3	4	5	6
Feeling slowed down	0	1	2	3	4	5	6
Feeling like "in a fog"	0	1	2	3	4	5	6
"Don't feel right"	0	1	2	3	4	5	6
Difficulty concentrating	0	1	2	3	4	5	6
Difficulty remembering	0	1	2	3	4	5	6
Fatigue or low energy	0	1	2	3	4	5	6
Confusion	0	1	2	3	4	5	6
Drowsiness	0	1	2	3	4	5	6
More emotional	0	1	2	3	4	5	6
Irritability	0	1	2	3	4	5	6
Sadness	0	1	2	3	4	5	6
Nervous or Anxious	0	1	2	3	4	5	6
Trouble falling asleep (if applicable)	0	1	2	3	4	5	6
Total number of symptoms:						of 22	
Symptom severity score:						of 132	
Do your symptoms get worse with physical activity?						Y	N
Do your symptoms get worse with mental activity?						Y	N
If 100% is feeling perfectly normal, what percent of normal do you feel?							

If not 100%, why?

_____

_____

_____

Please hand form back to examiner

3

STEP 3: COGNITIVE SCREENING
Standardised Assessment of Concussion (SAC)[4]

ORIENTATION

What month is it?	0	1
What is the date today?	0	1
What is the day of the week?	0	1
What year is it?	0	1
What time is it right now? (within 1 hour)	0	1
Orientation score		of 5

IMMEDIATE MEMORY

The Immediate Memory component can be completed using the traditional 5-word per trial list or optionally using 10-words per trial to minimise any ceiling effect. All 3 trials must be administered irrespective of the number correct on the first trial. Administer at the rate of one word per second.

Please choose EITHER the 5 or 10 word list groups and circle the specific word list chosen for this test.

I am going to test your memory. I will read you a list of words and when I am done, repeat back as many words as you can remember, in any order. For Trials 2 & 3: I am going to repeat the same list again. Repeat back as many words as you can remember in any order, even if you said the word before.

List	Alternate 5 word lists					Score (of 5)		
						Trial 1	Trial 2	Trial 3
A	Finger	Penny	Blanket	Lemon	Insect			
B	Candle	Paper	Sugar	Sandwich	Wagon			
C	Baby	Monkey	Perfume	Sunset	Iron			
D	Elbow	Apple	Carpet	Saddle	Bubble			
E	Jacket	Arrow	Pepper	Cotton	Movie			
F	Dollar	Honey	Mirror	Saddle	Anchor			
				Immediate Memory Score		of 15		
				Time that last trial was completed				

List	Alternate 10 word lists					Score (of 10)		
						Trial 1	Trial 2	Trial 3
G	Finger	Penny	Blanket	Lemon	Insect			
	Candle	Paper	Sugar	Sandwich	Wagon			
H	Baby	Monkey	Perfume	Sunset	Iron			
	Elbow	Apple	Carpet	Saddle	Bubble			
I	Jacket	Arrow	Pepper	Cotton	Movie			
	Dollar	Honey	Mirror	Saddle	Anchor			
				Immediate Memory Score		of 30		
				Time that last trial was completed				

Name:	
DOB:	
Address:	
ID number:	
Examiner:	
Date:	

CONCENTRATION

DIGITS BACKWARDS

Please circle the Digit list chosen (A, B, C, D, E, F). Administer at the rate of one digit per second reading DOWN the selected column.

I am going to read a string of numbers and when I am done, you repeat them back to me in reverse order of how I read them to you. For example, if I say 7-1-9, you would say 9-1-7.

Concentration Number Lists (circle one)					
List A	List B	List C			
4-9-3	5-2-6	1-4-2	Y	N	0
6-2-9	4-1-5	6-5-8	Y	N	1
3-8-1-4	1-7-9-5	6-8-3-1	Y	N	0
3-2-7-9	4-9-6-8	3-4-8-1	Y	N	1
6-2-9-7-1	4-8-5-2-7	4-9-1-5-3	Y	N	0
1-5-2-8-6	6-1-8-4-3	6-8-2-5-1	Y	N	1
7-1-8-4-6-2	8-3-1-9-6-4	3-7-6-5-1-9	Y	N	0
5-3-9-1-4-8	7-2-4-8-5-6	9-2-6-5-1-4	Y	N	1
List D	List E	List F			
7-8-2	3-8-2	2-7-1	Y	N	0
9-2-6	5-1-8	4-7-9	Y	N	1
4-1-8-3	2-7-9-3	1-6-8-3	Y	N	0
9-7-2-3	2-1-6-9	3-9-2-4	Y	N	1
1-7-9-2-6	4-1-8-6-9	2-4-7-5-8	Y	N	0
4-1-7-5-2	9-4-1-7-5	8-3-9-6-4	Y	N	1
2-6-4-8-1-7	6-9-7-3-8-2	5-8-6-2-4-9	Y	N	0
8-4-1-9-3-5	4-2-7-9-3-8	3-1-7-8-2-6	Y	N	1
		Digits Score:			of 4

MONTHS IN REVERSE ORDER

Now tell me the months of the year in reverse order. Start with the last month and go backward. So you'll say December, November. Go ahead.

Dec - Nov - Oct - Sept - Aug - Jul - Jun - May - Apr - Mar - Feb - Jan	0 1
Months Score	of 1
Concentration Total Score (Digits + Months)	of 5

4

STEP 4: NEUROLOGICAL SCREEN

See the instruction sheet (page 7) for details of
test administration and scoring of the tests.

Can the patient read aloud (e.g. symptom check-list) and follow instructions without difficulty?	Y	N
Does the patient have a full range of pain-free PASSIVE cervical spine movement?	Y	N
Without moving their head or neck, can the patient look side-to-side and up-and-down without double vision?	Y	N
Can the patient perform the finger nose coordination test normally?	Y	N
Can the patient perform tandem gait normally?	Y	N

BALANCE EXAMINATION

Modified Balance Error Scoring System (mBESS) testing⁵

Which foot was tested (i.e. which is the non-dominant foot)	☐ Left ☐ Right

Testing surface (hard floor, field, etc.) _____

Footwear (shoes, barefoot, braces, tape, etc.)_____

Condition	Errors
Double leg stance	of 10
Single leg stance (non-dominant foot)	of 10
Tandem stance (non-dominant foot at the back)	of 10
Total Errors	of 30

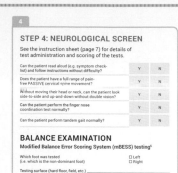

Name:	_____
DOB:	_____
Address:	_____
ID number:	_____
Examiner:	_____
Date:	_____

5

STEP 5: DELAYED RECALL:

The delayed recall should be performed after 5 minutes have
elapsed since the end of the Immediate Recall section. Score 1
pt. for each correct response.

*Do you remember that list of words I read a few times earlier? Tell me as many words
from the list as you can remember in any order.*

	Time Started	

Please record each word correctly recalled. Total score equals number of words recalled.

_____
_____
_____

Total number of words recalled accurately:	of 5	or	of 10

6

STEP 6: DECISION

Domain	Date & time of assessment:		
Symptom number (of 22)			
Symptom severity score (of 132)			
Orientation (of 5)			
Immediate memory	of 15 of 30	of 15 of 30	of 15 of 30
Concentration (of 5)			
Neuro exam	Normal Abnormal	Normal Abnormal	Normal Abnormal
Balance errors (of 30)			
Delayed Recall	of 5 of 10	of 5 of 10	of 5 of 10

Date and time of injury:_____

If the athlete is known to you prior to their injury, are they different from their usual self?
☐ Yes ☐ No ☐ Unsure ☐ Not Applicable
(If different, describe why in the clinical notes section)

Concussion Diagnosed?
☐ Yes ☐ No ☐ Unsure ☐ Not Applicable

If re-testing, has the athlete improved?
☐ Yes ☐ No ☐ Unsure ☐ Not Applicable

**I am a physician or licensed healthcare professional and I have personally
administered or supervised the administration of this SCAT5.**

Signature:_____

Name:_____

Title:_____

Registration number (if applicable):_____

Date:_____

**SCORING ON THE SCAT5 SHOULD NOT BE USED AS A STAND-ALONE
METHOD TO DIAGNOSE CONCUSSION, MEASURE RECOVERY OR
MAKE DECISIONS ABOUT AN ATHLETE'S READINESS TO RETURN TO
COMPETITION AFTER CONCUSSION.**

CLINICAL NOTES:

_____

_____

_____

_____

Name:	_____
DOB:	_____
Address:	_____
ID number:	_____
Examiner:	_____
Date:	_____

_____

_____

_____

_____

_____

_____

_____

_____

_____

_____

✂ ·

CONCUSSION INJURY ADVICE

(To be given to the person monitoring the concussed athlete)

This patient has received an injury to the head. A careful medical examination has been carried out and no sign of any serious complications has been found. Recovery time is variable across individuals and the patient will need monitoring for a further period by a responsible adult. Your treating physician will provide guidance as to this timeframe.

If you notice any change in behaviour, vomiting, worsening headache, double vision or excessive drowsiness, please telephone your doctor or the nearest hospital emergency department immediately.

Other important points:

Initial rest: Limit physical activity to routine daily activities (avoid exercise, training, sports) and limit activities such as school, work, and screen time to a level that does not worsen symptoms.

1) Avoid alcohol

2) Avoid prescription or non-prescription drugs without medical supervision. Specifically:

a) Avoid sleeping tablets

b) Do not use aspirin, anti-inflammatory medication or stronger pain medications such as narcotics

3) Do not drive until cleared by a healthcare professional.

4) Return to play/sport requires clearance by a healthcare professional.

Clinic phone number: _____

Patient's name: _____

Date / time of injury: _____

Date / time of medical review: _____

Healthcare Provider: _____

Contact details or stamp

INSTRUCTIONS

Words in *Italics* **throughout the SCAT5 are the instructions given to the athlete by the clinician**

Symptom Scale

The time frame for symptoms should be based on the type of test being administered. At baseline it is advantageous to assess how an athlete "typically" feels whereas during the acute/post-acute stage it is best to ask how the athlete feels at the time of testing.

The symptom scale should be completed by the athlete, not by the examiner. In situations where the symptom scale is being completed after exercise, it should be done in a resting state, generally by approximating his/her resting heart rate.

For total number of symptoms, maximum possible is 22 except immediately post injury, if sleep item is omitted, which then creates a maximum of 21.

For Symptom severity score, add all scores in table, maximum possible is 22 x 6 = 132, except immediately post injury if sleep item is omitted, which then creates a maximum of 21x6=126.

Immediate Memory

The Immediate Memory component can be completed using the traditional 5-word per trial list or, optionally, using 10-words per trial. The literature suggests that the Immediate Memory has a notable ceiling effect when a 5-word list is used. In settings where this ceiling is prominent, the examiner may wish to make the task more difficult by incorporating two 5–word groups for a total of 10 words per trial. In this case, the maximum score per trial is 10 with a total trial maximum of 30.

Choose one of the word lists (either 5 or 10). Then perform 3 trials of immediate memory using this list.

Complete all 3 trials regardless of score on previous trials.

"I am going to test your memory. I will read you a list of words and when I am done, repeat back as many words as you can remember, in any order." The words must be read at a rate of one word per second.

Trials 2 & 3 MUST be completed regardless of score on trial 1 & 2.

Trials 2 & 3:

"I am going to repeat the same list again. Repeat back as many words as you can remember in any order, even if you said the word before."

Score 1 pt. for each correct response. Total score equals sum across all 3 trials. Do NOT inform the athlete that delayed recall will be tested.

Concentration

Digits backward

Choose one column of digits from lists A, B, C, D, E or F and administer those digits as follows:

Say: *"I am going to read a string of numbers and when I am done, you repeat them back to me in reverse order of how I read them to you. For example, if I say 7-1-9, you would say 9-1-7."*

Begin with first 3 digit string.

If correct, circle "Y" for correct and go to next string length. If incorrect, circle "N" for the first string length and read trial 2 in the same string length. One point possible for each string length. Stop after incorrect on both trials (2 N's) in a string length. The digits should be read at the rate of one per second.

Months in reverse order

"Now tell me the months of the year in reverse order. Start with the last month and go backward. So you'll say December, November ... Go ahead"

1 pt. for entire sequence correct

Delayed Recall

The delayed recall should be performed after 5 minutes have elapsed since the end of the Immediate Recall section.

"Do you remember that list of words I read a few times earlier? Tell me as many words from the list as you can remember in any order."

Score 1 pt. for each correct response

Modified Balance Error Scoring System (mBESS)[5] testing

This balance testing is based on a modified version of the Balance Error Scoring System (BESS)[5]. A timing device is required for this testing.

Each of 20-second trial/stance is scored by counting the number of errors. The examiner will begin counting errors only after the athlete has assumed the proper start position. The modified BESS is calculated by adding one error point for each error during the three 20-second tests. The maximum number of errors for any single condition is 10. If the athlete commits multiple errors simultaneously, only

one error is recorded but the athlete should quickly return to the testing position, and counting should resume once the athlete is set. Athletes that are unable to maintain the testing procedure for a minimum of five seconds at the start are assigned the highest possible score, ten, for that testing condition.

OPTION: For further assessment, the same 3 stances can be performed on a surface of medium density foam (e.g., approximately 50cm x 40cm x 6cm).

Balance testing – types of errors

1. Hands lifted off iliac crest	3. Step, stumble, or fall	5. Lifting forefoot or heel
2. Opening eyes	4. Moving hip into > 30 degrees abduction	6. Remaining out of test position > 5 sec

"I am now going to test your balance. Please take your shoes off (if applicable), roll up your pant legs above ankle (if applicable), and remove any ankle taping (if applicable). This test will consist of three twenty second tests with different stances."

(a) Double leg stance:

"The first stance is standing with your feet together with your hands on your hips and with your eyes closed. You should try to maintain stability in that position for 20 seconds. I will be counting the number of times you move out of this position. I will start timing when you are set and have closed your eyes."

(b) Single leg stance:

"If you were to kick a ball, which foot would you use? [This will be the dominant foot] *Now stand on your non-dominant foot. The dominant leg should be held in approximately 30 degrees of hip flexion and 45 degrees of knee flexion. Again, you should try to maintain stability for 20 seconds with your hands on your hips and your eyes closed. I will be counting the number of times you move out of this position. If you stumble out of this position, open your eyes and return to the start position and continue balancing. I will start timing when you are set and have closed your eyes."*

(c) Tandem stance:

"Now stand heel-to-toe with your non-dominant foot in back. Your weight should be evenly distributed across both feet. Again, you should try to maintain stability for 20 seconds with your hands on your hips and your eyes closed. I will be counting the number of times you move out of this position. If you stumble out of this position, open your eyes and return to the start position and continue balancing. I will start timing when you are set and have closed your eyes."

Tandem Gait

Participants are instructed to stand with their feet together behind a starting line (the test is best done with footwear removed). Then, they walk in a forward direction as quickly and as accurately as possible along a 38mm wide (sports tape), 3 metre line with an alternate foot heel-to-toe gait ensuring that they approximate their heel and toe on each step. Once they cross the end of the 3m line, they turn 180 degrees and return to the starting point using the same gait. Athletes fail the test if they step off the line, have a separation between their heel and toe, or if they touch or grab the examiner or an object.

Finger to Nose

"I am going to test your coordination now. Please sit comfortably on the chair with your eyes open and your arm (either right or left) outstretched (shoulder flexed to 90 degrees and elbow and fingers extended), pointing in front of you. When I give a start signal, I would like you to perform five successive finger to nose repetitions using your index finger to touch the tip of the nose, and then return to the starting position, as quickly and as accurately as possible."

References

1. McCrory et al. Consensus Statement On Concussion In Sport – The 5th International Conference On Concussion In Sport Held In Berlin, October 2016. British Journal of Sports Medicine 2017 (available at www.bjsm.bmj.com)

2. Maddocks, DL; Dicker, GD; Saling, MM. The assessment of orientation following concussion in athletes. Clinical Journal of Sport Medicine 1995; 5: 32-33

3. Jennett, B., Bond, M. Assessment of outcome after severe brain damage: a practical scale. Lancet 1975; i: 480-484

4. McCrea M. Standardized mental status testing of acute concussion. Clinical Journal of Sport Medicine. 2001; 11: 176-181

5. Guskiewicz KM. Assessment of postural stability following sport-related concussion. Current Sports Medicine Reports. 2003; 2: 24-30

CONCUSSION INFORMATION

Any athlete suspected of having a concussion should be removed from play and seek medical evaluation.

Signs to watch for

Problems could arise over the first 24-48 hours. The athlete should not be left alone and must go to a hospital at once if they experience:

- Worsening headache
- Drowsiness or inability to be awakened
- Inability to recognize people or places
- Repeated vomiting
- Unusual behaviour or confusion or irritable
- Seizures (arms and legs jerk uncontrollably)
- Weakness or numbness in arms or legs
- Unsteadiness on their feet.
- Slurred speech

Consult your physician or licensed healthcare professional after a suspected concussion. **Remember, it is better to be safe.**

Rest & Rehabilitation

After a concussion, the athlete should have physical rest and relative cognitive rest for a few days to allow their symptoms to improve. In most cases, after no more than a few days of rest, the athlete should gradually increase their daily activity level as long as their symptoms do not worsen. Once the athlete is able to complete their usual daily activities without concussion-related symptoms, the second step of the return to play/sport progression can be started. The athlete should not return to play/sport until their concussion-related symptoms have resolved and the athlete has successfully returned to full school/learning activities.

When returning to play/sport, the athlete should follow a stepwise, medically managed exercise progression, with increasing amounts of exercise. For example:

Graduated Return to Sport Strategy

Exercise step	Functional exercise at each step	Goal of each step
1. Symptom-limited activity	Daily activities that do not provoke symptoms.	Gradual reintroduction of work/school activities.
2. Light aerobic exercise	Walking or stationary cycling at slow to medium pace. No resistance training.	Increase heart rate.
3. Sport-specific exercise	Running or skating drills. No head impact activities.	Add movement.
4. Non-contact training drills	Harder training drills, e.g., passing drills. May start progressive resistance training.	Exercise, coordination, and increased thinking.
5. Full contact practice	Following medical clearance, participate in normal training activities.	Restore confidence and assess functional skills by coaching staff.
6. Return to play/sport	Normal game play.	

In this example, it would be typical to have 24 hours (or longer) for each step of the progression. If any symptoms worsen while exercising, the athlete should go back to the previous step. Resistance training should be added only in the later stages (Stage 3 or 4 at the earliest).

Written clearance should be provided by a healthcare professional before return to play/sport as directed by local laws and regulations.

Graduated Return to School Strategy

Concussion may affect the ability to learn at school. The athlete may need to miss a few days of school after a concussion. When going back to school, some athletes may need to go back gradually and may need to have some changes made to their schedule so that concussion symptoms do not get worse. If a particular activity makes symptoms worse, then the athlete should stop that activity and rest until symptoms get better. To make sure that the athlete can get back to school without problems, it is important that the healthcare provider, parents, caregivers and teachers talk to each other so that everyone knows what the plan is for the athlete to go back to school.

Note: If mental activity does not cause any symptoms, the athlete may be able to skip step 2 and return to school part-time before doing school activities at home first.

Mental Activity	Activity at each step	Goal of each step
1. Daily activities that do not give the athlete symptoms	Typical activities that the athlete does during the day as long as they do not increase symptoms (e.g. reading, texting, screen time). Start with 5-15 minutes at a time and gradually build up.	Gradual return to typical activities.
2. School activities	Homework, reading or other cognitive activities outside of the classroom.	Increase tolerance to cognitive work.
3. Return to school part-time	Gradual introduction of school work. May need to start with a partial school day or with increased breaks during the day.	Increase academic activities.
4. Return to school full-time	Gradually progress school activities until a full day can be tolerated.	Return to full academic activities and catch up on missed work.

If the athlete continues to have symptoms with mental activity, some other accommodations that can help with return to school may include:

- Starting school later, only going for half days, or going only to certain classes
- More time to finish assignments/tests
- Quiet room to finish assignments/tests
- Not going to noisy areas like the cafeteria, assembly halls, sporting events, music class, shop class, etc.
- Taking lots of breaks during class, homework, tests
- No more than one exam/day
- Shorter assignments
- Repetition/memory cues
- Use of a student helper/tutor
- Reassurance from teachers that the child will be supported while getting better

The athlete should not go back to sports until they are back to school/learning, without symptoms getting significantly worse and no longer needing any changes to their schedule.

Sport concussion assessment tool - 5th edition

Br J Sports Med published online April 26, 2017

Notes

Lake Louise Score for the Diagnosis of Acute Mountain Sickness

A diagnosis of acute mountain sickness (AMS) is based on the following:
- A rise in altitude within the last 4 days
- Presence of a headache
  PLUS
- Presence of at least one other symptom
- A total score of 3 or more from the questions in the self-report questionnaire

SELF-REPORT QUESTIONNAIRE

Add together the individual scores for each symptom to get the **total score.**

Headache	No headache	0
	Mild headache	1
	Moderate headache	2
	Severe headache, incapacitating	3
Gastrointestinal symptoms	None	0
	Poor appetite or nausea	1
	Moderate nausea and/or vomiting	2
	Severe nausea and/or vomiting	3
Fatigue and/or weakness	Not tired or weak	0
	Mild fatigue/weakness	1
	Moderate fatigue/weakness	2
	Severe fatigue/weakness	3
Dizziness/ light-headedness	Not dizzy	0
	Mild dizziness	1
	Moderate dizziness	2
	Severe dizziness, incapacitating	3
	TOTAL SCORE:	

Total Score of:

- 2 to 4 = mild AMS
- 5 or more = moderate to severe AMS

Note:

- Do not ascend with symptoms of AMS.
- Descend if symptoms are not improving or are getting worse.
- Descend if symptoms of high-altitude cerebral edema or high-altitude pulmonary edema develop.

Contingency Supplies for Wilderness Travel

Basic categories to consider:
- Navigation
- Sun protection
- Illumination
- Repair kit and tools/power
- First-aid supplies
- Fire starter
- Nutrition (extra food)
- Hydration (safe water)
- Insulation (clothing/sleeping bag)
- Emergency shelter

ITEM	DESCRIPTION, QUANTITY (NO.; WEIGHT)*	COMMENT
1. Whistle	Nonmetal, shrill (1 oz)	Emergency signal (bursts of 3)
2. Knives	A sturdy folding or straight knife (3–8 oz)	e.g., Swiss Army knife
3. Maps	Trail and topographic (1 oz) (as needed per group)	Plastic coated or with cover
4. Global positioning system (GPS) Personal locator beacon (i.e., person emergency locator transmitter)	Lightweight, portable (4–6 oz)	Carry spare batteries Not a replacement for map
5. Compass, fluid-filled	2-degree gradations (1–2 oz)	Know area declination
6. Headlamp	LED most efficient; lithium or alkaline spare batteries attachment (1; 3–6 oz)	Headlamp superior to flashlight for rescue and medical procedures

ITEM	DESCRIPTION, QUANTITY (NO.; WEIGHT)*	COMMENT
7. Sunglasses (and spare sunglasses)	With side and nose blocks; polycarbonate or glass lens (1–3 oz)	>99% UVB filtering; >85% light absorption
8. Rescue and survival guide	Condensed (3–6 oz) (1 per group)	Learn basic air-to-ground signals
9. Pencil and paper	Waterproof paper preferred (2 oz)	
10. Multipurpose tool ("multitool")	Lightweight model	
11. Accident report forms	Waterproof preferred (1 oz) (2 per group)	
12. Toilet paper, small roll	One (1 oz)	Store in plastic bag
13. Personal locator beacon (PLB)	4–16 oz	Must be registered online before travel
14. Matches, waterproof, windproof	"Strike-anywhere" type (12; 1 oz)	Store in plastic bag or commercial (waterproof) match container
15. Spare bulb, batteries	(1–3 oz)	Store in plastic bag
16. Closed-cell foam pads	0.3 × 0.3 m (1 × 1 ft) sections (1–3; 3 oz)	e.g., Ensolite; to insulate stove, seats, use as cervical collar or splint pads
17. "Space" blanket	142.2 × 212.4 cm (56 × 84 in) (2–3; 1 oz)	Emergency insulation (replace every 3 years)
18. Surveyor's trail tape	Bright color, 15.2 m (50 ft) (1 oz) (per group)	Trail, avalanche site markers
19. Utility cord	Nylon, 7.6–15.2 m (25–50 ft) (2 oz)	Shelter; utility
20. Heat source	Candle; fuel tabs (1 or 2; 2 oz)	

ITEM	DESCRIPTION, QUANTITY (NO.; WEIGHT)*	COMMENT
21. Emergency toboggan kit	Variable (per 2–3 persons)	Convert skis and poles; e.g., NSP
22. Goggles	Rose or amber (4 oz)	Double lens, polarized preferred
23. Avalanche transceiver	(8 oz); e.g., Pieps, Skadi, Ortovox	Use in avalanche terrain
24. Scraper	Metal edged (1 oz)	Ice and wax removal
25. Shovel	Lexan or aluminum (16–32 oz) (per 1–3 persons)	
26. Face mask	Leather, silk, or synthetic (1 oz)	
27. Aerial flares; ground smoke bombs	Red smoke, (2–4; 1 oz) (per group)	Rescue signal
28. Bungee elastic cords with hooks	15.2–30.5 cm (6–12 in) (1–2; 1 oz)	Pack compression; lash equipment to pack
29. Swami belt	2.5-cm (1-in) webbing, 3–6.1 m (10–20 ft) (4–8 oz)	Waist, seat harness
30. Carabiner, locking type	Aluminum, (2–3; 3 oz)	Climbing or rappel harness; rope brake; Prusik handle
31. Rescue pulley	Small (1–2; 2 oz)	Cliff, crevasse rescue
32. Rope, Perlon or Goldline	5.5–9 mm (0.22–0.35 in), 15.2–22.9 m (50–75 ft) (8–16 oz) (per group)	Rescue, evacuation
33. Magnifying lens	8–15 × (1 oz) (per group)	Snow crystal examination; map reading; splinter removal; fire starter
34. Altimeter	6.1-m (20-ft) accuracy (2 oz) (per group)	Altitude orienteering; barometric changes
35. Saw	Wire or blade (2–15 oz) (per 1–4 persons)	Fuel or shelter (cuts wood, snow, ice)

Continued

ITEM	DESCRIPTION, QUANTITY (NO.; WEIGHT)*	COMMENT
36. Extra food and energy bars	1-day supply (8–16 oz)	Prevent hypothermia, maintain energy in emergency
37. Extra clothing	Wool preferred	Sock doubles as mitten
38. Signal mirror	Unbreakable preferred (1 oz)	Learn to use before trip
39. Road flare	5-min, (1–3; 3 oz)	Rescue signal; emergency fire starter
40. Extra ski wax	Klister or two-wax system (3 oz)	If waxless skis, glide wax is sufficient
41. Emergency shelter	"Tube" tent, tarp, or bivi sack (3–16 oz)	May improvise with large plastic bags
42. Water bottles	0.47 L (1 pint), metal container preferred (18 oz) or 1-L (1.1 quart) Lexan type	Metal canteen can be heated directly, quantity dependent on trip type
43. Thermometer, outdoor	In protective case (0.5 oz) (per group)	Snow, water, air temperature
44. Lens antifogger	Liquid or stick (1 oz)	For glasses, goggles
45. Climbing skins, adhesive	"Skinny" type (11–16; 26 oz)	Urgent snow climbing on skis, or slowing ski descent

*Quantity is per person per trip, unless otherwise specified; weight given is per individual item, in ounces (35.2 oz = 1 kg = 2.2 lb).
LED, Light-emitting diode; *NSP*, US National Search and Rescue Plan; *UVB*, ultraviolet B.

Repair Supplies for Wilderness Travel

- Duct tape. Carry several yards of high-thread count duct tape rolled over on itself, or wound around ski poles, kayak paddles, water bottles. Fix tears in clothing, tents, sleeping bags, broken ski poles, skins that are peeling off skis, etc.
- Headlamp
- Parachute cord
- Cable ties (large and small)
- Extra plastic hardware (e.g., cord locks, Fastex buckles, D rings)
- Safety pins
- Hot-melt glue stick (do not need the gun, just a cigarette lighter)
- Cigarette lighter
- Heavy-duty needle, thimble, or sewing awl
- Nylon thread (size #69)
- Multitool or screwdrivers (flat and Phillips No. 2)
- Wire (e.g., braided steel, such as picture-hanging wire); paper clips
- Awl (on multifunction knife). Useful if you need to punch holes for repairs or fabricate improvised rescue devices (e.g., toboggan)
- Glue (e.g., two-component epoxy)
- Seam sealer (e.g., Seam Grip adhesive; repairs, strengthens, and waterproofs); can be used to patch a Therm-a-Rest pad
- Adhesive ripstop nylon (and alcohol swabs)
- Tent pole splint (hollow aluminum tube)
- Knife sharpener
- Portable, lightweight reading glasses (if needed)

BACKCOUNTRY SKIING OR CLIMBING

- Camping stove repair kit (varies with brand of stove and includes parts like jet cleaning wire and O-rings)
- Spare bale and screws (for repair of ski binding)
- P-Tex ski base repair
- Spare ski tip (if lightweight or fragile skis)
- Extra ski pole basket
- Spare crampon wrench and/or Allen wrench
- Crampon file

AIRWAY/BREATHING/CIRCULATION

- CPR mouth barrier or pocket mask
- Oral and nasopharyngeal airways
- Bag-valve-mask device
- Endotracheal tube(s), laryngeal mask airway, King airway
- Chest tube set (Heimlich valve, McSwain dart)
- Cricothyrotomy set (Cricothyrotomy cannula or catheter [e.g., Abelson cannula] or prepackaged cricothyrotomy kit)
- Oxygen and administration device (e.g., nasal cannula, face mask)
- Suction device (mechanical)
- Stethoscope
- Pulse oximetry device
- Angiocatheters (22 to 14 gauge), IV insertion kits, extension tubing, pressure bags
- Intraosseous needle kit or device (e.g., EZ-IO handheld driver) and adult needles (15 gauge × 25 mm [1 inch])
- Intravenous solutions (e.g., normal saline, lactated Ringer)
- Manufactured tourniquet for life-threatening bleeding (e.g., combat application tourniquet [CAT], SWAT-T, SAM XT Extremity Tourniquet)

WOUND MANAGEMENT

- Alcohol-based gel for hand sanitation
- Germicidal soap
- Nitrile examination gloves
- Antiseptic towelettes
- Syringe (20-mL) for irrigating with 18-gauge catheter tip
- Lidocaine, 0.5% to 2% solution for injection
- Xeroform or Vaseline gauze
- Wound-closure adhesive strips
- Disposable skin stapler and remover
- Tissue adhesive (e.g., Dermabond)
- Suture materials, needle driver, and tissue forceps
- Tincture of benzoin
- Scalpel with No. 11 blade
- Cotton-tipped applicators
- Blister care materials (e.g., Moleskin and Molefoam)

BANDAGES, SPLINTS, AND SLINGS

- Safety pins
- Trauma shears
- Adhesive cloth tape

- Dressings, bandages, Kerlix bandages, Kling bandages
- 10.2 × 10.2 cm (4 × 4 inch) sterile dressing pads
- SAM Splints (15 × 110 cm [4.4 × 36 inch])
- 4″ compression bandages (e.g., ACE wrap)
- Hemostatic dressings (e.g., QuickClot)
- Trauma dressings (e.g., Israeli trauma bandage)

OVER-THE-COUNTER MEDICATIONS AND REMEDIES
- Acetaminophen (Tylenol)
- Aloe vera gel
- Antibiotic or antiseptic ointment (e.g., bacitracin)
- Diphenhydramine (Benadryl)
- Famotidine (Pepcid)
- Glycerin rectal suppositories
- Hemorrhoid ointment or witch-hazel pads
- High–sun protection factor (SPF) sunscreen and lip balm
- Hydrocortisone cream 1%
- Ibuprofen (e.g., Advil, Motrin), 200 mg
- Loperamide (Imodium A-D)
- Meclizine (e.g., Antivert or Bonine)
- Omeprazole (Prilosec)
- Oxymetazoline (Afrin) or phenylephrine (Neo-Synephrine or Sinex)
- Pseudoephedrine (Sudafed)
- Ranitidine (Zantac 75)
- Simethicone (Mylanta II antacid)
- Antifungal foot cream (e.g., tolnaftate)

PRESCRIPTION MEDICINES
- For allergic reactions and anaphylaxis: epinephrine (e.g., EpiPen or Twinject), diphenhydramine (Benadryl)
- β-Adrenergic agonist metered-dose inhaler (for asthma, anaphylactic reaction)
- Oral opiate combinations (e.g., oxycodone-acetaminophen)
- Parenteral opiates (e.g., morphine, Dilaudid, fentanyl)
- Ondansetron 4-mg sublingual dissolving tablets and IV preparation
- Diphenhydramine oral (for allergic reactions, mild sedation, or insomnia)
- Oral and parenteral corticosteroid (e.g., prednisone, dexamethasone)
- For high altitude: acetazolamide (Diamox), dexamethasone (Decadron), sildenafil (Viagra)
- For respiratory, soft tissue, gastrointestinal, and other infections: oral antibiotics (see Appendix J)
- Intravenous antibiotics (see Appendix J)

MISCELLANEOUS ITEMS
- Notebook and pencil
- Plastic zippered bags (for snow; sprain and contusion treatment)

- Thermometers (low reading for cold weather and high altitude; regular for hot weather)
- Tourniquet
- Nasal packing material (e.g., Rhino Rocket)
- Foley catheter, gloves, lubricant, clamp, and plug
- Urine pregnancy test
- Urine test "dip" strips
- Gamow Bag for travel to high altitude
- Small pulse oximeter for travel to high altitude
- Cavit (dental temporary filling)
- Paraffin (dental wax) stick
- Sterile water for reconstituting medications
- Duct tape (e.g., for repair, splinting, improvisation)

Antimicrobials

Amoxicillin: adult dose, 500 mg q12h or 250 mg PO q8h; pediatric dose, 45 mg/kg/day PO divided q8h for mild to moderate infections or 90 mg/kg/day PO divided q8h or q12h for severe infections or otitis media

Amoxicillin/clavulanate (Augmentin): adult dose, 500 to 875 mg PO q12h; pediatric dose, 25 to 45 mg/kg PO divided q12h. For otitis media in children, use the higher dose

Ampicillin: adult dose, 500 mg PO q6h; pediatric dose, 50 to 100 mg/kg/day PO divided q6h, max 1000 mg/day

Artemether–lumefantrine: adult dose, 4 tablets (20 mg artemether with 120 mg lumefantrine) PO q12h for 3 days for treatment of uncomplicated acute falciparum malaria, or following parenteral therapy for severe falciparum malaria; pediatric dose: <3 years but >5 kg, 1 tablet PO q12h for 3 days; 3 to 8 years, 2 tablets PO q12h for 3 days; 9 to 14 years, 3 tablets PO q12h PO for 3 days

Artesunate: adult dose, 200 mg PO daily for 3 days; pediatric dose: 2 to 11 months, 25 mg PO daily for 3 days; 1 to 5 years, 50 mg PO daily for 3 days; 6 to 13 years, 100 mg PO daily for 3 days

Azithromycin (Zithromax): adult dose, 500 mg PO once on day 1, then 250 mg PO daily for 4 additional days; pediatric dose, 10 mg/kg PO on day 1, then 5 mg/kg PO daily for 4 additional days

Cefadroxil (Duricef): adult dose, 500 mg to 1 g PO q12h. For pharyngitis, to eradicate group A *Streptococcus*, an acceptable dose is 1 g PO daily for 10 days. Pediatric dose: for skin infections, 30 mg/kg/day PO daily or divided q12h for 10 days

Cefdinir (Omnicef): adult dose, 300 mg PO q12h for 10 days; pediatric dose up to 12 years, 14 mg/kg/day PO daily or divided q12h for 5 to 10 days

Cefixime: adult dose, 400 mg PO daily or 200 mg PO q12h; pediatric dose, 8 mg/kg/day PO daily or divided q12h; no refrigeration needed; discard 14 days after the dry powder is reconstituted with water

Cefuroxime axetil: adult dose, 500 mg PO q12h; pediatric dose up to 12 years, 30 mg/kg/day PO divided q12h

Cefpodoxime (Vantin): adult dose, 200 mg PO q12h for 10 to 14 days for pneumonia, 400 mg PO q12h for 7 to 14 days for skin and/or soft tissue infection; pediatric dose 2 months to 12 years, 10/mg/kg/day PO daily or divided q12h for 7 to 14 days

Cephalexin (Keflex): adult dose, 250 mg PO q4-6h or 500 mg PO q12h; pediatric dose, 25-50 mg/kg/day PO divided q6h or 50-100 mg/kg/day PO divided q6h for severe infections

Chloramphenicol: adult dose, 3 to 4 g PO daily divided q6h to q8h for the treatment of typhoid fever or rickettsial infections; pediatric dose, 50 mg/kg/day PO divided q6h to q8h. *This medication is not readily available in the United States. Its use should be limited to treatment of severe infections only when no other effective medication is available*

Chloroquine (Aralen): adult dose, 500 mg PO once weekly for prevention; 1000 mg PO once, then 500 mg PO after 6 to 8 hours, then 500 mg PO once daily for 2 consecutive days for treatment of acute malaria; pediatric dose, 10 mg/kg of base PO daily on day 1 and 2, 5 mg/kg of base PO daily on day 3 for the treatment of acute malaria

Ciprofloxacin (Cipro): adult dose, 500 mg PO q12h for 3 days to treat infectious diarrhea; 500 mg PO q12h for bone, skin, and soft tissue infections. *Consider risks vs benefits in pregnant women given possible increased risk of spontaneous abortion.*

Clarithromycin (Biaxin): adult dose, 250 to 500 mg PO q12h; pediatric dose, 15 mg/kg/day PO divided q12h for 7 to 14 days

Clindamycin (Cleocin): adult dose, 150 to 450 mg PO q6h; pediatric dose, 8 to 16 mg/kg/day suspension PO divided q6h to q8h

Dicloxacillin: adult dose, 125 to 500 mg PO q6h, max 2 g/day; pediatric dose, 12.5 to 50 mg/kg/day PO divided q6h if <40 kg

Doxycycline (Vibramycin): adult dose, 100 mg PO q12h for treatment or once daily for prevention of infectious diarrhea, 100 mg PO q12h for treatment of Rocky Mountain spotted fever, skin infections, and urinary tract infections; pediatric dose, 4.4 mg/kg PO divided q12h. *Do not give to pregnant women or children up to age 7 years* because this drug may cause permanent dark discoloration of the teeth

Erythromycin: adult dose, 250 mg PO q6h or 500 mg PO q12h; pediatric dose, 30 to 50 mg/kg/day PO divided q6h, max 4 g/day

Erythromycin/sulfisoxazole (Pediazole): pediatric dose, 50 mg/kg based on the erythromycin component divided q6h

Fleroxacin: adult dose, 400 mg PO daily for 3 days for the treatment of infectious diarrhea or complicated urinary tract infection

Fluconazole (Diflucan): adult dose, 150 mg PO daily

Levofloxacin (Levaquin): adult dose, 250 to 750 mg PO/IV daily

Metronidazole (Flagyl): adult dose, 250 to 500 mg q8h; pediatric dose, 15 mg/kg/day PO divided q8h for 7 to 10 days for giardiasis, 35 to 50 mg/kg/day PO divided q8h for 10 days for acute amebic dysentery. *Do not drink alcohol when taking this medication and for 3 days afterward. The interaction would cause severe abdominal pain, nausea, and vomiting*

Nitazoxanide (Alinia): adult dose 500 mg PO q12h for 3 days; pediatric dose: 1 to 3 years, 100 mg PO; 4 to 11 years, 200 mg PO q12h for 3 days

Noroxin: adult dose, 400 mg PO q12h for 1 to 3 days for traveler's diarrhea

Ofloxacin: adult dose, 300 to 400 mg PO q12h for 7 to 10 days

Phenoxymethyl penicillin (Pen-Vee K): adult dose, 250 to 500 mg PO q4-6h; pediatric dose: 2 to 6 years, 125 mg PO q6-8h; 6 to 10 years, 250 mg PO q6-8h. For pharyngitis, to eradicate the group A *Streptococcus*, an acceptable adult dose is 1 g PO q12h for 10 days

Quinine: adult dose 650 mg PO q8h for 7 days for malaria in chloroquine-resistant areas

Tetracycline: adult dose, 500 mg PO q6h. *Do not give to pregnant women or children up to age 7 years* because this drug may cause permanent dark discoloration of the teeth

Trimethoprim with sulfamethoxazole (Bactrim or Septra double strength): adult dose, 1 tablet (80 mg trimethoprim with 400 mg sulfamethoxazole) PO q12h for infectious diarrhea or urinary tract infection, 1 tablet PO daily for prevention of traveler's diarrhea; pediatric dose in children 8 years or older, 25 to 50 mg/kg/day PO divided q6h

MEDICATIONS

- Moxifloxacin 0.5% drops
- Tetracaine 0.5% drops
- Prednisolone 1% drops
- Moxifloxacin 400 mg tabs
- Levofloxacin 500 mg tabs
- Bacitracin ointment
- Prednisone 20 mg tabs
- Artificial tears
- Scopolamine 0.25% drops
- Diclofenac 0.1% drops
- Pilocarpine 2% drops

MISCELLANEOUS

- Penlight with blue filter
- Fluorescein strips
- Cotton-tipped applicators
- Metal eye shield
- Tape (1 inch wide, plastic or nylon)
- Near-vision card
- Wound closure strips ($\frac{1}{4}$ inch wide)
- Magnifying glass
- Fine forceps

Recommended Oral Antibiotics for Prophylaxis of Domestic Animal and Human Bite Wounds

Although universal antibiotic prophylaxis is not recommended, antibiotics reduce the rate of infection due to certain animal bites, especially cat bites that produce a puncture wound and are difficult to irrigate. Prophylaxis is also warranted in certain high-risk wounds, including the following:

- Deep puncture wounds (especially due to cat bites)
- Wounds with associated crush injury or devitalized tissue
- Wounds on the hand(s), feet, or near a bone or joint
- Bite wounds in compromised individuals (e.g., immuno-compromised, asplenia, diabetes)

If patients are to receive antimicrobial prophylaxis, the first dose should be given as soon as possible after the injury.

FOR ESTABLISHED INFECTIONS WHEN THE ORGANISMS ARE KNOWN

Treat according to specific antibiotic sensitivities of cultured organism(s).

WHEN ORGANISMS ARE UNKNOWN (DOG AND MOST OTHER BITES)

ANTIBIOTIC	RECOMMENDED ADULT DOSE	RECOMMENDED CHILD DOSE*
Agent of Choice		
Amoxicillin-clavulanate	875/125 mg twice daily	22.5 mg/kg per dose (amoxicillin component) two times daily (maximum 875 mg amoxicillin and 125 mg clavulanate per dose)
Alternate Combination Regimens		
One of the Following Agents With Anaerobic Coverage		
Metronidazole	500 mg three times daily	10 mg/kg per dose three times daily
Or:		
Clindamycin	450 mg three times daily	10 mg/kg per dose three times daily

ANTIBIOTIC	RECOMMENDED ADULT DOSE	RECOMMENDED CHILD DOSE*
Plus One of the Following Agents With Coverage Against Pasteurella multocida		
Doxycycline	100 mg twice daily	Not for use in children <8 years old
Trimethoprim-sulfamethoxazole	160/800 mg (1 DS tab) twice daily	4 to 5 mg/kg (trimethoprim component) per dose twice daily
Penicillin V potassium	500 mg four times daily	12.5 mg/kg per dose four times daily
Cefuroxime	500 mg twice daily	10 mg/kg per dose twice daily
Levofloxacin	750 mg once daily	Use with caution in children <18 years of age; if unable to tolerate other choices: <5 years old: 10 mg/kg per dose twice daily (maximum 750 mg daily) ≥5 years old: 10 mg/kg per dose once daily (maximum 750 mg daily)
Moxifloxacin	400 mg once daily	Use with caution in children

*Child dose should not exceed recommended adult dose.
Modified from Marvin Harper: Clinical manifestations and initial management of animal and human bites. In Danzl D, Wolfson A, editors: *UpToDate,* Waltham, Massachusetts, 2017, UpToDate.

Therapy for Parasitic Infections

ETIOLOGIC AGENT	ADULT TREATMENT	PEDIATRIC TREATMENT AND ALTERNATIVES
Giardia lamblia	Tinidazole, 2000 mg single dose *or*	Children: tinidazole, 50 mg/kg single dose
	Nitazoxanide, 500 mg twice daily for 3 days *or*	Children Age 1–4 yr: nitazoxanide, 100 mg twice daily for 3 days
		Children Age 4–11 yr: nitazoxanide, 200 mg twice daily for 3 days
	Metronidazole, 250 mg three times daily for 5–7 days or 2 g/day in a single dose for 3 days (high dose has more side effects) *or*	Children: metronidazole, 15 mg/kg/day divided three times daily for 5–7 days
	Albendazole, 400 mg single dose or daily for 5–7 days (single dose less effective) *or*	Children: albendazole, 10–15 mg/kg daily for 5–7 days
	Diloxanide (Furamide), adults and children age 12 yr and older: 500 mg three times daily for 5–10 days	Children up to age 12 yr: diloxanide, 20 mg/kg/day in three divided doses for 5–10 days

ETIOLOGIC AGENT	ADULT TREATMENT	PEDIATRIC TREATMENT AND ALTERNATIVES
Entamoeba histolytica	**Treatment for asymptomatic cyst excretion**	
	Iodoquinol, 650 mg three times daily for 20 days *or*	Children: iodoquinol, 10–13.3 mg/kg three times daily for 20 days
	Paromomycin, 500 mg three times daily for 7 days	Children: paromomycin, 25 mg/kg/day in three doses for 7 days
	Treatment of diarrhea	
	Metronidazole, 750 mg three times daily for 5–10 days *or*	Children: metronidazole, 50 mg/kg/day in three doses for 10 days
	Tinidazole, 1000 mg twice daily for 3 days *or*	Children: tinidazole, 50 mg/kg/day in three doses for 3 days
	Secnidazole, 2000 mg single dose	Children: secnidazole, 30 mg/kg/day single dose
	Followed by:	
	Iodoquinol, 650 mg three times daily for 20 days *or*	Children: iodoquinol, 30–40 mg/kg/day (max 2 g) PO in three daily doses for 20 days
	Paromomycin, 500 mg three times daily for 7 days	Children: paromomycin, 25–35 mg/kg/day orally in three daily doses/day for 7 days

ETIOLOGIC AGENT	ADULT TREATMENT	PEDIATRIC TREATMENT AND ALTERNATIVES
Dientamoeba fragilis	Paromomycin, 25–35 mg/kg/day orally in three daily doses for 7 days *or*	Children: paromomycin, 25–35 mg/kg/day orally in three daily doses for 7 days
	Metronidazole, 500–750 mg orally three times daily for 10 days *or*	Children: metronidazole, 30–50 mg/kg/day orally three times daily for 10 days
	Iodoquinol, 650 mg orally three times daily for 20 days	Children: iodoquinol, 30–40 mg/kg/day (max 2 g) PO in three daily doses for 20 days
Balantidium coli (symptomatic)	Tetracycline, 500 mg four times daily for 10 days *or*	Children: metronidazole, 35–50 mg/kg/day in three divided doses for 5 days
	Metronidazole, 750 mg three times daily for 5–10 days *or* Iodoquinol, 650 mg three times daily for 20 days	Children: iodoquinol, 30–40 mg/kg/day (max 2 g) in three doses for 20 days
Entamoeba polecki	Metronidazole, 250 mg q8h for 10 days for adults	Children: metronidazole, 35–50 mg/kg/day in three divided doses for 5 days

Continued

ETIOLOGIC AGENT	ADULT TREATMENT	PEDIATRIC TREATMENT AND ALTERNATIVES
Blastocystis hominis (symptomatic)	Nitazoxanide, 500 twice daily for 3 days *or*	Children: nitazoxanide Age 12–47 mo: 100 mg (5 mL) twice daily for 3 days Age 4–11 yr: 200 mg (10 mL) twice daily for 3 days
	Metronidazole, 750 mg three times daily for 5–10 days	Children: metronidazole, 35–50 mg/kg/day in three divided doses for 5 days
Cryptosporidiosis	Nitazoxanide, 500 mg twice daily for 3 days	Children: nitazoxanide
	In severe cases or patients with AIDS, consider:	Age 12–47 mo: 100 mg (5 mL) twice daily for 3 days
	Nitazoxanide, 500 mg twice daily for 2 weeks	Age 4–11 yr: 200 mg (10 mL) twice daily for 3 days
	Paromomycin, 500–750 mg three times daily or four times daily for 2 weeks	Adult alternatives: Azithromycin, 1200 mg daily for 4 weeks Albendazole, 400 mg twice daily for 7–14 days
Isospora belli	TMP/SMX, 160 mg/800 mg q6h for 10 days, followed by same dose q12h for 3 wk *or* Pyrimethamine, 75 mg daily with folinic acid 10 mg daily for 2 wk	

ETIOLOGIC AGENT	ADULT TREATMENT	PEDIATRIC TREATMENT AND ALTERNATIVES
Cyclosporiasis	TMP/SMX, 160 mg/800 mg twice daily to four times daily for 7 days In patients with AIDS, follow with: TMP/SXZ, 160 mg/800 mg three times per week	Children: TMP/SMX, 5 mg/25 mg/kg/day for 7 days
Angiostrongylus cantonensis	Mebendazole, 100 mg q12h for 5 days for adults	Children: mebendazole, 100 mg q12h for 5 days
Ascaris lumbricoides	Mebendazole, 100 mg q12h for 3 days or 500 mg once for adults	Children: mebendazole, 100 mg q12h for 3 days
Babesia spp.	Azithromycin, 500 mg on day 1; 250 mg on days 2–7 and atovaquone 750 mg q12h for 7 days	Children: azithromycin, 10 mg/kg on day 1; 5 mg/kg on days 2 to 6–9 Children: atovaquone, 20 mg/kg q12h for 7–10 days
Schistosoma	Praziquantel, 40–60 mg/kg/day once or divided q12h to q8h for 1 day	Children: praziquantel, 20 mg/kg two to three times daily for 1 day
Microsporidiosis	Albendazole, 400 mg twice daily for 2–4 weeks In patients with AIDS: follow with chronic suppression	

Continued

ETIOLOGIC AGENT	ADULT TREATMENT	PEDIATRIC TREATMENT AND ALTERNATIVES
Tapeworms: *Diphyllobothrium latum* (fish), *Taenia saginata* (beef), *Taenia solium* (pork), *Dipylidium caninum* (dog)	Praziquantel, 5–25 mg/kg once for adults and for children	Children: praziquantel, 5–25 mg/kg orally once
Strongyloides stercoralis	Ivermectin, 200 mcg/kg orally once	Children: Ivermectin, 200 mcg/kg orally once
Trichomonas vaginalis	Metronidazole, 2 g once; or 250 mg q8h for 7 days for adults	Children: metronidazole, 15 mg/kg/day divided q8h for 7 days
Trichuris trichiura (whipworm)	Mebendazole, 100 mg q12h for 3 days for adults	Children: mebendazole, 100 mg q12h for 3 days
Trypanosoma gambiense	Hemolymphatic stage: pentamidine isethionate, deep IM 4 mg/kg once daily for 7–10 days Meningoencephalitic stage: eflornithine, IV infusion over 2 hr 400 mg/kg/day divided q6h for 14 days	Children: eflornithine, <12 yr, 600 mg/kg/day divided q6h for 14 days

ETIOLOGIC AGENT	ADULT TREATMENT	PEDIATRIC TREATMENT AND ALTERNATIVES
Trypanosoma rhodesiense	Hemolymphatic stage: suramin, slow test dose of 100 mg IV is first given to detect possible idiosyncratic reactions. If tolerated, 1 g should be given on the initial day of treatment and 3, 7, 14, and 21 days later. Meningoencephalitic stage: melarsoprol slow IV, 2–3.6 mg/kg daily for 3 days. After 1 week with no drug given, additional injections of 3.6 mg/kg/day IV for 3 days are given. Repeat again after 1 week with no drug given.	
Trypanosoma cruzi	Nifurtimox, 8–10 mg/kg/day divided q8h for 120 days for adults	

AIDS, Acquired immunodeficiency syndrome; *IM*, intramuscular; *IV*, intravenous; *TMP/SMX*, trimethoprim/sulfamethoxazole.

Suggested Basic Contents of a Survival Kit for Temperate to Cold Weather

Persons traveling to remote areas or locations from which rescue would be difficult should develop the habit of carrying, at the very least, a minimal survival kit consisting of basic equipment for shelter, fire, and signaling. Each person in the group should have his or her own basic survival kit.

ITEM	APPROXIMATE WEIGHT IN GRAMS (OUNCES)
Fire-Building Equipment	
Two waterproof screw-top match containers filled with REI or UCO stormproof matches	57 (2)
Candle	43 (1.5)
Fire starter (e.g., cotton impregnated with petroleum jelly) in a waterproof container, such as an additional match container	28 (1)
Metal match	14 (0.5)
Knife: Swiss Army knife (consider a camping model with a saw, file, scissors, and so on; made by Victorinox)	142 (5)
Alternative: Leatherman tool with wire-cutting pliers, file, one serrated and two regular blades, saw, and scissors	227 (8)
Shelter-Building Equipment	
⅛ inch braided nylon cord or parachute cord, 30.48 m (100 feet)	113 (4)
Rip-stop waterproof nylon tarp, approximately 2.4 × 3 m (8 × 10 feet) with grommets around the edges	55.3 (19.5)
Alternatives:	
Tarp (blue and crinkly; laminated polyethylene weave)	737 (26)
or	

ITEM	APPROXIMATE WEIGHT IN GRAMS (OUNCES)
One or two large, heavy-duty (3- to 4-mil), orange or royal blue plastic bags, 0.9 × 1.7 m (3 × 5.5 feet)	255–5100 (9–18)
Folding saw or small rigid saw (e.g., 18-inch Dandy saw)	340 (12)
Signaling and Navigating Equipment	
Headlamp or flashlight with spare bulb and batteries (a good choice is a headlamp with both light-emitting diode and bulb options; the light-emitting diode light uses up much less electricity but is more diffuse and does not cast a long beam; the bulb is brighter and casts a longer beam but uses much more electricity)	212 (7.5)
Plastic pealess whistle on a lanyard	14 (0.5)
Small notebook and pencil	43 (1.5)
Small roll of orange surveyor's tape	57 (2)
Glass signaling mirror with sighting device	57 (2)
Miscellaneous	
Metal pot with bale that contains emergency food of choice (e.g., tea, soup mix, power bars, small can of mixed nuts, trail mix)	964 (334)
Metal cup with handle (for heating liquid by putting the cup at the edge of a fire)	85 (3)
Plastic or Lexan spoon	14 (0.5)
Toilet paper	43 (1.5)
Sunscreen with sun protection factor of 30 or more	113 (4)
Lip balm with sun protection factor of 30 or more	14 (0.5)
Insect repellent (e.g., *N,N*-diethyl-meta-toluamide)	113 (4)
First-aid kit, one per party (see Chapter 61)	701 (25)
Canteen (1–1.5 L [34–50 fl oz] when full; stainless steel or plastic)	1091–1446 (38.5–51.0)

Continued

ITEM	APPROXIMATE WEIGHT IN GRAMS (OUNCES)
Sunglasses, preferably polarized, with side shields	57 (2)
Light raingear (e.g., laminated [Gore-Tex] pants and jacket with hood)	879 (31)
Repair kit that is adapted to the type of travel (e.g., ski, snowshoe, kayak) and that includes the following:	
Small needle-nosed pliers with wire-cutting feature (if Leatherman tool not carried)	85 (3)
Small crescent wrench	57 (2)
Small screwdriver with multiple tips	156 (5.5)
Picture wire	28 (1)
Fiberglass tape, standard roll	85 (3)
Duct tape, small roll	28 (1)
Steel wool for shimming (e.g., ski binding repair)	28 (1)
Assorted nuts, bolts, and screws	43 (1.5)
Total weight of repair kit	510 (18)
Total weight of basic survival equipment (not including shovel, snow saw, backpack, or cold weather fourth layer of clothing	Approximately 6520–7087 g (230–250 oz) or 6.5–7 kg (14–16 lb)
Other Useful Equipment for Consideration	
Nondigital watch	
Altimeter	
Magnifying glass	
Two sets of correct coins for pay phone; calling card	
Light pair of leather gloves (hand protection)	
Water disinfection equipment: chemicals (e.g., Potable Aqua) or filter	
Thermometer (plastic alcohol type clipped to the outside of the pack)	

ITEM	APPROXIMATE WEIGHT IN GRAMS (OUNCES)
Spare eyeglasses	
Electronic communication and navigation equipment:	
Cell phone (if service is available in the area)	
Global positioning system unit	
Personal locator beacon (i.e., person emergency locator transmitter)	
Pepper spray (to repel bears, moose, and so on)	
Usual day-trip items to be added:	
Small insulated drink canister of hot or cold drink	
Lunch	
Binoculars	
Camera	

In addition to basic survival items from Appendix L, carry the following:

- Spare clothing for severe weather (at least four layers total)
  - Hat, neck gaiter, and neoprene face cover or balaclava
  - Spare mittens
- Snow shovel: small grain-scoop type with detachable handle
- Snow saw (consider this for above-timberline travel and potential igloo building; should have a 227-g [8-oz] capacity)
- Three-quarter-length piece of open- or closed-cell foam mattress or Therm-a-Rest mattress
- Sleeping bag
- Bivouac sack
- Small stove and fuel
- In avalanche terrain:
  - Avalanche transmitter beacon and receivers for each party member
  - Avalanche probe poles or ski poles that join to form a probe for each party member

Sample Desert Survival Kit

In addition to basic survival items from Appendix L, carry the following:

- Fold-up steel shovel with short handle
- Items for construction of four solar stills:
  - Four sheets of clear plastic, 1.8 × 1.8 m (6 × 6 feet), reinforced in center by cross of duct tape
  - Four pieces of surgical tubing, 1.8 to 2.4 m (6 to 8 feet) long
  - Four 1-L (1.1-quart) plastic bowls
  - One 19-L (5-gallon) water jug, full (when space and weight conditions permit)
- One 1-L (1.1 quart) wide-mouth bottle for use as urinal
- Large sun hat, wide-brim hat, and/or cotton cravat, bandana, or large handkerchief for fashioning a head covering
- Spare sunglasses
- Heavy leather gloves
- Goggles
- Light rifle or target pistol
- Metal cup
- Hard candy
- Water filter or iodine-derived water disinfection chemicals
- Mosquito head net

- Trail shoes (1 pair)
- Camp boots (1 pair)
- Special cleats (e.g., Covell Ice Walker Quick Clip Cleats)
- Socks, lightweight cotton or thin nylon (3 pairs)
- Hat (1)
- Pullover garment, polyester (1)
- Shirts, cotton
  - Long sleeved (2)
  - Short sleeved (2)
- Pants; lightweight cotton, Supplex, or Taslan lined with mesh underwear (2 pairs)
- Undergarments
  - Underpants, lightweight polyester mesh (3)
  - Sports bra, cotton or cotton-Lycra blend mesh (2)
- Poncho, nylon (1)
- Flannel sheet
- Hammock or Therm-a-Rest
- Mosquito net
- Backpack for porter
- Personal backpack
- Antifogging solution for eyeglasses
- Batteries
- Binoculars
- Camera equipment and film
- Campsuds or other biodegradable soap
- Candles, dripless
- Cup (Lexan polycarbonate)/plate (melamine)
- Duct tape, 1 small roll
- Ear plugs
- Fishing supplies
- Garbage bags
  - 30-gallon size (4)
  - 13-gallon size (4)
- Headlamp
- Inflatable cushion
- Insect repellent
- Laminated maps
- Machete (Collins style)
- Waterproof matches or butane piezo ignition lighter
- Pen
- Toilet paper

- Leatherman or similar pocket survival tool
- Polycarbonate wide-mouth bottles (2)
- Razor/battery-operated shaver
- Spoon or spork
- Sport sponge
- Sunglasses
- Umbrella
- Whistle, plastic
- Zipper-lock bags
  - Gallon size (5)
  - Quart size (5)
  - Pint size (5)
- Dry bags
- Wide-mouth 1-L water bottles (2)

Vehicle Cold Weather Survival Kit

In addition to basic survival items from Appendixes L and M, take the following:

- Sleeping bag or two blankets for each occupant
- Extra winter clothing, including snow boots, wool or fleece hat, and mittens for each occupant
- Emergency food
- Two 36-hour candles in a can
- Waterproof and windproof matches in a waterproof container
- Space blanket
- First-aid kit (see Appendix G)
- Spare doses of personal medications—enough for 3 or more days
- Two plastic water jugs, full
- Large, heavy-duty, zipper-lock plastic bags
- Extra toilet paper
- Citizens band radio or cell phone
- Flashlight with extra batteries and bulb (if light-emitting diode, spare bulb not applicable)
- Battery booster cables
- Tire chains
- Snow shovel
- Tow chain or strap, at least 6.1 m (20 feet) long
- Small sack of sand
- Tool kit
- Gas line deicer
- Signal flares
- Extra quart of oil (place some in a hubcap and burn it for an emergency smoke signal)
- Long rope
- Carbon monoxide detector
- Axe
- Folding saw
- Full tank of gas

Experts generally recommend that individuals in a vehicle caught in a snowstorm stay inside the vehicle. It is the best source of shelter available. Minimizing exposure is important. In a severe storm, going outside the car to find firewood, and then maintaining the fire, would be nearly impossible.

If in deep and accumulating snow, it is important NOT to run the car engine and heater for warmth. The exhaust pipe(s) can become blocked by blowing/drifting snow, causing carbon monoxide to enter the car. The candles will provide adequate heat in combination with the sleeping bags and extra clothing for 72 hours.

Some authorities recommend running the engine for a few minutes to operate the vehicle's heater, then having a quiet period until the temperature drops. If this technique is used, it is necessary to check the exhaust pipe(s) before running the motor, for the reason stated earlier.

After the storm abates and it becomes safe to exit the vehicle, flares and smoke from a fire (e.g., burning oil in a hubcap) can be used for signaling as needed.

EQUIPMENT

Assorted adhesive bandages
Butterfly bandages or Steri-Strips
Gauze pads
Cotton-tipped applicators
Gauze roll
Nonadherent dressings
Tape
Moleskin, Spenco 2nd Skin, or New-Skin
Eye patches
Triangular bandage or sling
Elastic bandage
Povidone-iodine solution 10% (use to cleanse wounds and disinfect water)
Antiseptic wipes (benzalkonium chloride)
Antibacterial soap
Tincture of benzoin
Alcohol wipes
Lightweight malleable splint (SAM splint)
Needles (assorted sizes)
Safety pins
Syringe, 20 to 35 mL (for wound irrigation)
Plastic catheter or irrigation tip, 18-gauge (for wound irrigation)
Bulb syringe
Digital oral thermometer
Rectal thermometer for infants <3 mo
Scissors
Tweezers
Sunscreen waterproof cream, sun protection factor at least 15
Insect repellent (no more than 35% N,N-diethyl-3-methylbenzamide [DEET])
First-aid book
Whistle for child
Identification card with basic health information (past medical history, medications, allergies, blood type, weight, immunizations)
Surgical stapler, suture material, and suturing supplies
2-Octyl cyanoacrylate (Dermabond) tissue glue

MEDICATIONS

MEDICATION	INDICATION	DOSE
Topical Medications		
Antiseptic ointment (e.g., bacitracin or polymyxin)	Superficial skin infections	Apply as directed qd to tid
Topical corticosteroid (e.g., 1% hydrocortisone)	Contact or atopic dermatitis, insect bites, sunburn	Apply to affected areas bid to tid (use sunscreen aggressively; avoid >1% corticosteroid on face)
Antifungal cream (e.g., clotrimazole or miconazole)	Yeast at diaper area, groin, scalp, feet; ringworm	Apply bid for 7–10 days and for several days after rash has resolved
Desitin cream	Sunblock, diaper-area erythema	Apply thick coat as sunscreen or thin coat for diaper area
Permethrin (Elimite)	Scabies, lice, treatment for clothing and mosquito netting	Apply 5% cream from chin to soles of feet and wash after 8–14 hr; do not use in children <2 mo of age or on eyes, nose, mouth
Anesthetic eye drops (e.g., proparacaine)*[†]	Removal of superficial ocular foreign body	1 drop in affected eye for removal of foreign body; must patch eye for protection for at least 1 hr
Antibiotic eye ointment (e.g., erythromycin)[†] or drops (e.g., polymyxin B sulfate plus trimethoprim [Polytrim])[†]	Purulent conjunctivitis, suspected corneal abrasion	Ointment: thin line upper lid margin tid to qid Drops: 1 drop every 3 h for 7 days
Antipyrine-benzocaine otic drops[†]	Ear pain (otitis externa or media); avoid if <3 mo or tympanic membrane rupture suspected	3–4 drops in affected ear every 2–3 h as needed to relieve pain

Continued

MEDICATION	INDICATION	DOSE
Oral Medications		
Diphenhydramine 12.5 mg/5 mL elixir 25- or 50-mg capsules	Allergy symptoms, pruritus, insomnia, nausea, motion sickness	1.25 mg/kg/dose every 6 h (up to 25–50 mg/dose); may cause paradoxic restlessness in children
Acetaminophen 80 mg/0.8 mL drops 160 mg/5 mL elixir 80- and 160-mg chewable tabs	Fever control, pain	15–20 mg/kg every 4–6 h up to 650 mg/dose
Ibuprofen 40 mg/1 mL drops 100 mg/5 mL elixir 50- or 100-mg chewable tabs 100- or 200-mg caplets	Fever control, pain, antiinflammatory	10 mg/kg/dose every 8 h up to 600 mg/dose
Dimenhydrinate (Dramamine) 12.5 mg/5 mL elixir 50-mg chewable tabs	Motion sickness	1–1.5 mg/kg/dose 1 h before departure and every 6 h after; may cause drowsiness
Oral Antibiotics (as Appropriate for Age of Child)		
Amoxicillin[†]	Acute otitis media, sinusitis, pharyngitis, pneumonia	80 mg/kg/day in divided dose bid for 10 days if <5 yr or for 5 days if >5 yr
		125- or 250-mg chewable tabs
		250-mg capsule

MEDICATION	INDICATION	DOSE
Amoxicillin-clavulanate (Augmentin)[†]	Penicillin-resistant organisms, acute otitis media, sinusitis, animal bites	80 mg/kg/day in divided dose bid
		200- and 400-mg chewable tabs
		200 and 400 mg/5 mL elixir
Azithromycin (Zithromax)[†]	Acute otitis media, sinusitis, pharyngitis, pneumonia, traveler's diarrhea, skin infections, animal bites	10 mg/kg on day 1, then 5 mg/kg/day for 4 days
		125 and 250 mg/5 mL elixir
		250-mg tabs (best)
Ciprofloxacin (Cipro)[†]	Not first line <18 yr due to adverse effects: urinary tract infection, traveler's diarrhea, wounds acquired in an aquatic environment	20–30 mg/kg/day in divided dose bid up to 500 mg bid
		100-, 200-, 500-mg tabs
Trimethoprim-sulfamethoxazole (Septra)[†]	Suspected methicillin-resistant *Staphylococcus aureus* skin infection 80/400 SS tab; 160/800 DS tab	8–10 mg trimethoprim/kg/day in divided dose bid
		>2 mo old
Oseltamivir (Tamiflu)[†]	Influenza treatment (12 mg/mL susp 30-, 45-, 75-mg caps)	Not recommended <3 mo old; treat for 5 days
		3–12 mo: 3 mg/kg/dose twice daily
		>12 mo or <15 kg: 30 mg bid
		15–23 kg: 45 mg bid
		24–40 kg: 60 mg bid
		>40 kg: 75 mg bid

Continued

MEDICATION	INDICATION	DOSE
Other Preparations		
Epinephrine (premeasured)[†] 0.15 mg EpiPen Jr 0.3 mg EpiPen	Anaphylaxis, severe asthma	0.15 mg intramuscularly up to 15 kg (33 lb); 0.3 mg intramuscularly if >15 kg (>33 lb)
Oral rehydration packet	Dehydration	
Foreign Travel		
Loperamide 1 mg/5 mL 1 mg caps	Nonbloody diarrhea, minimally febrile, significant diarrhea older than age 2 yr	13–20 kg (29–44 lb): 1 mg tid 20–30 kg (44–66 lb): 2 mg bid >30 kg (>66 lb): 2 mg tid
Ondansetron (Zofran) ODT[†] 4 mg tab	Nausea/vomiting, dehydration	6 mo–1 yr: 1 mg 1–4 yr: 2 mg >4 yr: 4 mg
Travel to High Altitude		
Acetazolamide (Diamox)[†] 30 or 50 mg/mL suspension 125-mg tab	Recurrent acute mountain sickness despite graded ascent	5 mg/kg/day divided bid up to 250 mg/day

*Administration of this medication by other than trained medical personnel is strongly discouraged, given the risk of overuse and subsequent worsening of eye injury; if significant eye irritation persists, medical attention must be sought to evaluate for corneal injury.

[†]Available by prescription only.

Note: Chewable tablets, if tolerated by the child, weigh less than liquids and can be crushed and hidden in soft foods for administration.

R Drug Stability in the Wilderness

ENVIRONMENTAL FACTORS INFLUENCING DRUG STABILITY

The main environmental factors affecting drug stability are temperature, light, and humidity. Additives included with a medication can preserve or, under certain conditions, diminish a drug's efficacy during long-term storage.

Extreme temperatures and light can cause medications to spontaneously decompose, reassemble, or react with air, contaminants, or a drug's otherwise inactive ingredients. Exposure to high humidity can decrease a drug's rate of dissolution, the bottleneck step in bioavailability of drugs taken by mouth. Common additives, such as bicarbonate or D_5W, and dilution can drastically reduce robustness and durability of some medications in extreme environments.

Manufacturers generally recommend little variation in storage temperatures. Brief excursions into temperatures below the minimum or beyond the maximum recommended temperatures for a given drug are often acceptable, so long as two conditions are met: (1) the drug is not exposed to a maximum temperature constituting excessive heat for a period longer than 24 hours and (2) the mean kinetic temperature (MKT), or average temperature, for the drug remains at or below the maximum temperature of its ideal range. These less commonly known rules for excursions ease medical fieldwork related to wilderness emergency situations of short duration by minimizing the amount of artificial cooling absolutely necessary in the field, depending on the drugs involved.

EXPIRATION DATES AND SHELF LIFE

The United States Pharmacopeia (USP) requires manufacturers to list a drug's shelf life as the time during which a drug's potency (or concentration of active product) is guaranteed to be 90% to 110% of its listed potency (or concentration). Expiration dates are based on the shelf life of a drug under ideal, manufacturer-suggested conditions of temperature, humidity, light exposure, and packaging integrity. When stored in environments that do not correlate with those listed by the manufacturer, the printed expiration date no longer indicates whether a drug is potent. For this reason, multiple studies have evaluated the rate and extent of degradation and loss of potency for numerous drugs under various circumstances. Tropical climates pose difficulty for drugs susceptible to heat and humidity.

PACKAGING

Where drugs are stored significantly influences their stability and safety. Packaging can shield drugs from environmental assaults but only when conditions optimize the packaging's performance. For example, glass or plastic syringes containing medication, such as epinephrine, for immediate use may develop hairline cracks when frozen, leading to leakage and compromising stability and sterility of the remaining drug.

Independent of environmental conditions, packaging can negatively influence a drug's stability by leaching chemicals into drugs, absorbing drugs, and reacting with medications. These effects may reduce efficacy of stored medications and increase potential for their toxicity. Polyvinylchloride (PVC) is known to contain toxic compounds that may seep into drugs in trace amounts; the most infamous is the carcinogen diethylhexyl phthalate, which represents 30%–80% of the weight of fluid-filled bags (for infusion) and intravenous (IV) tubing that contain PVC.

Regarding small pill storage, certain pill containers maintain pill integrity more than do others. One study demonstrated that Medidose pill packs maintained atenolol's bioavailability more effectively than did either blister packs or refillable pill containers at 25°C (77°F), but the converse was true at 40°C (104°F) and 75% humidity. Place such pill packs in a water-sealed, light-tight container not containing PVC. Brands such as SealLine, Seattle Sports, Dry Pak, and Sea to Summit offer bags that meet these requirements.

STERILITY

Some drugs must be mixed with buffer or saline solutions prior to use. When preparing these solutions, caution should be taken to ensure sterile formulation. Brief exposures of less than 4 hours to air do not appear to compromise sterility. No significant difference existed between sterility of saline infusion solutions used immediately and those repackaged up to 72 hours prior to use.

STORAGE

The site selected to store medications affects drugs' stability either by shielding them from extremes of environment or by increasing the chance that they will be exposed to those extremes. Air conditioning and refrigeration, humidifiers and desiccants, and light control can create a stable environment for medications. Short of an ongoing energy source to power climate-controlled storage, all storage systems eventually fail in one or more ways to protect medication from ambient environmental conditions. Furthermore, storage systems can actively damage drugs. For example, storage containers can prolong exposure to high temperatures if they are overinsulated in heated environments or can create an environment that is too arid when air conditioning is used, destabilizing drugs, such as certain formulations of epinephrine.

Vehicular storage is convenient in many wilderness and tactical settings. It offers a mobile source of medications and potential power supply for artificial cooling. Air ambulances expose the drugs they carry to environmental extremes that are similar to those of ground ambulances.

HOW TO READ THE DRUG LIST

The following list summarizes stable conditions for drugs most likely to be included in field or tactical medical kits. The list offers options for similar types of drugs, depending on the particular requirements of the users.

Certain terms are used for brevity's sake. *Room temperature* is defined as 15°C to 30°C (59°F to 86°F). *Controlled room temperature* is defined as 20°C to 25°C (68°F to 77°F). *Excessive heat* is defined as temperature exceeding 40°C (104°F).

Packaging and inert compounds used with a medication may vary, especially for generic drugs. In all cases, information from the manufacturer should supplement the following guide.

Deviation from the manufacturer's recommendations is the decision of the treating medical professional and not recommended by the authors of this Appendix. Medications are generally listed by their generic names. Mention of trade names does not imply endorsement.

Availability in the United States is subject to Food and Drug Administration (FDA) and Drug Enforcement Agency (DEA) regulations and annotated as **OTC** (over-the-counter), **Rx** (prescription required), DEA Schedule (**S II to S IV**), or **NA** (not available in the United States).

DRUG LIST
Acetaminophen Capsules, Tablets, Oral Solution, and Suppositories (OTC)

Store capsules, tablets, and the oral solution at a controlled room temperature. Most are fairly stable in light, moisture, and heat, but high humidity should be avoided for gel-coated capsules. High humidity and light should be avoided for oral-dissolving and chewable tablets. Excessive heat (≥40°C [104°F]) should be avoided for extended-release tablets. Solid forms of acetaminophen remain stable for 3 years, and liquid forms remain stable for 2 years from the date of manufacture. Store suppositories at 8°C to 25°C (46°F to 77°F).

Acetaminophen With Codeine Tablets and Oral Solution (S III)

Store tablets and the solution in light-resistant containers at a controlled room temperature.

Acetaminophen With Hydrocodone Tablets and Oral Solution (S II)

Store tablets and the solution in light-resistant containers at a controlled room temperature.

Acetazolamide Tablets, Extended-Release Capsules, Oral Solution, and Injection (Rx)

Store tablets and extended-release capsules at a controlled room temperature. Brief excursions to 15°C to 30°C (59°F to 86°F) are permitted for tablets. Dry powder for the injection solution should be stored in an unopened vial at a controlled room temperature. Powder reconstituted with 5 mL sterile water is stable for 12 hours at room temperature and is stable for 3 days if refrigerated at 2°C to 8°C (36°F to 46°F).

An extemporaneous formulation can be prepared in three ways:

To prepare a solution of acetazolamide 50 mg/mL, crush 20 acetazolamide 250-mg tablets in 25 mL glycerin or distilled water. Add flavored syrup or 2 : 1 simple syrup or flavored syrup to bring the total volume to 100 mL. Shake well before use. This solution should be stored under refrigeration and is stable for 1 week.

To prepare a solution of acetazolamide 5 mg/mL, crush two acetazolamide 250-mg tablets in 7 mL polyethylene glycol 400, 53 mL propylene glycol, 15 mL 70% sorbitol solution, 15 mL 85% sucrose solution, 1 mL sweet syrup, 0.5 mL ethanol, and 8 mL of 0.1 M citrate to achieve a total volume of 100 mL.

The solution can be prepared in a concentration of acetazolamide 25 mg/mL by crushing 10 acetazolamide 250-mg tablets in 50 mL Ora-Sweet and 50 mL Ora-Plus. Store the solution in an opaque container at room temperature. This solution remains stable for 60 days.

Acetic Acid Otic Solution (OTC)

Store the solution in an airtight, light-resistant container at room temperature. Protect from heat.

Albuterol Tablets, Syrup, and Inhaled Formulation (Rx)

Store tablets at 2°C to 25°C (36°F to 77°F). Store extended-release tablets at 15°C to 30°C (59°F to 86°F). Store syrup at 2°C to 30°C (36°F to 86°F). Store capsules for inhalation at room temperature.

For the inhalation route, be certain that albuterol is at room temperature prior to use. For the nebulization route, store albuterol solution for inhalation 0.083% (Proventil), 0.5% (Ventolin), and 0.42% or 0.21% (Accuneb) at 2°C to 25°C (36°F to 77°F). Accuneb nebulized solution must be used within 1 week after removal from the foil pouch. In the pouch, Ventolin Nebules inhalation solution can be stored at 2°C to 8°C (36°F to 46°F) for up to 6 months and remains stable at room temperature for 14 days.

Store albuterol aerosol inhalers containing chlorofluorocarbon propellants at room temperature. Store albuterol sulfate aerosol inhalers containing hydrofluoroalkane (HFA) propellants out of direct sunlight at 15°C to 25°C (59°F to 77°F). To avoid bursting, do not exceed 49°C (120°F). Do not puncture or incinerate. If infrequently used, Ventolin HFA is stable for 6 months from removal from the pouch. Store Ventolin HFA canisters with the mouthpiece down. If frequent nebulization is required, 200 µg/mL of albuterol sulfate inhalation solution in normal saline remains stable for 7 days at room temperature or under refrigeration when placed in polyvinyl chloride or polyolefin bags, polypropylene syringes and tubes, or borosilicate glass tubes.

Aloe Vera Gel, Ointment, and Laxatives (OTC)
Store gel, ointment, and laxatives away from excessive heat and prolonged strong direct light.

Antacids (OTC)
Store aluminum hydroxide and magnesium hydroxide (often called milk of magnesia) products in tightly sealed containers at a controlled room temperature. Store calcium carbonate conventional tablets at 15°C to 30°C (59°F to 86°F). Store calcium carbonate chewable tablets below 25°C (77°F). Protect all products from light, moisture, and excessive heat. Do not freeze.

Aspirin Tablets, Oral Solution, and Suppositories (OTC)
Store tablets and solution in tightly sealed, light-resistant containers at room temperature. Protect from moisture. Store suppositories in the original sealed wrapper at 2°C to 15°C (35°F to 59°F). Do not freeze. Protect from light, moisture, and excessive heat. Discard aspirin if a strong vinegar odor is present, because potency may be significantly decreased.

Atenolol Tablets (Rx)
Store tablets in light-resistant containers at a controlled room temperature.

Atropine Injection and Ophthalmic Solution (Rx)
Store ophthalmic and injection solutions in light-resistant containers at room temperature. To prevent contamination, do not touch the applicator tip directly to the eyes or skin. Atropine sulfate 1 mg/mL injection solutions in Tubex (0.5- and 1-mL) packaging have been shown to remain stable for 3 months. Atropine methyl nitrate 10 mg/mL solutions have been shown to remain stable for 6 months. Inspect the solution prior to administration for the presence of particulate matter, cloudiness, or discoloration, and discard if present. Do not freeze.

Azithromycin Tablets, Oral Solution, Injection, and Ophthalmic Solutions (Rx)
Store tablets at room temperature. Store dry powder for reconstitution below 30°C (86°C). After reconstitution, store suspension at 5°C to 30°C (41°F to 86°F) and discard after use. After reconstitution, store extended-release solution at a controlled room temperature

and use at room temperature. Do not refrigerate or freeze. The solution remains stable for 12 hours. Shake oral azithromycin suspension before use, and do not take simultaneously with antacids containing aluminum or magnesium. The injection solution remains stable for 24 hours if stored at 30°C (86°F) or for 7 days if stored under refrigeration below 5°C (41°F). Store ophthalmic solution in an unopened bottle under refrigeration at 2°C to 8°C (36°F to 46°F) and at 2°C to 25°C (36°F to 77°F) once opened. The solution remains stable for 14 days.

Bacitracin Topical Formulation (OTC)
Store the aqueous topical formulation at 2°C to 8°C (36°F to 46°F) for up to 1 week. Store the nonaqueous topical formulation at room temperature for 3 days and for longer periods if stored in an anhydrous base, such as lanolin and paraffin.

Bismuth Subsalicylate Tablets and Oral Solution (OTC)
Store tablets and suspension in tightly sealed containers at room temperature. Protect from direct light and excessive heat. Do not freeze the suspension.

Bupivacaine Injection (Rx)
Store the injection solution at a controlled room temperature. Protect solutions containing epinephrine from light. Bupivacaine hydrochloride 1.25 mg/mL in 0.9% sodium chloride injection solution in disposable polypropylene syringes is stable for 32 days at 3°C to 23°C (37°F to 73°F).

Calcium Chloride, Calcium Gluceptate, and Calcium Gluconate Injection (Rx)
Store injection solutions of calcium chloride, calcium gluceptate, and calcium gluconate at room temperature. Sterile solutions of calcium in water are indefinitely stable.

Calendula Topical Formulation (OTC)
Protect from heat, moisture, and direct light.

Ceftriaxone Injection (Rx)
Store dry powder for solution preparation in a light-resistant container at or below 25°C (77°F). Dry powder for injection solutions should not be combined with diluents containing calcium, such as Ringer or Hartmann solution, because there will be particulate formulation. After constitution, intramuscular (IM) solutions in water or normal saline remain stable for 2 days at 25°C (77°F) and for 10 days refrigerated at 4°C (39°F) in a concentration of 100 mg/mL; however, at a concentration of 250 mg/mL, such solutions remain stable for only 24 hours at 25°C (77°F) and 3 days refrigerated at

4°C (39°F). IV solutions at concentrations of 10, 20, and 40 mg/mL remain stable for 2 days at 25°C (77°F) and for 10 days refrigerated at 4°C (39°F). Do not refrigerate injection solutions that contain 5% dextrose and 0.9% or 0.45% sodium chloride diluent solutions. IV solutions of ceftriaxone that contain 5% dextrose and 0.9% sodium chloride solution can be frozen at −20°C (−4°F) in PVC or polyolefin containers and remain stable for 26 weeks. Thaw at room temperature before use, and discard any unused, thawed solution.

Cephalexin Capsules, Tablets, and Oral Solution (Rx)
Store capsules at room temperature. The suspension is stable for 14 days under refrigeration.

Charcoal, Activated (OTC)
Store activated charcoal in an airtight container. Sealed aqueous suspensions are stable for 1 year.

Ciprofloxacin Tablets, Capsules, Oral Solution, Injection, Ophthalmic Solution, and Otic Solutions (Rx)
Store tablets below 30°C (86°F). Store extended-release tablets at 25°C (77°F). Brief excursions are permitted at room temperature. Store microcapsules and diluent for oral suspensions below 25°C (77°F). Do not freeze. After reconstitution, the solution should be stored below 30°C (86°F); it remains stable for 14 days. Store ophthalmic solution in original vials at 2°C to 25°C (36°F to 77°F). Protect from light and excessive heat. Do not freeze tablets or oral and ophthalmic solutions. Store otic solution in a light-resistant container at room temperature of 15°C to 25°C (59°F to 77°F).

Crotalidae Antivenom (Rx)
Store vials at 2°C to 8°C (36°F to 46°F). Do not freeze. Use within 4 hours of reconstitution.

Deet (*N,N*-Diethyl-*Meta*-Toluamide, Diethyltoluamide)-Containing Insect Repellent (OTC)
Store the repellent below 49°C (120°F). Store away from heat and flames.

Dermabond (2-Octyl Cyanoacrylate) Topical Skin Adhesive (Rx)
Store the adhesive below 30°C (86°F). Discard if the package is open or has been tampered with. Discard the excess after use because the adhesive hardens on exposure to air. Protect from moisture and direct heat.

Dexamethasone Tablets and Oral, Injection, Implantation, Intravitreal, and Ophthalmic Solutions (Rx)

Store tablets in a light-resistant container at a controlled room temperature. Protect from moisture. Store the oral solution in the original bottle, and dispense only with the supplied calibrated dropper at a controlled room temperature. Once opened, the oral solution remains stable for 90 days. Discard if precipitation forms. Store the implantation, intravitreal, and ophthalmic solutions at room temperature. Extemporaneous formulations remain stable for 91 days.

Dextrose Oral Solution (OTC) and Injection (Rx)

Store oral solution in a well-filled, airtight container. For injection, do not exceed 25°C (77°F). Do not freeze or expose to extreme heat. Discard if cloudy prior to use and discard any unused portions once open.

Diazepam Tablets, Oral Solution, Suppositories, and Injection (S IV)

Store tablets, oral solution, and suppositories at room temperature. Protect from light, heat, and moisture. Do not freeze the oral solution. Suppositories are stable for 8 months at 40°C (104°F) and can withstand at least three freeze-thaw cycles. Brief excursions are permitted to room temperature. Store the injection solution at a controlled room temperature. Do not refrigerate.

Diltiazem Tablets, Oral Solution, and Injection (Rx)

Store tablets at 25°C (77°F). Brief excursions are permitted to 15°C to 30°C (59°F to 86°F). Avoid excess humidity. An extemporaneous formulation of a 1-mg/mL solution can be prepared using 250 mg diltiazem (2.5 mL of diltiazem hydrochloride stock solution) combined with dextrose, fructose, mannitol, sorbitol, or sucrose to a volume of 250 mL. A solution of 12-mg/mL diltiazem can be prepared by crushing 16 tablets of 90-mg diltiazem in 10 mL of 1:1 mixtures of Ora-Plus with either Ora-Sweet or Ora-Sweet SF or in 1:4 mixtures of flavored syrup with simple syrup and then bringing the solution to a total volume of 120 mL. Protect from light.

Diphenhydramine Tablets, Oral Solution (OTC), and Injection (Rx)

Store at a controlled room temperature in a light-resistant container. Do not freeze oral and injection solutions.

Domeboro (Acetic Acid and Aluminum Acetate) Otic Solutions (OTC)

Store otic solutions in a tightly sealed container at either room temperature or under refrigeration. Protect from direct light, heat, and moisture. Do not freeze.

Dopamine Hydrochloride Injection (Rx)

Store the injection in a light-resistant container. Discard if the injection has yellow-brown discoloration or if pH outside of the 4.0 to 6.4 range is detected, because these are indications of decomposition. Dopamine 6.4 mg/mL in 5% dextrose injection is stable at a controlled room temperature for up to 24 hours in ambient humidity and in the presence of light.

Doxycycline Capsules, Tablets, Oral Solution, and Injection (Rx)

Store capsules and tablets in light-resistant containers at room temperature. Store doxycycline hyclate delayed-release tablets in light-resistant containers at a controlled room temperature. Brief excursions are permitted at room temperature. Store lyophilized powder in a light-resistant container at a controlled room temperature. Refrigerate in a light-resistant container immediately after reconstitution, or dilute the injection solution to 0.1 to 1 mg/mL within 12 hours after reconstitution, where it will remain stable for up to 48 hours at 25°C (77°F) and 72 hours at 4°C (39°F). Avoid direct sunlight during storage and infusion. Infusions of doxycycline made with lactated Ringer or 5% dextrose in lactated Ringer diluents must be used within 6 hours of reconstitution to ensure stability. Solutions of 10 mg/mL doxycycline in sterile water can be frozen and stored at −20°C (−4°F) and remain stable for up to 8 weeks. Avoid excess heat after thawing and discard any unused thawed solution.

EMLA (Lidocaine/Prilocaine) Topical Formulation (Rx)

Store EMLA at room temperature. Do not freeze. Discoloration does not necessarily indicate lack of stability. Precipitate indicates that the solution is not stable.

Epinephrine Injection and Topical, Inhaled, and Intranasal Formulations (Rx)

Store injection ampules at 5°C to 25°C (41°F to 77°F). Do not freeze. Injection ampules stored at 38°C (100°F) will last less than 3 months at low humidity (15%) and less than 4 months at high humidity (85%). An extemporaneous formulation of a topical anesthetic solution can be prepared with 2.25 mg/mL of racemic epinephrine hydrochloride, 40 mg/mL of lidocaine hydrochloride, 5 mg/mL of tetracaine hydrochloride, and 0.63 mg/mL of sodium metabisulfite. Store this topical solution in a light-resistant container at 18°C (64°F) for no more than 4 weeks, and at 4°C (39.2°F) for up to 26 weeks. Store the epinephrine inhaler at a controlled room temperature. Do not exceed 49°C (120°F). Do not puncture or incinerate the inhaler. Store the intranasal solution in a light-resistant container at 15°C to 25°C (59°F to 77°F). Do not freeze.

Erythromycin Tablets, Oral Solution, and Topical Ointment (Rx)

Store tablets and oral solution at less than 30°C (86°F). Reconstituted granules must be used within 10 days. Reconstituted erythromycin ethyl succinate solution must be used within 14 days if kept at room temperature. Reconstituted EryPed solution should be stored at less than 25°C (77°F) and used within 35 days. Refrigeration of the suspension is encouraged for the best taste. Optimal stability is maintained at pH above 6.0, with significant decomposition at or below pH of 4.0. Store the topical ointment at less than 27°C (81°F).

Famotidine Tablets (OTC) and Injection (Rx)

Store regular and chewable tablets at a controlled room temperature. Brief excursions for chewable tablets to room temperature are permitted. Protect from moisture. Store injection vials in a light-resistant container at 2°C to 8°C (36°F to 46°F).

Fentanyl Oral Lozenges, Sublingual Tablets, Sublingual Spray, Buccal Film, Injection, and Intranasal Formulation (Rx)

Store oral lozenges, sublingual tablets, sublingual spray, and buccal film at a controlled room temperature. Brief excursions to room temperature are permitted. Protect from moisture. Do not freeze. Store the injection solution in a light-resistant container at a controlled room temperature. Store the intranasal canister in a light-resistant container at 2°C to 25°C (36°F to 77°F).

Fluocinolone Acetonide Topical Ointment, Otic Solution, and Shampoo (Rx)

Store topical cream, ointment, and shampoo at room temperature. Do not freeze. Store the otic solution at a controlled room temperature.

Furosemide Tablets, Solution, and Injection (Rx)

Store tablets and solution in light-resistant containers at 25°C (77°F). Brief excursions are permitted to 15°C to 30°C (59°F to 86°F). Protect from moisture. Store the injection solution in a light-resistant container at room temperature. Discard all types of furosemide if discoloration occurs.

Glucagon Injection (Rx)

Store dry powder in a light-resistant container at a controlled room temperature. Do not freeze. Powder remains stable for 24 months. Use the injection solution immediately after reconstitution and discard unused portions.

Haloperidol Tablets and Injection (Rx)

Store tablets in a tightly closed, light-resistant container at a controlled room temperature. Store the injection solution in a light-resistant container at room temperature. Do not freeze.

Hydrocortisone Tablets, Solution, Injection, and Topical Cream (Rx)

Store tablets, oral solution, injection, and topical cream at room temperature in the original container. Protect from light, moisture, and heat. Do not freeze oral solution or injections.

Hydromorphone Tablets, Solution, Suppositories, and Injection (S II)

Store tablets, solution, suppositories, and injectables in light-resistant containers at a controlled room temperature. Excursions are permitted to 15°C to 30°C (59°F to 86°F). Slight yellow discoloration of the injection liquid does not affect potency.

Ibuprofen Tablets and Solution (OTC)

Store tablets at a controlled room temperature and solution at room temperature.

Insulin (Regular) Injection and Inhaled Formulation (Rx)

Store subcutaneous and IV injections in a light-resistant container refrigerated at 2°C to 8°C (36°F to 46°F). Do not freeze. Store open vials at room temperature for up to 31 days. Store inhalers refrigerated at 2°C to 8°C (36°F to 46°F). Store at room temperature for up to 10 days. Discard unused cartridges from an open blister pack strip after 3 days.

Intravenous Solutions (D₅W, NS, LR, D₅NS, and Other Admixtures)

Store solutions below 90°C (194°F) and preferably at room temperature for ease of use. Pure sodium chloride and lactated Ringer solutions at concentrations used in medicine are unlikely to show precipitation at 0°C (32°F) or if frozen for 3 months.

Ivermectin Tablets (Rx)

Store below 30°C (86°F).

Kaletra (Lopinavir/Ritonavir) Tablets (Rx)

Store tablets at a controlled room temperature. Brief excursions are permitted at room temperature. Once the tablet container is opened or tablets are exposed to high humidity, tablets remain stable for up to 2 weeks.

Ketoconazole Tablets, Shampoo, Foam, and Gel (Rx)

Store tablets in light-resistant containers at a controlled room temperature. Protect from heat and moisture. Store shampoo in a light-resistant container below 25°C (77°F). Store foam in a light-resistant container at a controlled room temperature. Do not refrigerate. Avoid direct light. Store foam at a controlled room temperature with excursions permitted to room temperature.

Store drops in a tightly sealed container below 30°C (86°F).

Lemon Grass (Cymbogogon) Citronella Oil Topical Formulation (OTC)

Store at room temperature. Protect from heat, moisture, and direct light.

Levetiracetam Tablets, Oral Solution, and Injection (Rx)

Store immediate-release tablets, extended-release tablets, and oral solution at 25°C (77°F). Brief excursions are permitted at room temperature. The injection diluted in solution in a polyvinyl chloride bag is stable for at least 24 hours. Discard the unused portion of the vial after opening.

Levofloxacin Tablets, Solution, Injection, and Ophthalmic Formulation (Rx)

Store tablets at 15°C to 30°C (59°F to 86°F). Store oral solution at 25°C (77°F). Brief excursions are permitted at 15°C to 30°C (59°F to 86°F). The injection solution remains stable for 72 hours if stored at or below 25°C (77°F). Injection solution can be diluted in plastic or glass containers and then frozen at −20°C (−4°F), where it remains stable for up to 6 months. Thaw slowly (no hot water baths or microwaves) at 25°C (77°F) or under refrigeration at 8°C (46°F). Use immediately after thawing. Do not refreeze. Store flexible containers of premixed solutions in a light-resistant container at or below 25°C (77°F). Avoid excessive heat and do not freeze. Store levofloxacin 0.5% and 1.5% ophthalmic solutions at 15°C to 25°C (59°F to 77°F).

Lidocaine Injection and Topical, Intradermal, and Ophthalmic Solutions (Rx)

Store injection solution in a light-resistant container at room temperature. Do not freeze. Do not reuse "one-time-use" injection bottles, because they lack methylparaben preservative. Store topical gel and jelly at a controlled room temperature. Store viscous topical preparation, topical patches, and intradermal powder in sealed original packaging at room temperature at 15°C to 30°C (59°F to 86°F).

Lidocaine/Epinephrine/Tetracaine (LET) Topical Solution (Rx)

Store solution in a light-resistant container. The solution remains stable at 18°C (64°F) for 4 weeks and at 4°C (39°F) for 26 weeks.

Lindane (Gamma-Hexachlorocyclohexane) Lotion and Shampoo (Rx)

Store lotion and shampoo at a controlled room temperature.

Loperamide Hydrochloride Capsules (OTC)

Store capsules at 15°C to 25°C (59°F to 77°F). Placing the contents of 10 of the 2-mg capsules in hard fat, such as suet, leaf lard, or fatback lard, and rolling into shape can create rectal suppositories of 20 mg loperamide.

Lorazepam Tablets, Oral Solution, and Injection (S IV)

Store tablets in a tightly sealed container at a controlled room temperature. Store oral solution at 2°C to 8°C (36°F to 46°F). Discard opened bottle after 90 days. Store IM and IV solutions in light-resistant containers at 2°C to 8°C (36°F to 46°F).

Malarone (Atovaquone/Proguanil) Tablets (Rx)

Store in a light-resistant container at a controlled room temperature. Brief excursions to room temperature are permitted.

Mebendazole Tablets (Rx)

Store at 15°C to 25°C (59°F to 77°F).

Metoprolol Tablets, Oral Solution, and Injection (Rx)

Store tablets at a controlled room temperature. Brief excursions are permitted to room temperature. An extemporaneous oral suspension solution can be created by combining 12 crushed 100-mg metoprolol tablets with a small amount of Ora-Sweet, Ora-Sweet SF, or Ora-Plus and bringing the volume to 120 mL with water. The suspension remains stable for 60 days under refrigeration. Shake well before use. Store injection ampules in tight, light-resistant, moisture-free containers at a controlled room temperature.

Metronidazole Capsules, Tablets, and Injection (Rx)

Store capsules at 15°C to 25°C (59°F to 77°F). Store extended-release tablets at a controlled room temperature. Brief excursions are permitted to room temperature. Store injection solution in a light-resistant container at room temperature.

Midazolam Oral Solution and Injection (S IV)

Store oral solution at a controlled room temperature. Brief excursions are permitted to 15°C to 30°C (59°F to 86°F). Store injection solution at a controlled room temperature. Injection solution may be stored for at least 28 days at 3°C to 25°C (37°F to 77°F).

Modafinil Tablets (S IV)

Store tablets at a controlled room temperature.

Morphine Sulfate Tablets, Epidural Suspension, and Injection (S II)

Store tablets in light-resistant containers at a controlled room temperature. Excursions are permitted to room temperature.

Store epidural extended-release suspension under refrigeration at 2°C to 8°C (36°F to 46°F). Do not freeze. Unopened vials remain stable for 30 days at a controlled room temperature. Do not return vials to the refrigerator once they have been stored at room temperature. Solution withdrawn from the vial can be stored at room temperature for up to 4 hours prior to administration. After that, all withdrawn solution should be discarded.

Store injection solution in the original carton at a controlled room temperature. Brief excursions are permitted to 15°C to 30°C (59°F to 86°F). Do not freeze. Discard any unused solution.

Pain cocktails containing preservatives without alcohol or chloroform water will remain stable for 3 weeks after compounding.

Moxifloxacin Tablets, Oral Solution, Injection, and Ophthalmic Route (Rx)

Store tablets and injection solution at a controlled room temperature. Brief excursions are permitted to 15°C to 30°C (59°F to 86°F). Do not refrigerate injection solution because precipitate forms. Extemporaneous oral suspension can be formed to create 60 mL of 20 mg/mL moxifloxacin hydrochloride by combining three crushed 400-mg tablets with 30 mL of Ora-Plus, Ora-Sweet, or Ora-Sweet SF. When stored in a light-resistant amber plastic bottle, oral suspension remains stable for 90 days if stored at 23°C to 25°C (73°F to 77°F). Store 0.5% moxifloxacin ophthalmic solution at 2°C to 25°C (36°F to 77°F).

Mupirocin Topical Formulation (Rx)

Store cream and ointment at a controlled room temperature. Do not freeze cream.

Nalbuphine Hydrochloride Injection (Rx)

Store injection solution in a light-resistant container at a controlled room temperature.

Naloxone Hydrochloride Injection (Rx)

Store injection solution ampules and vials in original containers at a controlled room temperature. Use infusion solutions within 24 hours of opening. For Evzio, store between 15°C and 25°C (59°F and 77°F). Brief excursions are permitted to 4°C to 40°C (39°F to 104°F).

Neosporin Ointment (OTC)

Store ointment in the original container with the cap tightly sealed at room temperature. Protect from light, moisture, and heat.

Nifedipine Capsules, Tablets, Oral Solution, and Injection (Rx)

Store capsules in a light-resistant container at 15°C to 22°C (59°F to 77°F). Store tablets in a light-resistant container below 30°C (86°F). An extemporaneous formulation of an oral solution can be made by combining five nifedipine 10-mg tablets and soaking them in a small amount of 1% hypromellose for 5 minutes and then bringing the total volume to 50 mL with 1% hypromellose. Package 1-mg/mL extemporaneous suspension in single-dose syringes stored in opaque black plastic bags. Solution remains stable for 28 days at 6°C or 22°C (43°F or 72°F).

Store injection solution in a light-resistant container below 25°C (77°F). Because the infusion is extremely light sensitive, the solution retains its potency for 1 hour in daylight and 6 hours in artificial light. Do not remove the vial from the container until immediately before use.

Nitroglycerin Capsules, Sublingual Tablets and Sprays, Injection, Patches, and Topical Formulation (Rx)

Store capsules at room temperature. Store sublingual tablets and sprays at a controlled room temperature. Protect tablets from moisture. Sprays may have brief excursions to room temperature. Store concentrated nitroglycerin for injection solution in a light-resistant container at room temperature. Injection solutions in polyolefin containers can be stored at room temperature for at least 24 hours. Premixed nitroglycerin in either normal saline or 5% dextrose can be stored for 48 hours at room temperature and 7 days under refrigeration. The extemporaneous formulation of solutions with a concentration of 0.035 to 1 mg/mL in glass containers remains stable for 70 days at room temperature and 6 months under refrigeration. Store transdermal patches at room temperature. Store topical ointment at a controlled room temperature.

Ofloxacin Tablets, Injection, Ophthalmic Solution, and Otic Solution (Rx)

Store tablets in a tightly sealed container below 30°C (86°F). Store single-use vials and premixed bottles of injection solution in light-resistant containers at room temperature. Brief exposure to temperatures up to 40°C (104°F) are permitted. Do not freeze. In diluted concentrations between 0.4 and 4 mg/mL and stored in a glass or plastic container, solution remains stable for 14 days under refrigeration at 5°C (41°F), or for 6 months frozen at −20°C (−4°F). Solution will remain stable for up to 14 days under refrigeration at 2°C to 8°C (36°F to 46°F) after thawing. Do not use hot water or a microwave oven for rapid thawing. Store ophthalmic and otic solutions at 15°C to 25°C (59°F to 77°F).

Penicillin G Procaine Injection (Rx)

Store at 2°C to 8°C (36°F to 46°F). Avoid freezing. Injection is stable for 7 days at 25°C (77°F) and 1 day at 40°C (104°F). Wycillin remains stable for 6 months if stored at room temperature.

Penicillin GK and G Sodium Injection (Rx)

Store penicillin GK vials at a controlled room temperature. Once they have been diluted, refrigerate for up to 7 days. Once prepared, penicillin G solutions remain stable and free from allergenic components for 24 hours at room temperature or under refrigeration. At a concentration of 40 million units/L, more than 90% potency was retained for 1 month for penicillin GK, and for 39 days for penicillin G when stored in PVC containers at −20°C (−4°F), and for 70 days for penicillin G under refrigeration.

Phenobarbital Tablets, Solution, and IM and IV Injections (S IV)

Store tablets, oral solution, and IM and IV injection solutions in tightly sealed light-resistant containers at a controlled room temperature. Protect oral solution and tablets from moisture. Slight discoloration is allowable. Discard the solution if there is more discoloration or any precipitation.

Phenylephrine Injection and Ophthalmic Solution (Rx) and Nasal Spray (OTC)

Store injection solution in a light-resistant container at a controlled room temperature. Brief excursions to room temperature are permitted. Once it has been diluted, the solution is stable for 4 hours at room temperature and 24 hours if refrigerated. Store nasal spray in light-resistant containers at room temperature. Refrigerate ophthalmic solution. Discard all forms of phenylephrine if brown discoloration occurs or a precipitate forms.

Phenytoin Capsules, Tablets, Oral Solution, and Injection (Rx)

Store capsules, tablets, and oral solution at a controlled room temperature. Keep extended-release tablets and oral solution in a light-resistant container. Do not freeze oral solution. Store phenytoin sodium injection solution at a controlled room temperature. The solution is usable while clear or faintly yellow. Discard if the solution becomes hazy or if a precipitate forms and persists at room temperature. Because phenytoin is more stable in saline than in dextrose, use or discard phenytoin in 5% dextrose solution within 2 hours of mixing.

Polysporin Ointment (Rx)

Store at room temperature. Do not freeze.

Potassium Permanganate Astringent Solution (OTC)

Store solution in a tightly sealed container at 15°C to 30°C (59°F to 86°F).

Povidone-Iodine Solution (OTC)

Store solution at a controlled room temperature. Brief excursions are permitted to 15°C to 30°C (59°F to 86°F).

Prednisone Tablets and Oral Solution (Rx)

Store tablets and oral solution at a controlled room temperature. Brief excursions to room temperature are permitted. Extemporaneous formulations should be stored at room temperature or under refrigeration, and remain stable for 1 to 2 months.

Prochlorperazine Capsules, Tablets, Oral Solution, and Injection (Rx)

Store capsules, tablets, and solution in tightly closed light-resistant containers at room temperature. Slight yellow discoloration is acceptable. Discard if more discoloration develops. If preparing an IV admixture, use it immediately or dissolve the prochlorperazine in a dextrose solution and store under refrigeration in a light-resistant container. Prochlorperazine 5 mg/mL or 10 mg/2 mL retained 100% potency when stored at room temperature in Tubex containers for 3 months.

Promethazine Capsules, Tablets, Solution, Injection, and Suppositories (Rx)

Store capsules, tablets, and oral and injection solutions in a light-resistant container at a controlled room temperature. Light pink discoloration of white promethazine tablets does not indicate significant loss of potency. Discard the solution if color or precipitate develops. Refrigerate suppositories. Suppositories remain stable at room temperature for 2 weeks and under refrigeration for weeks.

Pseudoephedrine and Pseudoephedrine/Triprolidine Capsules and Tablets (OTC)

Store capsules and tablets in light-resistant containers at 15°C to 25°C (59°F to 77°F). Protect them from moisture.

Rocuronium Injection (Rx)

Store at 2°C to 8°C (36°F to 46°F). Do not freeze. Injection solutions can be stored at a controlled room temperature for 60 days. Open vials should be used within 30 days.

Sildenafil Tablets (Rx)

Store tablets at a controlled room temperature. Brief excursions are permitted to room temperature.

Simethicone Capsules, Tablets, Drops, and Ultrasound Suspension (OTC)

Store capsules, tablets, and drops in a light-resistant container below 40°C (104°F) and preferably at room temperature. Do not freeze.

Sodium Bicarbonate Tablets, Injection, and Suppositories (Rx)

Store tablets at room temperature. Do not refrigerate. Store injection solution at a controlled room temperature in an airtight container to stop the solution from changing to sodium carbonate. Brief exposure to 40°C (104°F) does not affect stability or potency.

Sodium Sulfacetamide Tablets, Cream, Lotion, Ointment, and Ophthalmic Route (Rx)

Store tablets and cream in light-resistant containers at 15°C to 30°C (59°F to 86°F). Do not freeze vaginal cream. Store 10% sulfacetamide topical lotion and ointment at room temperature. The lotion will remain stable for 4 months. Do not freeze. Store ophthalmic solution in a light-resistant container at 8°C to 15°C (46°F to 59°F). Discard if it becomes darkened.

Succinylcholine Injection (Rx)

Store at 2°C to 8°C (36°F to 46°F). The injection solution is stable at a controlled room temperature for 14 days. Once it has been diluted, discard within 24 hours.

Tetanus Toxoid, Tetanus Toxoid/Diphtheria/Acellular Pertussis, and Hyperimmune Tetanus Globulin Vaccine Solutions (Rx)

Store vaccine solutions at 2°C to 8°C (36°F to 46°F). Do not freeze. The solutions are stable for 72 hours at a controlled room temperature.

Tetracaine Hydrochloride Ophthalmic Solution (Rx)

Store ampules in light-resistant containers at 2°C to 8°C (35.6°F to 46.4°F) to prevent oxidation and crystallization. Tetracaine hydrochloride remains stable for 3 days at room temperature and retains the original manufacturer's expiration date if returned to refrigeration. For topical "LET" solution information, see the Lidocaine/Epinephrine/Tetracaine entry.

Tetracycline Capsules, Tablets, Oral Solution, Injection, and Topical Ointment (Rx)

Store capsules, tablets, oral solution, and topical ointment in light-resistant containers at room temperature. Reconstituted solutions are stable for 12 hours, and tetracycline hydrochloride is stable in 5% dextrose and water for 6 hours. Do not use outdated products, because they may cause proximal renal tubular acidosis and Fanconi syndrome.

Trimethoprim/Sulfamethoxazole (80 mg/400 mg) Tablets, Oral Solution, and Injection (Rx)

Store tablets, oral solution, and unopened injection vials at a controlled room temperature. Protect tablets from moisture. Store oral solution in a light-resistant container. Injection solution, including 80 mg trimethoprim in 100 mL D_5W, is stable for 4 hours, but will last longer if it is more dilute. Vials drawn into a polypropylene syringe will remain stable for 60 hours. Do not refrigerate. Do not inject intramuscularly. Discard if cloudiness or precipitation develops.

Truvada (Emtricitabine/Tenofovir) Tablets (Rx)

Store in a tightly closed container at 25°C (77°F). Brief excursions are permitted at room temperature.

Zinc Salts (OTC)

Store zinc salts in an airtight, nonmetallic container. An extemporaneous formulation of an oral solution can be made up for zinc sulfate by combining 22 g of zinc sulfate powder with 250 mL of flavored syrup and bringing the total volume to 500 mL with purified water. The solution of 10 mg/mL zinc remains stable for 60 days under refrigeration or for 12 months after addition of a paraben concentrate for a final zinc concentration of 0.5%.

Zolpidem Tablets, Sublingual Tablets, and Spray (S IV)

Store sublingual, immediate-release, and extended-release tablets and oral spray in a light-resistant container at a controlled room temperature. Protect from light and moisture. Brief excursions are permitted to temperatures of 15°C to 30°C (59°F to 86°F). Do not freeze.

Species		Manufacturer, Antivenom	Approximate Average Initial Dose (Reference)
Latin Name	**English Name**		
Acanthophis spp.	Death adder	CSL* Death Adder or polyvalent antivenom	1–3 vials
Bitis arietans, Africa	Puff adder	Sanofi-Pasteur ("Fav-Afrique" or "Favirept") polyvalent[†]; SAVP[‡] polyvalent; ICP[§] EchiTAb-plus-ICP	80 mL
Bitis arietans, Middle East	Puff adder	NAVPC[‖] polyvalent snake antivenom	80 mL
		Vacsera polyvalent or anti-viper venom antiserum	80 mL
Bothrops asper	Terciopelo	ICP[§] polyvalent, LBS[¶] Antivipmyn TRI	5–20 vials
Bothrops atrox	Common lancehead	Butantan, FED** Antibotropico polyvalent	2–12 vials
Bothrops bilineatus	Papagaio	Butantan polyvalent	2–4 vials
Bothrops jararaca	Jararaca	Butantan polyvalent	2–12 vials[††]
Bothrops lanceolatus, B. caribbaeus	Lesser Antillean fer de lance	Sanofi-Pasteur Bothrofav	2–6 vials

Species		Manufacturer, Antivenom	Approximate Average Initial Dose (Reference)
Latin Name	English Name		
Bungarus caeruleus	Common krait	Indian manufacturers[tt] polyvalent	100 mL
Bungarus candidus	Malayan krait	TRC[tt] Malayan Krait Antivenin monovalent or neuro-polyvalent	50 mL
Bungarus fasciatus	Banded krait	TRC[tt] Banded Krait Antivenin	
		Monovalent or neuro-polyvalent	50 mL
Bungarus multicinctus	Chinese krait	Shanghai Vaccine & Serum Institute	
		Antivenom of Bungarus multicinctus	
		Blyth Taiwan	5 vials
		NIPM Taipei Naja-Bungarus antivenin	5 vials
Calloselasma (Agkistrodon) rhodostoma	Malayan pit viper	TRC[tt] Malayan Pit Viper Antivenin monovalent or hemato-polyvalent	100 mL
Cerastes spp.	Desert (horned) vipers	NAVPC[||] polyvalent	30–50 mL
		Vacsera anti-viper or polyvalent	30–50 mL
Crotalus durissus	Tropical rattlesnakes	Butantan or FED** Anticrotalico or Antibotropico-crotalico	5–20 vials

Species		Manufacturer, Antivenom	Approximate Average Initial Dose (Reference)
Latin Name	*English Name*		
Crotalus simus	Central American	ICP§ LBS¶ polyvalent	5–15 vials
Cryptelytrops albolabris, C macrops see below *Trimeresurus (Trimeresurus) albolabris* etc.	Green pit vipers	TRC†† Green Pit Viper Antivenin or hemato-polyvalent	100 mL
Daboia (Vipera) palaestinae	Palestine viper	Rogoff Medical Research Institute, Tel Aviv, Palestine viper monovalent	50–80 mL
Daboia (Vipera) russelii, D siamensis	Russell's vipers	Myanmar Pharmaceutical Factory, monovalent	80 mL
		Indian manufacturers‡‡ polyvalent	100 mL
		TRC†† Russell's Viper	
		Antivenin monovalent or hemato-polyvalent	50 mL
Dendroaspis spp.	East/South African mambas	SAVP‡ Dendroaspis or polyvalent antivenoms	50–100 mL
Dispholidus typus	African boomslang	SAVP‡ Boomslang antivenom	1–2 vials

Continued

Species		Manufacturer, Antivenom	Approximate Average Initial Dose (Reference)
Latin Name	*English Name*		
Echis spp., Africa	Saw-scaled or carpet	SAVP[†], Echis, monovalent	20 ml
	Vipers	Sanofi-Pasteur ("Fav-Afrique")[†]	100 mL
		MicroPharm Echi-TAb G	1 vial
		ICP[§] EchiTAb-plus-ICP	3 vials
Echis spp., Middle East	– – – – – – – – –	NAVPC[‖] polyvalent snake antivenom	50 mL
		Vacsera polyvalent and anti-viper	
		Venom antiserum	50 mL
Echis carinatus, India	– – – – – – – – –	Indian manufacturers[¶] polyvalent	50 mL
Gloydius (Agkistrodon) blomhoffii	Chinese Mamushi	Shanghai Vaccine & Serum Institute	5 vials
		Mamushi antivenom	
Hydrophiinae	Sea snakes	CSL* Sea Snake Antivenom	1–10 vials
Lachesis spp.	Bushmasters	ICP[§] polyspecific, FED** Antibotropico laquetico, Butantan Antiofidico	10–20 vials
Micropechis ikaheka	New Guinean small-eyed snake	CSL* polyvalent antivenom	?2 vials

Species		Manufacturer, Antivenom	Approximate Average Initial Dose (Reference)
Latin Name	*English Name*		
Micrurus corallinus, M. frontalis	Brazilian coral snakes	Butantan "Antielapidico"	1–5 vials
M. nigrocinctus, M. mipartitus, M. multifasciatus	Central American coral snakes	ICP[§] monovalent	1–5 vials
Naja kaouthia	Monocellate Thai cobra	TRC[††] Cobra Antivenin monovalent or neuro-polyvalent	100 mL
Naja naja, N. oxiana	Indian cobras	Indian manufacturers[‡‡] polyvalent	100 mL
Naja haje, N. anchietae, N. annulifera, N. melanoleuca, cobras, N. nivea, N. senegalensis	African neurotoxic	SAVP2 and Sanofi-Pasteur[†] polyvalent	100 mL
Naja haje (Middle East)	Egyptian cobra	Vacsera polyvalent venom antiserum	100 mL
Naja haje arabica	Arabian cobra	NAVPC[‖] Bivalent Naja/Walterinnesia or polyvalent snake antivenom	100 mL
Naja nigricollis, N. mossambica, etc.	African spitting cobras	SAVP[‡] and Sanofi-Pasteur polyvalent[†] ICP[§] Echi-TAb G	100 mL

Continued

Species		Manufacturer, Antivenom	Approximate Average Initial Dose (Reference)
Latin Name	*English Name*		
Naja nubiae	Egyptian spitting cobra	Vacsera polyvalent venom antiserum	100 mL
Naja siamensis, N. sumatrana	Indo-Chinese and other SE Asian spitting cobras	TRC[††] neuro-polyvalent antivenom	100 mL
Notechis scutatus	Tiger snake	CSL* Tiger Snake or polyvalent antivenom	1–3+ vials
Ophiophagus hannah	King cobra	TRC[††] King Cobra antivenin or neuro-polyvalent	100–200 mL
Oxyuranus scutellatus	Australian/ Papuan taipans	CSL* polvalent (or Taipan) antivenom	1–6+ vials
Pseudonaja species	Australian brown snakes	CSL* Brown Snake or polyvalent antivenom	1–6+ vials
Pseudechis spp.	Australian black snakes	CSL* Black Snake Antivenom	1–3 vials
Rhabdophis tigrinus	Japanese yamakagashi	Japanese Snake Institute, Nitta-gun	1–2 vials
R. subminiatus	SE Asian red-necked keelback	Yamakagashi antivenom	

Species		Manufacturer, Antivenom	Approximate Average Initial Dose (Reference)
Latin Name	English Name		
Trimeresurus (Trimeresurus) albolabris, T. macrops	Green pit vipers	TRC[††] Green Pit Viper Antivenin or hemato-polyvalent	100 mL
Vipera berus and other European Vipera	European adder	"ViperaTAb" MicroPharm Fab monovalent Sanofi-Pasteur Viperfav	100–200 mg 4 mL
Walterinnesia aegyptia	Black desert cobra	NAVPC[‖] Bivalent Naja/ Walterinnesia or polyvalent snake antivenom	50 mL

*Commonwealth Serum Laboratories, Parkville, Australia.
[†]Sanofi-Pasteur announced that they have stopped production of FavAfrique and FaviRept antivenoms.
[‡]South African Vaccine Producers, formerly SAIMR, Johannesburg.
[§]Instituto Clodomiro Picado, San Jose, Costa Rica.
[‖]National Antivenom and Vaccine Production Center, National Guard Health Affairs, Riyadh, KSA.
[¶]Laboratorios Bioclon, Silanes, Mexico.
**Fundação Ezequiel Dias, Belo Horizonte, Brazil.
[††]Thai Red Cross Society, Bangkok.
[‡‡]Indian Manufacturers: Bharat Serums and Vaccines, Mumbai, Biological E (Evans), Vins Bioproducts, Hyderabad.

Index

Page numbers followed by "*f*" indicate figures, "*t*" indicate tables, and "*b*" indicate boxes.

A

ABC (airway, breathing, and circulation), 643
Abdomen
    frostbite on skin of, P1*f*
    movement of, in airway assessment, 119, 121*f*
Abdominal pain
    lower, 351–353
    in malaria, 568
Abortion, spontaneous, 344–345
Abrasions, 233–245
    from coral, 665
    corneal, 379–380
        contact lens-related, 380–381
    definition of, 244–245
    first-aid supplies for, care of, 234*b*
    general treatment of, 234*b*, 244–245
Abscess
    apical, 403, 404*f*
    Bartholin's, 351
    vulvovaginal, 351
Abuse, substance, disorders due to, 414
Acclimatization, 9–11
    to hot environment, 53–54, 790
ACDU mnemonic, 895
Ace wrap, 269
Acepromazine maleate, 874
    in trek animals, 881*t*–886*t*
        with laminitis, 874
Acetaminophen
    for acute mountain sickness, 3
    for cluster headache, 326
    for dehydration headache, 327
    dosage recommendations for, 296*t*–297*t*
    for high-altitude headache, 1
    in medical kit
        for wilderness travel, 819*t*–843*t*
        for women, 347*t*–348*t*
    for migraine headache, 326
    with narcotic analgesics, 295
    in pain management first-aid kit, 284*b*
    during pregnancy, 363*t*–369*t*
    for pyelonephritis, 337
    storage and stability of
        capsules, tablets, oral solution, and
            suppositories, 945

Acetaminophen *(Continued)*
    with codeine tablets and oral solution, 945
    with hydrocodone tablets and oral solution, 945
Acetazolamide
    for acclimatization to high altitudes, 10–11
    for acute angle-closure glaucoma, 378
    allergic reaction to, 10
    for high-altitude illness, 2, 7
        in children, 856
    for hyphema, 390
    during pregnancy, 363*t*–369*t*
    for prevention of high-altitude pulmonary
        edema, 6
    tablets, extended-release capsules, oral
        solution, and injection, storage and
        stability of, 946
    in wilderness medical kit, 819*t*–843*t*
Acetic acid solution
    for bristleworm irritation, 673
    for jellyfish sting, 668
    otic solution, storage and stability of, 946, 951
    for otitis externa, 701–702
    for sea bather's eruption, 670
    for sea cucumber irritation, 672
Acetylsalicylic acid. *see* Aspirin
Achilles tendon, ruptured, 247–248
Achromycin. *see* Tetracycline
Acid burn, 68
Acidosis, in malaria, 572*t*
ACR. *see* Active core rewarming
Acromioclavicular joint separation, 185–187, 187*f*
Activated carbon, for water disinfection, 551
Activated charcoal
    for paralytic shellfish poisoning, 685
    storage and stability of, 949
    for tetrodotoxin fish poisoning, 684
    in trek animals, 883*t*–886*t*
    for water disinfection, 552*t*
Active core rewarming (ACR), 41
Activity level, wet bulb globe temperature
    and, 52*t*
Acular. *see* Ketorolac

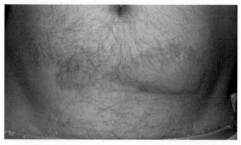

PLATE 1 A Nordic skier with first-degree frostbite (central pallor having cleared after rewarming) of the abdominal skin; despite wearing a parka, this skier reported having skied for 90 minutes in −23.3°C (−10°F) temperature, unaware that his shirt had come untucked from his trousers. (Courtesy Luanne Freer, MD.)

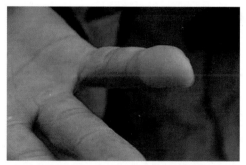

PLATE 2 A climber with second-degree frostbite of the fifth finger sustained after only several seconds exposure to −45.6°C (−50°F) wind chill when gloves were briefly removed to handle placement of a carabiner to the fixed rope. Clear bullae developed after rewarming. (Courtesy Luanne Freer, MD.)

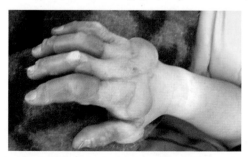

PLATE 3 A climber with second-, third-, and fourth-degree frostbite of the hand. Note fingers 1 through 4 with hemorrhagic bullae over the areas of third-degree injury, clear bullae over the dorsum of the hand with second-degree injury, and deeply violaceous and unblistered fourth-degree injury of the distal phalanx of the fifth finger. (Courtesy Luanne Freer, MD.)

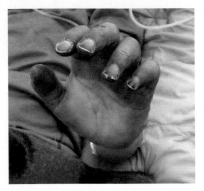

PLATE 4 A climber with fourth-degree or full-thickness frostbite injury just hours after rewarming. Note absence of any blistering. Fingers are insensate, and capillary refill is absent. (Courtesy Luanne Freer, MD.)

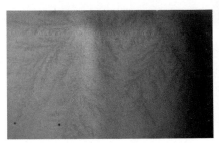

PLATE 5 Lichtenberg figure (pathognomonic sign of lightning injury that resolves spontaneously and needs no treatment). (Courtesy Mary Ann Cooper, MD.)

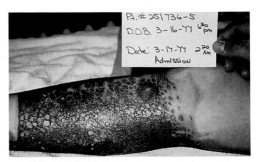

PLATE 6 Punctate burns from lightning injury. (Courtesy Arthur Kahn, MD.)

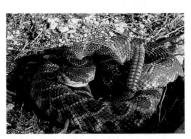

PLATE 7 Southern Pacific rattlesnake (*Crotalus viridis helleri*) is one of nine subspecies of western rattlesnakes (*C. viridis* spp.). (Courtesy Michael Cardwell/Extreme Wildlife Photography.)

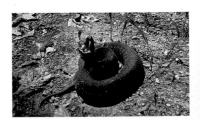

PLATE 8 Cottonmouth water moccasin (*Agkistrodon piscivorus*). The open-mouthed threat gesture is characteristic of this semiaquatic pit viper. (Courtesy Sherman Minton, MD.)

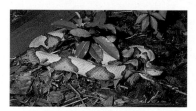

PLATE 9 Southern copperhead *(Agkistrodon contortrix contortrix)* has markings that make it almost invisible when lying in leaf litter. (Courtesy Michael Cardwell and Carl Barden Venom°Laboratory.)

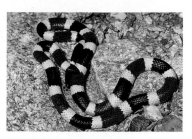

PLATE 10 Sonoran coral snake *(Micruroides euryxanthus)* is also known as the Arizona coral snake. No documented fatality has followed a bite by this species. (Courtesy Michael Cardwell and Jude McNally.)

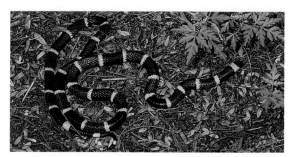

PLATE 11 Texas coral snake *(Micrurus fulvius tener)* has a highly potent venom but is secretive, and bites are uncommon. (Courtesy Michael Cardwell and the Gladys Porter Zoo.)

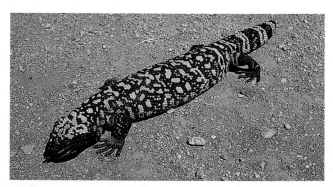

PLATE 12 Gila monster *(Heloderma suspectum)* is one of only two known venomous lizards and the only species found in the United States. (Courtesy Michael Cardwell/Extreme Wildlife Photography.)

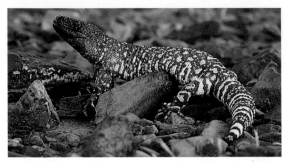

PLATE 13 Mexican beaded lizard *(Heloderma horridum)* is located south of the Gila monster's range in Mexico. (Courtesy Michael Cardwell/Extreme Wildlife Photography.)

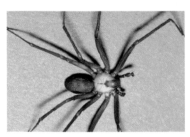

PLATE 14 Brown recluse spider *(Loxosceles recluse)*. (Courtesy Indiana University Medical Center.)

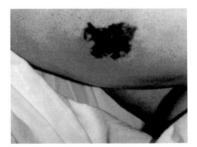

PLATE 15 Brown recluse spider bite after 24 hours, with central ischemia and rapidly advancing cellulitis. (Courtesy Paul S. Auerbach, MD.)

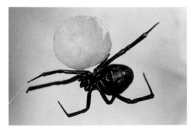

PLATE 16 Adult female black widow spider *(Latrodectus mactans)* with a fresh egg case. (Courtesy Michael Cardwell & Associates.)

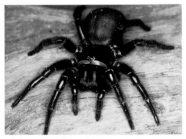

PLATE 17 Funnel-web spider *(Atrax* species) wearing a wedding ring. (Courtesy Sherman Minton, MD.)

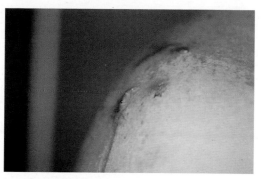

PLATE 18 Lateral view of three lesions caused by infestation with *Dermatobia hominis* larva. The nodules were initially assumed to be furunculosis. A central breathing aperture is present in each nodule. Serosanguineous fluid is draining from two of the nodules. Larval spiracles are visible emerging from the uppermost nodule. (Courtesy Brewer TF, Wilson ME, Gonzalez E, Felsenstein D: Bacon therapy and furuncular myiasis. *JAMA* 270:2087, 1993.)

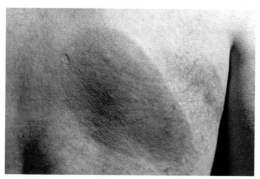

PLATE 19 Rash of erythema migrans. (Courtesy Paul Auerbach, MD.)

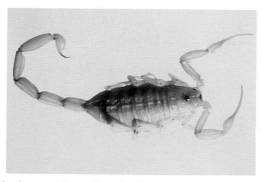

PLATE 20 Centruroides exilicauda (*Centruroides sculpturatus*), the bark scorpion of Arizona.

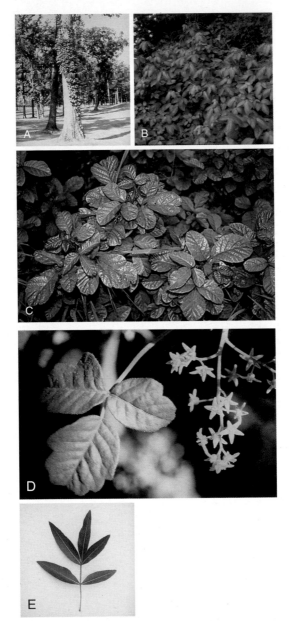

PLATE 21 Plants in the *Toxicodendron* genus. **A,** Poison ivy. **B,** Poison ivy growing as a sea of vines. **C,** Poison oak. **D,** Poison oak, close up. **E,** Poison sumac.

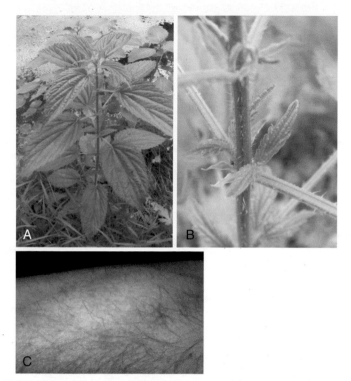

PLATE 22 **A,** Stinging nettle. **B,** Close-up view of the stinging nettle spines. **C,** Urticarial papules induced after contact with the stinging nettle.

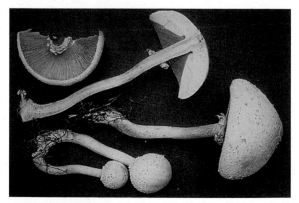

PLATE 23 *Chlorophyllum molybdites.* A gastrointestinal irritant. (Courtesy Roger Phillips, rogersmushrooms.com.)

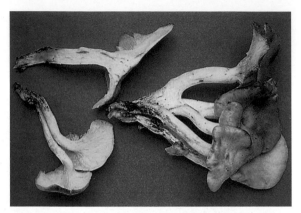

PLATE 24 *Omphalotus olearius* (jack-o'-lantern mushroom). A gastrointestinal irritant. (Courtesy Roger Phillips, rogersmushrooms.com.)

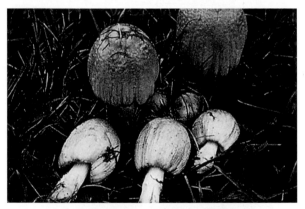

PLATE 25 Inky cap *(Coprinus atramentarius)*. (Courtesy Orson J. Miller, PhD.)

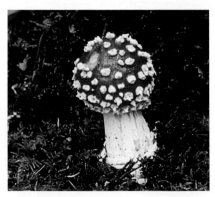

PLATE 26 *Amanita muscaria.*

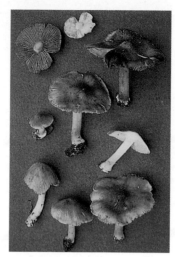

PLATE 27 *Inocybe cookei.* Contains muscarinic toxins. (Courtesy Roger Phillips, rogersmushrooms.com.)

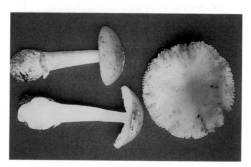

PLATE 28 *Amanita pantherina.* Contains the neurotoxins ibotenic acid and isoxazole derivatives. (Courtesy Roger Phillips, rogersmushrooms.com.)

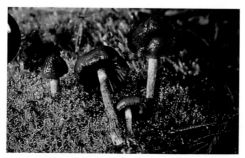

PLATE 29 *Psilocybe caerulipes.*

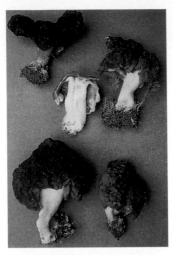

PLATE 30 *Gyromitra esculenta.* Contains the hepatotoxin gyromitrin. (Courtesy Roger Phillips, rogersmushrooms.com.)

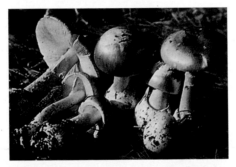

PLATE 31 Death cap (*Amanita phalloides*).

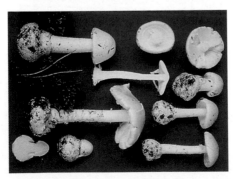

PLATE 32 *Amanita virosa.* Causes delayed hepatotoxicity. (Courtesy Roger Phillips, rogersmushrooms.com.)

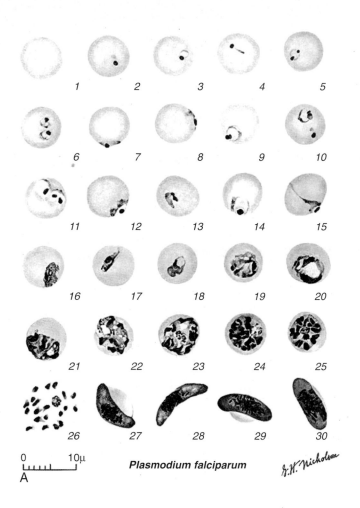

0   10μ

Plasmodium falciparum

G.W. Nicholson

A

PLATE 33 Malaria thin blood smears. **A,** Thin smears, *Plasmodium falciparum.*

Continued

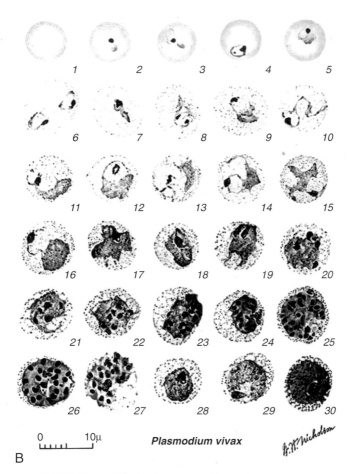

Plasmodium vivax

0 ___ 10μ

B

PLATE 33, cont'd   B, Thin smears, *Plasmodium vivax.*

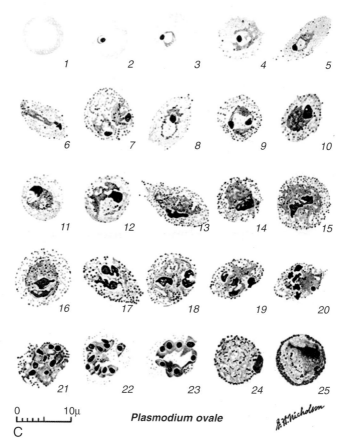

1   *2*   *3*   *4*   *5*

6   *7*   *8*   *9*   *10*

11   *12*   *13*   *14*   *15*

16   *17*   *18*   *19*   *20*

21   *22*   *23*   *24*   *25*

0   10µ   **Plasmodium ovale**   *F. H. Nicholson*

C

PLATE 33, cont'd C, Thin smears, *Plasmodium ovale*.

Continued

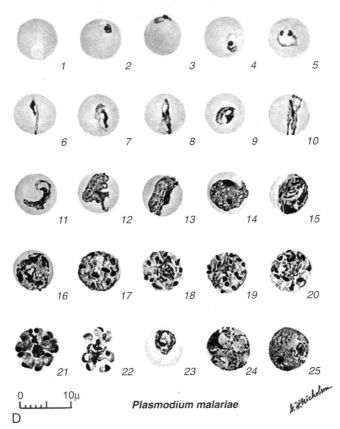

1 2 3 4 5

6 7 8 9 10

11 12 13 14 15

16 17 18 19 20

21 22 23 24 25

0   10μ

Plasmodium malariae

D

PLATE 33, cont'd D, Thin smears, *Plasmodium malariae*. (All images from http://www.dpd.cdc.gov/dpdx/HTML/ImageLibrary/Malaria_il.htm. **A–D,** from Coatney GR, Collins WE, Warren M, Contacos PG: *The primate malarias*, Bethesda, Md, 1971, U.S. Department of Health, Education, and Welfare.)

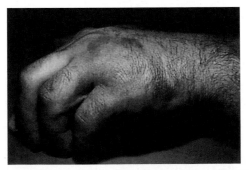

PLATE 34 Typical appearance of *Erysipelothrix rhusiopathiae* skin infection. (Photograph by Paul S. Auerbach, MD.)

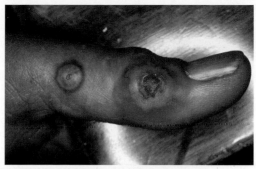

PLATE 35 Seal finger secondary to *Mycoplasma*. (Courtesy Edgar Maeyens Jr, MD.)

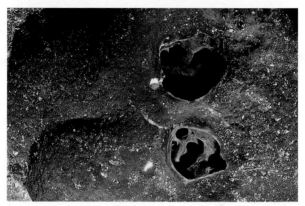

PLATE 36 Pacific fire sponge. (From Norbert Wu, with permission. http://www.norbertwu.com.)

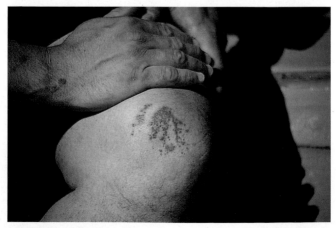

PLATE 37 Fernlike hydroid "print" on the knee of a diver. (Photograph by Paul S. Auerbach, MD.)

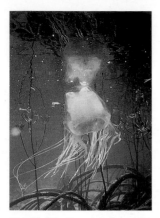

PLATE 38 Box jellyfish *(Chironex fleckeri)*, swimming just beneath the surface of the water. (Courtesy John Williamson, MD.)

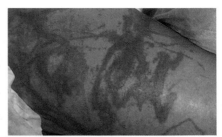

PLATE 39 Intense necrosis (here at 48 hours) is typical of a severe box jellyfish *(Chironex fleckeri)* sting. Skin darkening can be rapid with cellular death. (Courtesy John Williamson, MD.)

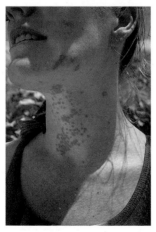

PLATE 40 Sea bather's eruption on the neck of a diver in Cozumel, Mexico. (Photograph by Paul S. Auerbach, MD.)

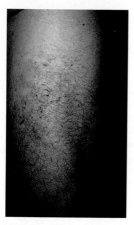

PLATE 41 Thigh of the author demonstrating multiple sea urchin punctures from black sea urchins *(Diadema)*. Within 24 hours the black markings were absent, indicative of spine dye without residual spines. (Photograph by Ken Kizer, MD.)

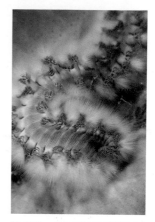

PLATE 42 The chitinous spines of a bristleworm are easily dislodged into the skin of an unwary diver. (Copyright Stephen Frink.)

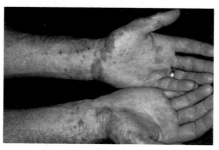

PLATE 43 Sea moss dermatitis. Dermatitis of palms and forearms from a moving sea moss entangled in nets. (Courtesy Edgar Maeyens Jr, MD.)

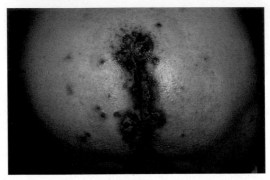

PLATE 44 *Microcoleus lyngbyaceus* causes rare and extreme superficial necrosis and inflammation secondary to dermonecrotic toxins. (Courtesy Edgar Maeyens Jr, MD.)

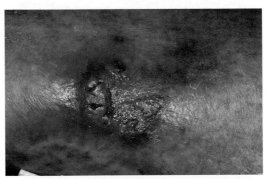

PLATE 45 Protothecosis of anterior leg. (Courtesy Edgar Maeyens Jr, MD.)

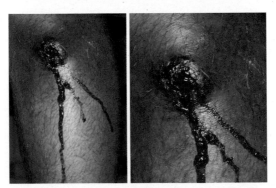

PLATE 46 Human pythiosis. Suppurative necrotizing cellulitis of *Pythium insidiosum* infection.

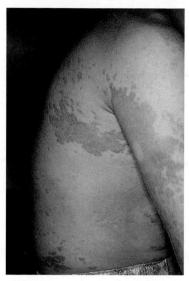

PLATE 47 Aquagenic urticaria. Pruritic punctate and perifollicular wheals characteristic of the rash of aquagenic urticaria. (Courtesy Edgar Maeyens Jr, MD.)

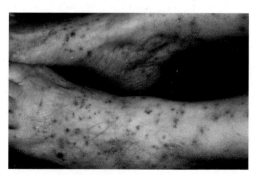

PLATE 48 Schistosome cercarial dermatitis of the feet and ankles. (Courtesy Edgar Maeyens Jr, MD.)

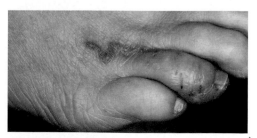

PLATE 49 Cutaneous larva migrans. (Courtesy Edgar Maeyens Jr, MD.)

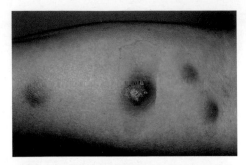

PLATE 50 Nodular lymphangitis from *Mycobacterium marinum*. (Courtesy Edgar Maeyens Jr, MD.)

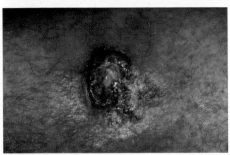

PLATE 51 *Aeromonas hydrophila*. Trauma-induced necrotic ulcer of the anterior leg of a fisherman. (Courtesy Edgar Maeyens Jr, MD.)

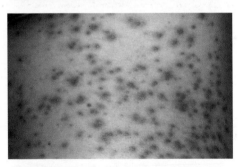

PLATE 52 Hot tub folliculitis. (Courtesy Edgar Maeyens Jr, MD.)

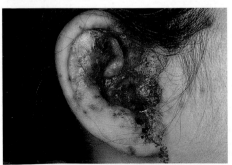

PLATE 53 Malignant otitis externa. (Courtesy Edgar Maeyens Jr, MD.)